Methods in Molecular Biology™

Series Editor
John M. Walker
School of Life Sciences
University of Hertfordshire
Hatfield, Hertfordshire, AL10 9AB, UK

For other titles published in this series, go to
www.springer.com/series/7651

Analgesia

Methods and Protocols

Edited by

Arpad Szallasi

Department of Pathology and Laboratories, Monmouth Medical Center, Long Branch, NJ, USA

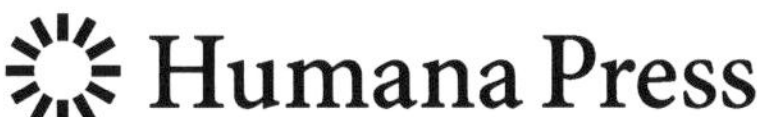

Editor
Arpad Szallasi, MD, Ph.D.
Department of Pathology and Laboratories
Monmouth Medical Center
Long Branch, NJ
USA
aszallasi@sbhcs.com

ISSN 1064-3745 e-ISSN 1940-6029
ISBN 978-1-60327-322-0 e-ISBN 978-1-60327-323-7
DOI 10.1007/978-1-60327-323-7
Springer New York Dordrecht Heidelberg London

Library of Congress Control Number: 2010924278

Cover illustration: Inset image: Distribution and concentration of mu-opioid receptors, the site of action of the opiate analgesics, in the human brain. This is a three-dimensional representation, that shows the concentration in color coding from lower (blue, green) to highest (red). Mu-opioid receptors were quantified using positron emission tomography and the selective radiotracer [11C]carfentanil. The receptor maps were superimposed over a magnetic resonance image of the same subject. Provided by Dr. Jon-Kar Zubieta.
Background image: Adapted from Figure 3 of Chapter 26.

Printed on acid-free paper

Humana Press is a part of Springer Science+Business Media (www.springer.com)

Foreword

We congratulate the editor, Dr. Arpad Szallasi, for enlisting outstanding experts active in important areas of pain research to contribute to this book and for the breadth of topics presented – from the molecular level to clinical application.

Freedom from pain is argued by some to be a fundamental human right. Despite tremendous breakthroughs in our understanding of the biological basis of pain perception and the treatment of pain, freedom from pain cannot be guaranteed. More research that builds upon the current knowledge base will advance the realization of this right for all.

Creativity is essential for scientific investigation, but tools are required to test the validity of creative thought. This book provides a cross discipline view of techniques used to investigate the biological basis for pain perception and to discover new treatments. The techniques themselves reflect great creativity and have strengths and weaknesses. Description in this book of techniques used in pain research by scientists who use them, and in some cases developed or improved them, provide readers of the book the opportunity to benefit from the experience of the authors and to participate in advancing the goal of freedom from pain for everyone.

Gabor Racz ***James E. Heavner***

Preface

Analgesia: no pain, lot to gain

Ancient Greeks considered diseases to be penalties sent by gods. Indeed, the English word "pain" has its origin in the Greek word *poine* ("penalty"). The word analgesia is derived from the Greek adjective *analgetos* ("not sensing pain") that, in turn, stems from the verb *alego*, meaning "to care, look after". Modern medical dictionaries define analgesia as (1) absence of sensibility to pain, or (2) the relief of pain without loss of consciousness.

Chronic pain is a complex phenomenon, which continues to remain undertreated in the majority of affected patients and thus represents a significant unmet medical need. For any given analgesic drug, the NNT (number needed to treat) number is estimated to be as low as one in seven. Such clinical value (beneficial only in 15% of treated patients) would be unacceptably low for any other disease. Not surprisingly, the medical management of chronic pain remains frustrating both for patients and their clinicians.

Chronic pain is rampant, affecting a major segment of the population. In the US, an estimated 50 million adults are suffering from chronic pain. Chronic pain, however, is not only a health problem. Many patients are in their productive age: the loss of work hours due to pain has grave implications for the economy. As the population is graying, the prevalence of chronic pain is expected to rise. The term "pain epidemic" is hardly unjustified. The US market for treatment of chronic pain is expected to nearly double from today's $2.6 billion to $5.1 billion in the next ten years. This represents opportunities for the pharmaceutical industry but may strain the resources of the healthcare system. The world-wide prevalence of chronic pain in unknown, but the global pain market was reported to generate total sales of $34 billion in 2007.

Most existing analgesic drugs (painkillers) are derivatives of natural products that had been introduced into clinical practice on a largely empirical basis. The current Decade of Pain Control and Research (2001–2010) has, however, witnessed major changes in analgesia research, progressing from a system level to cellular, subcellular, and molecular. Breakthrough advances in biomedical technologies have allowed us to develop a better understanding of the mechanisms by which pain is generated, transmitted, modulated, and perceived. Genomics ("brain on a chip") and proteomics have been applied to identify genes and their products that change during pain and thus may represent novel targets for pharmacological manipulation. These genes as pain targets are validated by generation of knockout mice, site-specific mutation, silencing by RNA interference, or knock-down by antisense methods. Cell lines heterogously expressing these genes are generated and used to screen compound libraries for lead analgesic molecules. Then drug candidates are tested in animal models of pain for analgesic activity. Gene transfer by viral vectors represents an attractive alternative strategy for the delivery of antinociceptive substances. Molecular neurosurgery (targeted neurodegeneration by neurotoxins) is another approach for permanent pain relief.

The molecular mechanisms that underlie drug tolerance, dependence, and individual sensitivity are beginning to be understood. Receptor heterogeneity secondary to single nucleotide polymorphism (SNPs) is believed to play an important role. SNPs, however, are not the only source of genetic variability. Copy number variation (CNV) is now emerging as a new source of genomic variation. Indeed, CNVs are now thought to include more nucleotides than SNPs. It is now generally accepted that one size does not fit all: chronic pain patients need individualized therapeutic decisions, a concept popularized in the media as personalized medicine. Enhanced analytic strategies, like microarrays, array-based comparative genomic hybridization and microfluidic chips, may make pain theranostics, the fusion of diagnostics and therapeutics, a reality.

It is hoped that these discoveries will eventually lead to individualized analgesia protocols. Furthermore, new techniques explore low affinity interactions of anesthetics and analgesics with proteins that cannot be detected by traditional binding methodology. Finally, fMRI (functional magnetic resonance imaging) technology creates a unique opportunity for "virtual reality analgesia" by the effects of analgesic drugs on brain functions.

This volume offers comprehensive coverage of molecular analgesia research methods from target discovery through target validation and clinical testing to tolerance and dependence. Emerging receptor classes as targets for analgesic drugs and innovative analgesic strategies are discussed in separate chapters. From the molecular research bench through the animal laboratory to the bed-side, this book is for all those scientists and clinicians who are interested in what the increasingly molecular future has in store for analgesia research.

I used a paraphrase of the title of Robert Herrick's poem ("No pain, no gain") in the title of this preface thus it is fitting to close my writing with another poem of his:

96. To Critics
I'll write, because I'll give
You critics means to live;
For should I not supply
The cause, th' effect would die.

Arpad Szallasi

Contents

Contributors

ANNA-MARIA ANESTI • *BioVex Inc., Woburn, MA, USA*

ALEXANDRU BABES • *Department of Physiology and Biophysics, University of Bucharest, Bucharest, Romania*

SILVIA BENEMEI • *Department of Preclinical and Clinical Pharmacology, Headache Center, University of Florence, Florence, Italy*

EDWARD J. BILSKY • *Department of Pharmacology, University of New England College of Osteopathic Medicine, Biddeford, ME, USA*

JANEL M. BOYCE-RUSTAY • *Neuroscience Research, Global Pharmaceutical Research and Development, Abbott Laboratories, Abbott Park, IL, USA*

KATA BÖLCSKEI • *Analgesic Research Laboratory, University of Pécs, Gedeon Richter Plc., Pécs, Hungary*

DANIEL C. BROOM • *Branford, CT, USA*

JASON C. CALDWELL • *Department of Anesthesiology, Duke University Medical Center, Durham, NC, USA*

NORMA ALEJANDRA CHASSEING • *Instituto de Biologia y Medicina Experimental, CONICET, Buenos Aires, Argentina*

PHILIP CHENG • *Center for Neurosensory Disorders, University of North Carolina, Chapel Hill, NC, USA*

STEPHEN A. COOPER • *Senior VP Clinical and Medical Affairs (retired), Palm Beach Gardens, FL, USA*

MARIA FLORENCIA CORONEL • *Faculdad de Ciencias Biomedicas, Universidad Austral, Buenos Aires, Argentina*

DANIEL N. CORTRIGHT • *Science Foundry LLC, Orange, CT, USA*

RICARDO A. CRUCIANI • *Research Division, Department of Pain Medicine and Palliative Care, Beth Israel Medical, Center Institute for Non-Invasive Brain Stimulation of New York, New York, NY, USA; Departments of Neurology and Anesthesiology, Albert Einstein College of Medicine, Bronx, NY, USA*

WILLIAM P. DAILEY • *Department of Chemistry, University of Pennsylvania School of Arts and Sciences, Philadelphia, PA, USA*

CANDICE DAVIDOFF • *Integral Molecular, Inc., Philadelphia, PA, USA*

FRANCESCO DE CESARIS • *Department of Preclinical and Clinical Pharmacology, Headache Center, University of Florence, Florence, Italy*

PAUL J. DESJARDINS • *Senior VP Clinical and Medical Affairs, Wyeth Consumer Healthcare, Madison, NJ, USA*

LUDA DIATCHENKO • *Center for Neurosensory Disorders, Carolina Center for Genome Sciences, University of North Carolina, Chapel Hill, NC, USA*

ELISA DOMINGUEZ • *Faculty of Medicine Pitié-Salpêtrière, Brain and Spinal Cord Research Institute, INSERM UMRS 975, Pain Group, Paris, France*

BENJAMIN J. DORANZ • *Integral Molecular, Inc., Philadelphia, PA, USA*
RODERIC G. ECKENHOFF • *Department of Anesthesiology and Critical Care, University of Pennsylvania School of Medicine, Philadelphia, PA, USA*
ANDERS B. ERIKSSON • *Department of Molecular Pharmacology, AstraZeneca R&D, Södertälje, Sweden*
MICHAEL J.M. FISCHER • *Institute of Physiology and Pathophysiology, University of Erlangen – Nuremberg, Erlangen, Germany*
NARASIMBAN GAUTAM • *Departments of Anesthesiology and Genetics, Washington University School of Medicine, St. Louis, MO, USA*
PIERANGELO GEPPETTI • *Department of Preclinical and Clinical Pharmacology, Headache Center, University of Florence, Florence, Italy*
SRABONI GHOSE • *Genionics AG, Schlieren, Switzerland*
PAVEL GRIS • *Center for Neurosensory Disorders, University of North Carolina, Chapel Hill, NC, USA*
KENNETH M. HARGREAVES • *Departments of Endodontics, Pharmacology, Physiology and Surgery, University of Texas Health Science Center, San Antonio, TX, USA*
MASAKAZU HAYASHIDA • *Department of Anesthesiology, Saitama Medical University International Medical Center, Hidaka, Japan*
DENNIS HELLGREN • *Department of Disease Biology, AstraZeneca R&D, Södertälje, Sweden*
PRISCA HONORE • *Neuroscience Research, Global Pharmaceutical Research and Development, Abbott Laboratories, Abbott Park, IL, USA*
MICHAEL J. IADAROLA • *Neurobiology and Pain Therapeutics Section, National Institute of Dental and Craniofacial Research, National Institutes of Health, Bethesda, MD, USA*
SOICHIRO IDE • *Department of Pharmacology, Graduate School of Pharmaceutical Sciences, Hokkaido University, Sapporo, Japan*
KAZUTAKA IKEDA • *Division of Psychobiology, Tokyo Institute of Psychiatry, Tokyo, Japan*
LEÓN D. ISLAS • *Departamento de Fisiología, Faculdad de Medicina, Universidad Nacional Autónoma de México, Mexico City, Mexico*
MICHAEL F. JARVIS • *Neuroscience Research, Global Pharmaceutical Research and Development, Abbott Laboratories, Abbott Park, IL, USA*
MIA KARPITSCHKA • *Walter-Brendel Institute for Surgical Research, Ludwig-Maximilian's University, Munich, Germany*
ASMA KHAN • *Department of Endodontics, University of North Carolina, Chapel Hill, NC, USA*
HYANGIN KIM • *Department of Anesthesia and Critical Care, Massachusetts General Hospital Center for Translational Pain Research, Harvard Medical School, Boston, MA, USA*
IGOR KISSIN • *Department of Anesthesiology, Perioperative and Pain Medicine, Brigham and Women's Hospital, Harvard Medical School, Boston, MA, USA*
HELENA KNOTKOVA • *Research Division, Department of Pain Medicine and Palliative Care, Beth Israel Medical Center, Institute for Non-Invasive Brain Stimulation of New York, New York, NY, USA; Department of Neurology, Albert Einstein College of Medicine, Bronx, NY, USA*

HISASHI KOGA • *Laboratory of Medical Genomics, Department of Human Genome Technology, Kazusa DNA Research Institute, Kisarazu, Japan*
MARTIN E. KREIS • *Department of Surgery, Hospital Grosshadern, Ludwig-Maximilian's University, Munich, Germany*
JOHANNES J. KRUPP • *Department of Molecular Pharmacology, AstraZeneca R&D, Södertälje, Sweden*
WILLIAM R. LARIVIERE • *Departments of Anesthesiology and Neurobiology, University of Pittsburgh School of Medicine, Pittsburgh, PA, USA*
WILLIAM MAIXNER • *Center for Neurosensory Disorders, Carolina Center for Genome Sciences, University of North Carolina at Chapel Hill, Chapel Hill, NC, USA*
JIANREN MAO • *Department of Anesthesia and Critical Care, Massachusetts General Hospital Center for Translational Pain Research, Harvard Medical School, Boston, MA, USA*
SERENA MATERAZZI • *Department of Preclinical and Clinical Pharmacology, Headache Center, University of Florence, Florence, Italy*
DAVID J. MATSON • *Amgen Inc., Cambridge, MA, USA*
ALICE MEUNIER • *Pitié-Salpêtrière Hospital, Brain and Spinal Cord Research Institute, INSERM UMRS 975, Neuron-Glia Interactions Group, Paris, France*
MASABUMI MINAMI • *Department of Pharmacology, Graduate School of Pharmaceutical Sciences, Hokkaido University, Sapporo, Japan*
JAMES R. MINER • *Department of Emergency Medicine, Hennepin County Medical Center, University of Minnesota Medical School, Minneapolis, MN, USA*
KENDALL MITCHELL • *Neurobiology and Pain Therapeutics Section, National Institute of Dental and Craniofacial Research, National Institutes of Health, Bethesda, MD, USA*
JAMES G. MODIR • *Department of Anesthesiology, University of California (UCSD), San Diego, CA, USA*
JEFFREY S. MOGIL • *Department of Psychology, Alan Edwards Center for Research on Pain, McGill University, Montreal, QC, Canada*
PHIL G. MORGAN • *Center for Developmental Therapeutics, Seattle Children's Research Institute, Seattle, WA, USA; Department of Anesthesiology & Pain Medicine, University of Washington, Seattle, WA, USA*
ANDREA G. NACKLEY • *Center for Neurosensory Disorders, University of North Carolina, Chapel Hill, NC, USA*
MAKOTO NAGASHIMA • *Department of Surgery, Toho University Sakura Medical Center, Sakura, Japan*
ROMINA NASSINI • *Department of Preclinical, and Clinical Pharmacology, Headache Center, University of Florence, Florence, Italy*
S. STEVENS NEGUS • *Department of Pharmacology and Toxicology, Virginia Commonwealth University, Richmond, VA, USA*
PAOLA NICOLETTI • *Department of Preclinical and Clinical Pharmacology, Headache Center, University of Florence, Florence, Italy*
DAISUKE NISHIZAWA • *Division of Psychobiology, Tokyo Institute of Psychiatry, Tokyo, Japan*
CHRISTOPHER NOTO • *Department of Anesthesiology, Mount Sinai School of Medicine, New York, NY, USA*

Marco Pappagallo • *Department of Anesthesiology, Mount Sinai School of Medicine, New York, NY, USA*

Gail Pereira Do Carmo • *School of Social and Behavioral Sciences, Marist College, Poughkeepsie, NY, USA*

Gábor Pethő • *Department of Pharmacology and Pharmacotherapy, Faculty of Medicine, University of Pécs, Pécs, Hungary*

John Pierson • *Center for Neurosensory Disorders, University of North Carolina, Chapel Hill, NC, USA*

Michel Pohl • *Pitié-Salpêtrière Hospital, Brain and Spinal Cord Research Institute, INSERM UMRS 975, Neuron–Glia Interactions Group, Paris, France*

Peter W. Reeh • *Institute of Physiology and Pathophysiology, University of Erlangen – Nuremberg, Erlangen, Germany*

Gordon Reid • *Department of Physiology, University College, Cork, Ireland*

Nichole A. Reisdorph • *Department of Immunology, National Jewish Health, University of Colorado, Denver, CO, USA*

Richard Reisdorph • *Departments of Pediatrics and Immunology, National Jewish Health, University of Colorado, Denver, CO, USA*

Tamara Rosenbaum • *Departamento de Biofísica, Instituto de Fisiología Celular, Universidad Nacional Autónoma de México, Mexico City, Mexico*

Joseph Rucker • *Integral Molecular, Inc., Philadelphia, PA, USA*

Deepak Kumar Saini • *Department of Anesthesiology, Washington University School of Medicine, St. Louis, MO, USA*

Susanne K. Sauer • *Institute of Physiology and Pathophysiology, University of Erlangen – Nuremberg, Erlangen, Germany*

Margaret M. Sedensky • *Center for Developmental Therapeutics, Seattle Children's Research Institute, Seattle, WA, USA; Department of Anesthesiology & Pain Medicine, University of Washington, Seattle, WA, USA*

William K. Sietsema • *Regulatory Consulting and Submissions, Kendle International Inc., and College of Pharmacy, University of Cincinnati, Cincinnati, OH, USA*

Sidney A. Simon • *Department of Neurobiology, Center for Neuroengineering, Duke University Medical Center, Durham, NC, USA*

Dario Siniscalco • *Department of Experimental Medicine, Section of Pharmacology "L. Donatelli," Second University of Naples, Naples, Italy*

Ichiro Sora • *Division of Psychobiology, Department of Neuroscience, Tohoku University Graduate School of Medicine, Sendai, Japan*

Louise M. Steele • *Center for Developmental Therapeutics, Seattle Children's Research Institute, Seattle, WA, USA*

Florian Steiner • *Genionics AG, Schlieren, Switzerland*

Glenn W. Stevenson • *Department of Psychology, University of New England, Biddeford, ME, USA*

Christian S. Stohler • *University of Maryland Dental School, Baltimore, MD, USA*

Backil Sung • *Department of Anesthesia and Critical Care, Massachusetts General Hospital Center for Translational Pain Research, Harvard Medical School, Boston, MA, USA*

ARPAD SZALLASI • *Department of Pathology and Laboratories, Monmouth Medical Center, Long Branch, NJ, USA; Drexel University College of Medicine, Philadelphia, PA, USA*

JÁNOS SZOLCSÁNYI • *Department of Pharmacology and Pharmacotherapy, Faculty of Medicine, University of Pécs, Pécs, Hungary*

URS THOMET • *Genionics AG, Schlieren, Switzerland*

W. DANIEL TRACEY, JR. • *Department of Anesthesiology, Duke University Medical Center, Durham, NC, USA*

MARCELO JOSE VILLAR • *Faculdad de Ciencias Biomedicas, Universidad Austral, Buenos Aires, Argentina*

MARK S. WALLACE • *Department of Anesthesiology, University of California (UCSD), San Diego, CA, USA*

JIN XI • *Department of Anesthesiology and Critical Care, University of Pennsylvania School of Medicine, Philadelphia, PA, USA*

KATHARINA ZIMMERMANN • *Institute of Physiology and Pathophysiology, University of Erlangen – Nuremberg, Erlangen, Germany*

JON-KAR ZUBIETA • *Departments of Psychiatry and Radiology, University of Michigan Medical School, Ann Arbor, MI, USA*

Chapter 1

Alternatives to Mammalian Pain Models 1: Use of *C. elegans* for the Study of Volatile Anesthetics

Louise M. Steele, Margaret M. Sedensky, and Phil G. Morgan

Abstract

Performing genetic studies in model organisms is a powerful approach for investigating the mechanisms of volatile anesthetic action. Striking similarities between the results observed in *Caenorhabditis elegans* and in other organisms suggest that many of the conclusions can be generalized across disparate phyla, and that findings in these model organisms will be applicable in humans. In this chapter, we provide detailed protocols for working with *C. elegans* to study volatile anesthetics. First, we explain how to fabricate chambers for exposing worms to these compounds. Then, we describe how to use the chambers to perform a variety of experiments, including behavioral assays, dose-response studies, and mutant screening or selection. Finally, we discuss a convenient strategy for performing mutant rescue assays. These methods are the building blocks for designing and interpreting genetic experiments with volatile anesthetics in *C. elegans*. Genetic studies in this simple, easy-to-use organism will continue to contribute to a more thorough understanding of anesthetic mechanisms, and may lead to the development and safer use of anesthetic agents.

Key words: *C. elegans*, Genetics, Animal models, Behavioral assays, Dose-response studies, Mutant screening, Mutant rescue, Volatile anesthetics

1. Introduction

Elucidating the molecular mechanisms of volatile anesthetic action has been one of the most challenging problems in biomedical research. One powerful approach for addressing questions in this field has involved performing genetic studies in organisms such as yeast, worms, flies, and mice (1, 2). Using genetics in a whole-animal system is appealing because no assumptions are made about the cellular components that *should* play a role in the mechanisms of action. By screening for mutations that alter

Arpad Szallasi (ed.), *Analgesia: Methods and Protocols*, Methods in Molecular Biology, vol. 617,
DOI 10.1007/978-1-60327-323-7_1, © Springer Science+Business Media, LLC 2010

the anesthetic response, the biology of the organism directs the researcher to the relevant molecules. Furthermore, because a high proportion of genes are conserved among these animals and humans, they can serve as models for understanding the molecular processes responsible for the effects of anesthetics on human patients.

In the 1970s, Sydney Brenner introduced the nematode, *Caenorhabditis elegans* (*C. elegans*), as a model for studying behavior (3). Brenner chose this 1 mm-long, nonparasitic roundworm primarily because it is a simple, inexpensive metazoan with some ideal features for genetic experiments. *C. elegans* is transparent, which allowed researchers to completely define its anatomy and determine its invariant cell lineage. Furthermore, *C. elegans* has a short generation time, a small genome with considerable homology to more complicated organisms, and the ability to produce hypomorphs by RNA interference (RNAi). The worm has a low forward mutation rate, with a single isogenic wild type strain. It usually exists as a self-fertilizing hermaphrodite, which can produce males for genetic crosses, and it can be frozen for storage in liquid nitrogen. A large number of mutants are easily obtained from a central stock center (*Caenorhabditis* Genetics Center; University of Minnesota, St. Paul). An extensive database that includes the sequence of the genome, information about available mutants, genetic and physical maps, a bibliography of publications, etc., is publicly accessible at www.wormbase.org.

Methods were developed in the 1980s for using *C. elegans* to study volatile anesthetic action. Under normal conditions, wild type *C. elegans* moves almost constantly. Morgan and Cascorbi (4) found that when *C. elegans* is exposed to anesthetics, there is an initial phase of increased locomotion, followed by uncoordinated motion that progresses to immobility. Motion returns quickly when the nematodes are removed from the anesthetic agent. These authors defined immobility as the anesthetic endpoint. Other behaviors have also been defined as endpoints, including radial dispersion (i.e., the ability of nematodes to move from a starting point in the center of a plate of agar toward a peripheral ring of food), inhibition of mating, loss of chemotaxis, uncoordination, changes in the rate of forward locomotion, and changes in the number of body bends per minute (5–9). Loss of mobility requires a higher concentration of anesthetic than do the other endpoints.

By using these behavioral assays, researchers have determined the anesthetic sensitivities of wild type and mutant worm strains. The results of such studies and of studies in other organisms suggest that changes in a broad range of membrane-associated components (1, 10–16) and the mitochondrial electron transport chain (17, 18) can change the behavior of animals in volatile anesthetics. Together, these data currently implicate the presynaptic neuron as a common functional target for volatile anesthetic agents. Intriguing similarities among results in yeast, worms, flies, and mice (1, 2) suggest that many of the findings obtained in model organisms can be generalized across disparate phyla. Indeed, similar observations have been made in humans (19, 20), which lends credence to the use of animal models for studies of anesthetic mechanisms.

The focus of this chapter is on techniques that are necessary to study anesthetic action in *C. elegans*. Methods for culturing and manipulating *C. elegans* have been described in detail elsewhere (3, 21). Here, we explain how to fabricate glass chambers to expose *C. elegans* to volatile anesthetics, and how to use the chambers to perform a variety of behavioral assays. In addition, we describe how to determine the anesthetic concentrations present in the chambers to construct dose-response curves. The curves enable one to determine and compare the half-maximal effective concentrations (EC_{50}s) of particular anesthetics in various worm strains. We cover how to screen or select for mutant worms that exhibit altered anesthetic sensitivities. Finally, we discuss a convenient approach for performing mutant rescue to confirm that a mutation of interest, rather than a linked genetic defect, is responsible for a worm's altered anesthetic phenotype. These protocols will be of value to researchers and clinicians who wish to perform such experiments and to those who wish to interpret literature in which *C. elegans* was used as a model for the study of anesthetic action.

2. Materials

2.1. Fabrication of Anesthetic Chambers

1. Containers (see criteria described in the text).
2. 18-gauge spinal needles, 3″ length (Becton-Dickinson, Franklin Lake, NJ).
3. High-strength epoxy. Avoid rapid-curing, lower-strength epoxies.
4. 2″ (1 1/16″ capacity) binder clips.
5. Foam weather stripping (0.5 cm thick × 3.2 cm wide × 5 cm long) (3/16″ thick × 1 1/4″ wide × 2″ long)
6. Male luer lock caps.
7. Window glass (6 mm thick) cut to the size of container.

2.2. Use of Anesthetic Chambers

1. Chambers.
2. 95% ethanol.

3. Vacuum grease (Fisher, Pittsburgh, PA).
4. 100-μl Hamilton syringe model #710 (Fisher).
5. Halothane (2-bromo-2-chloro-1,1,1-trifluoroethane, ≥99.0% (GC)) (Sigma, St. Louis, MO). Store the halothane at room temperature in a tightly capped, brown bottle to avoid evaporation and exposure to light. Use halothane in a well ventilated area.
6. Other volatile anesthetics currently in clinical use (and available by prescription only) include substituted ethers like isoflurane (FORANE, Abbott Laboratories, Abbott Park, IL), sevoflurane (ULTANE, Abbott Laboratories), and desflurane (SUPRANE, Baxter, Deerfield, IL). Historically useful agents include diethyl ether and chloroform. Cyclopropane, although once used clinically, is avoided even as an experimental agent due to its explosiveness.

2.3. Behavioral Assays

1. Chambers with accessories (see above).
2. Binocular dissecting microscope capable of up to 400× magnification with light source to illuminate samples from below.
3. Push-button counter with two counting units (VWR, West Chester, PA).
4. For most assays, nematodes are grown on 35-mm × 10-mm Petri plates (Fisher), several of which will fit in the chambers.
5. For radial dispersion assays, nematodes are transferred to 100-mm × 15-mm Petri plates (Fisher).
6. Isoamyl alcohol (Sigma).
7. Sodium azide (Sigma).
8. Detailed instructions for preparing Nematode Growth Medium (NGM), bacterial food source (*E. coli* strain OP50), and S. Basal buffer are described elsewhere (21).

2.4. Determining Anesthetic Concentration

1. Chambers and accessories (see above).
2. 30-ml BD Multifit™ glass syringe (Becton-Dickinson).
3. Three 3-way stopcocks, preferably metal, if much time will elapse between sampling the chamber and testing the anesthetic concentration (female luer to male luer and sidearm female luer) (Fisher).
4. Two 18-gauge spinal needles, 3″ length (Becton–Dickinson).
5. Gas chromatograph and a hydrophobic column of sufficient length to separate the very lipophilic anesthetics. (Many are available and no specific recommendation is necessary.)
6. 4-L sidearm vacuum flask (Fisher).
7. Vacuum tubing (Fisher).
8. Hemostats (Fisher).

9. Rubber stopper.
10. 100-μl Hamilton Microliter syringe model #710 (Fisher).
11. Vacuum source.

3. Methods

3.1. Fabrication of Anesthetic Chambers

In our laboratory, worms are exposed to volatile anesthetics in sealed, glass chambers (Fig. 1) that were made from glass lids for Corningware food storage containers. These lids are no

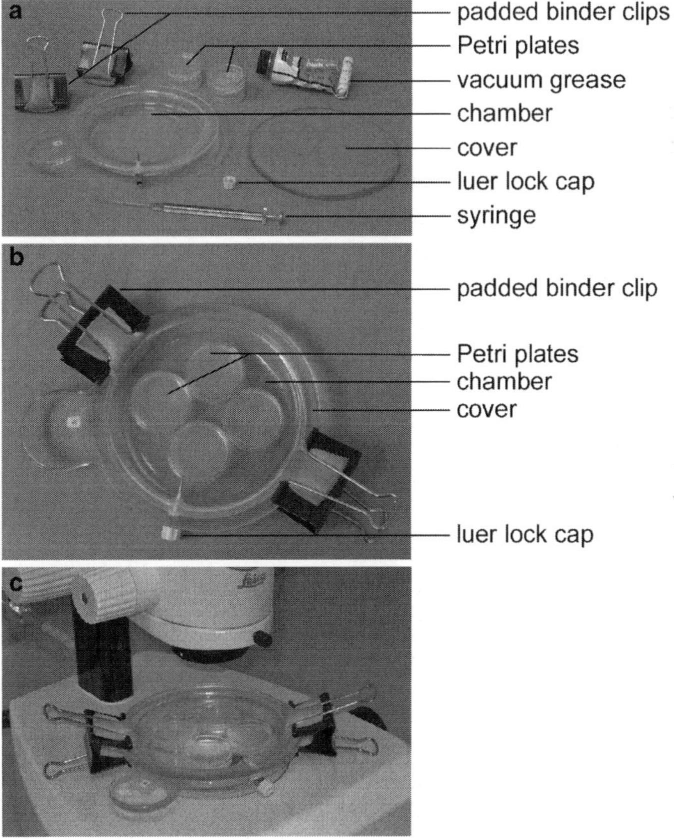

Fig. 1. Photographs of an anesthetic chamber. (**a**) An open chamber with accessories, including padded binder clips, luer lock cap, vacuum grease, Hamilton syringe, and worm plates. (**b**) Worm plates, without their lids, are placed in the chamber. The chamber is sealed with vacuum grease and binder clips are positioned on opposite sides of the chamber to hold the cover firmly in place. Immediately after anesthetic is dispensed through the injection port with a Hamilton syringe, a cap is placed on the luer lock. The chamber is shaken from side to side to distribute the anesthetic and then incubated until steady state is reached. (**c**) The chamber fits easily on the stage of a dissecting microscope. The transparency and uniform thickness of the glass chamber permit the worms to be viewed

longer easily available. A suitable chamber has the following characteristics:

1. The material should be clear glass (so that anesthetics do not dissolve the material and do not dissolve in the material) and of uniform thickness so that specimens in the chamber can be examined with a dissecting microscope.
2. The chamber must fit conveniently on a dissecting microscope stage. The height of the chamber should not exceed two inches.
3. The chamber must be deep enough to accommodate 35-mm × 10-mm Petri plates.
4. A cover will be placed on the chamber. The chamber should have a lip that can be used for clamping the cover to the body of the chamber.
5. There must be enough flat surface area where the chamber meets the cover to apply vacuum grease and clamps to ensure a seal that is as airtight as possible.

The steps required to fabricate the chambers will depend on the glassware that is chosen. The process that we followed is given here merely as an example (see Note 1).

1. The following steps may be performed by workers at a glass shop in your area. In our experience, glass craftsmen who are not familiar with the precision required for laboratory glassware produce chambers that are suboptimal.
   (a) If necessary, grind off any raised lips on the surface of the glassware that will meet the cover. This process has to be fairly precise, as it is impossible to get a good seal if the surface is not flat. Even small gaps will lead to a significant leakage of gas over time.
   (b) To create an injection port, drill a small hole (2-mm diameter) through the side of the glassware. If the glass is tempered, it must be reannealed first, as drilling will tend to shatter the chamber.
   (c) To create a cover for the chamber, cut a piece of window glass (about 6 mm thick) the same size as the glassware (14-cm diameter).
2. To complete the chamber, cut an 18-gauge spinal needle to a length of about 4 cm. Score or sand the outside of the needle to help form a bonding surface with the epoxy (see below).
3. Insert the needle through the hole with the luer lock on the outside of the glassware.
4. Fill the opening around the needle with slow-curing, high-strength epoxy to hold the needle in place and to form an airtight seal. The application of this epoxy is critical and must

be done carefully, or the needles will not be fixed. If the needles turn, anesthetic will escape the chamber.

5. Allow the epoxy to cure as directed on the package instructions.
6. Cut strips of foam weather stripping (0.5 cm thick × 3.2 cm wide × 5 cm long).
7. Adhere the foam to the jaws of 2″ binder clips. The foam will help prevent the clips from sliding off the chambers.
8. Obtain luer lock caps that will fit the needle hubs.
9. Check the chambers for leaks by injecting an anesthetic as described below, and by checking gas concentrations over time. If a chamber leaks, it most likely has a poor fit of the lid with the chamber bottom, or a loose injection port.

3.2. Use of Anesthetic Chambers

1. Clean the chamber cover with 95% ethanol to remove any residual vacuum grease that would interfere with viewing the worm specimens.
2. Apply a very thin coating of fresh vacuum grease to the surface of the chamber that will come in contact with the cover.
3. Remove the plastic lids from the worm plates that will be examined. If desired, use a felt-tipped pen to draw a grid on the bottom of the plates to help score worms.
4. Place the worm plates in the chamber. For our chambers, we grow nematodes on 35-mm plates.
5. Place the cover on the chamber by lowering it straight down onto the chamber to avoid spreading vacuum grease in the viewing area.
6. While applying downward pressure, turn the cover about a quarter of a turn to evenly distribute the vacuum grease.
7. Position two padded 2″ binder clips on opposite sides of the chamber to hold the cover firmly in place.
8. Use a Hamilton glass syringe calibrated in microliters to measure an appropriate amount of anesthetic.
9. Tilt the chamber so the worm plates slide away from the inlet.
10. Place the chamber on a benchtop or another flat surface.
11. Insert the syringe into the inlet and dispense the anesthetic (see Note 2).
12. Quickly withdraw the syringe from the inlet and immediately seal the inlet with a luer lock cap. Cover the inlet with your thumb while exchanging the syringe for the cap.
13. Invert the chamber and gently shake it from side to side to disperse the anesthetic.
14. Incubate the worms in the chamber until a steady-state behavioral effect is achieved (see Notes 3 and 4).

3.3. Behavioral Assays

A variety of behavioral assays are currently used to measure the anesthetic response in *C. elegans*, including assays for immobility, radial dispersion, chemotaxis, mating efficiency, velocity, and body bends (4–9). Other assays that have been used in the past measure defecation, pharyngeal pumping, egg laying, and mechanosensation and have been described in detail elsewhere (6, 22, 23). In this review, we will discuss only assays that are in common use in our laboratory: immobility, radial dispersion, chemotaxis and mating efficiency.

3.3.1. Immobility Assay

For immobility assays (4), young adult worms are used except when developmental assays are conducted (see Note 5). Worms must be well-fed (see Note 6).

1. Expose the worms to appropriate concentration(s) of anesthetic in sealed chambers until steady state is achieved (see Note 3).
2. If room temperature is not 20–22°C, keep the chambers in a 20°C incubator.
3. For halothane and other anesthetics that are denser than room air, shake the sealed chamber briefly every 10 min to mix the anesthetic with the room air in the chamber.
4. Place the sealed chamber on the stage of a dissecting microscope and examine the worms at about 160× magnification. If condensation forms on the glass cover, consider incubating the chambers stacked on top of each other.
5. Without opening the chamber, score the worms as mobile or immobile. A worm is considered immobile if it does not move its body for a period of ten seconds. If a worm remains motionless or moves only its head during that time frame, it is immobile. If a worm does move its body during that time frame, even if only to writhe in place, it is mobile.

3.3.2. Radial Dispersion Assay

Radial dispersion assays measure the worms' ability to move from a starting point at the center of an agar plate out to a peripheral ring of food (6, 7).

1. Use 1 ml of S. Basal to wash well-fed, young adult worms off plates into 1.5 ml microcentrifuge tubes (see Notes 5 and 6).
2. Rinse the worms twice with 1 ml of S. Basal.
3. Rinse the worms once with 1 ml of distilled water.
4. Resuspend the worms in 100 μl of distilled water.
5. Dispense 10-μl aliquots (containing 50–100 worms) onto the center of a 100-mm plate seeded with a narrow ring (about 5 mm) of *E. coli* along the outer edge of the plate. Use an inoculating loop to spread the ring the night before performing the test so that a visible lawn is present.

6. Immediately place the plates in a sealed chamber and add an appropriate amount of anesthetic. These plates are so large that only one plate will fit in a chamber. Do not shake the chamber until the water droplet containing the worms has dried.
7. After the droplet containing the worms has dried (usually within 5 min), shake the chamber from side to side.
8. Incubate the worms in the chamber for 45 min at room temperature.
9. Determine the percent of worms reaching the ring of bacteria.
10. Compare the results in step 9 to a control plate treated identically but without anesthetic added. This is especially important when testing mutant strains that will vary in their ability to reach the ring of bacteria in the absence of anesthetic.

3.3.3. Chemotaxis Assay

Chemotaxis assays measure the ability of worms to move from a starting point to a spot of chemoattractant near the edge of the plate (5, 6).

1. Use a felt-tipped pen to mark three 1-cm diameter circles on the underside of a 100-mm unspread plate. The circles should be about 0.5 cm from the edge of the plate, and they should form an equilateral triangle.
2. In the center of one circle, spot a chemoattractant, such as 1 μl of isoamyl alcohol, with 1 μl of 1 M sodium azide. The sodium azide will immobilize worms that enter the chemoattractant zone so they will remain there to be counted.
3. As a control, spot 1 μl of 1 M sodium azide in the center of another circle.
4. The third circle, which should be equidistant from the other two, is the starting point for the worms. Wash, dispense, and anesthetize the worms as directed for radial dispersion assays. No *E. coli* lawn is used for these plates unless the lawn is the chemoattractant.
5. Incubate the worms in the anesthetic for 45 min at room temperature.
6. Count the worms to determine a "chemotaxis index" according to the equation, (A–C)/T, where A is the number of worms within the attractant zone, C is the number of worms within 5 mm of the control zone, and T is the total number of worms on the plate.

3.3.4. Mating Efficiency Assay

Mating efficiencies can be estimated by performing the following assay (6, 9):

1. Spread 35-mm plates with a relatively small area of bacterial lawn.
2. On five plates, plate 10 young adult males and two hermaphrodites with a visible marker such as *dpy-11(e224)*.

3. Place the plates in a chamber and add an appropriate concentration of anesthetic.
4. Take a sample of gas from the chamber to measure the anesthetic concentration at the beginning of the experiment by gas chromatography as described in the next section, "Determining Anesthetic Concentrations."
5. Ensure that the chamber is well-sealed.
6. Incubate the chamber for 24 h at 20°C.
7. To verify that the chamber did not leak during the incubation, take another sample of gas from the chamber to measure the anesthetic concentration at the end of the experiment.
8. Open the chambers and remove the male worms from the plates.
9. Allow the offspring to develop for 3 or 4 days at 20°C in room air.
10. Calculate the "mating index" for each chamber as the fraction of plates with cross progeny.

3.4. Determining Anesthetic Concentration

The capacity of each anesthetic chamber differs slightly. Therefore, for experiments in which the concentration of anesthetic in a chamber must be known precisely, gas chromatography is used to analyze samples of gas taken from each chamber. The concentration of anesthetic is determined by comparison to a known standard.

3.4.1. Collection of Gas Samples

After an experiment is complete, and before opening the anesthetic chambers, collect and analyze a sample of gas from each chamber as follows:

1. Remove the luer lock cap from the inlet and immediately cover the inlet with your thumb.
2. Remove your thumb from the inlet and immediately connect a 30-ml gas-tight syringe into the inlet.
3. Move the syringe plunger in and out a few times to mix the gas in the chamber again.
4. Draw a 10-ml sample of gas into the syringe and close the valve on the syringe.
5. Remove the syringe from the chamber and immediately cover the inlet with your thumb.
6. Remove your thumb from the inlet and immediately replace the luer lock cap.
7. Analyze the sample according to the operating instructions for the particular gas chromatograph that is used.
8. Expect a large peak of nitrogen and oxygen (air) followed by a smaller peak of anesthetic. Less hydrophobic anesthetics

(isoflurane, diethylether) will elute more quickly than gases like halothane and may be difficult to separate from the large air peak.

9. Note the area under the anesthetic peak. This area is proportional to the concentration of anesthetic and represents the value of $A_{unknown}$ in the equation in Subheading 3.4.2, step 20.

3.4.2. Preparation of a Known Standard

1. Choose a rubber stopper that will fit a 4-L sidearm vacuum flask.
2. Insert two 3.5-inch spinal needles through the rubber stopper and attach stainless steel 3-way stopcocks to the needles.
3. Use parafilm to seal the sidearm of the flask.
4. Determine the volume of the flask by completely filling it with water and capping the flask with the rubber stopper. Measure the amount of water to the nearest milliliter.
5. Allow the flask to dry completely and remove the parafilm from the sidearm.
6. Use a piece of vacuum tubing to connect the sidearm of the flask to a vacuum source.
7. Insert the stopper, close the stopcocks and apply a vacuum to the flask.
8. Use hemostats to clamp off the vacuum tubing as close to the sidearm as possible.
9. Turn off the vacuum and disconnect the tubing from the vacuum source.
10. Use a glass syringe graduated in microliters to measure the volume of anesthetic that will give the desired concentration of gaseous anesthetic in the flask (see Note 7). The gas concentration in the flask corresponds to $C_{standard}$ in the equation in step 20 below.
11. Hold the syringe needle in the opening of one of the stopcocks in the rubber stopper.
12. Open that stopcock, immediately insert the needle, and immediately inject the anesthetic. Keep the syringe in place for a second or two. Because of the lower air pressure in the flask, air will enter the flask and draw in the anesthetic.
13. Remove the needle, immediately close the stopcock and allow the anesthetic to volatilize.
14. After the anesthetic has volatilized, unclamp the tubing to allow the flask to reach atmospheric pressure. When air is no longer entering the flask, immediately reclamp the tubing as close to the sidearm as possible.

15. Invert the flask several times to mix the gases inside to achieve a uniform concentration of anesthetic.
16. Open the other stopcock on the flask and take a 10-ml sample of gas from the flask using an airtight glass syringe fitted with a stopcock. Close the stopcock on the syringe.
17. Remove the syringe from the flask and immediately close the stopcock on the flask.
18. Analyze the sample by following the operating instructions for the particular gas chromatograph that is used.
19. Expect a large peak of nitrogen and oxygen (air), followed by a smaller peak of anesthetic. Note the area under the anesthetic peak. This is A_{standard} in step 20. We make a fresh standard for each day of experimental assays.
20. Calculate the concentration of anesthetic in experimental chambers by comparison with the standard. The area under the anesthetic peak is proportional to the concentration of anesthetic in the sample.

$$C_{\text{standard}}/A_{\text{standard}} = C_{\text{unknown}}/A_{\text{unknown}}$$

where C equals the concentration of anesthetic, and A equals the area under the anesthetic peak observed on the gas chromatogram. Determine the concentration of anesthetic in each chamber by measuring the area for the experimental samples and solving the equation for C_{unknown}.

3.5. Dose–Response Curves

1. Prepare cultures of at least 100 synchronized, well-fed adult worms per plate (see Notes 5, 6, and 8).
2. Expose different plates of these worms to different concentrations of anesthetics in sealed chambers as described above.
3. Perform immobility assays as described above. The steady-state time should be determined before starting to gather dose-response data (see Note 3).
4. Determine the concentrations of anesthetic present in the chambers as described above.
5. Create a dose-response curve (Fig. 2) by plotting the percentage of worms that are immobilized (y) at each anesthetic concentration (x). Use a logistic regression to estimate the EC_{50} (the concentration at which half of the animals are anesthetized) and the slope of the curve. The precise values can be determined by the method first described by Waud (24). It may take multiple attempts to obtain data points at the characteristic steep part of the curve, especially for gases like diethyl ether that volatilize quickly.
6. Perform statistical analysis (*t*-test for two samples, ANOVA for multiple comparisons) to determine whether the EC_{50}s of various worm strains differ (24, 25).

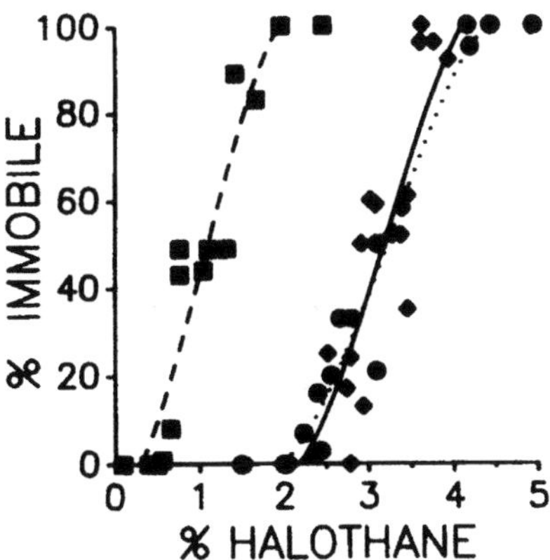

Fig. 2. Dose-response curves of wild-type N2 (♦) and mutant *unc-79* (■) and *unc-79; unc-9* (●) *C. elegans* in halothane. The curves compare the percentage of nematodes immobilized to the percent volumes (vol %) of halothane. From Morgan PG, Sedensky M, Meneely PM. (1990) Multiple sites of action of volatile anesthetics in *Caenorhabditis elegans. Proc. Natl. Acad. Sci.* U.S.A. **87,** 2965–2969

3.6. Screening/ Selecting for Mutants with Altered Anesthetic Sensitivity

A classic approach to identifying genes that may control response to a drug is to select or screen for resistance or hypersensitivity to that agent in mutagenized animals. Genes and gene products that cause the change can then be identified. It is important to keep in mind, however, that if multiple targets exist for volatile anesthetics, it could be difficult to obtain significant resistance by altering a single gene. Measuring anesthetic sensitivity essentially measures the EC_{50} of the most sensitive target. If multiple targets have similar EC_{50}s, then making one target resistant will simply unmask sensitivity of another target (of similar sensitivity). In addition, gene redundancy (multiple gene products sharing the same or overlapping function) may exist, which could make obtaining resistance difficult. However, genes of importance may be identified by screening for anesthetic hypersensitivity. In this case, the effects of making one target more susceptible to the anesthetic can be seen, despite gene redundancy or multiple overlapping targets. Making one target more sensitive will result in the animal becoming anesthetized at the new lower EC_{50}. With these caveats in mind, we describe protocols for screening and selection.

3.6.1. Screening

1. Prepare a large number of plates with about 100 mutagenized worms per plate.
2. Draw a 3×3 grid on the bottom of each plate with a felt-tipped pen.
3. Anesthetize the well-fed adult worms in anesthetic chambers as described above (see Notes 5, 6, and 9).
4. Without opening the anesthetic chambers, look at the worms with a dissecting microscope at about 160× magnification.

5. Look for worm(s) that are not moving (hypersensitive) and note their approximate location relative to the grid.
6. Remove the plate from the anesthetic chamber.
7. Immediately place the plate back under the microscope and use the grid pattern to facilitate finding the worm(s) of interest quickly and transfer them to a fresh plate.
8. Allow the worm(s) to recover in room air to verify that they remain alive and are capable of moving.

3.6.2. Selection

After mutagenesis, worms can be easily selected for survival in a lethal dose of anesthetic.

1. Prepare a large number of plates with about 100 mutagenized worms per plate.
2. Draw a 3×3 grid on the bottom of each plate with a felt-tipped pen.
3. Anesthetize the well-fed adult worms (see Notes 5 and 6) in anesthetic chambers as described above. Use a concentration of anesthetic that is known to be lethal for wildtype worms (see Note 2).
4. Without opening the anesthetic chambers, look at the worms with a dissecting microscope at about 160× magnification.
5. Look for worm(s) that are alive and note their approximate location relative to the grid.
6. Remove the plate from the anesthetic chamber.
7. Place the plate back under the microscope and use the grid pattern to facilitate finding the worm(s) of interest and transfer them to a fresh plate.

3.7. Mutant Rescue

Mutant rescue assays are performed to demonstrate that a phenotype is the result of a particular mutation and not of another linked genetic defect. Briefly, the assay involves microinjecting DNA into the gonad of the mutant worms, where it can be taken up by developing oocytes. If the injected DNA contains a wild-type copy of the mutated gene, then some of the offspring can be stably transformed to wild-type or "rescued." This technique has been completely described by Mello et al. (26, 27).

For studies of anesthetic sensitivity, it is generally necessary to score potentially rescued worms in a gaseous anesthetic as young adults. Therefore, unless the mutant animal displays an easily scored phenotype other than a changed behavior in an anesthetic, it is customary to co-inject a plasmid bearing an easily seen marker, such as the *rol-6* gene. The marker allows one to distinguish between transformed and nontransformed animals in room air. One can pick rollers to a fresh plate, make sure that they are well fed, and then test the worm's phenotype in anesthetic.

4. Notes

1. For similar experiments using larger animals (e.g., mice), we have used Lucite or other clear plastics and an anesthetic gas mixture from an anesthesia machine. This is usually done with a constant flow and can be sampled by gas chromatography as described for nematodes.
2. When injecting large volumes of anesthetic in their liquid form into a crowded chamber, it is important to take care not to drip any of the agent directly onto the plastic plates or allow it to fall directly on the worms. This can be problematic if the anesthetic does not volatilize rapidly. It is helpful to tilt the chamber until the plates slide away from the injection port. We usually aim to hit the lid of the chamber if the volume of anesthetic is large enough that volatilization is not immediate.
3. Volatile anesthetics differ significantly in the time necessary to reach steady state. The length of time required varies with the lipid solubility of the volatile anesthetic. The more lipid-soluble anesthetics are slower to reach steady state than are those that are less lipid soluble. The length of time required also depends on the endpoint being used, the specific chambers, and the size of the agar plates. Thus, time-course studies should be done to determine at what time steady-state effects are reached.
4. Preincubating the agar plates in the presence of anesthetic is an option that is advantageous when one wishes to limit the exposure time for the animals. For example, using immobility as an endpoint, halothane takes over an hour to reach steady state at room temperature in plates that have not been preequilibrated, so we typically assay the chamber at two hours. If plates are preincubated for 2 h in the presence of halothane at the same concentration used for screening and then worms quickly added, the assays reach steady state in the matter of a few minutes. Of course, the chambers need to be recharged with the desired amount of anesthetic after opening and adding nematodes.
5. The animals being scored should be young adults, i.e., within the first day of egg laying. The absolute age will vary with the mutant strain being studied. The EC_{50} in volatile anesthetics varies with age (younger worms are mildly resistant compared to older worms).
6. Sensitivity to volatile anesthetics is strongly affected by nutritional status. Starved worms are decidedly resistant compared to well-fed animals. This resistance is not fully restored to normal by subsequent feeding. Once animals have been allowed to starve, one must wait until the subsequent generation for measuring anesthetic sensitivity.

7. Choose a concentration for the standard that is in the range of that being used in the chambers during that day's experiment. Then use the following formula to calculate the volume of liquid anesthetic that must be injected into the flask to generate that concentration of gaseous anesthetic in the flask:

$$V = [\{(C_{\text{standard}} \times V_f) / 22.4\text{L}\} \times mw] / p$$

where V=volume of anesthetic injected (mls)
C_{standard}=chosen concentration of the anesthetic in the flask
V_f =volume of flask
mw=molecular weight of anesthetic
p=density of anesthetic (g/ml)
The derivation of this formula is presented here:

The percent (which you choose) of gaseous anesthetic in the flask is $C_{\text{standard}} = V_g / V_f$,

where Vg is the volume of anesthetic gas at standard temperature and pressure (STP=20°C and 1 atm).

Since 1 mole of anesthetic will vaporize to 22.4 L at STP, then $V_g = f_A \times 22.4$ L,
where f_A is the fraction of a mole of anesthetic injected.

Since $f_A = (V \times p)/mw$, then $C_{\text{standard}} = (\{(V \times p)/mw\} \times 22.4 \text{ L})/V_f$.

Rearranging this equation to solve for V yields the formula above. We inject 0.497 ml of halothane into our 4.390-L flask, which gives a 2.4% halothane standard.

8. It is important to tightly synchronize cultures for dose-response curves. We prefer that worm cultures for dose-response curves are grown from eggs laid within a 4–6 h time window. It is best if the bacterial lawn does not go to the extreme edge on these plates in order to keep the worms in easy view when scoring for immobility.

9. Use a preselected concentration of a particular anesthetic. For example, in 2% halothane, wild type worms move well. Any worms that are not moving in this dose of halothane are either hypersensitive to the anesthetic, immobilized in room air, or dead. Conversely, screening for resistance would require injecting halothane to a concentration of about 4%, and looking for animals that are still moving.

Acknowledgments

This work was supported by NIH grants GM 45402 and GM 58881.

References

1. Humphrey JA, Sedensky MM, Morgan PG (2002) Understanding anesthesia: making genetic sense of the absence of senses. Hum Mol Genet 11:1241–1249
2. Steele LM, Morgan PG, Sedensky MM (2007) Genetics and the mechanisms of action of inhaled anesthetics. Curr Pharm 5:125–141
3. Brenner S (1974) The genetics of *Caenorhabditis elegans*. Genetics 77:71–94
4. Morgan PG, Cascorbi HF (1985) Effect of anesthetics and a convulsant on normal and mutant *Caenorhabditis elegans*. Anesthesiology 62:738–744
5. Bargmann CI, Hartwieg E, Horvitz HR (1993) Odorant-selective genes and neurons mediate olfaction in *C. elegans*. Cell 74:515–527
6. Crowder CM, Shebester LD, Schedl T (1996) Behavioral effects of volatile anesthetics in *Caenorhabditis elegans*. Anesthesiology 85: 901–912
7. Epstein HF, Isachsen MM, Suddleson EA (1976) Kinetics of movement of normal and mutant nematodes. J Comp Physiol 110:317–322
8. Hawasli AH, Saifee O, Liu C, Nonet ML, Crowder CM (2004) Resistance to volatile anesthetics by mutations enhancing excitatory neurotransmitter release in *Caenorhabditis elegans*. Genetics 168:831–843
9. Hodgkin J (1983) Male phenotypes and mating efficiency in *Caenorhabditis elegans*. Genetics 103:43–64
10. Campagna JA, Miller KW, Forman SA (2003) Mechanisms of actions of inhaled anesthetics. N Engl J Med 348:2110–2124
11. Franks NP, Lieb WR (1994) Molecular and cellular mechanisms of general anaesthesia. Nature 367:607–614
12. Heurteaux C, Guy N, Laigle C, Blondeau N, Duprat F, Mazzuca M, Lang-Lazdunski L, Widmann C, Zanzouri M, Romey G, Lazdunski M (2004) TREK-1, a K^+ channel involved in neuroprotection and general anesthesia. EMBO J 23:2684–2695
13. Nash HA, Scott RL, Lear BC, Allada R (2002) An unusual cation channel mediates photic control of locomotion in *Drosophila*. Curr Biol 12:2152–2158
14. Rajaram S, Spangler TL, Sedensky MM, Morgan PG (1999) A stomatin and a degenerin interact to control anesthetic sensitivity in *Caenorhabditis elegans*. Genetics 153: 1673–1682
15. Sonner JM, Vissel B, Royle G, Maurer A, Gong D, Baron NV, Harrison N, Fanselow M, Eger EI 2nd (2005) The effect of three inhaled anesthetics in mice harboring mutations in the GluR6 (kainate) receptor gene. Anesth Analg 101:143–148
16. van Swinderen B, Saifee O, Shebester L, Roberson R, Nonet ML, Crowder CM (1999) A neomorphic syntaxin mutation blocks volatile-anesthetic action in *Caenorhabditis elegans*. Proc Natl Acad Sci U S A 96:2479–2484
17. Falk MJ, Kayser EB, Morgan PG, Sedensky MM (2006) Mitochondrial complex I function modulates volatile anesthetic sensitivity in *C. elegans*. Curr Biol 16:1641–1645
18. Kayser EB, Morgan PG, Sedensky MM (1999) GAS-1: a mitochondrial protein controls sensitivity to volatile anesthetics in the nematode *Caenorhabditis elegans*. Anesthesiology 90: 545–554
19. Liem EB, Lin CM, Suleman MI, Doufas AG, Gregg RG, Veauthier JM, Loyd G, Sessler DI (2004) Anesthetic requirement is increased in redheads. Anesthesiology 101:279–283
20. Morgan PG, Hoppel CL, Sedensky MM (2002) Mitochondrial defects and anesthetic sensitivity. Anesthesiology 96:1268–1270
21. Stiernagle T (2006). Maintenance of *C. elegans*. In: WormBook (ed) The *C. elegans* Research Community. WormBook, doi10.1895/wormbook.1.101.1, http://www.wormbook.org
22. Chalfie M, Sulston J (1981) Developmental genetics of the mechanosensory neurons of *Caenorhabditis elegans*. Dev Biol 82:358–370
23. Liu DW, Thomas JH (1994) Regulation of a periodic motor program in *C. elegans*. J Neurosci 14:1953–1962
24. Waud DR (1972) On biological assays involving quantal responses. J Pharmacol Exp Ther 183:577–607
25. DeLean A, Munson PJ, Rodbard D (1978) Simultaneous analysis of families of sigmoidal curves: application to bioassay, radioligand assay, and physiological dose-response curves. Am J Physiol 235:E97–E102
26. Mello C, Fire A (1995) DNA transformation. Methods Cell Biol 48:451–482
27. Mello CC, Kramer JM, Stinchcomb D, Ambros V (1991) Efficient gene transfer in *C. elegans*: extrachromosomal maintenance and integration of transforming sequences. EMBO J 10:3959–3970

Chapter 2

Alternatives to Mammalian Pain Models 2: Using *Drosophila* to Identify Novel Genes Involved in Nociception

Jason C. Caldwell and W. Daniel Tracey Jr.

Abstract

Identification of the molecules involved in nociception is fundamental to our understanding of pain. *Drosophila*, with its short generation time, powerful genetics and capacity for rapid, genome-wide mutagenesis, represents an ideal invertebrate model organism to dissect nociception. The fly has already been used to identify factors that are involved in other sensory systems such as vision, chemosensation, and audition. Thus, the tiny fruit fly is a viable alternative to mammalian model organisms. Here we present a brief primer on techniques used in screening for thermal and/or mechanical nociception mutants using *Drosophila*.

Key words: *Drosophila*, Larva, Multidendritic neuron, Thermal nociception assay, Mechanical nociception assay, Screen, Behavior

1. Introduction

An organism's ability to sense and respond to the sensory cues from the surrounding environment is essential for its survival. In particular, there has been significant research aimed at unveiling the molecular players that contribute to the detection of noxious stimuli and the development and maintenance of the pain-sensing neurons collectively called the nociceptors.

Drosophila melanogaster is emerging as a promising invertebrate model organism for the study of nociception. The highly branched *Drosophila* nociceptive MULTIDENDRITIC (md) neurons tiling the larval body wall are functionally and morphologically

Arpad Szallasi (ed.), *Analgesia: Methods and Protocols*, Methods in Molecular Biology, vol. 617, DOI 10.1007/978-1-60327-323-7_2, © Springer Science+Business Media, LLC 2010

analogous to the vertebrate nociceptive neurons whose branched, naked nerve endings likewise tile the skin (1). Although the evolutionary distance between flies and humans is vast, there is already some compelling evidence that suggests that the nociceptive molecular machinery is, at least in part, conserved among invertebrates and vertebrates (2, 3). The implication of these molecular players in nociception has laid the early groundwork for our understanding of the machinery at work in this specialized and essential sensory system. There are numerous other as yet unidentified molecules, both in vertebrates and invertebrates, that contribute to the normal function of the nociceptive neurons and *Drosophila* is emerging as a premiere system to uncover these players.

Two behavioral assays have been developed to probe nociceptive function in *Drosophila* larvae (1). These animals exhibit a robust nocifensive escape behavior in response to noxious mechanical or thermal challenges within physiologically and biologically relevant ranges. During escape locomotion, the larvae rotate around the long body axis in a corkscrew-like fashion. In contrast, normal locomotion of the undisturbed larvae involves rostral to caudal waves of muscle contraction. The nocifensive behavioral output is highly stereotyped and genetically encoded and can therefore be used as a measure of normal nociceptive neuron function. This, coupled with the fact that *Drosophila* possesses a simplified nervous system that is readily amenable to sophisticated, large-scale, high-throughput genetic dissection, makes it possible to rapidly determine the molecules responsible for conferring mechanosensory and thermosensory function to the nociceptors. With respect to this final point, we will briefly describe the major techniques to generate mutants in *Drosophila* that can be subsequently tested in the thermal and/or mechanical nociception assays (described below).

This mutagenesis primer is in no way exhaustive, but does highlight the most commonly used techniques that fall under three main categories: irradiation, chemical, and genetic mutagenesis. The specific details of these techniques are not included, as they would be far beyond the scope of this work, but a brief summary of the technique as well as the original citation(s) are included.

Irradiation. Flies can be irradiated with either γ- or X-rays to produce lesions in the genome (4). This technique has somewhat fallen out of favor since the resulting chromosomal aberrations can be quite large and complex. Nevertheless, large rearrangements or deletions can be cytologically mapped with the larval salivary gland polytene chromosome preparation (4) and further refined with Southern Blot. In the post-genome era, homozygous viable deletions can also be mapped using genomic tiling arrays.

Chemical Mutagenesis. Ethylmethanesulfonate (EMS) mutagenesis is well-established and routine form of chemical mutagenesis that is extraordinarily convenient because it simply involves feeding a standard dose of EMS to male flies and following a proscribed mating scheme (5). EMS is a powerful mutagen that causes G/C-to-A/T transition point mutations at a very high rate (75–100%) but other mutations, such as deletions, are possible although at a vastly low rate (4, 6–8). Similar to EMS mutagenesis, ethylnitrosurea (ENU) mutagenesis can likewise be used to generate mutants. ENU typically causes A-to-T transversion and A/T-to-G/C transition point mutations, but it is far less effective than EMS (4). The trade-off for efficient generation of mutants and subsequent screening for your phenotype of interest is the time-consuming task of mapping the mutation. Rough genetic mapping is typically performed with the *Drosophila* Deficiency Kit (http://flystocks.bio.indiana.edu/Browse/df-dp/dfkit-info.htm) and once the region is narrowed, finer mapping can be carried out with smaller deficiency strains available from the Bloomington Stock Center Kit, Exelixis Deficiency Kit or the DrosDel Kit (9–12) and, ultimately, PCR sequencing the gene or denaturing HPLC (8) on mutagenized flies must be used to identify the specific mutation. Finally, as the cost and speed of sequencing entire genomes has substantially improved, it is now possible that mutant strains can be fully sequenced to identify the causative mutation (13).

Genetic Mutagenesis. Transposable Elements (TEs), also known as mobile genetic elements, are perhaps a Drosophilist's most important genetic tool. There are literally thousands upon thousands of fly strains that harbor individual TEs – such as P-elements, piggyBac elements, and Minos elements (12, 14, 15), to name a few – that have been inserted randomly into the genome to disrupt many of the ~14,000 predicted *Drosophila* genes (16). Several groups have initiated large-scale projects (12, 17–22) to randomly insert different TEs into the *Drosophila* genome and altogether these transposable element strains are estimated to disrupt roughly 65% of the genes in the fly genome; there are also private collections that likely increase the coverage to a small degree.

These thousands of strains are publicly available and potentially mutate novel pain genes. Indeed, a screen of one such collection of 1,500 randomly inserted EP (20) P-element strains for thermal nociception defects was used to isolate the nociception gene *painless* (1). The advantage of transposable element mutagenesis is that the precise insertion site of a given TE has been pre-determined and therefore the gene underlying the phenotype is known. If the insertion site of a given TE is unknown, it can easily be determined, by inverse PCR using primers directed against the P-element sequence.

While these random TE insertions cause a loss-of-function phenotype, a clever design feature of the EP type P-element can be used to reveal a gain-of-function phenotype. In other words, with a routine genetic tool (the Gal4/UAS system, see Brand and Perrimon 1993 for details), the gene in which the TE is inserted can be over-expressed in a tissue-, cell- or stage-specific manner (18, 20, 23, 24).

If a given TE strain that is inserted into a gene has a mild nociception phenotype, it is likely that the insertion is only a hypomorphic allele. The advantage of P-elements, however, is that they can be readily mobilized by introduction of a transposase enzyme (25, 26) or, as discussed above, irradiation, to produce flanking deletions into a gene of interest (27, 28). These deletions vary in size, but it is possible to precisely define the breakpoints caused by the lesion using a combination of Southern Blot and PCR. Even though the frequency of flanking deletions generated by transposase-mediated imprecise excision from a P-element is fairly low, this is still the most efficient and commonly used technique to generate stronger or null alleles of a given gene; a few similar but less well known techniques (*cis* or *trans* hybrid-element insertion and hobo deletion-generator) have also been developed (11, 29, 30). With P-element mobilization, many excision events will be precise, and these events often revert to the original phenotype lending further support to the idea that the gene where the P-element is inserted is indeed responsible for the defect. Interestingly, the piggyBac TEs do not generate flanking deletions when mobilized (only precise excisions), but these elements are engineered with so-called FRT sites that allow for the rapid generation of precise custom-made deletions at or around a gene of interest that can easily be confirmed by PCR (9, 10, 12).

There are several other TE constructs that were used to create new collections and have features that can likewise uncover novel gene functions including: (1) gene disruption by insertion of GT1 (19, 31) or SUPor-P P-elements (these can also be used to make imprecise excisions) and (2) so-called "Gal4 enhancer trapping" (17, 23, 32, 33). In enhancer trap strains, candidate genes are isolated based on their expression in a tissue of interest.

The techniques discussed above are useful for performing unbiased screens for candidate genes, however, there are also genetic tools available for disrupting a specific gene. It is likely that a gene of interest – perhaps one that is a fly homologue of a human gene implicated in pain states – will have TEs inserted in or near it. This can be determined by searching FlyBase (http://www.flybase.org), and, if TEs are available, though a number of the public Stock Centers (http://flybase.org/static_pages/allied-data/stock_collections.html), the genetic mutagenesis techniques outlined above can be performed in those cases. Recall, however, that ~35% of the genes in the fly genome do not have TE alleles, and in those cases a few additional approaches (discussed below) can be taken to generate mutants.

RNA interference (RNAi) is another powerful tool that can be used to knock down genes in *Drosophila*. In brief, gene regulation in vivo by RNAi involves the production of double stranded RNAs (dsRNAs) that are processed into small interfering RNAs (siRNAs) by the Dicer riboendonuclease, and these siRNAs in turn guide degradation of their complementary mRNA through Argonaute, which is a catalytic component of RNA-Induced Signaling Complex. Initially, dsRNAs were generated and microinjected into *Drosophila* embryos, but this technique is labor intensive and invasive, dosage is difficult to control, and the injected dsRNAs may not interfere with later development. In order to circumvent these pitfalls, inverted repeats – used to create dsRNAs – have been cloned into P-element vectors for nearly 90% of the *Drosophila* genes ((34) and http://flyrnai.org/). These dsRNA-containing P-element vectors were stably incorporated into individual fly strains (~22,000; some are duplicates for the same gene) and made publically available (http://www.vdrc.at). These P-elements have been designed to drive expression of a given dsRNA under strict tissue-, cell-, and stage-specific control, as alluded to above (23, 24, 34). We have used a subset of these RNAi strains to systematically knock out/knock down the various *Drosophila* ion channel subunits specifically in the larval md neurons and have screened this collection for defects in thermal and mechanical nociception. Potential disadvantage in this type of screen is that false-positives may occur due to promiscuous off-targeting of the processed siRNA and false-negatives may occur due to incomplete knock-down of a given gene. Nevertheless, the ease of screening with RNAi is a strong advantage to traditional screen and verification of RNAi phenotypes by creation of genetic mutants is relatively straightforward.

Homologous recombination has been used routinely in eukaryotic organisms to target and replace a wild type copy of a gene with a mutant version created in the lab or to simply delete the gene altogether. Until recently, gene targeting was not possible in *Drosophila* but two techniques, ends-in and ends-out (replacement) gene targeting, have been developed (35–39).

2. Materials

2.1. General

1. Distilled water.
2. 60 × 15 mm Polystyrene Petri Dish.
3. DVD Handycam Camcorder with DVD-R Recordable Media (Sony, Tokyo, Japan).

4. MZ6 Stereomicroscope (Leica, Wetzlar, Germany).
5. MM99 Adaptor S/N: 1658 (Martin Microscope, Easley, SC).
6. Ace Light Source with Dual Gooseneck Fiber Optic Light Guide (Schott, Elmsford, NY).

2.2. Thermal Nociception Assay

1. Variable Autotransformer/Digital Voltmeter (Variac, Ceveland, OH) 120 VAC, Single Phase Input, 0-120 VAC Output, 12A.
2. BAT-12 Thermocouple (Physitemp, Clifton, NJ).
3. MLT1402 T-type Ultra Fast Thermocouple Probe (IT-23).
4. Soldering iron with a copper tip shaped into a chisel 0.6 mm wide outfitted with the thermocouple lead wire under the copper tip.

2.3. Mechanical Nociception Assay

1. Glass pipettes.
2. Nylon Monofilament fishing line (Shakespeare Omniflex 6 lb test, diameter 0.009 inch [0.23 mm]).
3. Weighing scale.

3. Methods

Once a station to test nociceptive function in larvae has been built, and after some practice, the behavioral assays (1) are straightforward, rapid, and reproducible. It is important to empirically calibrate your thermal nociception probe such that 80–90% of control animals respond in one second or less.

3.1. Fly Husbandry

1. Flies are maintained on typical *Drosophila* media at 25°C with 70% humidity and 12:12 Light:Dark Cycle.

3.2. Thermal Nociception Assay

1. Six virgin females are mated to three males, and the adults are transferred into new food vials on the fifth day.
2. Third instar wandering larvae (those which are no longer in the food but are actively crawling on the walls of the vial) are gently washed from the food vials into Petri dishes with distilled water on the fifth day (see Note 1).
3. Larvae are tested at room temperature (21–23°C) in Petri dishes containing water shallow enough to allow the ventral cuticle of animals to make contact with the dish (see Note 2).
4. The soldering iron probe is heated to the desired temperature by adjusting the voltage on the Variac and is monitored on the digital readout on the thermocouple (see Note 3).

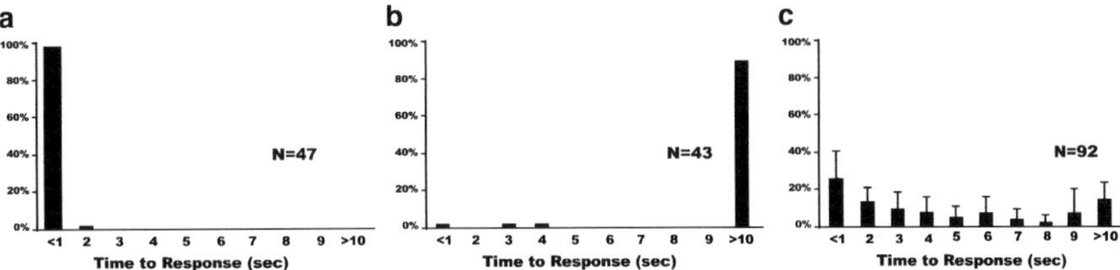

Fig. 1. In control animals (**a**), nearly 100% of the larvae initiate nocifensive rolling in response to a 46°C probe. In contrast, strains where the multidendritic nociceptive neurons are genetically silenced with tetanus toxin (**b**, md-Gal4; UAS-TNT-E), most of these animals do not respond to the thermal stimulus. Similarly, *painless* (1) mutants (**c**) exhibit significantly different average rolling latencies compared to controls at 46°C. Reprinted from reference (1)

5. With the video camera running (see Note 4), the heated probe is gently placed against the lateral surface of abdominal segments 4, 5, or 6 until the animal completes a 360° roll along the dorsal–ventral axis (see Note 5).
6. Videos are played back and the latency to roll in response to the probe is calculated with a digital stopwatch http://tools.arantius.com/stopwatchanalyzed (see Note 6). Response latencies are separated into 11 bins (<1 s, <2, 3, 4...10 s, >10 s).
7. Data are graphed as percentage of larvae that fall into each bin (Fig. 1) and are analyzed by comparing average latency of wild type controls and a given experimental genotype by *T*-test.

3.3. Mechanical Nociception Assay

1. Crosses and handling of larvae are performed as described above for the thermal nociception assay. Furthermore, the larva selected for testing should be relatively stationary and in an aqueous environment as described above.
2. The noxious mechanical stimulus is delivered to the dorsal midline of a wandering third instar larva. To deliver the mechanical stimulus, a 50 mN Von Frey Fiber (see Note 7) is used to rapidly jab the larva midway along the anterior posterior axis (see Note 8). The fiber is held perpendicular to the larva and rapidly depressed downward (effectively squashing the larvae against the surface of the Petri dish).
3. By varying the length of the Von Frey Fiber, it is possible to deliver forces of greater or lesser intensity and to generate a response curve (see Note 9).
4. Data are graphed as percent of larvae that initiate rolling in response to a particular intensity of mechanical stimulation. The data are analyzed by *T*-test comparing wild type controls to a given experimental genotype.

4. Notes

1. The stage of the larvae is important; they should be opaque wandering third instar (108–120 h after egg laying).
2. It is important to perform the behavioral assay in an aqueous environment (the larvae must be wet but not floating). For reasons that are not fully understood, escape locomotion is not readily elicited if the larvae are dry. One possible explanation may be that the selective advantage of rotational escape locomotion is most significant when the larvae are buried in the food (and wet).
3. Monitoring the temperature of the probe is very critical. The BAT-12 thermocouple from Physitemp is outfitted with an IT-23 thermocouple probe to the tip of the soldering iron (the thermocouple is attached using a small drop of solder). The temperature at the tip of the soldering iron is lower than the temperature on the shaft, so measuring temperature as close to the tip of the soldering iron as possible is very important. It is also important to "rest" the probe for a few seconds to let it reheat between animals as the temperature of the probe dips slightly when the tip is placed in the aqueous environment.
4. The *Drosophila* behavioral assay for thermal nociception is a population measurement. At 46°C, the probe is close to the threshold temperature for eliciting the behavior, therefore a distribution of response latency will be evident. To obtain a precise population measurement of latency, the behavior must be video recorded and then documented off-line.
5. It is also important to stimulate animals when they are relatively stationary (with mouth hooks moving as if feeding). If the animals are moving rapidly with peristalsis, they are reluctant to initiate escape locomotion in response to noxious heat. The stimulation should be applied near the middle of the anterior/posterior axis in abdominal segment 4, 5 or 6. The larvae appear to have behavioral options that depend upon the somatotopic location of the noxious heat stimulus. Stimulation near posterior does not robustly elicit escape locomotion in wild type since they can escape by moving forward. In addition, if the stimulation is applied too close to the head, the larvae have a tendency to turn away with their head to escape rather than rotate.
6. Stopwatch outputs of the response times of individual larvae are recorded in a spreadsheet format. Off-line analysis is performed by an observer and is the most time-consuming aspect of the assay.

7. Von Frey fibers can be homemade by attaching nylon monofilament to glass pipettes that have been bent in a Bunsen Burner to form a right angle. To make a 50 mN probe, the monofilament fishing line (Shakespeare Omniflex 6 lb test, diameter 0.009 inch [0.23 mm]) is first cut to make a short piece of 18 mm in length. The 18 mm long filament is then glued to the bent glass pipette such that 8 mm of the fiber protrudes from the end, and 10 mm anchors the fiber to the pipette. The exact force delivered by an individual fiber will vary slightly among fibers as the fiber becomes more flexible with prolonged use. To precisely measure the maximum force delivered by a particular Von Frey fiber, the fibers are used to depress a balance until the fishing line begins to bend. The force measured on the balance just prior to bending represents the maximum force exerted. The force in grams is converted to milliNewtons through multiplication by a factor of 9.8 (i.e., Gravity). For example, a fiber that generates a force of 1 g delivers a maximum force of 9.8 mN.
8. The stimulus should be delivered as instantaneously as possible, so that the larva is immediately released from it. Following such a stimulus, the wild type larvae will be observed to briefly pause movement (for approximately one second), and the nocifensive escape behavior will initiate after this pause. We typically observe nocifensive behavior in 75% of trials using a 50 mN Von Frey fiber in wild type strains. In contrast, strains that harbor mutations that interfere with mechanical nociception show infrequent escape behavior following the 50 mN stimulus.
9. Although the *painless* mutant, for example, shows significantly reduced nociception responses to a 50 mN stimulus, nocifensive responses can still be elicited by 100 mN of force. The latter result suggests that this mutant is not defective in the motor output.

References

1. Tracey WD Jr, Wilson RI, Laurent G, Benzer S (2003) *painless*, a *Drosophila* gene essential for nociception. Cell 113:261–273
2. Dhaka A, Viswanath V, Patapoutian A (2006) TRP ion channels and temperature sensation. Annu Rev Neurosci 29:135–161
3. Lumpkin EA, Caterina MJ (2007) Mechanisms of sensory transduction in the skin. Nature 445:858–865
4. Sullivan W, Ashburner M, Hawley RS (2000) *Drosophila* protocols. Cold Spring Harbor Laboratory Press, Cold Spring Harbor, New York
5. Lewis EB, Bacher F (1968) Method for feeding ethyl-methane sulfonate (EMS) to *Drosophila* males. Drosoph Inf Serv 43:193
6. Bokel C (2008) EMS screens: from mutagenesis to screening and mapping. Methods Mol Biol 420:119–138
7. Greene EA, Codomo CA, Taylor NE, Henikoff JG, Till BJ, Reynolds SH et al (2003) Spectrum of chemically induced mutations

from a large-scale reverse-genetic screen in Arabidopsis. Genetics 164:731–740

8. Bentley A, MacLennan B, Calvo J, Dearolf CR (2000) Targeted recovery of mutations in *Drosophila*. Genetics 156:1169–1173
9. Ryder E, Ashburner M, Bautista-Llacer R, Drummond J, Webster J, Johnson G et al (2007) The DrosDel deletion collection: a *Drosophila* genomewide chromosomal deficiency resource. Genetics 177:615–629
10. Ryder E, Blows F, Ashburner M, Bautista-Llacer R, Coulson D, Drummond J et al (2004) The DrosDel collection: a set of P-element insertions for generating custom chromosomal aberrations in *Drosophila melanogaster*. Genetics 167:797–813
11. Parks AL, Cook KR, Belvin M, Dompe NA, Fawcett R, Huppert K et al (2004) Systematic generation of high-resolution deletion coverage of the *Drosophila melanogaster* genome. Nat Genet 36:288–292
12. Thibault ST, Singer MA, Miyazaki WY, Milash B, Dompe NA, Singh CM et al (2004) A complementary transposon tool kit for *Drosophila melanogaster* using P and piggyBac. Nat Genet 36:283–287
13. Blumenstiel JP, Noll AC, Griffiths JA, Perera AG, Walton KN, Gilliland WD et al (2009) Identification of EMS-induced mutations in *Drosophila melanogaster* by whole genome sequencing. Genetics 182(1): 25–32
14. Metaxakis A, Oehler S, Klinakis A, Savakis C (2005) Minos as a genetic and genomic tool in *Drosophila melanogaster*. Genetics 171:571–581
15. Engels, W R (1989) P elements in *Drosophila melanogaster*. In: Berg, D. E. and Howe, M. M., (eds) *Mobile DNA*, pp. 437–484. American Society for Microbiology, Washington, DC
16. Adams MD, Celniker SE, Holt RA, Evans CA, Gocayne JD, Amanatides PG et al (2000) The genome sequence of *Drosophila melanogaster*. Science 287:2185–2195
17. Bier E, Vaessin H, Shepherd S, Lee K, McCall K, Barbel S et al (1989) Searching for pattern and mutation in the *Drosophila* genome with a P-lacZ vector. Genes Dev 3:1273–1287
18. Duffy JB (2002) GAL4 system in *Drosophila*: a fly geneticist's Swiss army knife. Genesis 34:1–15
19. Lukacsovich T, Asztalos Z, Awano W, Baba K, Kondo S, Niwa S et al (2001) Dual-tagging gene trap of novel genes in *Drosophila melanogaster*. Genetics 157:727–742
20. Rorth P (1996) A modular misexpression screen in *Drosophila* detecting tissue-specific phenotypes. Proc Natl Acad Sci U S A 93:12418–12422
21. Roseman RR, Johnson EA, Rodesch CK, Bjerke M, Nagoshi RN, Geyer PK (1995) A P element containing suppressor of hairy-wing binding regions has novel properties for mutagenesis in *Drosophila melanogaster*. Genetics 141:1061–1074
22. Bellen HJ, Levis RW, Liao G, He Y, Carlson JW, Tsang G et al (2004) The BDGP gene disruption project: single transposon insertions associated with 40% of *Drosophila* genes. Genetics 167:761–781
23. Brand AH, Perrimon N (1993) Targeted gene expression as a means of altering cell fates and generating dominant phenotypes. Development 118:401–415
24. Fischer JA, Giniger E, Maniatis T, Ptashne M (1988) GAL4 activates transcription in *Drosophila*. Nature 332:853–856
25. Laski FA, Rio DC, Rubin GM (1986) Tissue specificity of *Drosophila* P element transposition is regulated at the level of mRNA splicing. Cell 44:7–19
26. Robertson HM, Preston CR, Phillis RW, Johnson-Schlitz DM, Benz WK, Engels WR (1988) A stable genomic source of P element transposase in *Drosophila melanogaster*. Genetics 118:461–470
27. Daniels SB, McCarron M, Love C, Chovnick A (1985) Dysgenesis-induced instability of rosy locus transformation in *Drosophila melanogaster*: analysis of excision events and the selective recovery of control element deletions. Genetics 109:95–117
28. Voelker RA, Greenleaf AL, Gyurkovics H, Wisely GB, Huang SM, Searles LL (1984) Frequent imprecise excision among reversions of a P element-caused lethal mutation in *Drosophila*. Genetics 107:279–294
29. Cooley L, Thompson D, Spradling AC (1990) Constructing deletions with defined endpoints in *Drosophila*. Proc Natl Acad Sci U S A 87:3170–3173
30. Huet F, Lu JT, Myrick KV, Baugh LR, Crosby MA, Gelbart WM (2002) A deletion-generator compound element allows deletion saturation analysis for genomewide phenotypic annotation. Proc Natl Acad Sci U S A 99:9948–9953
31. Lukacsovich T, Yamamoto D (2001) Trap a gene and find out its function: toward functional genomics in *Drosophila*. J Neurogenet 15:147–168

32. Bellen HJ (1999) Ten years of enhancer detection: lessons from the fly. Plant Cell 11: 2271–2281
33. Manseau L, Baradaran A, Brower D, Budhu A, Elefant F, Phan H et al (1997) GAL4 enhancer traps expressed in the embryo, larval brain, imaginal discs, and ovary of *Drosophila*. Dev Dyn 209:310–322
34. Dietzl G, Chen D, Schnorrer F, Su KC, Barinova Y, Fellner M et al (2007) A genome-wide transgenic RNAi library for conditional gene inactivation in *Drosophila*. Nature 448:151–156
35. Maggert KA, Gong WJ, Golic KG (2008) Methods for homologous recombination in *Drosophila*. Methods Mol Biol 420: 155–174
36. Gong WJ, Golic KG (2003) Ends-out, or replacement, gene targeting in *Drosophila*. Proc Natl Acad Sci U S A 100:2556–2561
37. Rong YS, Titen SW, Xie HB, Golic MM, Bastiani M, Bandyopadhyay P et al (2002) Targeted mutagenesis by homologous recombination in *D. melanogaster*. Genes Dev 16:1568–1581
38. Rong YS, Golic KG (2001) A targeted gene knockout in *Drosophila*. Genetics 157: 1307–1312
39. Rong YS, Golic KG (2000) Gene targeting by homologous recombination in *Drosophila*. Science 288:2013–2018

Chapter 3

Animal Models of Acute Surgical Pain

Hyangin Kim, Backil Sung, and Jianren Mao

Abstract

Animal models of tissue injury have been used to investigate the mechanisms of pain. Here, we describe a variety of animal models that have been used to mimic acute surgical pain in human subjects, which include the plantar, tail, and gastrocnemius incision models. We also provide discussion on animal models of laparotomy, thoracotomy, visceral pain, and bone injury. Preclinical studies using these models have provided insights into the mechanisms and causes of acute surgical pain as well as the treatment options to control postsurgical pain.

Key words: Acute surgical pain, Incision, Visceral pain, Laparotomy, Thoracotomy, Osteotomy

1. Introduction

Pain is an important defensive mechanism that includes both sensory and emotional experience. Surgical pain is an important type of acute pain. Acute surgical injury induces peripheral and central sensitization leading to an enhanced nociceptive process (1). Managing acute surgical pain is of high clinical significance because satisfactory management of acute surgical pain could decrease the morbidity and mortality following operation (2, 3). Furthermore, there will be adverse consequences if acute surgical pain is not adequately relieved. For example, severe surgical pain may lead to postoperative delirium (4) and immune suppression (5). The management of perioperative pain is very important to reduce infection and metastasis as well (6).

To manage surgical pain, effective analgesia is necessary (7–9) and new investigative treatment options must be developed to meet this challenge. Understanding the basic mechanisms underlying surgical pain could aid the innovative development of new tools to manage postsurgical pain. Due to the limitations of the

Arpad Szallasi (ed.), *Analgesia: Methods and Protocols*, Methods in Molecular Biology, vol. 617,
DOI 10.1007/978-1-60327-323-7_3,

experimental approaches that are inherent to studying surgical pain in human subjects, animal models of acute pain should be considered as an alternative that could help investigate the pathogenesis and the treatment option of surgical pain (10). Recently, several animal models have been developed to investigate the mechanism of pain and provide new information on the treatment of pain. The pathophysiology of acute pain is now better understood owing to the development of such animal models. Each of these animal models may mimic a specific clinical condition of acute surgical pain. This chapter summarizes the animal models of acute surgical pain currently used in the pain research field.

2. Materials

2.1. Experimental animals

1. Adult male Sprague-Dawley rats weighing 250–350 g are housed (lights on from 7:00 am to 7:00 pm) with water and food ad libitum.
2. Pentobarbital.

2.2. Surgical Tools

1. Scissors, straight and curved, Forceps, Mosquito, Hemostat, Retractor, Clipper, Staples, Needle and needle holder (FST, Heidelberg, Germany).
2. Blade holder and surgical blade 22/11.
3. Suture, Silk, Nylon, and Chromic gut.
4. High intensity illuminator; Fiber-Lite MI-150 (Dolan-Jenner, Andover, MA).

2.3. von Frey Filaments

1. The standard Semmes–Weinstein set of von Frey hairs (Stoelting, Wood Dale, IL).
2. The transparent plexiglass chamber (IITC, Woodland Hills, CA).
3. Customized wire-mesh plate.

2.4. Prevention of Infection

1. Dry sterilizer; the germ terminator, Germinator 500 (Cell point Inc. Rockville, MD).
2. Prophylaxis; Penicillin G, 30,000 IU (intramuscular injection).
3. Betadine solution (10% Povidone-iodine topical solution, Stamford, CT).
4. Antibiotic ointment (Bacitracin Zinc Ointment USP, Fougera & Co., New York, NY).

2.5. Maintenance of Body Temperature

1. Thermostatically controlled heating blanket (Leica, St.Louis, MO).
2. A digital electronic thermometer (Becton Dickinson, Franklin Lakes, NJ).

2.6. Preparation of Animal for Thoracotomy

1. Isoflurane and endotracheal catheter (14 gauge, 51-mm long Teflon IV catheter).
2. A small animal ventilator (model 683; Harvard Instruments, Holliston, MA).
3. A small self-retaining retractor (model SU-3146; Mueller, Mac Gaw Park, IL) with coated lubricant.
4. A 4-cm long piece of 0.047 inch diameter silicone rubber tubing.
5. The veterinary adhesive (VetBond; 3 M, St. Paul, MN).

2.7. Monitoring Pressure in the Visceral Distension Model

1. A balloon monitor by in-line pressure transducer (PX136 Omega Engineering, Stamford, CT).

2.8. Osteotomy Pain Model

1. A hand drill (drill bit diameter 1 mm; Plastic One Inc. Wallingford, CT).

3. Methods

Nociceptive responses in animals with incision models appears to mimic surgical pain in man (2). The incision involving the skin, fascia, and muscle induces pain behaviors at rest in response to nonnoxious stimuli (allodynia) (11). The pain behavior with mobilization, ambulation, and cough is more severe and longer lasting (12, 13). Moreover, the area of incision shows mechanical hyperalgesia (14) due to change in the nociceptive system. The sensitization of the primary afferent fiber occurs at the site of incision and is characterized by changes in the receptive field of WDR (wide dynamic range) neurons within the spinal cord dorsal horn (15). The primary hyperalgesia that occurs at the site of the incision is likely due to peripheral sensitization, whereas the secondary hyperalgesia observed in the nondamaged tissue surrounding the incisional site is due to central sensitization (11, 16).

Excitatory amino acids have been shown to be contributory to central sensitization (9, 17). In particular, the N-methyl-D aspartate (NMDA) receptor is critical for the development of central sensitization (18–22). Of interest, it has been demonstrated that activation of spinal NMDA receptors may not be a significant response to incision because intrathecal treatment with an NMDA receptor antagonist has only a minimal effects on pain behavior (23). In contrast, intrathecal treatment with a non-NMDA receptor antagonist appears to have a more marked effect on pain behavior (24).

Postoperative pain is often present at the site of the incision as well as in the area surrounding the incision (11, 16). The secondary hyperalgesia in the plantar incision model is, however, short lived (14, 25, 26). It has been reported that the degree of the secondary hyperalgesia changed with the size and degree of tissue damage (25, 27, 28). Accordingly, the gastrocnemius incision model was developed to produce more extensive tissue damage (29). In this model, the secondary hyperalgesia lasts 6–8 days, similar to the time course of surgical incisional pain in human subjects (29). If the muscle incision is made, the primary mechanical hyperalgesia lasts for 7 days and the secondary hyperalgesia develops 1 day after the incision from the 20 mm-incised skin, fascia, and muscle incision model (30).

Among different types of surgical pain, animal models of visceral pain differ from incision pain models. For example, visceral hyperplasia is rarely reported (31). Visceral pain models usually focus on the examination of both peripheral and deep pain. Deep pain could result from the direct injury to the internal organ and the gastrointestinal irritation to stimulate the visceral sensory afferent fibers (32). Although pain from the skin incision is the most important factor in acute surgical pain, pain from the muscles, viscera, and bones also contributes significantly to clinical pain conditions (33).

In general, less has been known about the visceral pain than somatic pain including acute surgical pain. There are several animal models of visceral pain. In rats, the ovariohysterectomy can be performed under anesthesia, which results in a reduced mechanical nociceptive threshold observed by a paw pressure test (34). In addition, unilateral nephrectomy can be used to investigate the influence of both surgical procedure and the consequence of nephrectomy (35). The reduction of food and water intake and the increase in spontaneous locomotor activity are observed in this model, which appears to be responsive to the opioid treatment (35). In a dog ovariohysterectomy model, nociception is observed by an algometer directly targeting the incisional wound including the reduced nociceptive threshold and/or vocalization (36). Overall, these models provide the opportunity to observe both postsurgical somatic and visceral pain behaviors via traditional nociceptive testing and other indicators such as food and water intake.

In the thoracotomy pain model, the affected costal nerve is stretched due to the procedure of thoracotomy, demonstrating long-tem allodynia after thoracotomy (37). The model appears to be mainly to assess somatic than visceral pain behavior, while the procedure itself mimics surgical thoracotomy in human subjects.

Pain resulting from the intra-abdominal pressure and/or distension of hollow visceral organs is an important contributing factor to postsurgical pain (38). Visceral pain is mediated through different afferent inputs (39) and the processing of visceral nociception is related to the sensory input and the change of autonomic nerve system (40). In this regard, the colorectal distension has been extensively used as a model of acute visceral nociception (41). Several animal studies have demonstrated that the colorectal distension is related to visceral pathological pain in human subjects (42).

Osteotomy or bone injury can induce severe "aching" pain (43). Patients suffering from bone pain are often treated with the analgesics including the nonsteroid anti-inflammatory drug and opioids (44, 45).

The aim of developing animal models of acute surgical pain is to offer experimental tools in search of the improved treatment of surgical pain in the clinical setting (46, 47). It should be noted, however, that animal models could entirely mimic clinical conditions of acute surgical pain for obvious reasons. Nonetheless, animal models of acute surgical pain may provide an important alternative to clinical pain research in order to understand the cellular and molecular mechanisms of pain and explore possible new treatment options for acute postsurgical pain.

3.1. Rat Model of Plantar Incision

1. Under anesthesia, a 1 cm longitudinal incision is made on the planter surface of a hindpaw. The depth of incision is through the skin and fascia. The starting point of incision is 0.5 cm from the proximal edge of the heel and extends toward the toe.
2. After the incision, the plantaris muscle is held and incised longitudinally with the origin and insertion of the muscle preserved.
3. Following hemostasis by gentle pressure, the site of the incision is closed in layers with 5–0 Nylon sutures (see Note 1).
4. Von Frey filament is applied to the area adjacent to the wound site on the foot pad to assess pain.

3.2. Rat Model of Gastrocnemius Incision

1. Under anesthesia, a 3 cm longitudinal incision is made on the midportion of the posterior surface in the hind limb. The starting point of incision is 1.0–1.5 cm from the edge of the heel and extends to the popliteal region.
2. After the skin and fascia incision, the gastrocnemius muscle is divided by blunt dissection, but the origin and insertion site of the muscle is undamaged.

3. The site of incision is sutured in layers.
4. Sutures are removed at postoperative day 3 and pain is assessed by von Frey filaments.

3.3. Rat Model of Tail Incision

1. Under anesthesia, a 0.1 cm or 0.2 cm longitudinal incision is made on the dorsal surface along the center of the tail. The depth of incision reaches the skin, fascia and/or muscle.
2. The site of incision is sutured in layers (see Note 2).

3.4. Rat Model of Laparotomy Pain

1. A 4 cm incision is made through the skin and muscle leading the exposure of abdominal viscera (see Note 3).
2. The viscera is gently manipulated for 2 min and postoperative food and water intake is observed.
3. Following the operative procedure, rats are administered buprenorphine and carprofen to minimize the change in food and water intake.
4. Rectal temperatures were taken daily using a digital electronic thermometer.

3.5. Subcostal Incision/Visceral Model

1. Under anesthesia, a 3 cm diagonal incision is made on one side about 0.5 cm below and parallel to the lowest rib through the peritoneal cavity (see Note 4).
2. The musculature is actively stretched.
3. The handling of the viscera is made through inserting an index finger into the peritoneal cavity.
4. A 10 cm long small intestine is exposed and vigorously handled by fingers.

3.6. Thoracotomy Pain

1. Rats were anesthetized with isoflurane and an endotracheal catheter with a Y-connector attached to a small animal ventilator.
2. In the rat, a 3 cm incision is made on the right lateral chest wall between the 4th and 5th ribs.
3. The ribs are retracted to expose the intercostal muscle.
4. The pleura is incised above the 5th rib.
5. The retractor is carefully placed under 4th and 5th ribs to make ribs separate 8 mm apart.
6. After the retraction period, the tube was inserted for removal of pleural air and the deep muscles covering the ribs were sutured with a secure apposition of tube (see Note 5).
7. The intrapleural pressure was restored with the aspiration of air from the pleural cavity with a 5-mL syringe (see Notes 6 and 7).

3.7. Visceral Distension Model

1. To induce the colorectal distension, a 6–7 cm long and 2–3 cm thick balloon catheter is inserted into the rat's anus. The catheter is flaccid and made of flexible latex.
2. The pressure within the balloon is steadily increased (see Note 8), and changes in the cardiovascular activation and contraction of abdominal muscle are observed as indication of pain.

3.8. Osteotomy Pain Model

1. Four steps of tissue damage are made including the periosteal membrane scrape, a hole through the tibia, aspiration of bone marrow from tibia, and a hole through the calcaneus (see Notes 9 and 10).
2. Soft tissue damage is made through drilling at the osteotomy site of 3 mm below the patella.

4. Notes

1. To minimize the inflammatory response on the site of incision, sutures were removed on postoperative day 2.
2. When the tail incision was made, a 10-mm longitudinal incision was sutured once with 4–0 Nylon, but twice for a 20-mm longitudinal incision.
3. During laparotomy, the temperature of animals was maintained at 37°C by using a heat lamp or a thermostatically controlled heating blanket.
4. In this model, the subcostal incision decreases the exploratory locomotor activity for up to 48 h after operation. The ambulatory and rearing movement is more sensitive than small movement such as grooming in this animal model.
5. When a model of thoracotomy was made, a 4-cm long piece (0.047 inch diameter) rubber tubing was put into the pleural space (1 cm inside) for preventing pneumothorax.
6. Then, the tube was removed from the pleural cavity, the site of the tubing removal was immediately sealed with adhesive.
7. Before the procedure, the rats were emptied the colon. Food except water was withheld for 20 h.
8. The balloon catheter was connected via a low-volume pressure transducer because a pressure of the balloon inside the colon indicated actual intracolonic pressure.
9. Of interest to note is that just scraping the periosteum does not produce mechanical hyperalgesia and allodynia in this model. But, aspiration of the bone marrow or having a hole made by drill results in mechanical hyperalgesia and allodynia.

10. In making bone injury, a hand driller was used to puncture the skin and soft tissue and to make a hole in bone. A 20-gauge needle was used to scrap the periosteal membrane.

References

1. Treede RD, Meyer RA, Raja SN, Campbell JN (1992) Peripheral and central mechanisms of cutaneous hyperalgesia. Prog Neurobiol 38:397–421
2. Brennan TJ, Zahn PK, Pogatzki-Zahn EM (2005) Mechanisms of incisional pain. Anesthesiol Clin North 23:1–20
3. Scott NB, Kehlet H (1988) Regional anaesthesia and surgical morbidity. Br J Surg 75:299–304
4. Vaurio LE, Sands LP, Wang Y, Mullen EA, Leung JM (2006) Postoperative delirium: the importance of pain and pain management. Anesth Analg 102:1267–1273
5. Beilin B, Shavit Y, Trabekin E, Mordashev B, Mayburd E, Zeidel A, Bessler H (2003) The effects of postoperative pain management on immune response to surgery. Anesth Analg 97:822–827
6. Page GG (2005) Surgery-induced immunosuppression and postoperative pain management. AACN Clin Issues 16:302–309
7. Collis R, Brandner B, Bromley LM, Woolf CJ (1995) Is there any clinical advantage of increasing the pre-emptive dose of morphine or combining pre-incisional with postoperative morphine administration? Br J Anaesth 74:396–399
8. Helmy SA, Bali A (2001) The effect of the preemptive use of the NMDA receptor antagonist dextromethorphan on postoperative analgesic requirements. Anesth Analg 92:739–744
9. Woolf CJ, Chong MS (1993) Preemptive analgesia – treating postoperative pain by preventing the establishment of central sensitization. Anesth Analg 77:362–379
10. Alonzo NC, Bayer BM (2002) Opioids, immunology, and host defenses of intravenous drug abusers. Infect Dis Clin North Am 16:553–569
11. Richmond CE, Bromley LM, Woolf CJ (1993) Preoperative morphine pre-empts postoperative pain. Lancet 342:73–75
12. Moiniche S, Dahl JB, Erichsen CJ, Jensen LM, Kehlet H (1997) Time course of subjective pain ratings, and wound and leg tenderness after hysterectomy. Acta Anaesthesiol Scand 41:785–789
13. Lavand'homme P (2006) Perioperative pain. Curr Opin Anaesthesiol 19:556–561
14. Zahn PK, Brennan TJ (1999) Primary and secondary hyperalgesia in a rat model for human postoperative pain. Anesthesiology 90:863–872
15. Zahn PK, Brennan TJ (1999) Incision-induced changes in receptive field properties of rat dorsal horn neurons. Anesthesiology 91:772–785
16. Stubhaug A, Breivik H, Eide PK, Kreunen M, Foss A (1997) Mapping of punctuate hyperalgesia around a surgical incision demonstrates that ketamine is a powerful suppressor of central sensitization to pain following surgery. Acta Anaesthesiol Scand 41:1124–1132
17. Woolf CJ, Costigan M (1999) Transcriptional and posttranslational plasticity and the generation of inflammatory pain. Proc Natl Acad Sci U S A 96:7723–7730
18. Woolf CJ, Thompson SW (1991) The induction and maintenance of central sensitization is dependent on N-methyl-D-aspartic acid receptor activation; implications for the treatment of post-injury pain hypersensitivity states. Pain 44:293–299
19. Coderre TJ, Melzack R (1992) The contribution of excitatory amino acids to central sensitization and persistent nociception after formalin-induced tissue injury. J Neurosci 12:3665–3670
20. Ma QP, Woolf CJ (1995) Noxious stimuli induce an N-methyl-D-aspartate receptor-dependent hypersensitivity of the flexion withdrawal reflex to touch: implications for the treatment of mechanical allodynia. Pain 61:383–390
21. Mao J, Sung B, Ji RR, Lim G (2002) Neuronal apoptosis associated with morphine tolerance: evidence for an opioid-induced neurotoxic mechanism. J Neurosci 22:7650–7661
22. Lim G, Wang S, Zeng Q, Sung B, Yang L, Mao J (2005) Expression of spinal NMDA receptor and PKCgamma after chronic morphine is regulated by spinal glucocorticoid receptor. J Neurosci 25:11145–11154
23. Pogatzki EM, Zahn PK, Brennan TJ (2000) Effect of pretreatment with intrathecal excitatory amino acid receptor antagonists on the

development of pain behavior caused by plantar incision. Anesthesiology 93:489–496

24. Zahn PK, Umali E, Brennan TJ (1998) Intrathecal non-NMDA excitatory amino acid receptor antagonists inhibit pain behaviors in a rat model of postoperative pain. Pain 74:213–223
25. Coderre TJ, Katz J (1997) Peripheral and central hyperexcitability: differential signs and symptoms in persistent pain. Behav Brain Sci 20:404–419
26. Millan MJ (1999) The induction of pain: an integrative review. Prog Neurobiol 57:1–164
27. Gilchrist HD, Allard BL, Simone DA (1996) Enhanced withdrawal responses to heat and mechanical stimuli following intraplantar injection of capsaicin in rats. Pain 67:179–188
28. Nozaki-Taguchi N, Yaksh TL (1998) A novel model of primary and secondary hyperalgesia after mild thermal injury in the rat. Neurosci Lett 254:25–28
29. Pogatzki EM, Niemeier JS, Brennan TJ (2002) Persistent secondary hyperalgesia after gastrocnemius incision in the rat. Eur J Pain 6:295–305
30. Weber J, Loram L, Mitchell B, Themistocleous A (2005) A model of incisional pain: the effects of dermal tail incision on pain behaviours of Sprague Dawley rats. J Neurosci Methods 145:167–173
31. Gebhart GF (2000) J.J. Bonica lecture–2000: physiology, pathophysiology, and pharmacology of visceral pain. Reg Anesth Pain Med 25:632–638
32. Habler HJ, Janig W, Koltzenburg M (1990) Activation of unmyelinated afferent fibres by mechanical stimuli and inflammation of the urinary bladder in the cat. J Physiol 425:545–562
33. Tong C, Conklin D, Eisenach JC (2006) A pain model after gynecologic surgery: the effect of intrathecal and systemic morphine. Anesth Analg 103:1288–1293
34. Lascelles BD, Waterman AE, Cripps PJ, Livingston A, Henderson G (1995) Central sensitization as a result of surgical pain: investigation of the pre-emptive value of pethidine for ovariohysterectomy in the rat. Pain 62:201–212
35. Flecknell PA, Liles JH (1991) The effects of surgical procedures, halothane anaesthesia and nalbuphine on locomotor activity and food and water consumption in rats. Lab Anim 25:50–60
36. Lascelles BD, Cripps PJ, Jones A, Waterman AE (1997) Post-operative central hypersensitivity and pain: the pre-emptive value of pethidine for ovariohysterectomy. Pain 73:461–471
37. Buvanendran A, Kroin JS, Kerns JM, Nagalla SN, Tuman KJ (2004) Characterization of a new animal model for evaluation of persistent postthoracotomy pain. Anesth Analg 99:1453–1460
38. Hogan Q (2002) Animal pain models. Reg Anesth Pain Med 27:385–401
39. Ness TJ, Metcalf AM, Gebhart GF (1990) A psychophysiological study in humans using phasic colonic distension as a noxious visceral stimulus. Pain 43:377–386
40. Grundy D, Al Chae ED, Aziz Q, Collins SM, Ke M, Tache Y, Wood JD (2006) Fundamentals of neurogastroenterology: basic science. Gastroenterology 130:1391–1411
41. Ness TJ, Gebhart GF (1988) Colorectal distension as a noxious visceral stimulus: physiologic and pharmacologic characterization of pseudaffective reflexes in the rat. Brain Res 450:153–169
42. Jensen FM, Madsen JB, Ringsted CV, Christensen A (1988) Intestinal distension test, a method for evaluating intermittent visceral pain in the rabbit. Life Sci 43:747–754
43. Fernyhough JC, Schimandle JJ, Weigel MC, Edwards CC, Levine AM (1992) Chronic donor site pain complicating bone graft harvesting from the posterior iliac crest for spinal fusion. Spine 17:1474–1480
44. Eskenazi J, Nikiforidis T, Livio JJ, Schelling JL (1976) Effect of paracetamol, mephenoxalone and their combination on pain following bone surgery. Eur J Clin Pharmacol 09:411–415
45. Evans PJ, McQuay HJ, Rolfe M, O'Sullivan G, Bullingham RE, Moore RA (1982) Zomepirac, placebo and paracetamol/dextropropoxyphene combination compared in orthopaedic postoperative pain. Br J Anaesth 54:927–933
46. Chapman CR, Casey KL, Dubner R, Foley KM, Gracely RH, Reading AE (1985) Pain measurement: an overview. Pain 22:1–31
47. Stanley KL, Paice JA (1997) Animal models in pain research. Semin Oncol Nurs 13:3–9

Chapter 4

Animal Models of Acute and Chronic Inflammatory and Nociceptive Pain

Janel M. Boyce-Rustay, Prisca Honore, and Michael F. Jarvis

Abstract

To facilitate the study of pain transmission and the characterization of novel analgesic compounds, an array of experimental animal pain models has been developed mainly in rodents. In these preclinical models, nociceptive pain can be measured by both spontaneous and evoked behaviors. Acute pain (seconds to hours) can be more easily measured, albeit still with some difficulty, by spontaneous behaviors (nocifensive behaviors such as licking, flinching), or by stimulation of the injured paw. Chronic pain (lasting at least several days) is most readily measured by evoked stimulation (thermal, mechanical, chemical). Experimental measures of evoked pain are well characterized and are analogous to clinical diagnostic methods. This chapter will focus on rodent models of inflammatory and nociceptive pain that are most used in our laboratory for identification of novel antinociceptive compounds in drug discovery.

Key words: Inflammatory pain, Animal models, Carrageenan, Complete Freund's adjuvant, Capsaicin, Thermal, Mechanical, Monoiodoacetate

1. Introduction

The conceptualization of the neurobiology of pain has undergone continuous refinement with increasing identification and characterization of multiple nociceptive targets and pathways (1–3). The psychophysical parameters used to describe nociceptive processing have thus been refined to differentiate acute withdrawal behaviors in response to dangerous (e.g. sharp or hot stimuli) stimuli in the environment (acute nociception) from increased sensitivity to mildly painful stimuli (hyperalgesia) or to otherwise innocuous stimuli (allodynia) (2). An increase in stimulus intensity in any sensory modality will eventually become noxious. Obviously, the sensation of noxious environmental stimuli

Arpad Szallasi (ed.), *Analgesia: Methods and Protocols*, Methods in Molecular Biology, vol. 617,
DOI 10.1007/978-1-60327-323-7_4, © Springer Science+Business Media, LLC 2010

(acute pain) is physiologically protective. However, following injury, this psychophysical function shifts such that previous noxious stimuli are now perceived as exceedingly painful (hyperalgesia). Additionally, tissue injury results in ongoing or spontaneous pain and the perception that normally nonnoxious stimuli are pain generating (allodynia). It is now well appreciated that distinct sensory mechanisms contribute to physiological pain and to pain arising from tissue damage (inflammatory or nociceptive pain). Nociceptive pain is caused by the ongoing activation of Aδ- and C-nociceptors in response to a noxious stimulus (injury, disease, inflammation). Under normal physiological conditions, there is a close correspondence between pain perception and stimulus intensity, and the sensation of pain is indicative of real or potential tissue damage. As the nervous system becomes sensitized (responding more strongly than normal to peripheral stimuli), in addition to spontaneous pain, nociceptive pain is also associated with evoked hyperalgesic and allodynic conditions (4–6). In general, nociceptive pain abates completely upon the resolution of injury if the disease process is controlled.

Tissue injury results in the release of pronociceptive mediators that sensitize peripheral nerve terminals (*peripheral sensitization*), leading to phenotypic alterations of the sensory neurons and increased excitability of the spinal cord dorsal horn neurons (*central sensitization*) (1, 7). Descending supraspinal systems modulate nociceptive responses (8). Consequences of peripheral sensitization are a lowering of the activation threshold of nociceptors and an increase in their firing rate. These changes result in the production of hyperalgesia and allodynia associated with nociceptive chronic pain. In addition, peripheral sensitization also plays an important role in the development and maintenance of central sensitization (8).

Central sensitization (long-lasting increases in dorsal horn and brain neuron excitability and responsiveness) is associated with spontaneous dorsal horn neuron activity, responses from neurons that normally respond only to low intensity stimuli (altered neural connections following sprouting of Aβ fibers to superficial laminae), expansion of dorsal horn neuron receptive fields, and reduction in central inhibition (9, 10). Central sensitization is associated with persistent pain, hyperalgesia, allodynia, and the spread of pain to uninjured tissue, i.e., secondary hyperalgesia due to increased receptor field of spinal neurons. In addition, it reflects a complex series of changes occurring in the spinal cord that may promote long-lasting increases in dorsal horn neuron excitability. Peripheral and central sensitization plays a role in nociceptive chronic pain. Thus, central sensitization also explains the observation that established pain is more difficult to suppress than acute pain because of the maladaptive changes that have taken place in the central nervous system (3, 11).

Glia, e.g. astrocytes and microglia, as well as infiltrating mast cells are involved in the generation and maintenance of central sensitization (12, 13).

Chronic pain is associated with a large variety of deranged patterns of neurotransmission at multiple levels of the neuroaxis with considerable target and pathway redundancy. Thus, in the absence of ongoing injury, chronic pain can be viewed as a disease in itself. The enhanced appreciation of the many neurochemical and neurophysiological alterations in neuronal function associated with chronic pain has led to the development of both new preclinical models of pain and a variety of potentially useful therapeutic interventions.

Animal models of acute pain allow the evaluation of the effects of potential analgesics on pain sensation/transmission in an otherwise normal animal. In addition, the same tests may be used to measure stimulus-evoked pain in animals with chronic inflammation or nerve injury. Usually, these tests rely on an escape behavior/withdrawal reflex or vocalization as an index of pain. The animals have control over the duration of the pain, that is, their behavioral response leads to termination of the noxious stimulus. Outlined below are more details on specific experimental materials and methods for the assessment of nociception in laboratory rodents. Experimental protocols are also provided that adapt appropriate behavioral endpoints to the measurement of hyperalgesia and allodynia in inflamed or nerve-injured rodents.

Methods to measure responses to thermal stimuli usually involve application of a noxious thermal stimulus (hot or cold) onto the paw of a rodent. Examples of noxious thermal stimuli are radiant heat, water bath (hot/cold), acetone application, and hot/cold plate. The main end point is a withdrawal response of the paw that is defined by a maximum cut off value in order to avoid tissue damage to the animal. Models have been developed to investigate acute thermal pain sensitivity, using various means of applying a noxious heat stimulus to the paw of rodents. More details on each thermal stimulus are described below.

The Hargreaves method utilizes a radiant heat source as pain-evoking stimuli that generated by a paw thermal stimulator (14). The temperature of the glass test surface is maintained at 30°C to prevent paw cooling and minimize sensitization artifacts. The heat source applied to the hind paw increases over time until it reaches a painful threshold (approximately 45°C). More specifics on how to run this model are included in Subheading 3 of this chapter.

Another thermal stimulus is a fixed temperature (hot or cold) water bath or a hot/cold plate. For the fixed temperature water bath, the animal must be restrained to assess the latency to withdrawal the hind limb from the water bath. While this method is not as common as other thermal pain methods, it does provide additional advantages and measurements. One of the advantages of this method is that the water bath can be set at various temperatures and it can be less sensitive to environmental conditions. However, this assay requires handling of the animals when testing for nociceptive behavior, making this measure highly dependent on experimenter experience/comfort handling/restraining animals by hand. The temperature of the water bath can be titrated to test either normal animals or inflamed animals. This method can also be used to test for reactivity to cold, using a 4 or 10°C water bath and recording latency to withdraw as an index of pain. The hot/cold plate test has the advantage of not requiring animal restraint. Additionally, unlike the fixed temperature water bath, the hot/cold plate does not require pre-handling to run the assay. Latency to licking, shaking of hind limbs or fore limbs in addition to latency to jump can be recorded and statistically analyzed for groups of animals. This assay can be difficult to standardize since the heat stimulus is not delivered in a controlled fashion. Possible sources of variability include differential exposure to the heated plate depending on how much weight the animal puts on each limb.

To further study inflammatory pain, various models have been developed to induce a localized inflammatory reaction by injecting various noxious chemical irritants/inflammogens e.g. formalin, carrageenan, or Complete Freud's Adjuvant (CFA) into the paw. Following the initial injection, pain can be measured minutes to days later, at the site of inflammation or away from the primary site of injury. Usually, the inflamed paw/joint becomes very sensitive to both thermal and mechanical stimuli, while the contralateral paw remains "normal". These models of more localized inflammation/ inflammatory pain have been widely used in pain research to test the effects of potential analgesic compounds but also in electrophysiological and gene expression studies to determine the plastic changes that initiate/maintain chronic inflammatory pain.

Models of nociceptive pain are defined as models of pain following tissue injury induced by trauma, surgery, or inflammation. Neuropathic pain can also result from inflammation around peripheral nerves. The most commonly used model is the chronic constriction injury (CCI, Bennett model) of the sciatic nerve model (15). Methods for inducing this injury as well as testing procedures are described in this chapter. As stated previously, spontaneous pain in these models is difficult to measure. Recently, models have been developed to mimic osteoarthritic (OA) pain observed in the clinic. Contrary to rheumatoid arthritis (RA) and the models of inflammatory pain, OA in the clinic and in animal models is not associated with a large amount of inflammation. In addition, to mimic more closely the clinical situation, pain evaluation in OA pain models relies on functional measures such as weight bearing or grip force of the affected limb rather than evaluation of withdrawal latencies to thermal or mechanical stimuli. Today, the more widely used model to measure and induce osteoarthritis are intra-articular administration of sodium monoiodoacetate into the knee (16). Iodoacetate injection into the knee/elbow joint cavity induced progressive joint degeneration and functional impairment (16) both of which are characteristic of clinical OA. Although the behavioral changes and histology both worsened over time, the majority of the pain responses were apparent within one week of surgery or iodoacetate injection.

2. Materials

2.1. Carrageenan Model

100 μl of a 1% (w/v) λ carrageenan solution (Sigma, St. Louis, MO) in phosphate buffered saline.

2.2. Complete Freund's Adjuvant Model

Complete Freund's Adjuvant (CFA) is mineral oil emulsion containing heat-killed tuberculosis basciteris (Sigma) diluted 1:1 in phosphate buffered saline.

2.3. Formalin Model

1. Formalin, 50 μl of a 5% (v/v) solution
2. Mirror
3. Stop watch
4. Transparent cages
5. Elevated mesh floor

2.4. Acetone Model

1. Acetone, 100 μl per animal
2. Six transparent mouse cages
3. Stop watch
4. Repeating pipettor
5. Elevated mesh floor

2.5. Capsaicin Model

1. Capsaicin (Sigma) is dissolved at 10 μg/10 μl in 10% ethanol and 2-hydroxypropyl BETA cyclodextrin
2. Six transparent mouse cages

2.6. Chronic Constriction Injury (CCI) Model

1. 5–0 chromic catgut sutures, with Petri dish to store sutures in saline
2. Sterile gauze, cotton swabs, and povidone-iodine solution
3. 70% alcohol, clippers (with size 40 blade), scalpel, 5–0 nylon sutures, wound clips, warming plate, and hemostat
4. Isoflurane anesthesia machine

2.7. Radiant Heat Source (Hargreaves) Method

Paw thermal stimulator (UARDG, University of California, San Diego, CA)

2.8. Fixed Temperature Water Bath, Hot or Cold Plate Method

1. Water bath, fixed to a temperature of 4–10°C or 45–50°C
2. Hot/cold plate (Columbus Instruments, Columbus, OH)

2.9. von Frey Monofilament Test Procedure

von Frey monofilaments (Stoelting, Wood Dale, IL)

2.10. Pin Prick Test Procedure

Safety pins

2.11. Grip Force Test Procedure

1. Monoiodoacetate (MIA) is dissolved at 60 mg/ml (w/v) in 0.05 ml in sterile saline.
2. 26 g needle.Grip force meter (DFE series Digital Force Gauge, Ametek, Largo, FL)

3. Methods

3.1. Carrageenan

1. On the day of testing, move rats from housing room to testing room at least 30 min prior to the onset of testing.
2. Rats are briefly restrained and administered 100 μl of a 1% λ-carrageenan solution into the intraplantar surface of the right hindpaw.
3. Rats are returned to the homecage. Behavioral testing occurs 2 h following carrageenan injection.
4. At predefined times, rats are injected with test compound and return to the homecage.
5. At the end of the pretreatment time, rats are then moved to the testing apparatus and allowed to acclimate for 15 min.
6. The thermal hyperalgesia is measured as described in the Hargreaves' method previously described in Subheading 2.7 (see Note 1).

3.2. Complete Freund's Adjuvant (CFA)

1. To make the CFA mixture, the CFA is brought to room temperature. Equal volumes of adjuvant and PBS are drawn up in separate syringes; air bubbles eliminated.
2. A 3-way stopcock is then placed between the two syringes.
3. The syringes are repeatedly drawn back and forth (approximately 35 repetitions) until the contents are emulsified.

4. 150 μl of CFA mixture is injected into the intraplantar surface of the right hindpaw with a 26 g needle.
5. Testing occurs 48 h following injection of CFA. Thermal hyperalgesia and mechanical allodynia can be both measured in CFA-treated rats. In the mechanical allodynia experiments, all rats are baselined for the paw withdrawal threshold. Only those rats that have a threshold score of ≤4.5 *g* are considered allodynic and used for pharmacological studies. See Subheading 3.7 for the thermal hyperalgesia testing method and Subheading 3.9 for the mechanical allodynia (von Frey filament) testing method.

3.3. Formalin

1. On the day of testing, move rats from housing room to testing room at least 30 min prior to the onset of testing.
2. Rats are acclimated to clear observation cages for at least 15 min. Four rats are tested at a time. Rats are positioned in the observation cages so that the hindpaw injected with formalin is always visible. It is advisable to elevate the observation cages and use mirrors below (see Note 2).
3. Following formalin injection (usually 5%/50 μl) into the dorsal or sometimes plantar surface of the rat hind paw, rats are returned to the observation cages.
4. Inject test compound at predetermined pretreatment time and return rats to the observation cages (see Note 3).
5. Phase I of the formalin response is defined as the period of time immediately following injection of formalin until 10 min after the formalin injection and corresponds to acute pain by direct activation of nociceptors by formalin.
6. Following a "quiet" period of little or no nocifensive behavior, the second phase of the formalin response can be observed (20–60 min postformalin injection) that corresponds to a more persistent inflammatory state.
7. Four rats are scored at a time, each for a 60 s period during a 5-min interval – 4 times over 20 min. Nociceptive behaviors that are scored (total time and total number) are flinching, licking, or biting the injected paw.
8. Repeat steps 2–6 until all subjects are tested.

3.4. Acetone

1. Move the rats from the housing room to the testing room at least 60 min before pretreatment or testing.
2. 15–20 min before the onset of testing, move 6 rats to acclimate in individual small plastic cages (mouse shoebox cage) inverted on an elevated mesh floor to acclimate to their new environment.
3. Apply a drop of cold acetone (100 μl) using an Eppendorf repipettor to the plantar surface of the right hind (ipsilateral)

paw (17) (see Note 4) and record the response of the rat. Note that the pipettor does not come in contact with the skin. Acetone produces a distinct cooling sensation as it evaporates. Normal rats will not respond to this stimulus or with a very small response (in amplitude and duration) while sensitized animals (e.g. neuropathic animals) will almost always respond with an exaggerated response (see Note 5).

4. Responses can be measured as the number of shakes/licking of hindpaw is counted for a set period of time or number of paw withdrawals (see Note 6).
5. This is repeated 5 times at 5 min intervals to obtain a baseline for each rat.
6. After the rats are selected based on their response to the baseline acetone stimulation, they are grouped and then dosed with either vehicle or test compound and then placed back in the cages on the wire mesh (see Note 7).
7. After the predetermined pretreatment time, acetone is again applied to the ipsilateral paw 5 times with 5 min between applications and the response of the rat is recorded.
8. Repeat steps 2–8 until all subjects are tested.

3.5. Capsaicin-Induced Acute and Secondary Pain

1. Move the rats from the housing room to the testing room at least 60 min before pretreatment or testing.
2. Rats are briefly retrained and administered capsaicin (intraplantar, i.pl.) at 10 μg/10 μl for secondary mechanical hypersensitivity and 2.5 μg/ul for acute capsaicin into the right hindpaw (see Note 8).
3. If testing acute nocifensive behaviors, 2 rats are tested at a time and licking, biting, and flinching behaviors are measured for (0–5 min) and cumulative scores are reported. If giving a drug treatment, this is administered before capsaicin injection since behavior is measured immediately after capsaicin (see Note 9).
4. If testing secondary pain, capsaicin is injected 3 h prior to testing is measured by mechanical testing (von Frey filaments), 3 h following injection of capsaicin Inject 6 rats at a time with capsaicin, so that rats can be tested for mechanical hypersensitivity in groups of 6 rats. Following injection return subjects to home cage.
5. Rats are then dosed with either vehicle or test compound and then placed back into the home cage for a predetermined pretreatment time. Continue to follow procedure listed in Subheading 3.9. von Frey monofilament testing procedure.

3.6. Chronic Constriction Injury (CCI)

1. Induce anesthesia by placing the rat in an induction chamber and delivering 4–5% isoflurane in oxygen at 3L/min. Once the rat has lost consciousness, remove it from the induction chamber and place the rat's nose in nose cone for delivery of anesthesia

during the surgical procedure. Maintain anesthesia with isoflurane at 1.5–3% and the oxygen level between 1 and 3 L/min.

2. Carefully clip the hair on the dorsal aspect of the right hind leg exposing the surgical area.
3. Clean the surgical area by wiping it with a sterile gauze soaked in 70% alcohol solution, wiping it down with sterile gauze in a circular motion to avoid contaminating the surgical field with hair. Repeat once more to ensure all hair is removed from the surgical field.
4. Prepare and sterilize the surgical area with povidone-iodine scrub/solution for 2–3 min contact time in order to sterilize the surgical area.
5. Place rat in nose cone where it will be still anesthetized during the procedure with the isoflurane flow.
6. Evaluate the rat's response to a toe pinch rat before incision to ensure that the rat is adequately anesthetized for surgery.
7. Following aseptic surgical techniques and using the scalpel blade make a 1.5 cm incision, where the dorsal to the pelvis and the biceps femoris and gluteous superficialis (right side) are separated.
8. Using the tip of the hemostat tool, place it on the exposed muscle and gently press down to make a small hole in the muscle to expose sciatic nerve.
9. Using gentle blunt dissection with forceps, expose/isolate the sciatic nerve with forceps.
10. Loosely ligate the nerves by 4 chromic gut (5–0, 1.5 metic, 18″ 45 cm) with <1 mm spacing in between by using forceps. (Note: Make sure knots are not too tight or too loose.)
11. Close the muscle layer (biceps femoris and gluteous superficialis) using a simple interrupted pattern with 5–0 nylon sutures.
12. Clip the incision site together using wound clips.
13. Inject warm sterile fluids (Lactated Ringers Solution or 0.9% saline (SC) solution (approximately 5–10 mL) to help prevent postoperative dehydration.
14. Allow the rat to recover from the effects of anesthesia (usually 10–15 min) on a 37°C warming plate.
15. Return rat to the home cage.
16. Rats are monitored daily and wound clips are removed 10–14 days post surgery.
17. Two and 3 weeks following surgery, rats can be tested for mechanical and cold allodynia and/or thermal hyperalgesia using methods described in this chapter.

3.7. Radiant Heat Source: Hargreaves Method

1. On testing day, move rats from the housing room to the testing room at least 30 min prior to onset of dosing and testing.
2. Inject carrageenan (Subheading 3.1.) into the dorsal surface of the hindpaw 2 h prior to testing if using a chemical inflammogen to induce hyperalgesia to a thermal stimulus and return to home cage. Do this in groups of 6 rats.
3. 60–90 min postcarrageenan injection, administer test compounds and return rats to home cage (see Note 10).
4. In each test session, each animal is habituated to the plastic chambers located on the glass surface of the paw thermal stimulator for 10 min prior to testing. This reduces the stress level of the test subjects when compared with the need for manual restraint in tail flick or immersion tests as described below (see Note 11).
5. Each animal is then tested in three sequential trials at approximately 5 min intervals to avoid sensitization of the response. For example, each rat is tested once on the ipsilateral paw, and then on the contralateral paw. This is repeated 3 times to get mean paw withdrawal latency for the ipsilateral and contralateral paws (see Note 12).
6. The paw withdrawal latency is recorded using a light beam that produces thermal stimulation on a very small region of the animal's paw. The stimulation ends when the animal withdrawals its paw.
7. In cases where the animal does not withdraw, the stimulation will last a maximum of 20 s to minimize tissue damage.
8. Remove rats from the plastic chambers and repeat the procedure for the remaining subjects.

3.8. Fixed Temperature Water Bath/Hot or Cold Plate

1. The water bath and hot/cold plate will take awhile to come to the desired temperature, so the apparatus should be turned on before moving the subjects into the testing room. For the hot/cold plate, it will take approximately 15–20 min to reach 55°C and 1 h to go from 20°C to 5°C (see Note 13).
2. Move rats from the housing to testing room at least 30 min prior to the onset of handling and testing (see Note 14).
3. If using neuropathic rats (e.g. CCI), the ipsilateral paw is baseline for paw withdrawal response to ensure allodynia in these rats. There is a maximum cut-off time of 20 s to prevent tissue injury and damage in either procedure.
4. In the hot/cold plate, use a clear acrylic cage with lid around the plate to prevent the rat from moving off of the plate.
5. Place the rat into the hot/cold plate and push the start button. Alternatively, restraint the rat and dip its paw into the fixed temperature water bath and start your timer.

6. Once the rat licks its paw (hot/cold plate) or withdraws its hindpaw from the water bath, push stop on the timer immediately remove rat from testing apparatus.
7. Manually record the time for withdrawal response.
8. Only take the allodynic rats to inject with compound for further testing.
9. Test compound is injected based on a predetermined pretreatment time and rats are placed back into their homecage.
10. Following the pretreatment, the rats are removed from the homecage and tested one at a time.
11. The withdrawal response of the ipsilateral paw/2 times for fixed temperature water bath and 1 time for hot/cold plate following compound administration is measured and recorded. The mean withdrawal time is used as the dependent variable for fixed temperature water bath.
12. A separate group of rats is used as a control to obtain the 100% value. There is a maximum cut-off time of 20 s to prevent tissue injury and damage in either procedure.
13. Repeat the procedure until all rats are tested.

3.9. von Frey Monofilaments Test Procedure

1. Move the rats from the housing room to the testing room at least 30 min before pretreatment or testing.
2. Rats used can be injected with CFA or capsaicin (see above for procedures for injection) or those that have undergone procedures to induce neuropathic pain (CCI, see above for surgical procedures).
3. Test compound is injected based on a predetermined pretreatment time and rats are placed back into their homecage (see Note 15). Six rats can be tested at a time.
4. 10 min before the onset of testing, move 6 rats to acclimate in individual inverted mouse cages on an elevated mesh floor.
5. Mechanical hypersensitivity is tested with von Frey monofilaments (see Note 16).
6. Responses are quantified as mechanical threshold can be determined using the up-down method (18) using the 0.41, 0.70, 1.20, 2.00, 3.63, 5.50, 8.50 and 15.10*g* von Frey monofilaments. Testing is initiated with the 2.00*g* von Frey monofilament.
7. Stimuli are presented for 6–8 s on the plantar surface of the hindpaw with several seconds between applications of monofilaments. A positive response is a paw withdrawal from the stimulus.
8. The monofilaments are presented in a consecutive order. If there is no response with a given monofilament, the next

highest *g* force monofilament is used. Likewise, if there is a response, the next lowest *g* force monofilament is used.

9. To determine the 50% threshold, six responses near the 50% threshold are needed for the calculation. The first monofilament used of the six for calculating the 50% threshold is the monofilament immediately preceding the first positive response. Four additional responses to monofilaments following the first positive response (up or down depending on the rat's response) are used to calculate the 50% threshold (see Note 17).
10. Two 50% threshold readings are recorded for each rat and are averaged to obtain a paw withdrawal threshold (*g*). The upper threshold limit is set to 15*g* (see Note 18).
11. Return rats to home cage and repeat procedure until all subjects are tested.

3.10. Pin Prick Testing Procedure

1. Pin prick to measure hyperalgesia can be tested immediately following von Frey monofilament testing (see Note 19).
2. The behavior can be measured by the duration of paw lifting in seconds following the pinprick application.
3. The application of the pinprick does not penetrate the skin and the maximum time for application is 15 s.

3.11. Grip Force Assessment

1. Under light isofluourane anesthesia, prepare the injection site by shaving the hair off around the knee joint and cleaning the area with alcohol swabs.
2. Inject sodium monoiodoacetate (3 mg, i.a.) injected at 0.05 ml in sterile sale into the knee/elbow joint cavity using a 26 G needle.
3. Use a sterile needle for each injection and do not reuse needles.
4. Immediately after the injection, allow the rat to recover from the effects of anesthesia (usually 10–15 min).
5. Return rat to the home cage.
6. Grip force is measured 21 days following MIA injection.
7. Use age matched naïve (non-MIA injected) rat as a control.
8. Grip force is used as a measure of fore limb and hindlimb neuromuscular performance. A computerized grip force meter (E-DPE-010, Ametek, Largo, FL) measures the amount of tensile force each rodent exerts against a wire mesh grid that is attached to a force transducer.
9. On the day of testing, move rats from housing room to testing room at least 30 min prior to the onset of testing.
10. Pretreat rats with test compound and return to the homecage (see Note 20).

11. At the end of the pretreatment time, test rats for grip strength one at a time.
12. The rat is gently held around its body, allowed to grasp the wire mesh grid with its fore paws/hind paws, and then gently pulled (~10 cm/s) away from the mesh.
13. The peak force exerted by the rodent before it releases its grasp is registered by a force transducer and recorded in grams. The rodent itself determines the force each rodent applies to the mesh grid. Therefore, the amplitude of force exerted is subject to factors such as hyperalgesia, which influence the behavioral performance of each rodent.
14. Three consecutive fore limb/hind limb grip force measurements (~10 s apart) are obtained for each rat at each time point; the average of these three measurements is used to represent each rodent's grip force for each time point (see Note 21).

4. Notes

1. We put paper towels the first half of the 15 min, so that the animals do not pee on the glass. Once the glass gets wet, it is impossible to get an accurate reading.
2. Use mirrors below and elevate the cages in a mesh floor. This makes the flinching behavior visible for easier scoring.
3. Morphine at 6 mg/kg, ip is typically used as the positive control in formalin.
4. A repeating pipettor that delivers 100 μl multiple times is much easier than using a syringe and delivers the acetone in a more uniform manner.
5. Chronic constriction Injury (CCI) rats show cold allodynia to a much greater extent than the Spinal Nerve Ligated (SNL) rats.
6. The following are the options for quantifying cold allodynia using acetone application. Both can be done at the same time in the same rats. For scoring, use a 0–3 scale where 0 = no response, 1 = 1 flinch of the paw, 2 = multiple flinches of the paw, 3 = multiple flinches of the paw with licking. For frequency, this is the number of times the rats respond to the acetone stimulus out of the 5 times being sprayed. The data for the scored rats is graphed as the median ± interquartile range. The frequency is graphed as %.
7. We typically use duloxetine at 30 mg/kg as a positive control in cold allodynia.

8. Doses of capsaicin can vary from 1 to 10 μg/10 μl injected to the ventral surface of the rat hind paw. The injection of capsaicin is immediately followed by an intense period of nocifensive behaviors that are usually recorded for 5 min following capsaicin injection (acute pain) or 3 h following injection of capsaicin with testing away from the injection site using mechanical stimuli (secondary mechanical hypersensitivity; SMH).
9. Acclimate rats for acute capsaicin for about 15 min in their testing cages. It is much easier to count flinching when the animals are not moving around. We typically use A-784168 (TRPV1 antagonist) at 100 μmol/kg as a positive control in capsaicin-induced nocifensive behaviors.
10. We typically use 30 mg/kg diclofenac as the positive control for thermal hyperalgesia.
11. Covering the front of the boxes with paper helps to prevent the rats from being affected (freezing) due to the presence of the experimenter.
12. The contralateral (uninjured) paw serves as control for the injured paw, which has proven a useful behavioral assessment in models of unilateral inflammation or nerve injury. The main advantage of this method versus the tail-flick assay is that both paws can be tested.
13. If the ambient temperature of the testing room is greater than 22°C, it may be difficult to reach 5°C using the hot/cold plate. Additionally, if the humidity is greater than 30%, condensation will form on the plate and make it difficult to obtain accurate readings.
14. If using the fixed temperature water bath, it is recommended that the rats are handled before testing. Handling for 5 min twice the day before the study helps to habituate the rats to the testing procedure and decreases experimental variability.
15. We typically use gabapentin at 100 mg/kg as the positive control when using von Frey monofilaments.
16. These are a series of hairs/nylon monofilaments of various thicknesses that exert various degrees of force when applied to the planter surface of the hind paw.
17. The formula and related tables needed to calculate the 50% *g* threshold are found in the Chapman et al (2004) methods paper. The formula for 50% *g* threshold = $(10^{(xf + k\delta)})/10{,}000$ where Xf = value (in log units) of the final von Frey hair used; *k* = tabular value (see Chapman Appendix) for the patter of positive/negative responses; and δ = mean difference (in log units) between stimuli.
18. Naïve rats will respond at approximately 15 g to stimulation with monofilaments. This is therefore set as the highest value.

19. This is similar to the pricking pain test done during the neurological exam in patients.
20. We typically use diclofenac at 30 mg/kg as the positive control in MIA-induced OA grip force assessment.
21. The body weight of the rat is factored into the final calculations.

Acknowledgments

Thank you to Gricelda Simler and Donna Gauvin for their insights into practical aspects in testing rodents in these models and to Elizabeth Cronin, Donna Gauvin, Heidi Shafford and La Geisha Lewis for clarification of methodological detail.

References

1. Scholz J, Woolf CJ (2002) Can we conquer pain? Nat Neurosci 5 Suppl:1062–1067
2. Cervero F, Laird JM (1996) Mechanisms of touch-evoked pain (allodynia): a new model. Pain 68:13–23
3. Millan MJ (1999) The induction of pain: an integrative review. Prog Neurobiol 57: 1–164
4. Coda B, Bonica J (2001). In: Bonica's management of pain. Lippincott, Baltimore, pp 222–240
5. Byers M, Bonica J (2001). In: Bonica's management of pain. Lippincott, Baltimore, pp 26–72
6. Meyer RA, Campbell JN, Raja SN (1985). In: Advances in pain research and therapy. Raven, New York, pp 55–71
7. Woolf CJ, Costigan M (1999) Transcriptional and posttranslational plasticity and the generation of inflammatory pain. Proc Natl Acad Sci U S A 96:7723–7730
8. Urban MO, Gebhart GF (1999) Supraspinal contributions to hyperalgesia. Proc Natl Acad Sci U S A 96:7687–7692
9. Woolf CJ (1983) Evidence for a central component of post-injury pain hypersensitivity. Nature 306:686–688
10. Woolf CJ, Thompson SW (1991) The induction and maintenance of central sensitization is dependent on N-methyl-D-aspartic acid receptor activation; implications for the treatment of post-injury pain hypersensitivity states. Pain 44:293–299
11. Woolf CJ, Salter MW (2000) Neuronal plasticity: increasing the gain in pain. Science 288:1765–1769
12. Watkins LR, Milligan ED, Maier SF (2001) Spinal cord glia: new players in pain. Pain 93:201–205
13. Tsuda M, Inoue K, Salter MW (2005) Neuropathic pain and spinal microglia: a big problem from molecules in "small" glia. Trends Neurosci 28:101–107
14. Hargreaves K, Dubner R, Brown F, Flores C, Joris J (1988) A new and sensitive method for measuring thermal nociception in cutaneous hyperalgesia. Pain 32:77–88
15. Ueda H (2006) Molecular mechanisms of neuropathic pain-phenotypic switch and initiation mechanisms. Pharmacol Ther 109:57–77
16. Fernihough J, Gentry C, Malcangio M, Fox A, Rediske J, Pellas T, Kidd B, Bevan S, Winter J (2004) Pain related behaviour in two models of osteoarthritis in the rat knee. Pain 112:83–93
17. Choi Y, Yoon YW, Na HS, Kim SH, Chung JM (1994) Behavioral signs of ongoing pain and cold allodynia in a rat model of neuropathic pain. Pain 59:369–376
18. Chaplan SR, Bach FW, Pogrel JW, Chung JM, Yaksh TL (1994) Quantitative assessment of tactile allodynia in the rat paw. J Neurosci Methods 53:55–63

Chapter 5

Noxious Heat Threshold Measured with Slowly Increasing Temperatures: Novel Rat Thermal Hyperalgesia Models

Kata Bölcskei, Gábor Pethő, and János Szolcsányi

Abstract

The conventional methods for the study of thermal pain in animals apply constant suprathreshold heat stimuli and measure the reflex latency of pain-avoiding reactions. The latency measured by these methods may greatly vary upon repeated measurements which is a major disadvantage concerning reliability. The presently introduced novel approach involves applying a slowly increasing thermal stimulus which allows determination of the noxious heat threshold i.e. the lowest temperature evoking pain-avoiding behaviour. An increasing-temperature hot plate and an increasing-temperature water bath are presented which are both suitable to determine the noxious heat threshold with high reproducibility. Acute thermal hyperalgesia models based on the drop of the heat threshold are also described for each equipment which proved to be highly sensitive to standard analgesics.

Key words: Noxious heat threshold, Increasing-temperature hot plate, Increasing-temperature water bath, Resiniferatoxin, Heat injury

1. Introduction

Owing to the subjective nature of pain experience, the study of nociception in animals is highly challenging and none of the presently employed nociceptive tests is ideal, principally in terms of reproducibility and pharmacological sensitivity (reviewed in (1)). In the present chapter, we introduce two novel methods with a new approach in the study of thermonociception which we consider to suit these requirements better.

The traditional methods for the study of thermonociception (constant temperature hot plate, tail-flick, plantar test) apply a constant suprathreshold heat stimulus and measure the reflex latency of nocifensive (pain-avoiding) reactions. The main disadvantage of these tests is that this latency may vary considerably

Arpad Szallasi (ed.), *Analgesia: Methods and Protocols*, Methods in Molecular Biology, vol. 617, DOI 10.1007/978-1-60327-323-7_5, © Springer Science+Business Media, LLC 2010

upon repeated measurements (e.g. due to sensitization or habituation) and, moreover, they can only detect reliably the antinociceptive action of opioids but not of cyclooxygenase inhibitors (1). These features can be attributed to several factors: (1) latency may be strongly influenced by factors unrelated to nociceptor responsiveness such as basal skin temperature, reaction time etc. (2) suprathreshold heat stimuli are more likely to cause tissue injury and (3) suprathreshold heat stimulation mainly activates Aδ nociceptors initiating faster reflexes than the slowly conducting C afferents, but Aδ nociceptors are less sensitive to therapeutic doses of analgesics (1).

Although the measurement of the heat threshold or heat-evoked ionic currents is a routine procedure in the in vitro electrophysiological study of nociceptive nerve fibres as well as the measurement of heat pain threshold in human experimental pain models, this approach for comparison has only been used in a few in vivo studies in animal tests of nociception (2, 3). By applying an increasing heat stimulus, the noxious heat threshold temperature (i.e. the lowest temperature evoking pain-avoiding behaviour) can be determined. Recently, we have validated two equipments which are suitable to determine the noxious heat threshold of conscious animals: the increasing-temperature hot plate (4) and the increasing-temperature water bath (5). In contrast to the conventional methods, these novel techniques yield remarkably reproducible threshold values upon repeated measurements which enhance their reliability. Acute thermal hyperalgesia models based on the decrease of the heat threshold induced by either the transient receptor potential vanilloid type 1 (TRPV1) receptor agonist, resiniferatoxin (RTX) or mild heat injury proved to be highly sensitive to standard analgesics. The most likely explanation of the excellent reproducibility and sensitivity is that the slow rate of heating mainly activates C-fibres and fails to alter nociceptor responsiveness. Noxious heat threshold measurement is therefore a promising new approach in animal studies of thermal nociception.

2. Materials

2.1. Equipment

1. Increasing-temperature (incremental) hot plate (Fig. 1a) (IITC Life Science, Woodland Hills, CA).
2. Increasing-temperature water bath (Fig. 1b) (Experimetria Ltd., Budapest, Hungary).

2.2. Animals

1. Female Wistar rats weighing 120–200 g are used (see Note 1). Animals are brought to the air conditioned laboratory at least

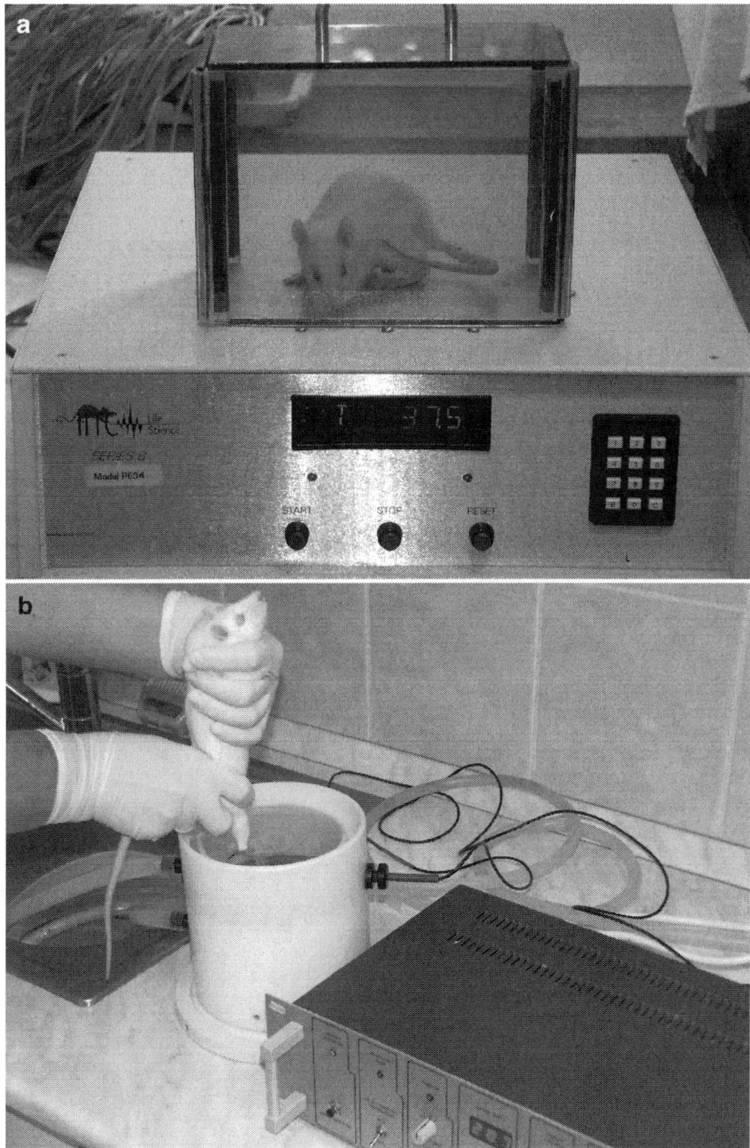

Fig. 1. The increasing-temperature hot plate (Panel **a**) and the increasing-temperature water bath equipment (Panel **b**)

a day before the experiment and they are provided with food and water ad libitum. In order to habituate them to the measurement's conditions, two threshold determinations are performed prior to the experiment (see Note 2).

2.3. Chemicals

1. Resiniferatoxin (Sigma, St. Louis, MO): a stock solution of 1 mg/mL is made with ethanol which is further diluted with saline to a concentration of 0.3 μg/mL.

3. Methods

The basis of the noxious heat threshold measurement is applying an increasing heat stimulus by slowly heating a metal plate or a water bath from subthreshold temperature until the appearance of nocifensive behaviour. The two equipments are both suitable to determine the noxious heat threshold with high reproducibility upon repeated measurements at intervals from 5 min to 1 day (see Fig. 2a, Fig. 3a and Note 3).

There are two major differences between the equipments: (1) on the hot plate only the plantar surface is exposed to heat,

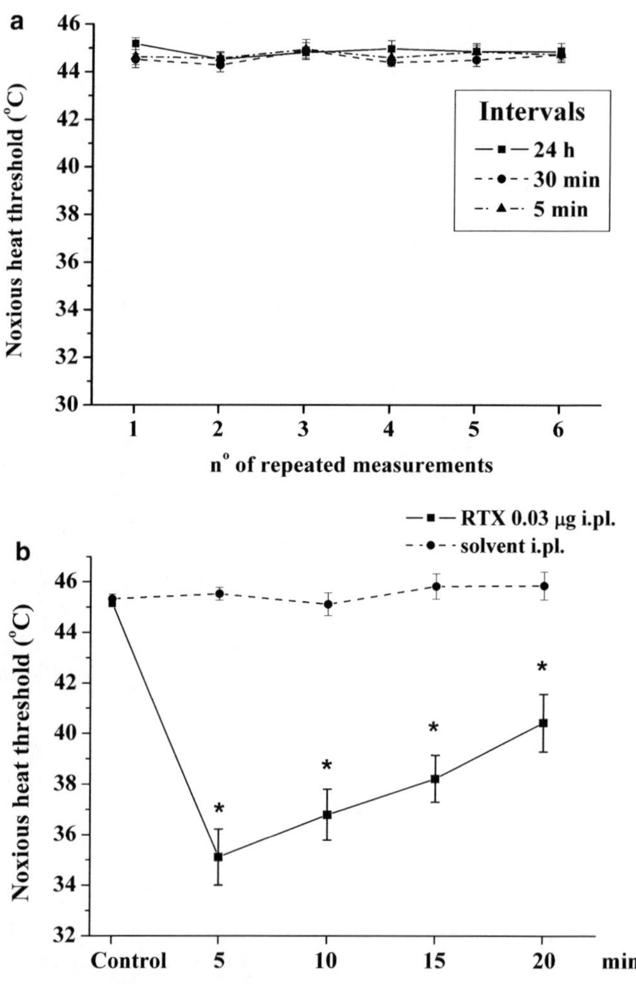

Fig. 2. Reproducibility of the noxious heat threshold measured by the increasing-temperature hot plate at intervals of 5, 30 min or 24 h (Panel **a**). Panel **b** shows the heat threshold drop induced by intraplantar RTX (0.03 μg i.pl.) determined by the increasing-temperature hot plate. The intraplantar injection of solvent fails to influence the heat threshold. Data are mean ± S.E.M. of 12–12 animals (modified figures from ref. 4)

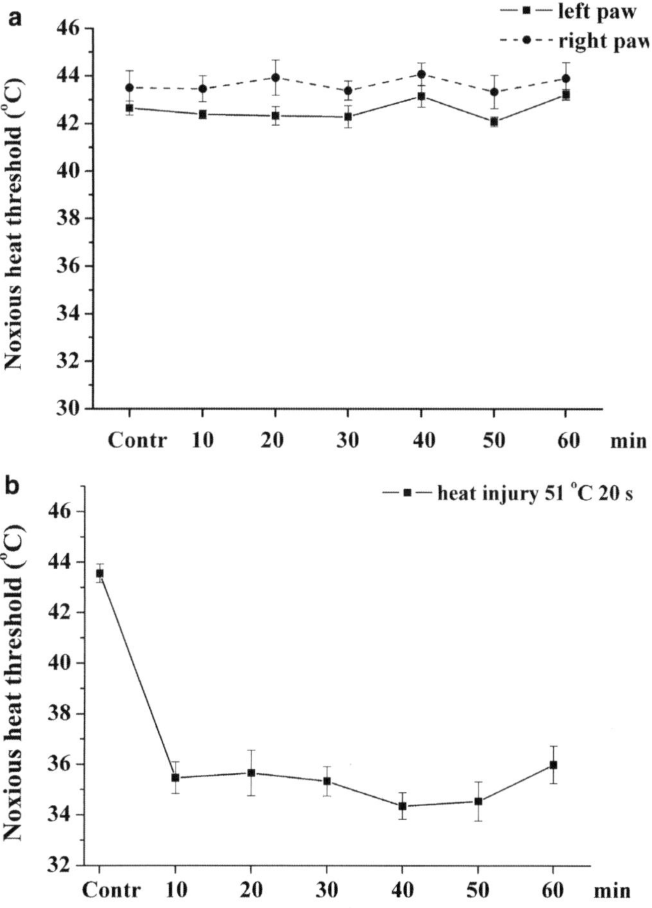

Fig. 3. Panel **a** shows the reproducibility of the noxious heat threshold measured by the increasing-temperature water bath at intervals of 10 min (modified figure from ref. 5). Panel **b** is a representative example of the heat threshold drop induced by mild heat injury (51°C 20 s) as measured by the increasing-temperature water-bath. Data are mean ± S.E.M. of 8–10 animals

while in the case of the water bath the whole paw is immersed; (2) rats move freely on the hot plate, but they are restrained when tested in the water bath. One must also consider that in the latter case, paw withdrawal from the water is a spinal reflex while the nocifensive behaviour of the freely moving rat involves supraspinal mechanisms.

The antinociceptive effect of drugs can be either investigated by the ability to increase the control noxious heat threshold; however, sensitivity to standard analgesics is enhanced when a heat threshold drop (thermal hyperalgesia) is induced. In the next section, the two sensitive thermal hyperalgesia models are also described, which have been validated using noxious heat threshold measurement.

3.1. Increasing-Temperature Hot Plate

1. The equipment consists of a steel plate (10 cm × 20 cm) with a microprocessor-controlled heating unit and a plexiglass observation chamber. The starting and cut-off temperatures can be set to any value from 0 to 70°C and the heating ramp is also adjustable (1–12°C/min). For control threshold measurements, the plate is heated up from 30°C at a rate of 12°C/min and the cut-off is set to 50°C. The animal is placed into the observation chamber and the heating is started immediately afterwards. Heating is stopped by the experimenter at the moment when the animal shows nocifensive behaviour (typically hind paw licking or shaking) involving any of the hind paws and the corresponding plate temperature is recorded as the noxious heat threshold of the animal.
2. By the interruption of heating, the plate is rapidly cooled back automatically to the starting temperature while the threshold temperature remains visible on the display. Due to the rapid cooling process, successive measurements can be performed at intervals of approximately 2 min. Two threshold measurements are performed at a 30-min interval for the same animal and the mean of the two values is considered the control noxious heat threshold.
3. For the induction of hyperalgesia, the ultrapotent TRPV1 receptor agonist RTX is used. The tested analgesic or its solvent is administered as a pretreatment either systemically or topically (intraplantarly – i.pl.). After a period of 30 min after intraperitoneal (i.p.) or 5 min after i.pl. injection, RTX is administered i.pl. (0.03 μg in a volume of 0.1 ml) and the animal is returned to the cage. Immediately after RTX injection, nocifensive behaviour (shaking and licking of the paw) of moderate intensity is observed, however it declines during the first 5 min (see Note 4). Meanwhile, the starting temperature of the plate is set to 25°C as the heat threshold may even drop below 30°C. Threshold measurements are repeated 5, 10, 15 and 20 min after injection. Typically, the heat threshold decreases by 8–10°C at the 5 min measurement and gradually returns to control (see Fig. 2b and Note 5).
4. For statistical analysis, threshold drop values are calculated for each time point by subtracting the measured threshold from the control value. Comparisons between the solvent- and drug-treated groups can be performed separately for each time point. Alternatively, the sum of threshold drops can also be statistically compared by adding all four threshold drop values to create an integrative parameter of the RTX effect. The model was validated by pretreatment with standard analgesics (morphine, diclofenac or paracetamol i.p.) to measure the inhibitory effect on RTX-induced heat threshold drop. The sensitivity of the test is reflected by their minimum effective doses (see Table 1) all of which proved to be remarkably low.

Table 1
Minimum effective doses of standard analgesics detected with noxious heat threshold measurement (ITHP – increasing-temperature hot plate; ITWB – increasing-temperature water bath)

	Minimum effective dose (mg/kg i.p.)			
	Morphine	Diclofenac	Paracetamol	Ibuprofen
Elevation of the noxious heat threshold (ITHP)	3	10	200	–
Inhibition of RTX-induced noxious heat threshold drop (ITHP)	1	1	100	–
Inhibition of heat injury-induced noxious heat threshold drop (ITWB)	0.3	0.3	30	10

The test was also suitable to show the systemic antinociceptive effect of novel potential analgesics such as the somatostatin receptor agonist TT-232 (6) or the local antihyperalgesic effect of the endocannabinoid anandamide (7).

5. Other hyperalgesic agents tested with the equipment are listed in Note 6.

3.2. Increasing-Temperature Water Bath

1. The equipment consists of a tap water-filled cylindrical container (12 cm inner diameter, 14 cm height) with a built-in heating unit in its bottom and a controlling unit. Two alternative starting temperatures (30 or 40°C) and three different heating rates (6, 12 or 24°C/min) can be set on the equipment. Typically, a starting temperature of 30°C and a heating rate of 24°C/min are chosen. For the threshold measurement, animals are lightly restrained allowing free movement of the hind limbs and one of the hind paws is immersed into the water and heating is started immediately afterwards. The controlling unit also has a display continuously showing the actual bath temperature measured by a thermocouple approximately at a depth to which the animal's paw is immersed in the water. When the rat withdraws its paw from the bath, heating is interrupted by a foot switch and the corresponding bath temperature remains on the display to be recorded which is considered as the noxious heat threshold of the given paw.
2. After each measurement, the water bath is cooled back to the starting temperature by pumping cold water into the container controlled by a feedback mechanism while the excess water is drained through a spillway. Successive measurements of rats can be performed at intervals of approximately 1.5 min. Two threshold measurements are performed at a 30-min interval for the same animal and the mean of the two values

is considered as the control noxious heat threshold of the tested paw.

3. For the induction of hyperalgesia, mild heat injury is used which involves exactly the same skin area which is stimulated in the water bath. Rats are anaesthetized with diethyl ether (in a chamber) or halothane (4%, via nose cone) and one of the hind paws is immersed in a constant, 51°C hot water bath for 20 s. After the paw is removed from the hot water, animals are returned to a cage lined with soft paper towel. They recover from anaesthesia within minutes and threshold measurements are performed 10 and 20 min after injury to confirm the development of heat threshold drop (see Fig. 3b). Anaesthesia itself does not influence the noxious heat threshold. Thermal hyperalgesia persists for up to 4 h afterwards. The tested analgesic or its solvent is administered as posttreatment (i.p. or i.pl.) after the 20-min measurement and its effect can be followed by repeated measurements at intervals of 10 min.

4. For statistical analysis, threshold drop values are calculated for each time point by subtracting the measured threshold from the control values. Comparisons between the solvent- and drug-treated groups can be performed separately for each time point after treatment. Alternatively, the sum of threshold drops can also be statistically compared by adding all threshold drop values to create an integrative parameter. The model was validated by administering standard analgesics (morphine, diclofenac, ibuprofen or paracetamol) as a posttreatment to measure the inhibitory effect on heat injury-induced heat threshold drop. Similarly to the previous test, this one also proved to be highly sensitive to detect the antihyperalgesic effect of the tested compounds whose minimum effective doses are shown in Table 1. Moreover, it was also suitable to detect the peripheral antihyperalgesic effect of morphine, diclofenac and ibuprofen after i.pl. administration of systemically ineffective doses (see ref. 5).

4. Notes

1. The reason for using female rats on the increasing-temperature hot plate is that in the case of male animals the skin of the scrotum (inevitably in contact with the hot plate) proved to be more sensitive than the paw which therefore produced a confounding effect. When developing the increasing-temperature water bath, we chose to continue the experiments with females to be able to compare the sensitivity of the two methods in the same gender.

2. In all experiments, the same experienced assistant handled all the animals. This is especially important and indispensable in the case of the increasing-temperature water bath as proper restraining is essential in this model. In the hands of an untrained experimenter, rats may be exposed to a variable level of restraint and consequent stress. For the same reason, escape attempts may also be confused with nocifensive paw withdrawal.

3. When applying the conventional testing methods such as the plantar test, authors frequently state that only animals having reproducible control responses are included in the study. It also has to be emphasized that due to the high reproducibility of the noxious heat threshold, no preselection of animals is required.

4. It is obvious that spontaneous nocifensive behaviour interferes with noxious heat threshold measurement, especially on the increasing-temperature hot plate as it cannot be distinguished from the heat-evoked nocifensive reaction. The experimenter must make sure that spontaneous paw licking or lifting is absent before starting the measurement.

5. It has been a surprising observation that the pattern of nocifensive behaviour on the increasing-temperature hot plate changed after the induction of hyperalgesia. During control measurements, paw licking was typically the first pain-avoiding response, but after RTX injection paw lifting was more frequently seen, and paw licking occurred only at higher plate temperatures (see ref. 4). We chose to accept paw lifting as an endpoint, first because it is also a clear-cut nocifensive reaction, and secondly because rats often held their paws in an elevated position after the first paw lifting reaction, thus avoiding further contact with the plate which made impossible to determine the threshold for the paw licking reaction.

6. Other compounds can also be applied to induce an acute heat threshold drop e.g. other TRPV1 receptor agonists such as *N*-oleoyl-dopamine (8) or 3-methyl-*N*-oleoyl-dopamine (7), as well as mediators which are known to sensitize nociceptors to heat (bradykinin, prostaglandin E_2, P2 purinoceptor agonists etc.). Surprisingly, we were unable to measure reliably the heat threshold lowering effect of the classical TRPV1 receptor agonist, capsaicin on the increasing temperature hot plate, most probably due to the very pronounced capsaicin-induced nocifensive reaction (see also Note 4). It is also noteworthy that no significant change of the noxious heat threshold was ever detected in subacute/chronic inflammatory models (e.g. carrageenan- or complete Freund's adjuvant (CFA)-induced inflammation) or in neuropathic pain models (Seltzer or Chung model).

References

1. Le Bars D, Gozariu M, Cadden SW (2001) Animal models of nociception. Pharmacol Rev 53:597–652
2. Hunskaar S, Berge OG, Hole K (1986) A modified hot-plate test sensitive to mild analgesics. Behav Brain Res 21:101–108
3. Farré AJ, Colombo M, Gutiérrez B (1989) Maximum tolerated temperature in the rat tail: a broadly sensitive test of analgesic activity. Methods Find Exp Clin Pharmacol 11:303–307
4. Almási R, Pethő G, Bölcskei K, Szolcsányi J (2003) Effect of resiniferatoxin on the noxious heat threshold temperature in the rat: a novel heat allodynia model sensitive to analgesics. Br J Pharmacol 139:49–58
5. Bölcskei K, Horváth D, Szolcsányi J, Pethö G (2007) Heat injury-induced drop of the noxious heat threshold measured with an increasing-temperature water bath: a novel rat thermal hyperalgesia model. Eur J Pharmacol 564:80–87
6. Szolcsányi J, Bölcskei K, Szabó Á, Pintér E, Pethő G, Elekes K, Börzsei R, Almási R, Szüts T, Kéri G, Helyes Z (2004) Analgesic effect of TT-232, a heptapeptide somatostatin analogue, in acute pain models of the rat and the mouse and in streptozotocin-induced diabetic mechanical allodynia. Eur J Pharmacol 498:103–109
7. Almási R, Szőke É, Bölcskei K, Varga A, Riedl Z, Sándor Z, Szolcsányi J, Pethő G (2008) Actions of 3-methyl-N-oleoyldopamine, 4-methyl-N-oleoyldopamine and N-oleoylethanolamide on the rat TRPV1 receptor in vitro and in vivo. Life Sci 82:644–651
8. Szolcsányi J, Sándor Z, Pethő G, Varga A, Bölcskei K, Almási R, Riedl Z, Hajós G, Czéh G (2004) Direct evidence for activation and desensitization of the capsaicin receptor by N-oleoyldopamine on TRPV1-transfected cell line, in gene deleted mice and in the rat. Neurosci Lett 361:155–158

Chapter 6

Locomotor Activity in a Novel Environment as a Test of Inflammatory Pain in Rats

David J. Matson, Daniel C. Broom, and Daniel N. Cortright

Abstract

Creating a robust and unbiased assay for the study of current and novel analgesics has been a daunting task. Traditional rodent models of pain and inflammation typically rely on a negative reaction to various forms of evoked stimuli to elicit a pain response and are subject to rater interpretation. Recently, models such as weight bearing and gait analysis have been developed to address these drawbacks while detecting a drug's analgesic properties. We have recently developed the Reduction of Spontaneous Activity by Adjuvant (RSAA) model as a quick, unbiased method for the testing of potential analgesics. Rats, following prior administration of an activity-decreasing inflammatory insult, will positively increase spontaneous locomotor exploration when given single doses of known analgesics. The RSAA model capitalizes on a rat's spontaneous exploratory behavior in a novel environment with the aid of computer tracking software to quantify movement and eliminate rater bias.

Key words: Pain, Inflammation, Behavior, Spontaneous activity, Complete Freund's adjuvant

1. Introduction

Valid preclinical evaluation of analgesic compounds has historically been challenging to achieve. Numerous models and behavioral tests for evaluating pain in rodents have been established and used widely for the testing of potential analgesics (1). The most commonly used tests involve evoking a "pain-like" nociceptive and/or aversive behavior and evaluating the effect of commonly used and potential analgesics to reverse this behavior. Such testing can be performed in rodents after the induction of sensory hypersensitivity (allodynia or hyperalgesia) by nerve injury or inflammation. Tests include measuring mechanical allodynia with von Frey (Semmes–Weinstein) monofilaments (2), mechanical

Arpad Szallasi (ed.), *Analgesia: Methods and Protocols*, Methods in Molecular Biology, vol. 617, DOI 10.1007/978-1-60327-323-7_6, © Springer Science+Business Media, LLC 2010

hyperalgesia with Randall–Selitto paw pressure apparatus (3), and thermal hyperalgesia with radiant heat (4).

Current behavioral endpoints present significant challenges for the development of novel analgesics. Firstly, they all to some degree rely on the subjectivity of the rater performing the test. For example, what is classified as a response to the mechanical or thermal stimulus being applied? This can be overcome somewhat by blinding the rater to the identity of each individual animal's treatment and randomizing the treatment groups throughout the experiment. Secondly, as these assays rely on an evoked input resulting in a behavioral outcome, test subjects require habituation and baseline testing to allow the animal to become accustomed to the testing procedure. Such activities often require time-consuming handling and baseline testing sessions resulting in less than optimal throughput if used in a drug screening paradigm. Thirdly, as these assays measure an evoked physical response (i.e. a nocifensive withdrawal of the hindpaw) and therefore an increase in behavioral responding, effects of test drugs on physical activity may produce changes in responding in the absence of analgesic activity (5). This is of particular concern as certain classes of analgesics, notably the opiates, affect locomotor activity in rodents. Indeed, when measuring a pain-stimulated response (acetic acid-induced abdominal stretching) and a pain-suppressed behavior (decreased consumption of a liquid), Stevenson and colleagues found a false positive effect of haloperidol, an antipsychotic agent, upon acetic acid induced stretching, but not upon the decreased consumption of a liquid (6). This result elegantly demonstrates the potential for falsely identifying locomotor modifying agents as potential analgesics when measuring pain-stimulating behavior and suggests a potential benefit from using pain-suppressing behavior as a measure of potential analgesia. Finally, most standard models of pain-like behavior, like many behavioral assays, act as surrogates for the clinical situation and demonstrate analgesia for currently known active mechanisms. The effect of compounds that act on novel mechanisms may be less clear in these assays and there is a chance that a novel compound may therefore be erroneously labeled as an analgesic when it is not or as a nonanalgesic when it actually is. This may partly stem from the problems of identifying an emotional endpoint in rodents. As clinical pain has a large subjective, emotional component, the testing of potentially novel analgesics by using an evoked, quantitative endpoint may not truly mirror the clinical response and therefore, may not be truly indicative of the analgesic potential of the specific compound. As stated above, these tests demonstrate analgesia with commonly used analgesics such as the opiates, nonsteroidal antiinflammatory drugs (NSAIDs), and anticonvulsants (gabapentin, pregabalin), all of which provide strong analgesic responses as measured by stimulus-evoked endpoints. However, the potential to falsely identify or completely miss new classes of analgesics remains. The addition of new assays to the existing standards may help minimize this risk.

In an attempt to address some of these issues, a variety of new models for evaluating pain-like behavior and the analgesic properties of compounds have been developed (7). Some models have evaluated unevoked measures of behavior, thus eliminating the necessity of a stimulus that may otherwise produce a potentially artificial behavior from the animal in order to obtain a quantifiable response. These tests include measures of weight bearing on injured compared to uninjured paws (8, 9). This assay involves the placement of each of the animal's hindpaws on a separate weight-sensitive pad that measures the weight the animal is placing on each hindpaw. Although useful and not directly evoked, it does require extensive habituation and baseline testing. This test has been pharmacologically validated with current analgesics providing reproducible effects and is therefore a valuable addition to the more traditional tests (9, 10). Gait analysis has also been used for measuring hypersensitivity and certain parameters of an animal's gait are modified in both neuropathic and inflammatory pain-like states in rats (11–15). Interestingly, the results of this test correlate with the results from the von Frey mechanical allodynia assay (15) suggesting great potential for the measurement of pain. However, to date, only 1–2 pharmacological agents have been evaluated in gait analysis paradigms. The lack of experimental results with commonly used analgesic agents in this type of test limits the utility of gait analysis in identifying analgesic drugs (11, 16).

We developed the reduction in spontaneous activity due to adjuvant (RSAA) assay (17) in an attempt to address the issues of using an evoked response. We aimed to utilize the spontaneous, unevoked and natural exploratory behavior of rats when placed in a novel environment as a way to measure the "comfort" of the rat in using injured hindlimbs to explore the novel environment. To do this, we used standard measures of locomotor activity.

2. Materials

2.1. Complete Freund's Adjuvant (CFA) Procedure

1. Complete Freund's Adjuvant (CFA) (Sigma, St. Louis, MO) stored at 4°C prior to use.
2. 0.9% sterile saline.
3. Male Sprague Dawley rats (Charles River, Kingston, NY) weighing 320 g at time of CFA injection.
4. One ml BD tuberculin syringes.
5. ½ inch 26-G PrecisionGlide beveled needles.
6. 2″ square gauze.

7. Towel or pad.
8. Isoflurane anesthesia vaporizer with nose cone and induction box (Vetequip, Pleasanton, CA).
9. Solid bottom cages with bedding.

2.2. Collagen-Induced Arthritis (CIA) Procedure

1. Highly purified type II Porcine Collagen (18) dissolved at 2 mg/ml in 0.05 M acetic acid. Store at 4°C in the dark for less than 1 week.
2. Incomplete Freund's Adjuvant (IFA) (Difco, Detroit, MI).
3. 0.9% Sterile saline.
4. Female Lewis rats (Harlan, Indianapolis, IN) weighing 150 g at time of first collagen injection.
5. 1 ml Hamilton syringes with luer lock tip.
6. ½ inch 26-G PrecisionGlide beveled needles.
7. 2″ square gauze.
8. Rodent restrainer.
9. Solid bottom cages with bedding.
10. Homogenizer (diameter: 5 mm or less).
11. 20 ml glass vials.
12. 1 ml BD tuberculin syringes.
13. 5 ml BD tuberculin syringes.
14. 1½ inch 20-G beveled needles.
15. Crushed ice.

2.3. Test Equipment

1. Digiscan-16 Animal activity monitor (model 1300JC/CCDigi, version 2.4, Omnitech Electronics, Columbus, OH). The Plexiglas testing box measures (41.25 × 41.25 × 30 cm). Each box should have at least 48 infrared photocell emitters and detectors (2.5 cm between sensors). 32 sensors should surround the perimeter of the box at the base to capture horizontal movement. 16 separate sensors should be set 13.5 cm above the floor to capture vertical rearing.
2. Cage bedding (thin layer on testing cage floor).
3. Versamax software version 4.0-125E (Accuscan Istruments, Columbus, OH) for measurement recording and analysis.
4. White noise generator capable of emitting 62 dB
5. Red light (60 W).
6. Testing room. This needs to be able to be completely shut off from other rooms in the facility. Ideally, it should have sound dampening materials on any common walls to prevent any inadvertent distractions during the test. All lights need to be able to be shut off.

3. Methods

3.1. CFA Injection Procedure

1. Remove CFA from the refrigerator 30 min prior to injection time and allow warming to room temperature.
2. Set up the anesthesia apparatus and charge the induction chamber (preferably in a fume hood or area with good ventilation). Set the vaporizer to between 3 and 4 L per minute with 5% isoflurane (see Note 1).
3. Mix the CFA to form a uniform suspension of the heat-killed mycobacteria. Be sure not to incorporate air into the adjuvant.
4. In the 1 ml syringe, draw up the CFA. Do not fill the syringe past 700 μl (see Note 2). Wipe excess CFA from the outside of the syringe with gauze.
5. Attach the ½″ 26G needle and remove any air.
6. Place a single animal in the induction chamber and monitor status until breathing is relaxed and even.
7. Once the animal is under anesthesia, move it onto a towel and attach the nose cone. The animal should be on its back with the head pointed to the right (for a right handed person).
8. Place a second animal in the induction chamber. Carefully monitor animal breathing to be sure that the animal is not in danger of respiratory distress. Animals should not be left in the induction chamber for any longer than 5 min.
9. Check the animal to make sure it is properly anesthetized by pinching the tail and looking for the loss of the reflex response.
10. With the middle finger and lower part of the thumb on the left hand, hold the lower leg and flex the tibia-femur joint to form a 120° angle.
11. With the pointer finger and the fingertip of the thumb on the left hand, hold the sides of the tibia-femur joint to stabilize the leg.
12. When the joint is flexed, there will be a small indentation on either side of the midline. The raised section on the midline is the ligament of the patella. Avoid damaging this ligament.
13. With the right hand, slide the needle between the bones into the tibia-femur joint space. You will feel the needle "pop" into the joint cavity. Be careful not to puncture through the other side of the joint space (see Notes 3 and 4).
14. Slowly inject 50 μl (50 μg) of CFA or saline into the joint space (see Notes 5). Use as little pressure on the syringe as possible (see Note 6).

15. Remove the needle and apply slight pressure to the injection site to help minimize any bleeding.
16. Repeat the procedure on the other knee.
17. Return the animal to its home cage and allow to it to fully waken.
18. Repeat steps 7–18 until all animals are injected.
19. Allow animals to develop inflammation for 48 h prior to testing.

3.2. CIA Injection Procedure (Slightly Modified from the Chondrex Inc. Protocol (18))

1. Remove the type II collagen from the freezer and allow warming to room temperature.
2. Place a 20 ml vial in the ice bath.
3. Add 5 ml of IFA to the vial.
4. Place the homogenizer probe into the IFA and mix at a slow speed.
5. Draw up 5 ml of the type II collagen with the 5 ml syringe with the 20G needle (see Note 7).
6. Start adding the Collagen to the IFA drop wise while mixing. Increase the mixing speed slightly while continuing to add the Collagen due to thickening of the emulsion.
7. Once all of the collagen has been added, slowly increase the speed to 30,000 rpm. Mix at that speed for 3 min. The end result will be a thick emulsion.
8. Test the stability of the emulsion. Partially fill a second 20 ml vial with approximately 10 ml of water. Take a 1 ml syringe and draw up a small amount of the emulsion. Place one drop of the emulsion on top of the water. A stable emulsion will remain as a solid drop on the surface of the water. If the emulsion breaks down, mix in a few drops of IFA and repeat.
9. Keep the emulsion on ice until you are ready to inject.
10. Draw up 0.8 ml of the emulsion into the Hamilton syringe. Be sure to remove any air from the syringe. Cap with a 26G needle.
11. Place an animal in the restrainer with the tail exposed.
12. Inject 0.4 ml of the emulsion (400 μg of collagen) subcutaneously in the tail (see Note 8). This should be about 2–3 cm from the base of tail. Hold the needle level with the tail, bevel up. After injection, apply slight pressure to the injection site to avoid leakage.
13. Place animal back in its home cage and return to the vivarium for 7 days.

14. On day 7 after initial injection, repeat steps 1–10 to make new collagen for the booster injection.
15. Give each animal a booster injection of the emulsion. Inject 0.2 ml of the emulsion (200 μg of collagen) subcutaneously in the tail. This should also be about 2–3 cm from the base of tail.
16. Return animals to their home cages and the vivarium for 14 days.

3.3. Test Procedure (48 h Post-CFA, 21 days Post-CIA)

1. Turn on white noise in testing room.
2. Turn on red light and turn off all other lights in the testing room.
3. Set up the Versamax software for the first run (see Note 9). At the very least specify the animal number. Set the total collection time to 15 min (see Note 10). The overall test session can be further broken down into bins if desired, but this is not necessary.
4. Scatter a thin layer of bedding on the bottom of the testing box and check to be sure the boxes are clean.
5. Transport the animals from the viviarium to a dosing room. This should be a separate room from the testing room. Allow at least 30 min to acclimate to the dosing room before testing.
6. Pretreat the animals with any desired test compound in the dosing room.
7. After the pretreatment time has elapsed, move the animals to the testing room and place them in their assigned testing box, one per box. It is permissible to test multiple animals in the same room at the same time.
8. After placing the animals in the box, flip the start switch to run on the front of the testing box to begin the test.
9. Leave the room while the test is being conducted.
10. After the 15 min test session is over, reenter the room and flip the start switches to off. Remove the animals from the testing room.
11. Reset the computer and proceed with any additional runs as above.
12. After the last run, remove the bedding from the testing boxes and replace with fresh bedding.
13. Data is typically presented as means with standard errors of measure. Overall analysis of the data determined using one-way analysis of variance. Follow-up post hoc tests are performed using Fisher's least significant difference with $p \leq 0.05$ (see Note 11).

4. Notes

1. The gas is set high to quickly put the animals under anesthesia. Once the injection procedure is mastered, animals will only be exposed to Isoflurane inhalation for less than 1 min. If the animal appears to be under anesthesia too deeply, turn down the Isoflurane to 3%. At Isoflurane levels under 2% the animal might not be deep enough under anesthesia and regain its reflex response to the injection.
2. With greater volumes, the syringe tends to jam or the plunger becomes hard to move due to the adjuvant. For the same reason, a new syringe should be used for each withdrawal. Only fill one syringe at a time. If syringes are preloaded, the heat-killed mycobacteria in the adjuvant will settle and result in a nonuniform suspension. Be sure to mix the CFA stock suspension before each withdrawal.
3. The entire ½″ needle does not need to be inserted for the tip of the needle to be within the intra-articular space.
4. Finding the appropriate injection site in the knee can be difficult. Needle insertion too far proximal or distal will result in hitting bones. This should be avoided as it can cause unwanted damage to the joint. The midline should also be avoided to limit damage to the ligaments as much as possible. Hold the needle perpendicular to the injection site and insert slowly. If any resistance is felt, pull back and move slightly toward the center of the joint. When in the correct location, the needle will slide easily into the joint space. If uncertain that the needle is in the correct place, slightly moving the needle in the correct position will move the joint naturally. Do not move the needle more than necessary as joint damage may occur.
5. The joint space can easily accommodate 50 μl of volume. Larger volumes are possible, if desired, but do not exceed 150 μl.
6. Filling the syringe takes time and can be messy as the adjuvant is “sticky”. For this reason, the syringe is preloaded to inject seven animals. If too much force is used on the plunger, the remaining CFA in the syringe will become compressed and obstruct the end of the syringe. Alternatively, occasionally a particle of the heat-killed mycobacteria will become stuck in the needle. If this occurs, gently pull back slightly on the plunger to move the orientation of the particle. Usually, this slight movement will allow the particle to pass thought the needle. Do not try to force the particle through the needle with more pressure as this might result in the needle separating from the syringe or clumping of the remaining heat-killed mycobacteria in the syringe.

7. This amount of collagen is used to dose around 40 animals. It is necessary to make a good deal more collagen emulsion than is needed. A lot of emulsion is lost on the outside of the syringe when wiping it clean after filling. There is also some emulsion that will not be able to be drawn into the syringe due to the emulsion sticking to the sides of the vial.
8. The original protocol from Chondrex Inc. recommends injection of 200 μg of collagen. There can be a large variation in CIA development between rat stains. This variation is also apparent in the same strain from different vendors. Under the conditions in our lab, we found that our suggested volume of collagen emulsion was needed to produce the expected level of arthritis.
9. There are many different companies that make locomotor tracking systems for rodents. The three measures most critical to the RSAA test are vertical rearing, movement time, and total distance traveled. Most systems do an adequate job tracking the horizontal movements and movement time of rodents. Vertical rearing is captured by the photocells above the floor of the testing box. On many systems, the height these photocells are set at are adjustable. The height that we used in our testing boxes gave us reproducible results on vertical rearing between studies.
10. Test sessions longer that 15 min are possible. The bulk of rodent exploratory behavior in a novel open field occurs in the first 15 min after test onset. Approximately after 30 min, the level of exploration of a naïve animal is greatly reduced when compared with the beginning of the test. Any benefit of exploration beyond 30 min is offset by inadvertent noise and variability in the data.
11. A typical CFA dose response curve is shown in Fig. 1. CFA administration greater than 50 μg/bilaterally does not significantly increase the therapeutic window for effect and might increase the dose of analgesic needed to see an analgesic result. At 50 μg of CFA bilaterally, morphine at 1 mg/kg and ibuprofen (IB) at 10 mg/kg will reliably attenuate nociceptive behaviors (see Fig. 2a). At doses of morphine greater than 1 mg/kg, its analgesic effect is reduced in association with an increasingly sedative profile (see Fig. 2b). Morphine and IB were repeatedly used as positive controls in every study. A positive control group run with each study is recommended to ensure that the model is working robustly and helps clarify any negative result of novel compounds. The RSAA will also discriminate against compounds that are excitatory in nature. Amphetamine will increase the locomotor behavior in measures of horizontal activity, but has no significant effect on vertical rearing (see Fig. 3a and b).

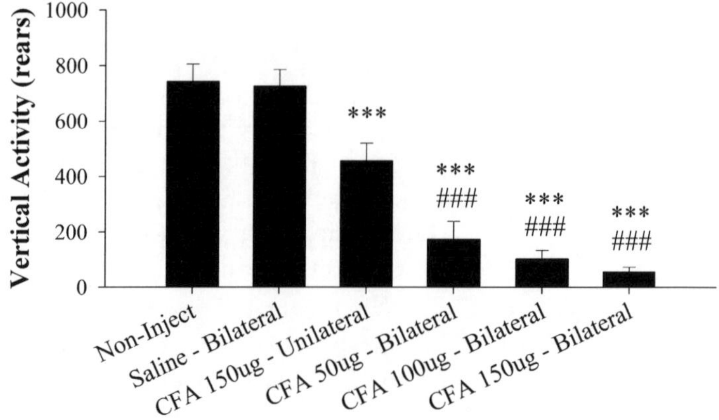

Fig. 1. Examples of the effect of bilateral knee injections of CFA on spontaneous locomotor activity in rats. CFA doses of 50 μg/50 μl/bilaterally and higher produced a significant reduction in rears compared with the noninjected group or the 150 μg/150 μl/unilateral group. Bars, mean rears ± S.E.M. ($n = 10$/group). *, $p < 0.05$; **, $p < 0.01$; or ***, $p < 0.001$ compared with the saline or noninjected groups. ###, $p < 0.001$ compared with the 150 μg of CFA unilateral injection group. Methods and full results are presented in Matson et al., 2007 (17). Figure reproduced from Matson et al., 2007 (17) with kind permission from the publisher

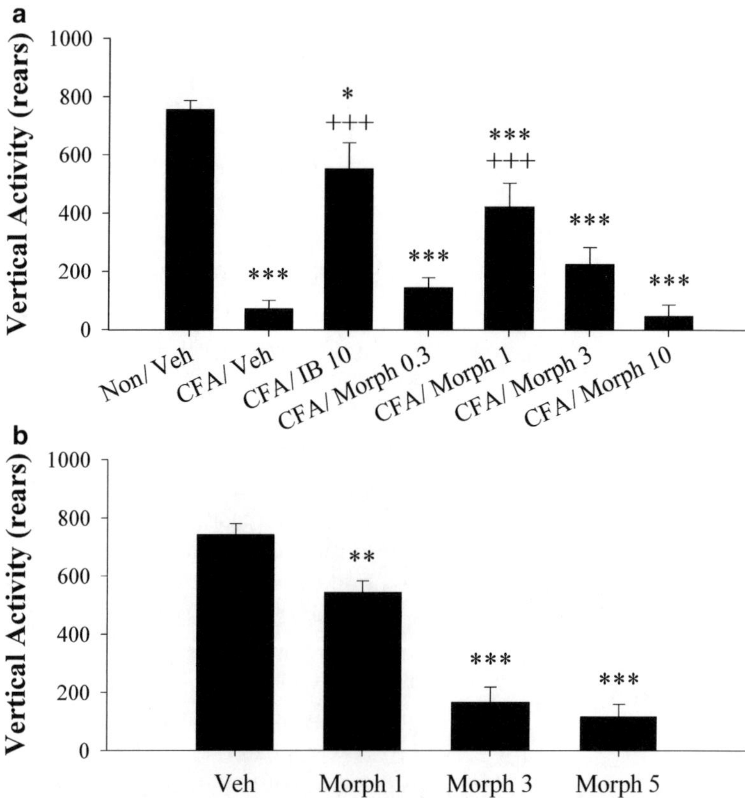

Fig. 2. (**a**) Effect of morphine on vertical activity in the RSAA model. Morphine dosed s.c. at 10 mg/kg was not significantly different from the CFA/vehicle group. The CFA/IB group was used as a positive control. (**b**) Morphine administered s.c. in a standard model of locomotor activity in untreated rats. Bars, mean rears ± S.E.M. ($n = 10$/group). *, $p < 0.05$; **, $p < 0.01$; or ***, $p < 0.001$ compared with the noninjected/vehicle or vehicle group. +++, $p < 0.001$ compared with the CFA/vehicle group. Methods and full results are presented in Matson et al., 2007 (17). Figure reproduced from Matson et al., 2007 (17) with kind permission from the publisher

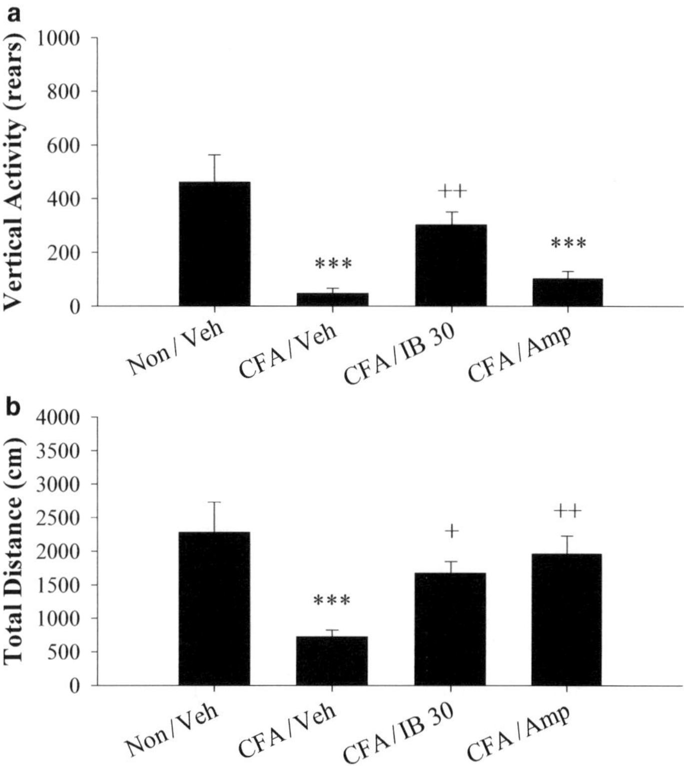

Fig. 3. The effect of amphetamine on vertical activity (**a**) and total distance (**b**) in the RSAA model. Amphetamine, administered i.p., did not increase vertical rearing above CFA/vehicle levels. Total distance was significantly increased over CFA/vehicle levels. Bars, mean rears or total distance traveled ± S.E.M. ($n = 10$/group). ***, $p < 0.001$ compared with the noninjected group. +, $p < 0.05$ or ++, $p < 0.01$ compared with the CFA/vehicle group. Methods and full results are presented in Matson et al., 2007 (17). Figure reproduced from Matson et al., 2007 (17) with kind permission from the publisher

References

1. Le Bars D, Gozariu M, Cadden SW (2001) Animal models of nociception. Pharmacol Rev 53:597–642
2. Chaplan SR, Bach FW, Pogrel JW, Chung JM, Yaksh TL (1994) Quantitative assessment of tactile allodynia in the rat paw. J Neurosci Methods 53:55–63
3. Randal L, Selitto J (1957) A method for measurement of analgesic activity on inflamed tissue. Arch Int Pharmacodyn Ther 111: 409–419
4. Hargreaves K, Dubner R, Brown F, Flores C, Joris J (1988) A new and sensitive method for measuring thermal nociception in cutaneous hyperalgesia. Pain 32:77–88
5. Negus SS, Vanderah TW, Brandt MR, Bilsky MR, Becerra L, Borsook D (2006) Preclinical assessment of candidate analgesic drugs: recent advances and future challenges. J Pharmacol Exp Ther 319:507–514
6. Stevenson GW, Bilsky EJ, Negus SS (2006) Targeting pain-suppressed behaviors in preclinical assays of pain and analgesia: effects of morphine on acetic acid-suppressed feeding in C57BL/6J mice. J Pain 7:408–416
7. Cortright DN, Matson DJ, Broom DC (2008) Assessing pain and analgesia in laboratory animals – new methods in drug discovery. Expert Opin Drug Discov 3(9):1099–1108
8. Whiteside GT, Harrison J, Boulet J, Mark L, Pearson M, Gottshall S, Walker K (2004) Pharmacological characterization of a rat model of incisional pain. Br J Pharmacol 141:85–91

9. Pomonis JD, Boulet JM, Gottshall SL, Phillips S, Sellers R, Bunton T, Walker K (2005) Development and pharmacological characterization of a rat model of osteoarthritis pain. Pain 114:339–346
10. Wilson AW, Medhurst SJ, Dixon CI, Bontoft NC, Winyard LA, Brackenborough KT, De Alba J, Clarke CJ, Gunthorpe MJ, Hicks GA, Bountra C, McQueen DS, Chessel IP (2006) An animal model of chronic inflammatory pain: pharmacological and temporal differentiation from acute models. Eur J Pain 10(6): 1099–1108
11. Clarke KA, Heitmeyer SA, Smith AG, Taiwo YO (1997) Gait analysis in a rat model of osteoarthrosis. Physiol Behav 62:951–954
12. Hamers FP, Lankhorst AJ, van Laar TJ, Veldhuis WB, Gispen WH (2001) Automated quantitative gait analysis during overground locomotion in the rat: its application to spinal cord contusion and transection injuries. J Neurotrauma 18:187–201
13. Coulthard P, Pleuvry BJ, Brewster M, Wilson KL, Macfarlane TV (2002) Gait analysis as an objective measure in a chronic pain model. J Neurosci Methods 116:197–213
14. Coulthard P, Simjee SU, Pleuvry BJ (2003) Gait analysis as a correlate of pain induced by carrageenan intraplantar injection. J Neurosci Methods 128:95–102
15. Vrinten DH, Hamers FF (2003) 'Catwalk' automated quantitative gait analysis as a novel method to assess mechanical allodynia in the rat; a comparison with von Frey testing. Pain 102:203–209
16. Simjee SU, Pleuvry BJ, Coulthard P (2004) Modulation of the gait deficit in arthritic rats by infusions of muscimol and bicuculline. Pain 109:453–460
17. Matson DJ, Broom DC, Carson SR, Baldassari J, Kehne J, Cortright DN (2007) Inflammation-induced reduction of spontaneous activity by adjuvant: a novel model to study the effect of analgesics in rats. J Pharmacol Exp Ther 320:194–201
18. Chondrex, Inc. Protocol for the successful induction of Collagen-Induced Arthritis in Rats, V1.2 (2006) Chondrex, Inc., Redmond, WA

Chapter 7

Rationale and Methods for Assessment of Pain-Depressed Behavior in Preclinical Assays of Pain and Analgesia

S. Stevens Negus, Edward J. Bilsky, Gail Pereira Do Carmo, and Glenn W. Stevenson

Abstract

Pain-depressed behavior can be defined as any behavior that decreases in rate, frequency, duration, or intensity in response to a putative pain state. Common examples include pain-related decreases in feeding, locomotion and expression of positively reinforced operant behavior. In humans, depression of behavior is often accompanied by a comorbid depression of mood. Measurements of pain-depressed behaviors are used to diagnose pain in both human and veterinary medicine, and restoration of pain-depressed behavior is often a priority of treatment. This article describes two strategies for integrating measures of pain-depressed behaviors into preclinical assays of pain and analgesia. Assays of pain-depressed behaviors may contribute both to improved translational efficiency in analgesic drug development and to new insights regarding the mechanisms and determinants of pain and analgesia.

Key words: Pain, Behavioral assay, Pain-depressed behavior, Feeding, Intracranial self-stimulation

1. Introduction

Preclinical behavioral assays of pain and analgesia necessarily include two elements: (a) a manipulation intended to produce a pain-like state (the independent variable), and (b) measurement of a response presumed to be indicative of that pain-like state (the dependent variable). In recent years, there have been significant advances in the methodology used to model acute, inflammatory, neuropathic and cancer pain states, and details of these methodologies are described elsewhere in this volume. However, the dependent measures in preclinical assays have been much slower to evolve (1–5). The most widely used measures fall into a category that we have described as "pain-stimulated behaviors," which can be defined as behaviors that increase in rate, frequency, duration

Arpad Szallasi (ed.), *Analgesia: Methods and Protocols*, Methods in Molecular Biology, vol. 617,
DOI 10.1007/978-1-60327-323-7_7, © Springer Science+Business Media, LLC 2010

or intensity in response to a putative pain state (3, 6). Common examples include withdrawal responses from stimuli that can be escaped (e.g. paw withdrawal from a mechanical or thermal stimulus) or stretching/flinching responses from stimuli that cannot be escaped (e.g. stretching responses elicited by intraperitoneal injection of noxious chemical stimuli). Although a focus on pain-stimulated behaviors can be useful for many applications, an exclusive reliance on these behaviors as dependent measures can be problematic for a number of reasons. These problems have been discussed at length elsewhere, and they include a difficulty in dissociating analgesia from motor impairment (3), a dissociation between expression of pain-stimulated behaviors and verbal reports of pain in some types of chronic pain in humans (7, 8), and mediation by neural substrates that may exclude or under-represent key brain areas involved in affective components of pain (9, 10).

As an alternative to the use of pain-stimulated behaviors as dependent measures, we and others have begun to explore strategies for incorporating *PAIN-DEPRESSED BEHAVIOR* into preclinical assays of pain and analgesia (11–16). "Pain-depressed" behaviors can be defined as any behavior that *decreases* in rate, frequency, duration or intensity in response to a noxious stimulus, and common examples include pain-related decreases in feeding, locomotion and expression of positively reinforced operant behavior. The use of pain-depressed behaviors as dependent variables may be associated with several advantages relative to the use of pain-stimulated behaviors. First, drugs or other manipulations that produce analgesia would be expected to *increase* pain-depressed behaviors, and as a result, true analgesia would be readily dissociable from motor impairment. Second, pain states that require clinical intervention are often associated with a depression of behavior rather than a stimulation of behavior, and in humans, pain-related depression of behavior is often accompanied by a comorbid depression of mood (17–20). Indeed, diagnostic tools that measure pain-related depression of behavior and mood are coming to play an increasingly prominent role in human medicine (21–23), and measures of functional impairment/depressed behavior are even more important for veterinary assessments of pain in animals (24). The utility of these measures of pain-depressed behavior in the clinical diagnosis of pain suggests that these measures may also be useful in preclinical research. Finally, a focus on pain-depressed behaviors could enable preclinical research on mechanisms and determinants of the affective components of pain (14, 25).

We have proposed that development of preclinical assays of pain-depressed behavior might best proceed in three systematic steps: (a) identification of conditions under which a target behavior occurs at a high and stable rate to provide a stable and sensitive behavioral baseline, (b) identification of conditions under which a putative pain state reliably depresses the rate of that target behavior, and (c) assessment of effects of candidate analgesic drugs or other manipulations on the rate of pain-depressed behavior. In addition, it is useful to conduct control experiments to assess the degree to which the drug or other manipulation alters (a) control, nondepressed rates of the target behavior in the absence of a pain state, and (b) rates of the target behavior depressed by a putative nonpainful manipulation. Under these circumstances, an optimal analgesic might be one that restores pain-depressed behavior without increasing baseline rates of that behavior in the absence of pain and without increasing rates of that behavior when it is depressed by nonpainful manipulations. We have pursued this strategy in developing two different assays of pain-depressed behavior in rodents, and methods for both assays are provided. The first assay measures feeding behavior in mice, and it has the advantage of requiring a modest experimental infrastructure and limited training of experimental subjects (6). The second assay measures intracranial self-stimulation (ICSS) in rats. ICSS has been used extensively to evaluate effects of experimental manipulations on motivated behavior (15, 25), and this technically more-demanding procedure may confer an advantage of heightened sensitivity in studies of pain-depressed behavior (14). In both assays, we have employed intraperitoneal injection of dilute acid to produce a pain state although other approaches could also easily be used (e.g. manipulations to model inflammatory, neuropathic, cancer or other pain states). In addition, we have evaluated the sensitivity of these procedures using the opioid analgesic morphine. Again though, a wide variety of other pharmacologic or nonpharmacologic manipulations could be used. One final caveat is also warranted. The use of these assays is in its infancy, and these procedures will be a topic of research in their own right. The Materials and Methods provided below should be considered as a starting point in the evolution of assays of pain-depressed behavior for preclinical research on pain and analgesia.

2. Materials

2.1. Acid-Depressed Feeding in Mice

1. Subjects: Adult male C57BL6/J Mice (e.g. Jackson Laboratories, Bar Harbor, ME) (see Notes 1 and 2)
2. Scale with resolution to 0.1 g suitable for weighing mice and feeding solutions
3. Observation cage (e.g. a clean, empty standard housing cage)
4. Vanilla-flavored Ensure™ protein drink

5. Wide flat dish capable of holding 8 ml (8.6 g) of Ensure (see Note 3)
6. Acetic acid solution
7. Injection supplies (syringes, saline for dilution of acid and drug solutions)

2.2. Acid-Depressed Intracranial Self-Stimulation (ICSS) in Rats

This procedure uses the same materials and methods for ICSS that have been described in detail previously (25). The reader is encouraged to refer to this excellent resource for a detailed description of the general methodology.

1. Subjects: Adult rats weighing approximately 300–350 g at the time of surgery (see Note 4)
2. Equipment for Operant Conditioning and ICSS Delivery
   (a) Rat operant conditioning stations housed in sound-attenuating chambers and equipped with at least one response lever, stimulus and house lights, ICSS stimulator, interface, and computer control equipment with software to operate ICSS experiments (e.g. Med Associates, St. Albans, VT) (see Note 5)
   (b) ICSS electrodes (e.g. MS303/1-AIU/SPC bipolar electrodes with one 0.25 mm insulated wire cut to 10 mm and one 0.125 mm uninsulated wire cut to 15 mm; Plastics One, Roanoke, VA)
   (c) Two-channel commutator to allow rat to rotate (e.g. SL2C, Plastics One; one per operant station)
   (d) Bipolar cables [one to connect ICSS stimulator to commutator (e.g. 305-491, Plastics One) and one to connect commutator to electrode (e.g. 305-305, Plastics One)] (see Note 6)
   (e) Oscilloscope to monitor ICSS (e.g. 2120B Dual Trace 30 MHZ Oscilloscope, BK Precision, Yorba Linda, CA 92887)
   (f) Ring stand, clamp holder and three pronged clamp to hold commutator above operant chamber (e.g. catalog numbers 11-474-207 Cast-iron L-shaped base support, 12621-250 Talon clamp holder, and 21570-126 three-pronged extension clamp, VWR International, Marietta, GA)
3. Equipment and Supplies for Surgical Implantation of Electrode
   (a) Rat stereotax (e.g. Model 900; Kopf Instruments, Tujunga, CA)
   (b) Electrode holder for stereotax (e.g. MH-300, Plastics One)
   (c) Skull screws (e.g. 0–80 × 1/8, Plastics One)

(d) Drill holder and drill bits to drill holes in skull for electrode and skull screws (e.g. DH-1 and D#56, Plastics One)

(e) Surgical supplies (e.g. anesthetic, atropine sulfate, antibiotic ointment, instruments (scalpel, hemostats), suture material; other supplies as required by institutional regulations for rodent surgery)

(f) Acrylic cement (e.g. catalog number 651006 Orthodontic resin powder and 651002 orthodonitic resin pink liquid, Dentsply Caulk, Densply International, Milford, DE)

4. Supplies for Experimental Manipulations (see Note 7)

3. Methods

3.1. Acid-Depressed Feeding in Mice

1. Mice are group housed under standard laboratory conditions. Access to food and water is controlled to optimize the likelihood of high, stable rates of feeding during daily feeding sessions. Specifically, a water bottle and the daily ration of mouse chow (8 g) are provided immediately after each daily session, and the water bottle and any uneaten food are removed 4 h before the next session. We tested mice during the light phase of the light-dark cycle.
2. Feeding sessions are conducted Monday–Friday beginning at 12:00 noon. For each session, mice are removed from their home cages, weighed and placed individually in observation cages equipped with a dish containing 8 ml (8.6 g) of liquid food (vanilla-flavored Ensure™ protein drink).
3. After a specified period of access (usually 30 min), mice are returned to their home cages, and the amount of Ensure consumed during the access period is determined by subtracting the weight of the dish at the end of the session from its weight at the beginning of the session. To control for any weight changes during the experiment, consumption is expressed as grams of liquid food consumed ÷ weight of the mouse in grams.
4. In our initial studies, mice were initially trained under these conditions until feeding stabilized (3 consecutive days with ≤20% variability in consumption). Testing was then initiated in three phases to (Phase 1) identify conditions that would generate high and stable rates of feeding, (Phase 2) identify conditions under which acetic acid would depress feeding, and (Phase 3) characterize the effects of morphine on acid-suppressed feeding and other control behaviors. The effects of the dopamine D2 receptor antagonist haloperidol were also examined as a representative nonanalgesic drug that impairs motor function.

5. During Phase 1, the concentration of Ensure (0–100% in water) and the duration of the access period (7.5–120 min) were manipulated. On the basis of our results, an Ensure concentration of 32% and access duration of 30 min were used for subsequent studies.
6. During Phase 2, feeding behavior was examined after intraperitoneal administration of acetic acid in the same group of mice. A range of acetic acid concentrations (0–1% in saline) and pretreatment times (0–240 min before the feeding session) were examined, and acetic acid was administered no more than once per week. On remaining days of each week, mice had access to 32% Ensure for 30 min. On the basis of these results, a concentration of 0.56% acetic acid given immediately before the feeding session (0 min pretreatment time) was used for subsequent studies.
7. During Phase 3, the effects of morphine and haloperidol were examined on acetic acid-suppressed feeding and a variety of other behaviors including (a) control rates of feeding determined without acid pretreatment, (b) rates of feeding suppressed by non-pain manipulations (substitution of water for Ensure, prefeeding subjects immediately prior to test session), and (c) expression of acetic acid-induced writhing, a pain-stimulated behavior.

Figure 1 shows selected results for effects of acetic acid alone or after pretreatment with morphine or haloperidol on a pain-stimulated behavior (writhing, top panels) or a pain-depressed behavior (feeding, bottom panels). Under baseline conditions in the absence of acetic acid treatment, animals displayed no writhing and relatively high and stable levels of feeding (~0.14 gram liquid food/gram of body weight) (see points above "BL" in all panels). Acetic acid produced a concentration-dependent increase in writhing and a decrease in feeding (left panels, bars over "Acid Alone" in right panels). Morphine attenuated both acid-stimulated writhing and acid-depressed feeding, whereas the nonanalgesic haloperidol decreased acid-stimulated writhing but failed to block acid-depressed feeding (right panels). The effects of morphine were time dependent and naltrexone reversible, and a dose of morphine that blocked acid-depressed feeding had little or no effect on baseline feeding or on feeding suppressed by other manipulations that did not involve noxious stimulation and pain (6). Overall, morphine produced antinociceptive effects in assays of both pain-stimulated and pain-depressed behavior, whereas the nonanalgesic drug haloperidol produced an antinociceptive effect only in the assay of pain-stimulated behavior. These results illustrate the utility of using complementary assays of pain-stimulated and pain-depressed behavior to evaluate candidate analgesics.

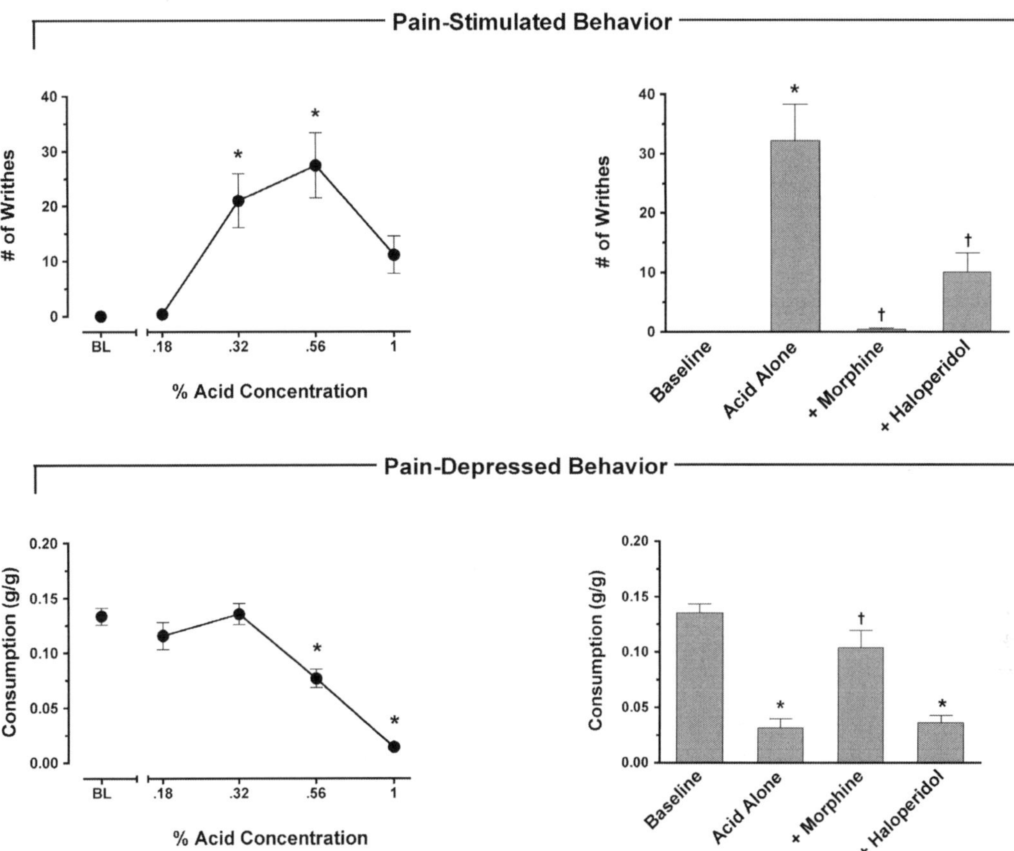

Fig. 1. Comparison of drug effects on pain-stimulated and pain-depressed behaviors in mice. Abscissae (*left panels*): % Acetic acid solution injected IP in mice. Points above "BL" show baseline in the absence of an IP injection. Abscissae (*right panels*): Treatment condition – baseline, 0.56% acetic acid alone (Acid Alone), 0.56% acetic acid + 1.0 mg/kg morphine (+morphine), 0.56% acetic acid + 1.0 mg/kg haloperidol (+haloperidol). Ordinates (*top panels*). # Writhes counted during observation period. Ordinates (*bottom panels*): Consumption of liquid food solution (gram consumed per gram body weight). All points/bars show mean ± SEM of 6–12 mice. * Indicates significantly different from "BL," $p < 0.05$. † Indicates significantly different from "Acid Alone," $p < 0.05$. Reprinted from (3) with permission from the Journal of Pharmacology and Experimental Therapeutics

3.2. Acid-Depressed Intracranial Self-Stimulation (ICSS) in Rats

1. Rats are typically ordered at a weight of approximately 250–275 g to allow some room for growth during an initial 1 week acclimation period before surgery.
2. Rats are singly housed to prevent inter-animal tampering with head-mounted ICSS electrodes, and they are given free access to food and water except during experimental sessions. We tested rats during the light phase of the light-dark cycle.
3. Electrodes are surgically implanted to target the medial forebrain bundle at the level of the lateral hypothalamus (see Note 8). In rats weighing 300–350 g, this can be achieved by securing the rat in the stereotax with level skull (i.e. bregma and lamda at identical dorso-ventral coordinates), and targeting

the electrode at 2.8 mm posterior to bregma, 1.7 mm lateral to the midsaggital suture, and 7.8 mm below dura.

4. Details of the anesthesia, surgical procedure and postoperative care should comply with institutional regulations. Briefly, the rat is anesthetized and secured in the stereotax, an incision is made in the scalp to expose the skull and the landmarks bregma and lamda, and holes are drilled in the skull to accommodate 3 or 4 skull screws and the electrode. Skull screws are placed before insertion of the electrode. When using the electrodes described above (MS303/1-AIU/SPC, Plastics One, Roanoke, VA), the thicker, insulated wire serves as the stimulating electrode, and it is inserted into the brain at the specified coordinates. The thinner, uninsulated wire serves as a ground, and this wire is wrapped around one or two of the skull screws.
5. Once the electrode is in place, it is secured with acrylic cement poured around the pedestal of the electrode and the skull screws.
6. After the acrylic cement dries, the incision is sutured, and the rat can be removed from the stereotax.
7. In our studies, training and testing for each rat have proceeded in three phases. The first phase (Lever Press Training) begins seven days after surgery, and daily sessions last 30–60 min (duration is not critical). Each lever press results in the delivery of a 0.5-s train of square wave cathodal pulses (0.1-ms pulse duration, 141 Hz), and stimulation is accompanied by the illumination of a 2-W "house" light located on the ceiling of the sound-attenuating chamber. Responses during the 0.5-s stimulation period do not earn additional stimulation. The stimulation intensity for each rat is set initially at 150 μA, and it is adjusted gradually to the lowest value that sustains a reliable rate of responding (≥20 responses/min) (see Notes 9 and 10).
8. In the second phase (Multiple-Frequency Training), daily sessions consist of multiple 15-min components. During each component, a descending series of 15 current frequencies (141–28 Hz in 0.05 log increments) is presented, with a 60-s trial at each frequency. Each frequency trial begins with a 5-s timeout period followed by 5 s of period of noncontingent stimulation (five 0.5 s pulses separated by 0.5 s intervals), which in turn is followed by a 50-s "response" phase during which stimulus lights are illuminated and each response produces electrical stimulation. Under these conditions, response rates are typically high during the initial high-frequency trials of each component, and responding declines to low rates as frequency declines (see Fig. 2). The intensity may again be adjusted during this phase so that the subject

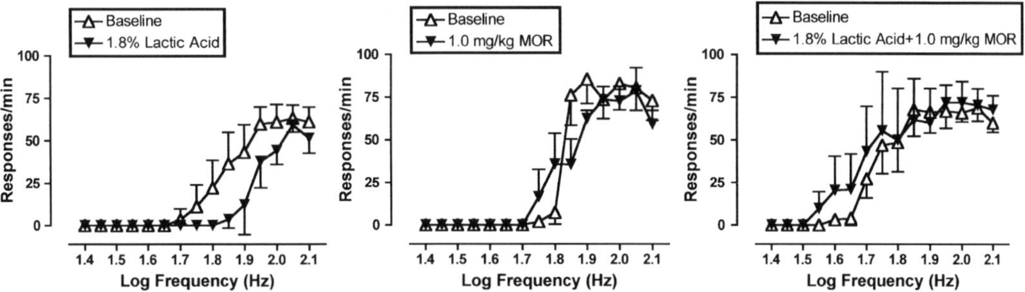

Fig. 2. Morphine effects on pain-depressed intracranial self-stimulation (ICSS) in rats. Abscissae: Frequency of electrical stimulation (log Hz). Ordinates: Response rate in responses/min. "Baseline" curves show data collected from the second and third baseline components conducted during each test session (the first component served as an acclimation period, and data were discarded). Test curves show data from the component of peak effect after delivery of each treatment. *Left panel* shows effects of 1.8% lactic acid delivered IP in a volume of 1 ml/kg. The center panel shows effects of 1.0 mg/kg morphine IP. The right panel shows effects of 1.0 mg/kg morphine administered as a pretreatment to lactic acid. All points show mean ± SEM from five rats

responds at high rates for the first 4–6 frequency trials and at lower rates for the remaining trials.

9. The third phase (Testing) begins once responding stabilizes under Multiple-Frequency Training. Test sessions consist of three consecutive "baseline" components followed by up to six consecutive "test" components, and experimental manipulations are introduced during an interval between the baseline and test components. Test sessions are conducted one or two times per week, with Multiple-Frequency Training sessions between test sessions.

Figure 2 shows illustrative results using this procedure to evaluate pain-depressed behavior. Each panel shows response rates as a function of log frequency for one test session in a group of five rats. During the baseline components at the beginning of each test session, there was a frequency-dependent increase in response rates. IP administration of 1.8% lactic acid (1 ml/kg injection volume) depressed ICSS as indicated by a rightward shift in the frequency-rate curve (Fig. 2, left panel). Notably, response rates were depressed at intermediate stimulus frequencies (i.e. 1.75–2.0 log Hz) but not at high frequencies (2.05–2.1 log Hz). These high response rates at high stimulus frequencies demonstrate that rats were still motorically capable of responding at high rates. Overall, these results suggest that a noxious stimulus (IP injections of 1.8% lactic acid) depressed responding by decreasing the reinforcing efficacy of brain stimulation rather than by decreasing the motoric ability of rats to respond.

The center panel of Fig. 2 shows that a relatively low dose of morphine (1.0 mg/kg IP) alone had little effect on ICSS. However, the right panel of Fig. 2 shows that pretreatment with this morphine dose completely blocked the effect of 1.8% lactic acid. Thus, pretreatment with a morphine dose that had no effect alone completely prevented lactic acid-induced depression of ICSS.

4. Notes

1. Mice, rats or subjects of a variety of other species could conceivably be used for this type of procedure. Mice were selected for these initial studies for two reasons: (a) they have been used extensively in assays of pain-stimulated behavior, including an assay of acetic acid induced stretching on which this assay is based, and (b) they are a useful species of experimental subject for genetic manipulations. In addition, we used young adult mice for our initial studies, but mice of different ages could conceivably be used for developmental studies.
2. Our initial studies were conducted using a repeated measures, within-subject design in which each mouse received all manipulations. This approach was taken to minimize animal usage, and animals displayed stable responses to repeated manipulations and little or no evidence of toxicity/pathology associated with repeated testing. However, studies proceeded at a relatively slow rate because acid injections were delivered no more often than once per week. It is likely that rate of throughput could be increased by using a between-subjects design in which each mouse received one acclimation session followed by one test session.
3. We used recycled caps from Starbucks™ bottled Frappuccino™ beverages. These had the advantage of being relatively wide and shallow with vertical side walls. These features were useful for minimizing spillage by promoting stability of the dish and facilitating access. To further promote stability, the dishes were secured to the floor of the observation cage with a putty adhesive (e.g. 3 M Scotch Removable Adhesive Putty).
4. Rats or mice are the species most often used for ICSS studies although other species could also be used. Rats were selected for these studies to build on the relatively large literature of ICSS studies with this species. In addition, we used young adult rats for our initial studies, but rats of different ages could conceivably be used for developmental studies although it would be necessary to adjust coordinates for electrode implantation to accommodate animals of various sizes.

5. Multiple vendors offer operant conditioning equipment. Med Associates offers operant conditioning stations for ICSS in both rats and mice, and these stations can be customized to include different types or numbers of response manipulanda, different stimulus light configurations, and devices for delivering different types of consequent stimuli (e.g. food pellets, liquid reinforcers). Med Associates also uses a proprietary programming language that is relatively accessible to nonspecialists, and Med Associates also has programmers who can write custom software.
6. The bipolar cable from commutator to electrode should be custom ordered at a length that will permit movement of rat throughout the operant chamber but without excessive slack. An appropriate length is the distance from the commutator (mounted in a fixed location above the chamber) to a corner of the chamber at floor level. In addition, it is necessary to attach this cable to the electrode in such a way that it delivers cathodal pulses to the target. To determine the cathodal wire in the bipolar cable, an ICSS program can be activated to deliver pulses while current amplitude is monitored by touching the red and black leads of an ammeter to the two pins at the end of the cable. If the sign of the current reading from each pulse is positive, the wire touching the black lead on the ammeter is the cathode, and the cable above this pin can be marked with an indelible marker for future reference. (If the sign of the current reading is negative, the leads of the ammeter can be switched to the opposite pins on the cable to generate a positive reading). The cathode should then be connected to the electrode port for the thick, insulated electrode.
7. In our initial studies, we used dilute lactic acid as the noxious stimulus, and morphine was evaluated for its ability to produce antinociceptive effects. These manipulations required lactic acid, sterile saline (for dilution of lactic acid and as vehicle for drug solutions), and syringes for delivery of solutions. Manipulations designed to model inflammatory, neuropathic or other pain states would obviously require different supplies.
8. In our initial studies, we targeted the medial forebrain bundle of the lateral hypothalamus because this region maintains high rates of ICSS and innervates cell bodies of the mesolimbic dopamine system, a neural system considered to be important in mediating behavior reinforced by various stimuli. However, other electrode targets may also be of interest, such as targets in pathways thought to be important in modulating pain (e.g. the periaqueductal gray).
9. During initial training, it is helpful to "shape" lever-press responding by delivering a stimulus pulse for successive approximations of the target behavior. Thus, for initial training

sessions, the rat is connected to the bipolar cable and allowed to explore the chamber while an observer operates a remote switch to deliver pulses. (e.g. for standard responses levers from Med Associates, the microswitch in the response lever can be operated from outside the chamber by inserting a paperclip through an access hole on the underside of the lever housing.) Initially, pulses can be delivered if the rat faces the lever. Subsequently, pulses can be delivered if the rat approaches or touches the lever. Ultimately, the rat will begin to press the lever on its own, and observer-delivered pulses are no longer necessary.

10. The effectiveness of intracranial stimulation as a reinforcer depends on the placement of the electrode. Although there is some room for error in electrode placement, larger displacements may place the electrode in contact with areas mediating motor effects, and stimulation may produce stereotyped motor responses, such as a turning of the head or lifting of the paw. In other cases, stimulation may promote seizures. In these cases, undesired effects of stimulation can sometimes be reduced or eliminated by reducing current intensity.

References

1. Blackburn-Munro G (2004) Pain-like behaviours in animals – how human are they? Trends Pharmacol Sci 25:299–305
2. Mogil JS, Crager SE (2004) What should we be measuring in behavioral studies of chronic pain in animals? Pain 112:12–15
3. Negus SS, Vanderah TW, Brandt MR, Bilsky EJ, Becerra L, Borsook D (2006) Preclinical assessment of candidate analgesic drugs: recent advances and future challenges. J Pharmacol Exp Ther 319:507–514
4. Vierck CJ, Hansson PT, Yezierski RP (2008) Clinical and pre-clinical pain assessment: are we measuring the same thing? Pain 135:7–10
5. Whiteside GT, Adedoyin A, Leventhal L (2008) Predictive validity of animal pain models? A comparison of the pharmacokinetic-pharmacodynamic relationship for pain drugs in rats and humans. Neuropharmacology 54:767–775
6. Stevenson GW, Bilsky EJ, Negus SS (2006) Targeting pain-suppressed behaviors in preclinical assays of pain and analgesia: effects of morphine on acetic acid-suppressed feeding in C57BL/6J mice. J Pain 7:408–416
7. Gracely RH, Petzke F, Wolf JM, Clauw DJ (2002) Functional magnetic resonance imaging evidence of augmented pain processing in fibromyalgia. Arthritis Rheum 46: 1333–1343
8. Skljarevski V, Ramadan NM (2002) The nociceptive flexion reflex in humans – review article. Pain 96:3–8
9. Price DD (2000) Psychological and neural mechanisms of the affective dimension of pain. Science 288:1769–1772
10. Price DD (2002) Central neural mechanisms that interrelate sensory and affective dimensions of pain. Mol Interv 2:392–402
11. Martin TJ, Buechler NL, Kahn W, Crews JC, Eisenach JC (2004) Effects of laparotomy on spontaneous exploratory activity and conditioned operant responding in the rat: a model for postoperative pain. Anesthesiology 101:191–203
12. Matson DJ, Broom DC, Carson SR, Baldassari J, Kehne J, Cortright DN (2007) Inflammation-induced reduction of spontaneous activity by adjuvant: a novel model to study the effect of analgesics in rats. J Pharmacol Exp Ther 320:194–201
13. Morgan D, Carter CS, Dupree JP, Yezierski RP, Vierck CJ (2008) Evaluation of prescription opioids using operant-based pain measures in rats. Exp Clin Psychopharmacol 16:367–375
14. Pereira Do Carmo G, Stevenson GW, Carlezon WA Jr, Negus SS (2009) Effects of pain- and analgesia-related manipulations on intracranial self-stimulation in rats: further studies on pain-depressed behavior. Pain 144:170–177

15. Reid LD (1987) Tests involving pressing for intracranial stimulation as an early procedure for screening the likelihood of addiction of opioids and other drugs. In: Bozarth MJ (ed) Methods of assessing the reinforcing properties of abused drugs. Springer, Berlin, pp 391–420
16. Roeska K, Doods H, Arndt K, Treede RD, Ceci A (2008) Anxiety-like behaviour in rats with mononeuropathy is reduced by the analgesic drugs morphine and gabapentin. Pain 139:349–357
17. Bair MJ, Robinson RL, Katon W, Kroenke K (2003) Depression and pain comorbidity: a literature review. Arch Intern Med 163: 2433–2445
18. Gureje O, Von Korff M, Kola L, Demyttenaere K, He Y, Posada-Villa J, Lepine JP, Angermeyer MC, Levinson D, de Girolamo G, Iwata N, Karam A, Guimaraes Borges GL, de Graaf R, Browne MO, Stein DJ, Haro JM, Bromet EJ, Kessler RC, Alonso J (2008) The relation between multiple pains and mental disorders: results from the World Mental Health Surveys. Pain 135:82–91
19. Jann MW, Slade JH (2007) Antidepressant agents for the treatment of chronic pain and depression. Pharmacotherapy 27:1571–1587
20. Lepine JP, Briley M (2004) The epidemiology of pain in depression. Hum Psychopharmacol 19(Suppl. 1):S3–S7
21. Cleeland CS, Ryan KM (1994) Pain assessment: global use of the Brief Pain Inventory. Ann Acad Med Singapore 23:129–138
22. Dworkin RH, Turk DC, Wyrwich KW, Beaton D, Cleeland CS, Farrar JT, Haythornthwaite JA, Jensen MP, Kerns RD, Ader DN, Brandenburg N, Burke LB, Cella D, Chandler J, Cowan P, Dimitrova R, Dionne R, Hertz S, Jadad AR, Katz NP, Kehlet H, Kramer LD, Manning DC, McCormick C, McDermott MP, McQuay HJ, Patel S, Porter L, Quessy S, Rappaport BA, Rauschkolb C, Revicki DA, Rothman M, Schmader KE, Stacey BR, Stauffer JW, von Stein T, White RE, Witter J, Zavisic S (2008) Interpreting the clinical importance of treatment outcomes in chronic pain clinical trials: IMMPACT recommendations. J Pain 9:105–121
23. Kerns RD, Turk DC, Rudy TE (1985) The West Haven-Yale Multidimensional Pain Inventory (WHYMPI). Pain 23:345–356
24. National Research Council (1996) Guide for the care and use of laboratory animals. National Academy Press, Washington, DC
25. Carlezon WA Jr, Chartoff EH (2007) Intracranial self-stimulation (ICSS) in rodents to study the neurobiology of motivation. Nat Protoc 2:2987–2995

Chapter 8

Animal Models of Orofacial Pain

Asma Khan and Kenneth M. Hargreaves

Abstract

Pain is one of the most common reasons for which patients seek dental and medical care. Orofacial pain conditions consist of a wide range of disorders including odontalgia (toothache), temporomandibular disorders, trigeminal neuralgia and others. Most of these conditions are either inflammatory or neuropathic in nature. This chapter provides an overview of the commonly used models to study inflammatory and neuropathic orofacial pain.

Key words: Inflammation, Neuropathic, Pain, Trigeminal, Orofacial, Dental, Pulpal, Periapical, Periradicular, Temporomandibular joint, TMD

1. Introduction

Orofacial pain conditions consist of a wide range of disorders including odontalgia, temporomandibular disorders, trigeminal neuralgia and others. Epidemiologic studies indicate that about 22 million people in the United States suffer from odontalgia (1). Studies evaluating the incidence of temporomandibular disorders have reported that about 9–15% of the population reports pain in this region (2, 3), although this may vary depending upon population studied (community vs. tertiary care centers) and case definitions. The peripheral mechanisms associated with orofacial pain conditions are generally similar to those seen elsewhere in the body. These similarities include the types of sensory neurons involved as well as the receptors, ion channels and signaling pathways that transduce, modulate, and propagate peripheral stimuli to the central nervous system (CNS). However, the innervation of the orofacial structures does have certain unique features. For example, some orofacial tissues, such as the dental pulp, lack innervation by larger diameter proprioceptive afferent fibers, and physiologic stimulation of these tissues only evokes the sensation

Arpad Szallasi (ed.), *Analgesia: Methods and Protocols*, Methods in Molecular Biology, vol. 617,
DOI 10.1007/978-1-60327-323-7_8, © Springer Science+Business Media, LLC 2010

of pain. In addition, several craniofacial structures (i.e., cornea, tooth pulp, vibrissal pad in rodents, etc) have no homolog elsewhere in the body and display unique innervation patterns. The peripheral and central organization and protein expression profile of the trigeminal system differs from that of the spinal system (4). In addition, as orofacial structures are involved in functions such as eating, drinking, and speech and the sensory homunculus of the cerebral cortex has considerable dedication for processing orofacial stimuli, the impact of orofacial pain can be significantly larger than that of pain elsewhere in the body.

Based on their pathophysiology, orofacial pain conditions can be classified into (1) dentinal hypersensitivity/inflammatory disorders (such as pulpitis and temporomandibular disorders) and (2) neuropathic disorders (such as trigeminal and post-herpetic neuralgias). Inflammatory orofacial pain conditions can be further subdivided into acute and chronic conditions. In this chapter, we provide an overview of the orofacial models of inflammatory and neuropathic pain along with detailed protocols of the commonly used animal models of orofacial pain. The protocol for retrograde labeling of sensory neurons innervating the orofacial tissues has been included separately as it can be used in models of inflammatory and neuropathic pain.

1.1. Dental Injury Model

Inflammation of the dental pulp or the periradicular tissues (the tissues surrounding the root of the tooth, aka periapical) induces moderate to severe pain. In the dental injury model, mechanical exposure of the tooth pulp with or without intrapulpal administration of bacteria or other irritants (e.g. capsaicin, mustard oil, or complete Freund's adjuvant) is used to induce pulpal and periradicular inflammation (5). Inflammatory changes in the pulp are detected as early as 24 h after the injury while detectable histological changes in the periradicular tissues take about 5 days to develop (6, 7). If an exposed pulp is left open to the oral environment, it results in infection and subsequent necrosis of the pulp and formation of a periradicular bony lesion (8). The active expansion of the periradicular lesion is maximal between 7 and 21 days after pulp exposure (9, 10). The outcome measures commonly used in this model are either the size of the periapical lesion, changes in expression of various inflammatory mediators or increased innervation density. One approach is to deeply anesthetize the animal, perform perfusion fixation, and then remove and decalcify the jaw bones with subsequent analysis using histomorphometry or immunohistochemistry (11–13). Another approach is to collect the periradicular tissues and analyze them for either protein or mRNA levels of various inflammatory mediators (14).

Complete Freund's adjuvant (CFA) is an emulsion containing heat-killed mycobacteria or mycobacterial cell wall components that elicits an intense inflammatory response. Injection of CFA in to the perioral skin, masseter muscle, or temporomandibular joint is used as a model of cutaneous or deep inflammation (15, 16). It induces thermal hyperalgesia and mechanical allodynia that persist for hours or days as well as expression of Fos, a marker of neuronal activity (17).

Injection of mustard oil (allyl iosothiocyanate) into the temporomandibular joint (TMJ) is used to study temporomandibular dysfunction (18–20). Mustard oil selectively activates the TRPA1 receptor expressed on trigeminal nociceptors (21). It induces significant nociceptive behaviors expressed as head flinching and rubbing of the orofacial tissues with a duration of about 45 min. Application of mustard oil to the dental pulp is used to study pulpal inflammation especially the central mechanisms associated with pulpitis (22, 23). Subcutaneous (s.c.) injection of formalin into the upper lip of rodents elicits both behavioral as well as electrophysiological responses (24-27). The behavioral response is biphasic with an early short lasting response (3-5 min) followed, after a quiescent period (10-15 min), by a prolonged tonic phase(20-40 min) (28).

The application of capsaicin (8-methyl-N-vanillyl-noneamid), the prototypical transient receptor potential vanilloid 1 (TRPV1) agonist, evokes neuropeptide release and induces primary and secondary hyperalgesia (29, 30). Intradental perfusion of capsaicin is a newly developed model used to evaluate the pulpal response to noxious stimuli (31, 32). It has also been applied to the cornea of the eye with measurement of TRPV1-mediated nocifensive behavior (33). The outcome measures in this model are either the nociceptive behavior displayed by the animal or the release of proinflammatory mediators from isolated tissues such as dental pulp (34, 35).

1.2. Neuropathic Pain by Chronic Constriction Injury (CCI) to the Infraorbital Nerve

Neuropathic pain conditions afflicting the orofacial tissues include postherpetic neuralgia, trigeminal neuralgia, glossopharyngeal neuralgia, and persistent idiopathic facial pain (aka atypical facial pain). Animal models used to study these conditions include chronic constriction injury (CCI) to the infraorbital nerve (36–38) and postherpetic neuralgia.

Behavioral changes in response to CCI of the infraorbital nerve develop in two phases (38). In the early phase (1–15 days post-op), the rats show increased face-grooming activity with face-wash strokes directed toward the injured area. During this phase, the responsiveness to mechanical stimuli is decreased. In the late phase (150–130 days post-op), the prevalence of face grooming is less as compared to the early phase though it remains significantly more than that in the controls. In this phase the rats show increased responsiveness to mechanical stimuli.

1.3. Retrograde Labeling of Neurons

Neuronal tracers are used to retrogradely label neurons innervating specific orofacial tissues. Florogold (FG) applied to exposed dentin diffuses into the pulp and labels pulpal afferents without inducing inflammation (39, 40). Injection of DiI (DiIC 18; 1,1′-dioctadecyl-3,3,3′,3′-tetramethylindocarbocyanine perchlorate) into orofacial structures (such as the masseter or the dental pulp) is yet another way to retrogradely label neurons (41–44).

2. Materials

2.1. Dental Injury Model

1. Adult Sprague-Dawley rats (weighing 175–300 g, males) rats or 8–11 week old C57bl/6 mice.
2. Anesthetic (e.g., sodium pentobarbital).
3. Round dental bur (size #2) or ultrasonic tip.
4. High speed dental drill or ultrasonic unit.
5. Surgical operating microscope or dental loupes.
6. Complete Freund's adjuvant (CFA) stock is suspended at 25 μg/50 μl in oil/saline.
7. Von Frey monofilaments.
8. Radiant heat source such as a high intensity projector lamp.
9. Strain gauge force transducer to measure bite force.
10. Mustard oil is prepared as a 20% solution in mineral oil.
11. Hamilton microsyringe with 30 gauge needle.
12. A temporary dental restorative material such as Cavit (3M ESPE, St Paul, MN).
13. Observation box: a glass chamber ($30 \times 30 \times 30$ cm^3) with mirrored sides.
14. Capsaicin is dissolved at 1 mg/mL in EtOH. Working solution is prepared by dilution in 100 μg/100 ml physiological saline/10% Tween-80.
15. Clamp, retractor, and bone rongeur.
16. Polyethylene tubing (PE 240, Outer diameter 0.095 inch).
17. Orthodontic stainless steel wire (0.01 inch).
18. Tigone tubing (internal diameter1/8 inch).
19. Vials for collection of perfusates.
20. Metal crown.

2.2. Chronic Constriction Injury to the Infraorbital Nerve

1. Adult Sprague-Dawley or Wistar rats (weighing 175–300 g, males).
2. Sterile saline.
3. Anesthetic (e.g., sodium pentobarbital).
4. Topical disinfectant (e.g., betadine).

5. Phytoestrogen-free rat chow.
6. Animal clippers.
7. Animal heating pad.
8. Dissecting microscope.
9. 4–0 chromic gut suture.
10. Rat toothed forceps.
11. Blunt tipped scissors.
12. Microscissors.
13. Sutures.

2.3. Retrograde Labeling of Neurons

1. Adult Sprague-Dawley rats (weighing 175–300 g, males).
2. Anesthetic (e.g., sodium pentobarbital).
3. Metal clamp.
4. Retractor.
5. Florogold: 5% Aqueous solution.
6. Water-repellant PAP Pen.
7. Dental high-speed drill with water coolant.
8. Dental bur (1/4 or 1/8 round).
9. Phosphoric acid containing gel (such as Tooth Conditioner Gel, L.D. Caulk Division, Dentsply Int., Inc., Milford, DE).
10. Syringe (5 μL) with a blunt tapered needle.
11. Light-cured restorative material (for example Fuji II, GC America, Inc., Alsip IL).
12. Temporary protective glaze.
13. DiI (5% w/v in dimethylformamide or dimethyl sulphoxide).
14. Electric hair clippers.
15. Eye ointment or petroleum jelly.
16. Nexaband formulated cyanoacrylate or sutures.
17. Hydrogen peroxide.
18. Syringe (10 μl) with 26 gauge needle.

3. Methods

3.1. Dental Injury Model

1. Anesthetize the animal.
2. Use the jaw retraction board to retract the mandible.
3. Expose the pulps of the molars using the high speed dental bur or ultrasonic tip.

4. Confirm the pulpal exposure using the surgical operating microscope or magnifying loupes.
5. Using a 30 gauge needle, inject CFA (50 μl; 0.025 mg) into the subcutaneous tissues of the upper lip or into the middle of the masseter muscle (see Note 1).
6. For experiments evaluating inflammation of the TMJ, identify the site of injection by palpating the zygomatic arch and condyle. Insert the needle into the skin at a point immediately inferior to the posterior–inferior border of the zygomatic arch and advance it until it contacts the posterior–lateral aspect of the condyle. After a gentle aspiration to rule out intravascular placement of the needle, inject CFA into the joint. Mustard oil may be administered in a similar fashion (see Note 2).
7. Evaluation of thermal hyperalgesia (using radiant heat) or mechanical allodynia (using von Frey filaments or a force transducer to measure bite force) can be done 24 h post-injection and may be continued up to 4 weeks after induction of inflammation (see Note 3). Most protocols involve using a restraint to permit access to the inflamed area.
8. When applying heat, use a rheostat to control the voltage applied to the lamp (which in turn controls the intensity of the heat stimulus). Use a stop watch to measure the time lapsed between initiation of heat application and the observed flinching or withdrawal response. Test each animal 3 times with a 5 min interval and calculate the mean withdrawal latency.
9. For evaluation of mechanical pain thresholds using Von Frey filaments, apply the filaments perpendicular to the inflamed site with force sufficient enough to cause the filament to bend. If the animal fails to respond, then use a von Frey filament of 1 log value greater and continue this process till a withdrawal response is elicited.
10. Bite force may also be used to measure mechanical allodynia. In this model, rats must be first trained to produce bite forces greater than 400 g prior to induction of inflammation. After induction of inflammation, the mean bite force and the success rates (ratio between bites exceeding 400 g to the total number of attempted bites) is a measure of mechanical allodynia.
11. To evaluate the release of proinflammatory mediators, anesthetize the rat and then use the clamp to fix the lower jaw of the rat to the metal bar. Nocifensory behavior can also be evaluated (see Notes 4 and 5).
12. Use the retractor to keep the mouth open.
13. Cut 2–2.5 mm of the incisal edges of the lower incisor and expose the dentin using the rongeurs.

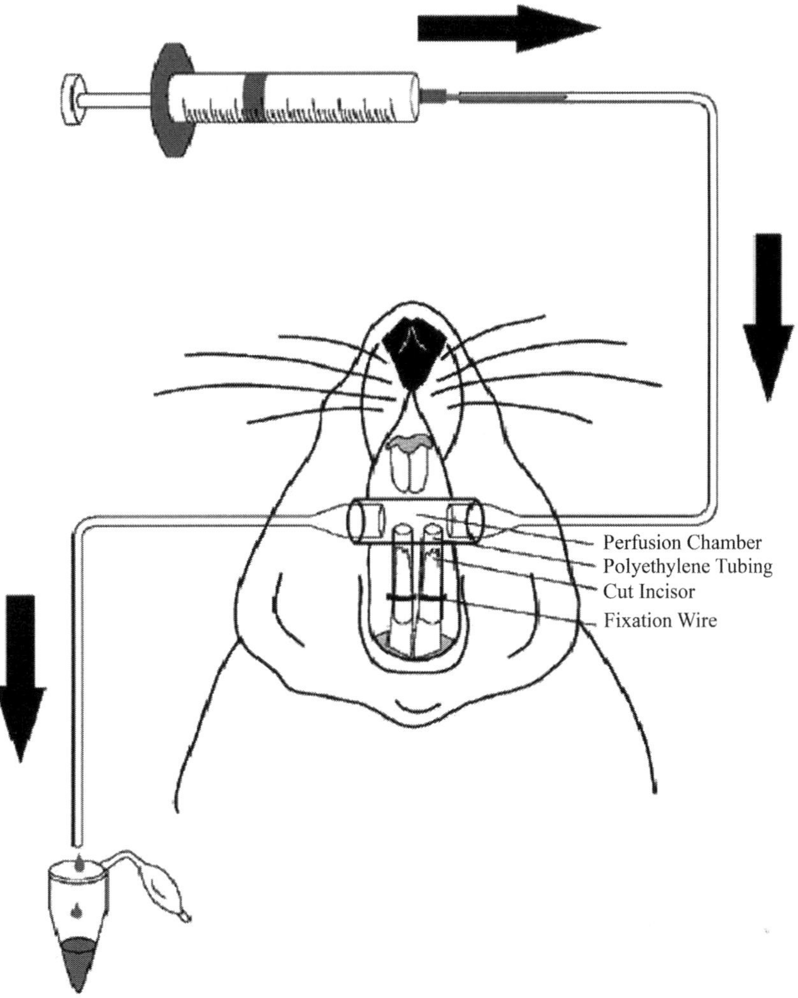

Fig. 1. Experimental setup for collection of perfusates following induction of pulpal inflammation. Reproduced from Chidiac et al., 2002 with permission from Elsevier Ltd

14. Wrap the polyethylene tubing around the tooth such that it extends to the gingival margin. Use the stainless steel wire to secure the tubing to the tooth (Fig. 1).
15. Place the perfusion chamber so that the upper end of the polyethylene tubing projects into it.
16. Attach a syringe to one end of the perfusion chamber and collection vials to the other end.
17. Expose the cut incisal edges of the teeth to capsaicin by placing it in the perfusion chamber for an hour.
18. Then, place sterile saline in the perfusion hour and change it every 40 min for 8 h.
19. The collected perfusates can then be analyzed for levels of inflammatory mediators released.

3.2. Chronic Constriction Injury to the Infraorbital Nerve

1. Anesthetize the animal and place it on a heating pad (see Note 6). A rectal thermometer may be used to avoid hypo- and hyperthermia.
2. Closely clip the fur over the snout and disinfect.
3. Make a midline incision over the snout and remove the connective tissue till the infraorbital nerve is exposed.
4. Pass a blunt probe under the nerve to release it from the underlying tissues.
5. Place two chromic gut sutures which have been soaked in sterile saline around the infraorbital nerve. The site of placement should be just distal to the inferior orbital foramen. Place the sutures such that they are 2 mm apart and tighten the sutures, so that the nerve is partially constricted (see Note 7).
6. Close the incision with 4–0 sutures.
7. Controls are rats where the infraorbital nerve is exposed but not ligated/transected.
8. Allow the animal to recover in a comfortable setting.
9. Behavioral testing of the animal is done prior to surgery and then ≥3 days after surgery. The tests include response to mechanical stimuli (see Note 8).

3.3. Retrograde Labeling of Neurons

1. Anesthetize the rat.
2. Use the clamp to fix the lower jaw of the rat to the metal bar.
3. Use the retractor to gain access to the maxillary molars.
4. Dry the mucosa around the maxillary teeth and use the PAP pen to coat the mucosa with a hydrophobic film. This prevents absorption of the tracer into the mucosa.
5. Use the high-speed dental hand piece drill to drill shallow cavities on the mesial and lingual surfaces of the maxillary first molar (see Note 9).
6. Apply the phosphoric acid containing gel to the cavity for 5 min to remove the smear layer.
7. Using sterile water, wash away the phosphoric acid.
8. Apply a droplet of the FG to the exposed dentin on the cavity floor and allow it to dry slightly.
9. Use the light cured resin to restore and seal the cavity.
10. Coat with the temporary glaze.
11. Allow the animal to recover in a comfortable setting.
12. Retrograde labeling of masseter afferents, coat the eyes of a rat under anesthesia with petroleum jelly or eye ointment to avoid irritation from hair.
13. Shave the hair overlying the masseter.
14. Use the topical disinfectant to disinfect the skin.

15. Using the scalpel, expose the masseter with a 1 cm incision parallel to the mouth line.
16. Use hydrogen peroxide to wipe away any blood.
17. Inject 1 μl of DiI into five different locations.
18. Cover the injection spots with petroleum jelly to prevent leakage.
19. Suture the incision closed or apply a drop of cyanaoacrylate to hold the margins of the incision together.

4. Notes

1. Handling of CFA can be an occupational hazard. The use of safety glasses and precautions to prevent accidental needle punctures is recommended.
2. Inject mustard oil into the TMJ in the same manner as that described for CFA. To induce inflammation of the dental pulp by mustard oil, anesthetize the animal and then use a bur and a high speed dental drill with a water coolant to expose the pulp of one of the maxillary molars. Apply mustard oil to the pulp and seal the cavity using a temporary dental restorative material.
3. When nociceptive behavior is used as an outcome measure, it must be remembered that all drug treatments that alter motor function can potentially confound the measure of nociception.
4. To evaluate nocifensive behavior, the experimental set up is exactly the same as described for neuropeptide release except that a metal crown is sealed on to the tooth instead of a perfusion chamber (Fig. 2).
5. Nociceptive behavior displayed by the animal consists of abnormal head movements including shaking of the head or lower jaw, placing the lower jaw on the floor or walls of the cage, and consistently rubbing the lower jaw with the foreleg. Once the animal recovers from the anesthetic, place it in an observation chamber and record the time spent displaying nociceptive behavior (head flinching and rubbing the ipsilateral face with hind- or fore- paw).
6. The use of ketamine must be avoided in models of neuropathic pain. N-methyl-D-aspartate (NMDA) receptors play an important role in the development of neuropathic pain. As ketamine is an N-methyl-D-aspartate (NMDA) receptor antagonist, its use could affect the development of neuropathic pain.
7. The lateral half of the ligated nerve fascicle may be transected and the median half spared.

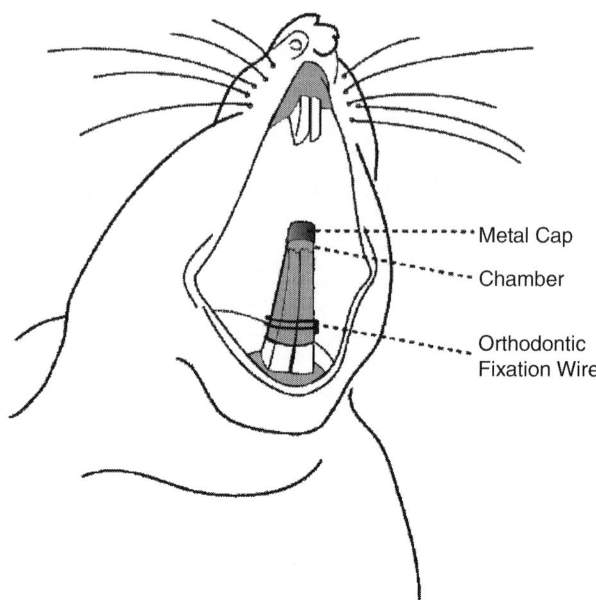

Fig. 2. Schematic diagram illustrating the placement of a metal cap over the mandibular incisors. Reproduced from Chidiac et al., 2002 with permission from Elsevier Ltd

8. Observation of free behavior such as frequency and duration of face grooming may also be used as indicators of sensory disturbances due to the nerve injury.
9. Do not deepen the cavity once the dentin is reached (dentin can be easily identified by its darker color as compared to enamel).

References

1. Lipton JA, Ship JA, Larach-Robinson D (1993) Estimated prevalence and distribution of reported orofacial pain in the United States. J Am Dent Assoc 124:115–121
2. Locker D, Slade G (1988) Prevalence of symptoms associated with temporomandibular disorders in a Canadian population. Community Dent Oral Epidemiol 16:310–313
3. Von Korff M, Dworkin SF, Le Resche L, Kruger A (1988) An epidemiologic comparison of pain complaints. Pain 32:173–183
4. Bereiter DA, Hargreaves KM, Hu JW (In press) Trigeminal mechanisms of nociception: peripheral and brainstem organization. In: Basbaum A, Bushnell C (eds) Handbook of the senses. vol 1
5. Byers MR, Narhi MV (1999) Dental injury models: experimental tools for understanding neuroinflammatory interactions and polymodal nociceptor functions. Crit Rev Oral Biol Med 10:4–39
6. Khayat BG, Byers MR, Taylor PE, Mecifi K, Kimberly CL (1988) Responses of nerve fibers to pulpal inflammation and periapical lesions in rat molars demonstrated by calcitonin gene-related peptide immunocytochemistry. J Endod 14:577–587
7. Kimberly CL, Byers MR (1988) Inflammation of rat molar pulp and periodontium causes increased calcitonin gene-related peptide and axonal sprouting. Anat Rec 222:289–300
8. Kakehashi S, Stanley HR, Fitzgerald RJ (1965) The effects of surgical exposures of dental pulps in germ-free and conventional laboratory rats. Oral Surg Oral Med Oral Pathol 20:340–349
9. Wang CY, Stashenko P (1991) Kinetics of bone-resorbing activity in developing periapical lesions. J Dent Res 70:1362–1366
10. Wang CY, Tani-Ishii N, Stashenko P (1997) Bone-resorptive cytokine gene expression in periapical lesions in the rat. Oral Microbiol Immunol 12:65–71

11. Byers MR, Taylor PE, Khayat BG, Kimberly CL (1990) Effects of injury and inflammation on pulpal and periapical nerves. J Endod 16:78–84
12. Kawashima N, Niederman R, Hynes RO, Ullmann-Cullere M, Stashenko P (1999) Infection-stimulated infraosseus inflammation and bone destruction is increased in P-/E-selectin knockout mice. Immunology 97:117–123
13. Tani-Ishii N, Wang CY, Stashenko P (1995) Immunolocalization of bone-resorptive cytokines in rat pulp and periapical lesions following surgical pulp exposure. Oral Microbiol Immunol 10:213–219
14. Kawashima N, Stashenko P (1999) Expression of bone-resorptive and regulatory cytokines in murine periapical inflammation. Arch Oral Biol 44:55–66
15. Ro JY (2005) Bite force measurement in awake rats: a behavioral model for persistent orofacial muscle pain and hyperalgesia. J Orofac Pain 19:159–167
16. Zhou Q, Imbe H, Dubner R, Ren K (1999) Persistent Fos protein expression after orofacial deep or cutaneous tissue inflammation in rats: implications for persistent orofacial pain. J Comp Neurol 412:276–291
17. Morgan JR, Gebhart GF (2008) Characterization of a model o chronic orofacial hyperalgesia in the rat: contribution of NaV 1.8. J Pain 9:522–531
18. Bereiter DA, Benetti AP (1996) Excitatory amino release within spinal trigeminal nucleus after mustard oil injection into the temporomandibular joint region of the rat. Pain 67:451–459
19. Bonjardim LR, da Silva AP, Gameiro GH, Tambeli CH, de Arruda F, Veiga MC (2009) Nociceptive behavior induced by mustard oil injection into the temporomandibular joint is blocked by a peripheral non-opioid analgesic and a central opioid analgesic. Pharmacol Biochem Behav 91:321–326
20. Haas DA, Nakanishi O, MacMillan RE, Jordan RC, Hu JW (1992) Development of an orofacial model of acute inflammation in the rat. Arch Oral Biol 37:417–422
21. Akopian A, Ruparel N, Jeske N, Hargreaves KM (2007) TRPA1 desensitization in sensory neurons is agonist-dependent and regulated by TRPV1-directed internalization. J Physiol 583:175–193
22. Chiang CY, Park SJ, Kwan CL, Hu JW, Sessle BJ (1998) NMDA receptor mechanisms contribute to neuroplasticity induced in caudalis nociceptive neurons by tooth pulp stimulation. J Neurophysiol 80:2621–2631
23. Zhang S, Chiang CY, Xie YF, Park SJ, Lu Y, Hu JW, Dostrovsky JO, Sessle BJ (2006) Central sensitization in thalamic nociceptive neurons induced by mustard oil application to rat molar tooth pulp. Neuroscience 142: 833–842
24. Clavelou P, Dallel R, Orliaguet T, Woda A, Raboisson P (1995) The orofacial formalin test in rats: effects of different formalin concentrations. Pain 62:295–301
25. Gilbert SD, Clark TM, Flores CM (2001) Antihyperalgesic activity of epibatidine in the formalin model of facial pain. Pain 89: 159–165
26. Porro CA, Cavazzuti M (1993) Spatial and temporal aspects of spinal cord and brainstem activation in the formalin pain model. Prog Neurobiol 41:565–607
27. Raboisson P, Bourdiol P, Dallel R, Clavelou P, Woda A (1991) Responses of trigeminal subnucleus oralis nociceptive neurones to subcutaneous formalin in the rat. Neurosci Lett 125:179–182
28. Raboisson P, Dallel R (2004) The orofacial formalin test. Neurosci Biobehav Rev 28: 219–226
29. Szolcsanyi J (2004) Forty years in capsaicin research for sensory pharmacology and physiology. Neuropeptides 38:377–384
30. Knotkova H, Pappagallo M, Szallasi A (2008) Capsaicin (TRPV1 Agonist) therapy for pain relief: farewell or revival? Clin J Pain 24:142–154
31. Chidiac JJ, Hawwa N, Baliki M, Safieh-Garabedian B, Rifai K, Jabbur SJ, Saade NE (2001) A perfusion technique for the determination of pro-inflammatory mediators induced by intradental application of irritants. J Pharmacol Toxicol Methods 46:125–130
32. Chidiac JJ, Rifai K, Hawwa NN, Massaad CA, Jurjus AR, Jabbur SJ, Saade NE (2002) Nociceptive behaviour induced by dental application of irritants to rat incisors: a new model for tooth inflammatory pain. Eur J Pain 6:55–67
33. Diogenes A, Patwardhan A, Ruparel N, Goffin A, Akopian A, Hargreaves KM (2006) Prolactin modulates TRPV1 in female rat trigeminal sensory neurons. J Neurosci 26:8126–8136
34. Bowles WR, Flores CM, Jackson DL, Hargreaves KM (2003) beta 2-Adrenoceptor regulation of CGRP release from capsaicin-sensitive neurons. J Dent Res 82:308–311
35. Hargreaves KM, Jackson DL, Bowles WR (2003) Adrenergic regulation of capsaicin-sensitive neurons in dental pulp. J Endod 29:397–399

36. Anderson LC, Vakoula A, Veinote R (2003) Inflammatory hypersensitivity in a rat model of trigeminal neuropathic pain. Arch Oral Biol 48:161–169
37. Henry MA, Freking AR, Johnson LR, Levinson SR (2007) Sodium channel Nav1.6 accumulates at the site of infraorbital nerve injury. BMC Neurosci 8:56
38. Vos BP, Strassman AM, Maciewicz RJ (1994) Behavioral evidence of trigeminal neuropathic pain following chronic constriction injury to the rat's infraorbital nerve. J Neurosci 14:2708–2723
39. Pan Y, Wheeler EF, Bernanke JM, Yang H, Naftel JP (2003) A model experimental system for monitoring changes in sensory neuron phenotype evoked by tooth injury. J Neurosci Methods 126:99–109
40. Wheeler EF, Naftel JP, Pan M, von Bartheld CS, Byers MR (1998) Neurotrophin receptor expression is induced in a subpopulation of trigeminal neurons that label by retrograde transport of NGF or fluoro-gold following tooth injury. Brain Res Mol Brain Res 61:23–38
41. Ambalavanar R, Moritani M, Haines A, Hilton T, Dessem D (2003) Chemical phenotypes of muscle and cutaneous afferent neurons in the rat trigeminal ganglion. J Comp Neurol 26:167–179
42. Eckert SP, Taddese A, McCleskey EW (1997) Isolation and culture of rat sensory neurons having distinct sensory modalities. J Neurosci Methods 77:183–190
43. Stephenson JL, Byers MR (1995) GFAP immunoreactivity in trigeminal ganglion satellite cells after tooth injury in rats. Exp Neurol 131:11–22
44. Sugaya A, Chudler EH, Byers MR (1995) Axonal transport of fluorescent carbocyanine dyes allows mapping of peripheral nerve territories in gingiva. J Periodontol 66: 817–821

Chapter 9

Migraine Models

Silvia Benemei, Francesco De Cesaris, Paola Nicoletti, Serena Materazzi, Romina Nassini, and Pierangelo Geppetti

Abstract

Migraine is a high prevalence disorder which affects a significant proportion of the general population, especially women during their central and more productive time of the life, thus causing severe disability. The genetic basis of the disease is unknown and the mechanism is poorly understood. The possibility that following a perturbation in the central nervous system, and particularly in the brainstem, trigeminal neurons become hyperexcitable and produce an uncontrolled release of sensory neuropeptides which eventually results in arterial vasodilatation and neuronal sensitization, has been gaining credit from studies in experimental animals and humans. In particular, experimental and clinical data with antagonists of the calcitonin gene-related peptide (CGRP) propose this molecule and its receptor as a major target for migraine treatment.

Key words: Migraine, Meninges, Neurogenic inflammation, Calcitonin gene-related peptide (CGRP), Trigeminal neurons, Blood flow, Neuropeptide

1. Introduction

Migraine is one of the commonest disorders in the general population and is characterized by severe headache associated with features other than pain (1). It affects around 18% of women and 7% of men (2) from infancy throughout adulthood, and causes severe disability and work loss (3) in a significant proportion of the population during the most productive time of the life. Although a genetic basis is considered for migraine (4), the specific gene(s) involved in the disease is(are) unknown. Therapy of migraine falls into two categories, acute and preventive. Nonsteroidal antiinflammatory drugs (NSAIDs) and triptans are mainly used for the acute treatment of the migraine attacks, whereas β-blockers, Ca^{2+} channel blockers, serotonin antagonists, and some antiepileptics are used for prophylaxis.

Arpad Szallasi (ed.), *Analgesia: Methods and Protocols*, Methods in Molecular Biology, vol. 617,
DOI 10.1007/978-1-60327-323-7_9,

The mechanism by which preventive treatments ameliorate migraine is poorly understood, and, except for the obvious inhibition of prostanoid ability of sensitizing sensory nerve terminals, the precise mechanisms by which NSAIDs and triptans are effective drugs in migraine attack remain elusive.

A subset of trigeminal neurons with C and A-δ fibres which express the transient receptor potential vanilloid 1 (TRPV1) channel and release centrally and peripherally the neuropeptides substance P (SP) and calcitonin gene-related peptide (CGRP), densely innervates arterial blood vessels in intra and extracranial structures (5). This trigeminovascular system has been proposed to contribute to migraine headache (6, 7). A large series of data obtained in experimental animals and in human beings and current clinical studies indicate that CGRP plays a major role in migraine mechanism and that CGRP receptor antagonists have a beneficial effect in the treatment of the migraine attack. Methods to assess CGRP release in tissue or body fluids have been developed by using radioimmunoassays or enzyme immunoassays.

Dura mater plasma extravasation in rodents is caused by stimuli, which act on sensory nerve terminals by releasing SP that, by interacting at tachykinin NK1 receptors, opens gaps between postcapillary venules, thus allowing the passage of macromolecules into the interstitial space. Evans blue dye (EBD) (8) is a di-azo compound widely used as a tracer to quantify vascular permeability because it binds plasma albumin when injected into the blood stream and leaves the circulation very slowly by diffusion. If the vascular permeability increases, EBD-marked albumin leaks out into tissues. Therefore, EBD concentration into the target tissue (the meninges in the present case) can be used as a marker for plasma extravasation (9).

Meningeal blood flow is a parameter useful to investigate intracranial vascular responses to chemical or physical stimuli which has been originally described (10) and further developed (11, 12) in animal models. Meningeal blood vessels diameter is another parameter assessed in order to identify intracranial vascular changes in various experimental settings (13). These two methods utilize a similar preparation, differing only for the signal detection systems as they measure two distinct parameters, and they could also be used simultaneously (13).

Cortical spreading depression (CSD) has been proposed by Aristides Leão in 1944 as a process involved in the mechanism of migraine (14). CSD is a self-propagating depolarization of neurons and glia, lasting approximately 1 min, associated with depressed neuronal electrical activity and changes in the distribution of ions between extra and intracellular space. Depolarization (induced by high K^+) results in ionic changes that spread in the cortical tissue. These changes are associated with a transient hyperemia in the cortex, pia and dura mater which are suggested to be associated with the underlying mechanism of migraine aura and attack (8).

Glyceryl trinitrate (GTN) is a nitric oxide donor which has long been known to induce headache (15). GTN is easy to administer, has a short half-life and well-known, mild and reversible side effects (16). After the original description by Sicuteri and coworkers (17) of a biphasic headache in migraine patients and in healthy subjects with a family history of migraine after infusion of GTN, additional studies have been performed in patients with migraine with or without aura with different GTN formulation including the sublingual administration (18, 19). Intravenous infusion of αCGRP causes a headache with a biphasic temporal profile, similar to that induced by GTN and histamine (17). CGRP stimulates intracellular production of cAMP and cGMP by NO signalling pathway (20, 21), and CGRP blood levels are elevated in external jugular vein during migraine attack (22). Finally, two newly developed CGRP antagonist, BIBN4096S (olcegepant) (23) and MK0974 (telcagepant) (24), have been reported to be beneficial in the acute treatment of migraine.

2. Materials

2.1. Neuropeptide Release from Tissue

1. Krebs' solution (KS): 119 mM NaCl, 25 mM $NaHCO_3$, 1.2 mM KH_2PO_4, 1.5 nM $MgSO_4$, 2.5 mM $CaCl_2$, 4.7 mM KCl 4.7, 11 mM d-glucose. Supplement KS with 0.1% (w/v) bovine serum albumin (BSA), 1 μM phosphoramidon and 1 μM captopril.
2. Krebs' solution Ca^{2+}-free medium (KSCaF): 119 mM NaCl, 25 mM $NaHCO_3$, 1.2 mM KH_2PO_4, 1.5 mM $MgSO_4$, 4.7 mM KCl, 11 mM d-glucose, 1 mM EDTA.
3. Human CGRP enzyme immunoassay kit for ELISA assay (SPI-bio, Montigny Le Bretonneux, France).
4. Ethanoic acid.

2.2. Radioimmunoassay (RIA) for CGRP-like Immunoreactivity (CGRP-LI)

1. Sep-pak C18 cartridges (Millipore, Billerica, MA).
2. Acetic buffer (AB): 4% (v/v) acetic acid in H_2O.
3. Elution buffer (EB): 90% (v/v) methanol and 10% (v/v) acetic acid.
4. Phosphate buffer (PB) 0.1 M at pH 7.4.
5. Antibody buffer (AbB) containing 7.5% polyethylene glycol.
6. CGRP antiserum (Peninsula, Belmont, CA).
7. Peptides.
8. ^{125}I-labeled CGRP (Amersham/GE Healthcare, Fairfield, CT).
9. Goat anti-rabbit antiserum (Analytical Antibodies, Milan, Italy).

2.3. Neurogenic Plasma Extravasation

1. Sodium pentobarbital (Sigma, St. Louis, MO) is dissolved at 60 mg/kg/L in sterile saline (see Note 1).
2. Evans' Blue Dye (EBD, Sigma) is dissolved at 30 mg/kg/L in sterile saline. Because EBD is a toxic compound that may cause cancer, the investigator should consider appropriate safety precautions, as wearing gloves and glasses to avoid direct contacts with the skin or mucosae.
3. Formaldehyde (Sigma). Because formaldehyde is a volatile toxic compound that may cause cancer, the investigator should consider appropriate safety precautions as well as work under a hood.

2.4. Meningeal Blood Flow

1. Sodium pentobarbital (Sigma) is dissolved at 60 mg/kg/L in sterile saline (see Note 1).
2. Modified synthetic interstitial fluid (SIF, pH 7.2): 135 mM NaCl, 5 mM KCl, 1 mM $MgCl_2$, 5 mM $CaCl_2$, 10 mM glucose, 10 mM Hepes. Make it fresh for each experimental session.
3. Laser Doppler Flowmeter (Perimed AB, Jarfalla, Sweden), with needle probe, data acquisition, and analysis software.
4. Microcamera (Sony DSP digital camera, MS50 objective, Japan) with video dimension analyser (V94) (Living Systems Instrumentation Inc., Burlington, VT).

2.5. Cortical Spreading Depression

1. Isoflurane (volatile anesthetic).
2. Ringer Solution (RS) which, when aerated with 95% oxygen and 5% carbon dioxide, reaches a pH of 7.3–7.4.
3. Glass micropipette (#2- 136 1 tip diameter, 24 pm, Supelco, Inc., Bellefonte, PA).
4. Axoprobe A-l amplifier system (Axon Instruments, Burlingame, CA).

2.6. Human Provocative Tests

1. Glyceryl trinitrate (NGT): 150 mg/ml solution.
2. Human αCGRP (hαCGRP).

3. Methods

3.1. Neuropeptide Release from Tissue

1. After terminal anesthesia, tissues (e.g. dorsal spinal cord, airways, urinary bladder) are rapidly removed and slices (0.4 μm) are prepared at 4°C using a tissue slicer.
2. Slices (~10–100 mg) are placed in 2 ml thermostated (37°C) chambers and superfused at a rate of 0.4 ml/min with oxygenated (95% O_2, 5% CO_2) KS.

3. After a 90 min stabilization period, slices are stimulated for 10 min.
4. In some experiments, slices are perfused with KSCaF, or sensory nerve terminals are desensitized to capsaicin by exposure to a high concentration of the drug (10 μM) for 20 min, 30 min before stimulation.
5. Fractions (4 ml) of superfusate are collected at 10 min intervals into ethanoic acid (final concentration 2 N) before, during, and after administration of stimulus and then freeze-dried, reconstituted with assay buffer and analyzed for CGRP immunoreactivity as described (25).
6. Peptide release is determined by subtracting basal levels from concentrations measured during and after exposure to the treatment. Neuropeptide concentrations are expressed as fmol of peptide per g per tissue per 20 min.

3.2. Radioimmunoassay (RIA) for CGRP-like Immunoreactivity (CGRP-LI)

1. Blood samples (5–8 ml) for the determination of CGRP are taken from antecubital or jugular vein and put into heparinized tubes maintained at 4°C. After centrifugation (15 min at 4°C), plasma is aliquoted and stored at −80°C until extraction.
2. Extraction is carried out in Sep-pak C18 cartridges activated with 5 ml of methanol and 10 ml of H_2O before loading with plasma to which 0.1 ml/min of HCl (1 N) have previously been added.
3. The precipitated samples are washed with 10 ml of H_2O followed by 10 ml of AB. Peptides are eluted with 5 ml of EB. Samples are then dried under a nitrogen stream and, after reconstitution with PB, they are stored at −80°C until assayed.
4. For CGRP-like immunoreactivity (CGRP-LI), radioimmunoassay aliquots (100 μl) of hCGRP (standard) or samples are incubated for 48 h at 4°C with the CGRP antiserum (100 μl). ^{125}I-CGRP (100 μl) is added and incubated for a further 48 h at 4°C.
5. After the addition of 1 ml of AbB with goat antirabbit antiserum (1:200) and normal rabbit serum (1:2,000), bound and free antigen are separated by centrifugation at 2,000×*g* for 30 min at 4°C. The coefficient of variation (CV) is <10% for values between 20 and 300 pg/ml. The interassay CV is 10%. Cross-reactivity of the antiserum is 100% for human CGRP-II and rat α- and β-CGRP, and 0.01% for human and salmon calcitonin.

3.3. Neurogenic Plasma Extravasation

1. After general anesthesia by an intraperitoneal injection of SP performed by the 2-men technique (see Note 2), animals (see Note 3) are placed on an automatic thermoregulated bed (see Note 4).

2. Animals are artificially ventilated by performing a tracheotomy incision, inserting a plastic cannula into the trachea and attaching the cannula to a rodent ventilator after selecting the physiological breathing rate for the chosen species.
3. After waiting for 10 min to let the animal stabilize, EBD and any test substance are injected into the jugular vein.
4. After waiting for the time necessary to test substance taking action, the animal is sacrificed with a lethal injection of *SP* (155 mg/kg).
5. After opening the thorax, an incision is performed in the right atrium for drainage and in the left ventricle to place a plastic cannula into the ascending aorta. Sterile saline is perfused via the left ventricle at 120 mm Hg for 2 minutes (see Note 5).
6. Following removal of the brain through an opening in the skull performed by the drill around the main diameter, the cranial cavity is thoroughly rinsed. The dura mater, after being carefully removed by screeching the skull internal superficies, is dried and weighted.
7. Dissected meninges are incubated in 1 ml of formaldehyde at room temperature for 24 h to extract the dye.
8. Evans blue is quantified by measuring the optical density of the formaldehyde extract at 620 nm and comparing the results with a standard curve of 0.05–25 μg/ml Evans blue in formaldehyde. Extravasation is expressed as ng of Evans blue per mg of dry weight (17).

3.4. Meningeal Blood Flow

1. Animals (see Note 6) are prepared (anesthesia, tracheotomy and thermoregulation) as described in the previous paragraph.
2. The femoral artery and vein are cannulated bilaterally to measure the mean arterial blood pressure (MABP) and to administrate test substances.
3. The animal is placed in the stereotaxic frame.
4. The skin covering the dorsal side of the head is divided by a sagittal section and pulled aside. Periosteum and the dorsal part of the masseter muscle are removed.
5. The skull is carefully opened by an electric drill while cooling it with SIF (4°C).
6. The dura mater is exposed performing one rectangular window of about 5 × 6 mm in the parietal bone. The cranial window is filled with SIF (see Note 7).
7. The needle type probe of the Laser Doppler Flowmeter is placed inside the filled cranial window 0.1 cm over a branch of the medial meningeal artery (MMA). Data are continuously displayed on a computer monitor by the specific software (Perisoft).

8. After reaching regular signal for at least 20 min, tests are initiated by administrating chosen stimuli according to the experimental design (see Note 8).
9. The microcamera is placed over a branch of the MMA and real-time image is displayed on a computer monitor. The diameter of the vessels is continuously measured by the video dimension analyser.
10. Your tests could be initiated by administrating chosen stimuli according to your experimental design (see Note 8).

3.5. Cortical Spreading Depression

1. General anesthesia of the animals (see Note 4) is obtained by isoflurane (5% for induction, 3% during surgical procedures) administered via a 20% oxygen-balance nitrogen air mixture and ventilation is mechanically assisted by inserting a tube via a tracheostomy.
2. A cannula is inserted into the femoral artery for arterial pressure recordings and blood samples assays.
3. Animals are placed in a stereotaxic frame. Stereotaxic ear bars should be avoided in order to minimize nociceptive stimulation. Rectal temperature should be maintained at $37 \pm 0.5°C$ using an automatic thermoregulated bed.
4. After parasagittal skin incision for approximately 1 cm long and 2–3 mm from the midline, the skull bone is scraped and cleaned up.
5. Two small (1–2 mm diameter) craniotomies are performed by a drill, paying attention not to damage the underlying tissues. Make the first hole 2 mm lateral and 3 mm anterior to the bregma (it will be the recording site) and the second one 6 mm posterior and 5 mm lateral to bregma (KCl application or electrical stimulation). Warm and clean the skull area with a preoxygenated RS at 37°C. The dura overlying the cortex should be gently removed and attention should be paid in order to avoid bleeding.
6. A plastic ring is glued with a resin around the craniotomies, which are filled with a preoxygenated RS in order to maintain the physiological conditions.
7. The cortex superfused with RS requires ~30 min to recover baseline conditions.
8. CSD is evoked by placing a cotton ball (2 mm diameter) soaked with 1 M KCl (see Note 9) on the pial surface and keeping moist by adding 5 μl of 1 M, KCl solution every 15 min.
9. The steady potential (DC) is recorded with glass micropipettes filled with 200 mM NaCl positioned on the pial surface through the anterior craniotomy. An Ag/AgCl reference electrode should be placed subcutaneously in the neck.

10. Recording microelectrodes are connected to an amplifier system and DC signals are reported. The number of KCl-induced CSDs should be counted for a standardized period of time (usually 2 h). Less than 5 mV amplitude shifts in extracellular DC potential are not included in the CSD count.

3.6. Human Provocative Tests

1. Increasing doses (0.25, 0.50, 1.00, 2.00 μg/kg/min) of GTN are given intravenously over 10 min, each administration being followed by a wash-out period with saline infusion.
2. GTN dose is adjusted per body weight and the duration of each wash-out period varies between 10 and 30 min.
3. Subjects are blind to saline or different GTN concentrations.
4. Blood pressure, heart rate, and skin temperatures in frontal region and on the pulp of the left first finger are recorded every 2 min.
5. Every 2 min, subjects are asked to score their headache on a scale from 0 to 10 (0 absent, 5 moderate, 10 worst) and to report pain localization, quality, aggravation by coughing, side effects.
6. After 1–8 weeks, another test is performed.
7. Headache intensity and characteristics, blood pressure and heart rate are recorded after 30 min of rest in supine position and every 10 min during infusion until 80 min after start of infusion.
8. Human αCGRP is infused intravenously for 20 min.
9. After discharge, headache intensity and characteristics are recorded by the patient every hour for the following 11 h.
10. Patient can take, in the following 11 h, sumatriptan tablets as needed.

4. Notes

1. Sodium pentobarbital is the suggested anesthetic for this technique because it acts in several minutes and minimizes the hemodynamic changes during the entire experiment procedure.
2. This procedure permits penetration into the peritoneal cavity without injuring viscera. If the injection has been performed in the correct manner, the animal should be under general anesthesia within 5 min. One-man procedure is less precise. During this technique, the operator holds the animal by the

skin of the back and neck in his left hand and injects into the same quadrant.

3. The current technique should be performed on 12 h fasted rodents.
4. Anesthesia level is assessed by testing corneal reflexes and motor responses to tail or inter-finger membrane pinch.
5. The extravasated dye is not removed by saline perfusion.
6. You can use different rodent species. Use male rats, indifferently Sprague-Dawley or Wistar, with body weight ranging 250–400 g in order to obtain an optimal cranial window.
7. During the whole experiment, the filling of the cranial window with SIF should be strictly checked.
8. Stimuli are physical, as electrical stimulation, or chemical. For electrical stimulation a parasagittal slit of about 2×6 mm to place the electrodes (wire diameter 0.2 mm, distance 1 mm, length of 4 mm) is performed. Wires must get in touch with the dural surface along their whole length parallel to the sagittal suture. The slit must be filled with a cotton pad soaked with liquid paraffin. Chemical stimuli could be given either intravenously or topically. After topical administration, you have to wash the cranial window with SIF in order to remove possible residuals before administration of the same or different substance.
9. Additional stimuli could be used to trigger CSD including, exposure to high concentrations of excitatory amino acids (26), direct electrical stimulation (27), direct cortical trauma (28).

References

1. (2004) The International Classification of Headache Disorders, 2nd edn. Cephalalgia 24:9–160
2. Lipton RB, Stewart WF, Diamond S, Diamond ML, Reed M (2001) Prevalence and burden of migraine in the United States: data from the American Migraine Study II. Headache 41:646–657
3. Burton WN, Conti DJ, Chen CY, Schultz AB, Edington DW (2002) The economic burden of lost productivity due to migraine headache: a specific worksite analysis. J Occup Environ Med 44:523–529
4. Ferrari MD (2008) Migraine genetics: a fascinating journey towards improved migraine therapy. Headache 48:697–700
5. Holzer P, Wachter C, Heinemann A, Jocic M, Lippe IT, Herbert MK (1995) Sensory nerves, nitric oxide and NANC vasodilatation. Arch Int Pharmacodyn Ther 329:67–79
6. Goadsby PJ (2005) Migraine pathophysiology. Headache 45:S14–S24
7. Geppetti P, Capone JG, Trevisani M, Nicoletti P, Zagli G, Tola MR (2005) CGRP and migraine: neurogenic inflammation revisited. J Headache Pain 6:61–70
8. Moskowitz MA, Macfarlane R (1993) Neurovascular and molecular mechanisms in migraine headaches. Cerebrovasc Brain Metab Rev 5:159–177
9. Saito K, Markowitz S, Moskowitz MA (1988) Ergot alkaloids block neurogenic extravasation in dura mater: proposed action in vascular headaches. Ann Neurol 24:732–737
10. Kurosawa M, Messlinger K, Pawlak M, Schmidt RF (1995) Increase of meningeal blood flow after electrical stimulation of rat dura mater encephali: mediation by calcitonin gene-related peptide. Br J Pharmacol 114: 1397–1402

11. Gerrits RJ, Stein EA, Greene AS (1998) Laser-Doppler flowmetry utilizing a thinned skull cranial window preparation and automated stimulation. Brain Res Brain Res Protoc 3:14–21
12. Dux M, Santha P, Jancso G (2003) Capsaicin-sensitive neurogenic sensory vasodilatation in the dura mater of the rat. J Physiol 552: 859–867
13. Petersen KA, Birk S, Doods H, Edvinsson L, Olesen J (2004) Inhibitory effect of BIBN 4096BS on cephalic vasodilatation induced by CGRP or transcranial electrical stimulation in the rat. Br J Pharmacol 143:697–704
14. Leao AA (1986) Spreading depression. Funct Neurol 1:363–366
15. Dalsgaard-Nielsen T (1955) Migraine diagnostics with special reference to pharmacological tests. Int Arch Allergy Appl Immunol 7:312–322
16. Ahlner J, Andersson RG, Torfgard K, Axelsson KL (1991) Organic nitrate esters: clinical use and mechanisms of actions. Pharmacol Rev 43:351–423
17. Sicuteri F, Del Bene E, Poggioni M, Bonazzi A (1987) Unmasking latent dysnociception in healthy subjects. Headache 27:180–185
18. Iversen HK, Olesen J, Tfelt-Hansen P (1989) Intravenous nitroglycerin as an experimental model of vascular headache. Basic characteristics. Pain 38:17–24
19. Sances G, Tassorelli C, Pucci E, Ghiotto N, Sandrini G, Nappi G (2004) Reliability of the nitroglycerin provocative test in the diagnosis of neurovascular headaches. Cephalalgia 24:110–119
20. de Hoon JN, Pickkers P, Smits P, Struijker-Boudier HA, Van Bortel LM (2003) Calcitonin gene-related peptide: exploring its vasodilating mechanism of action in humans. Clin Pharmacol Ther 73:312–321
21. Jansen-Olesen I, Mortensen A, Edvinsson L (1996) Calcitonin gene-related peptide is released from capsaicin-sensitive nerve fibres and induces vasodilatation of human cerebral arteries concomitant with activation of adenylyl cyclase. Cephalalgia 16:310–316
22. Goadsby PJ, Edvinsson L, Ekman R (1990) Vasoactive peptide release in the extracerebral circulation of humans during migraine headache. Ann Neurol 28:183–187
23. Olesen J, Diener HC, Husstedt IW, Goadsby PJ, Hall D, Meier U, Pollentier S, Lesko LM (2004) Calcitonin gene-related peptide receptor antagonist BIBN 4096 BS for the acute treatment of migraine. N Engl J Med 350:1104–1110
24. Ho TW, Mannix LK, Fan X, Assaid C, Furtek C, Jones CJ, Lines CR, Rapoport AM (2008) Randomized controlled trial of an oral CGRP receptor antagonist, MK-0974, in acute treatment of migraine. Neurology 70:1304–1312
25. Frobert Y, Nevers MC, Amadesi S, Volland H, Brune P, Geppetti P, Grassi J, Creminon C (1999) A sensitive sandwich enzyme immunoassay for calcitonin gene-related peptide (CGRP): characterization and application. Peptides 20:275–284
26. Kraig RP, Cooper AJ (1987) Bicarbonate and ammonia changes in brain during spreading depression. Can J Physiol Pharmacol 65:1099–1104
27. Ayata C, Jin H, Kudo C, Dalkara T, Moskowitz MA (2006) Suppression of cortical spreading depression in migraine prophylaxis. Ann Neurol 59:652–661
28. Echlin FA (1950) Spreading depression of electrical activity in the cerebral cortex following local trauma and its possible role in concussion. Arch Neurol Psychiatry 63: 830–832

Chapter 10

Experimental Models of Visceral Pain

Mia Karpitschka and Martin E. Kreis

Abstract

Visceral pain models are used to study afferent nerve traffic during noxious stimulation at the level of the visceral organ. This chapter provides details on several in vitro and in vivo models of organs in the gastrointestinal and genitourinary tract that use electrophysiological recordings of afferent nerve fibres in order to directly characterize stimulus-response relationships. These models can also be used to investigate stimulus–response patterns during physiological (nonpainful) stimulation of the visceral organs or during exposure to pathological stimuli, such as inflammatory mediators during inflammation of the visceral organ.

Key words: Visceral pain, Electrophysiology, Inflammation, Gastrointestinal tract, Genitourinary tract

1. Introduction

Visceral pain is transmitted via C-fibres to the central nervous system, while somatic pain is relayed by Aδ-fibres. The latter is characterized by well-localized, sharp or burning pain contrary to visceral pain, which is typically colicky, dull or aching, coming from ill-defined locations in the organ of origin. When studying somatic pain in animal models, the localization where the preparation stems from in the organism is of secondary importance since virtually the same mechanisms are relevant everywhere. This is different for visceral organs as each may be innervated by different populations of afferent nerve fibres; in addition, the relative content of subpopulations in afferent nerve bundles is variable.

In this chapter, different models of visceral pain arising from the genitourinary and gastrointestinal tracts are described. It is beyond the scope of this article to include all the available models

Arpad Szallasi (ed.), *Analgesia: Methods and Protocols*, Methods in Molecular Biology, vol. 617,
DOI 10.1007/978-1-60327-323-7_10, © Springer Science+Business Media, LLC 2010

or to describe models for all the visceral organs. Models may be classified as (1) those that employ direct electrophysiological afferent nerve recordings and (2) those that quantify stimulus–response patterns indirectly by behavioral changes. The latter are comparatively simple models, and therefore, have not been included in this chapter, electrophysiological recordings from visceral organs, however, are demanding and require a long learning curve at times.

In general, electrophysiological recordings from visceral organs to study pain may be undertaken in vitro or in vivo. While the in vivo approach ensures the viability of the organ recorded from, in vitro models have the advantage that confounding factors such as blood pressure and anaesthesia are eliminated. The appropriate model, therefore, needs to be chosen by considering and weighing the advantages and disadvantages of in vivo and in vitro preparations in the light of the aims and hypothesis of the planned investigation.

2. Materials

2.1. Small Bowel of Rat and Mouse In Vivo

1. Rats weighing about 300 g (e.g. male Sprague–Dawley rats from Harlan Industries, San Diego, CA) or mice weighing about 20 g (e.g. male C57BL/6 mice from Charles River, Sulzfeld, Germany) (see Note 1).
2. Heparinized catheter (200 U/ml heparin in saline) to cannulate the left carotid artery for arterial pressure recording. Keep heparin in a tightly closed container; store in a cool, dry, ventilated area before using it for catheter preparation.
3. Pentobarbitone sodium (e.g. Nembutal Sodium®, Abbott GmbH & Co KG, Wiesbaden, Germany) for intraperitoneal (i.p.) injection or intravenous infusion to produce anaesthesia in rats. The injectable product should be stored at room temperature.
4. Ketamine (Ketalar®, Park Davis, Caringbah, NSW, Australia), xylazine (e.g. Rompun®, Bayer, Botany, NSW, Australia) and acepromazine (e.g. Boehringer Ingelheim, Ingelheim, Germany) for intraperitoneal (i.p.) injection or intravenous infusion to produce anaesthesia in mice. Substances should be stored below 30°C (86°F).
5. 2-methyl-5-hydroxytryptamine (2-m-5-HT, e.g. Sigma-Aldrich, Castle Hill, NSW, Australia) to assess the viability of the preparation.
6. Heavy liquid paraffin (BDH, Poole, UK) prewarmed to a temperature of 37°C for electrical isolation within the nerve dissection area.

7. Rectal thermometer to monitor body temperature.
8. Homeothermic heating blanket (Harvard Apparatus, Holliston, Massachusetts, USA) to maintain body temperature.
9. A 20 mm diameter steel ring (dimensions for the mouse) to stabilize the intraoperative situs.
10. A pair of platinum wire recording electrodes, of about 0.25 mm diameter (e.g. Conatex, Neunkirchen, Germany).
11. Fine tip watchmaker's forceps and iris scissors (e.g. Fine Science Tools GmbH, Wesseling-Berzdorf, Germany).
12. Dissection microscope (e.g. model M900, D.F. Vasconcellos S.A., Sao Paulo, Brazil).
13. Fiber-optic light source (e.g. KL 2500 LCD, Schott, New York, NY) for illumination during nerve preparation.
14. Neurolog pressure amplifier NL108 (Digitimer, Welwyn, Garden City, UK) for arterial pressure recording.
15. 3.5 cm balloon (diameter 0.8 cm, CR Baird Inc., Kedah, Malaysia) to perform distensions of the jejunum.
16. A distension control device, e.g. computer-driven Barostat with Protocol PlusTM Deluxe software (Distender Series IIR, G & J Electronics, Ontario, Canada) to perform distensions of the jejunum.
17. Single channel 1902 amplifier (Cambridge Electronic Design, Cambridge, UK).
18. Micro 1401 interface (Cambridge Electronic Design).
19. PC running "Spike 2" software version 4.13 (Cambridge Electronic Design).

2.2. Small Bowel of the Rat and Mouse In Vitro

1. Rats weighing about 300 g (e.g. Male Sprague–Dawley rats from Harlan Industries) or mice weighing about 20 g (e.g. male C57BL/6 mice from Charles River) (see Note 1).
2. An organ bath consisting of two separate compartments was especially designed for this experimental method (1–3). All indicated values concerning the dimensions of the organ bath refer to experiments with the rat; for mouse experiments, the required dimensions are proportionately smaller (and not always indicated).

   The organ bath (see Fig. 1) consists of a milled perspex block with internal dimensions of about 80 mm × 60 mm and a depth of ca. 25 mm. The volume of the bath with the dissection platform in place should be about 45 cm^3 (for the mouse about 20 cm^3). Incorporated into the bath is a heating coil consisting of tungsten resistance wire coiled inside a thin-walled glass tube, inserted into the base of the bath and sealed with Sylgard (Dow Corning; Ajax Chemicals Pty Ltd, Auburn, NSW, Australia). The heater is controlled by the output from

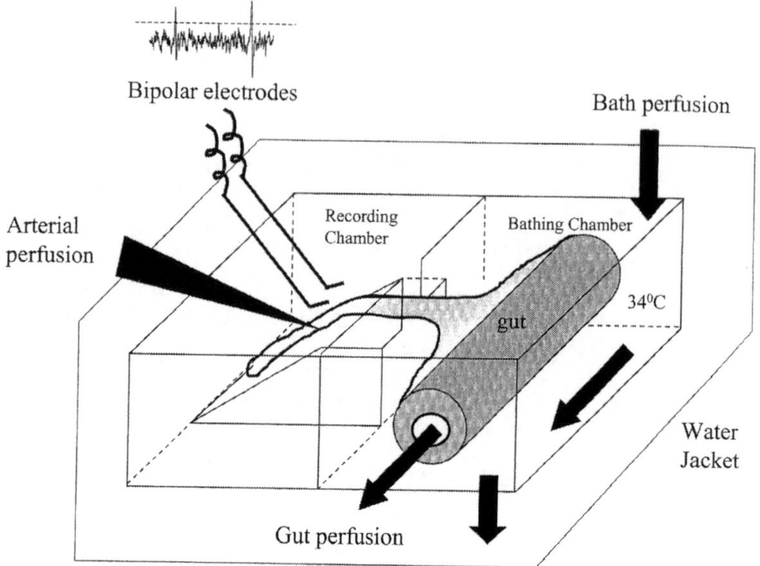

Fig. 1. Summary diagram and apparatus used to record afferent discharge (AD), vascular perfusion pressure (VPP), and gut perfusion pressure (GPP) simultaneously in a segment of rat jejunum in vitro

a homeothermic blanket controller (CFP Instruments, BioScience, UK) and regulated by a thermistor probe inserted just above the coil through a hole in the wall of the bath.

(a) One of the two compartments of the organ bath represents the *organ chamber*, in which the gut is placed. During experiment, this chamber is filled with Kreb's solution (saturated with O_2/CO_2 as described below) by means of an inlet port, allowing for serosal perfusion of the gut at a rate of 5–10 ml/min. The liquid level of the bath is controlled by means of a vertically adjustable outlet attached to a suction pump. The gut "tube" in the organ chamber is cannulated at both ends by a short length of glass cannulas (5 mm external diameter) passed through a hole in the wall of the bath, enabling perfusion through the gut lumen (Kreb's buffer, 1 ml/min). The aboral end of the segment under investigastion is connected to a pressure transducer (DTXPlus transducer, Ohmeda, Singapore) to record changes in intraluminal pressure (see Note 2).

(b) The second chamber of the organ bath, the *recording chamber*, represents a dissection platform for nerve preparation and forms a rectangular perspex block with internal dimensions of about 40 mm × 45 mm and a depth of ca. 8 mm. There is a 1 mm wide slit in the centre of the platform, through which the mesenteric arcade of the gut can be passed.

3. Kreb's solution: 117 mM NaCl, 4.7 mM KCl, 25 mM $NaHCO_3$, 1.2 mM NaH_2PO_4, 1.2 mM $MgCl_2$,11 mM glucose and 2.5 mM $CaCl_2$; pH maintained at 7.4 with 95% O_2/5% CO_2.
4. Modified Kreb's solution: Kreb's solution supplemented with 3% Dextran and 0.6 mM glutamine; superfused with 95% O_2/5% CO_2.
5. Pentobarbitone sodium (Abbott GmbH & Co KG) for intraperitoneal (i.p.) injection to produce anaesthesia. The injectable product should be stored at room temperature;

   Alternatively: Ketamine (e.g. Bioniche Pharma), xylazine (e.g. Bayer) and acepromazine (e.g. Boehringer Ingelheim) for intraperitoneal (i.p.) injection. Substances should be stored below 30°C (86°F).
6. Vaseline.
7. Heavy liquid paraffin (BDH) prewarmed to a temperature of 37°C for electrical isolation within the nerve dissection area.
8. A fine polyethylene cannula to cannulate the mesenteric artery for intravascular perfusion or drug administration via a peristaltic pump (Watson-Marlow, Falmouth, Cornwall, UK).
9. Pressure transducer (Transpac IV, Abbot Ireland, Sligo, Republic of Ireland) to monitor vascular perfusion pressure (VPP).
10. A pair of platinum wire recording electrodes, of about 0.25 mm diameter (e.g. Conatex).
11. Fine tip watchmaker's forceps and iris scissors (e.g. Fine Science Tools GmbH).
12. A dissection microscope.
13. Fiber-optic light source (Schott) for illumination during nerve preparation.
14. Neurolog headstage NL100 (Cambridge Electronic Design).
15. Neurolog preamplifier NL104 (Cambridge Electronic Design).
16. Neurolog filter NL125 (Cambridge Electronic Design).
17. Spike processor (e.g. Digitimer D130, Digitimer).
18. Oscilloscope (e.g. Tektronix TDS 210, Telektronix GmbH, Cologne, Germany).
19. Micro 1401 interface (Cambridge Electronic Design).
20. PC running "Spike 2" software version 4.13 (Cambridge Electronic Design).

2.3. Colon of the Rat In Vitro

1. Rats weighing 150–250 g (e.g. male Sprague–Dawley rats from Harlan Industries).
2. An organ bath was designed by Lynn et al. (4): it is laterally divided into two compartments (see Fig. 2).

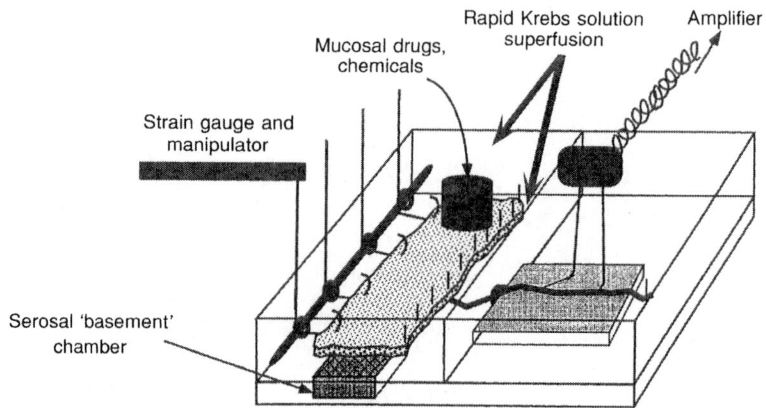

Fig. 2. Diagram of the organ bath used to record from colonic afferents. The bath has two compartments. The compartment on the left with two chambers holds the colon, which is opened out and placed mucosa side uppermost over the basement chamber. The distal colon is pinned down on the right (mesenteric) side. The left side is attached to a pulley system via silk thread. Modified Kreb's solution is superfused over both surfaces of the colon. Drugs are applied locally to the site of the receptive field which is isolated with a metal ring. Single fibre recordings are taken from the intermesenteric-lumbar splanchnic nerve bundle which has been passed through into the right-hand oil-filled compartment

(a) One compartment, the *colonic compartment*, is superfused with Kreb's solution and accommodates the colon. This compartment is further divided into two chambers, one above the other. The colon is mounted mucosal side up in the upper *mucosal chamber*, so that the serosal surface lies directly over the lower basement *serosal chamber*. The smaller *serosal chamber* therefore provides superfusion of Kreb's solution to the *serosal* surface of the colon, whilst the *mucosal chamber* above provides superfusion to the *mucosal* surface of the tissue. The colon is pinned down along the side closest to the nerves, and the opposite edge of the colon is attached at 1 cm intervals to silk threads, which are passed through a pulley system. Each thread can be attached to isometric or isotonic force transducers to measure local motility changes and to apply mechanical stimuli (see Note 17).

(b) The other compartment, the *recording compartment*, is filled with heavy liquid paraffin oil and contains the neurovascular bundle.

3. Modified Kreb's solution: 117.9 mM NaCl, 4.7 mM KCl, 25 mM $NaHCO_3$, 1.3 mM NaH_2PO_4, 1.2 mM $MgSO_4(H_2O)_7$, 2.5 mM $CaCl_2$; pH maintained at 7.4 with 95% O_2/5% CO_2.

   (a) For perfusion of the serosal chamber, 11.1 mM a-D-glucose, 3 μM indomethacin and 1 mM nifedipine are added to the modified Kreb's solution. The temperature of the Kreb's solution should be about 21 °C (see Note 16).

(b) For perfusion of the *mucosal chamber*, 3 μM indomethacin and 1 mM nifedipine are added to the modified Kreb's solution. Short-chain fatty acids butyrate (2 mM) and acetate (20 mM) are added as well (instead of glucose as for perfusion of the *serosal chamber*). The temperature of the Kreb's solution should be about 21°C (see Note 16).

(c) For dissection of the tissue, 1 mM sodium butyrate, 10 mM sodium acetate, 5.55 mM glucose, and 3 μM indomethacin are added to the modified Kreb's solution. The temperature of Kreb's solution should be ice-cold.

4. Ether to produce sedation in rats. Substance should be stored below 30°C (86°F).
5. Pentobarbitone sodium (Abbott GmbH & Co KG) for intraperitoneal (i.p.) injection to produce anaesthesia in rats. The injectable product should be stored at room temperature.
6. Pair of platinum wire recording electrodes, about 0.25 mm diameter (e.g. Conatex).
7. Fine watchmakers forceps and iris scissors (e.g. Fine Science Tools GmbH).
8. Dissection microscope (e.g. model M900) (D.F. Vasconcellos S.A.).
9. Fiber-optic light source (KL 2500 LCD) (Schott) for illumination during nerve preparation.
10. Biological amplifier (BA1, JRAK, Melbourne, Australia).
11. Scaling amplifier (SA1, JRAK).
12. Filter (F1 filter, JRAK).
13. Oscilloscope (e.g. Tektronix TDS 210, Telektronix GmbH).
14. Micro 1401 interface (Cambridge Electronic Design).
15. PC running "Spike 2" software version 4.13 (Cambridge Electronic Design).
16. Glass rods (tip contact area 6 mm^2).
17. Fine paint brushes.
18. Calibrated von Frey hairs (0.1–10 mN).
19. A 1 cm diameter ring for application of chemical substances.

2.4. Stomach of the Rat In Vivo

1. Rats weighing 400–500 g (e.g. male Sprague–Dawley rats from Harlan) (see Note 24).
2. Pentobarbitone sodium (Abbott GmbH & Co KG) for intraperitoneal (i.p.) injection to produce anaesthesia in rats. The injectable product should be stored at room temperature.
3. Pentobarbitone for intravenous (i.v.) infusion to maintain anaesthesia in rats.

4. 5% dextrose in saline to influence the mean arterial pressure.
5. Pancuronium bromide to paralyze the rat.
6. Nonreactive Wacker gel (Wacker Silicone, Adrian, MI).
7. Heavy liquid paraffin (BDH) prewarmed to a temperature of 37°C for electrical isolation within the nerve dissection area.
8. Homeothermic heating blanket (Harvard Apparatus) to maintain body temperature.
9. Overhead feedback-controlled heat lamp to maintain body temperature.
10. Teflon-coated, 40-gauge stainless steel wires stripped at the tips.
11. 2.0–2.5 cm long, 2–3 cm diameter flaccid, flexible latex balloon for phasic balloon gastric distension (GD).
12. Flexible plastic tubing (Tygon, Fisher Scientific Co., Pittsburgh, PA; 2.3 mm OD, 1.3 mm ID) for insertion into the cardia during fluid gastric distension.
13. Flexible plastic tubing (Fisher Scientific Co; 3.9 mm OD, 2.4 mm ID) for insertion into the pylorus during fluid gastric distension.
14. Pressure transducer (Transpac IV, Abbot Ireland) to measure blood pressure.
15. Pressure transducer (NL108T2, Digitimer) to record intragastric pressure.
16. A distension control device, e.g. computer-driven Barostat with Protocol PlusTM Deluxe software (Distender Series IIR, G & J Electronics, Ontario, Canada) to perform distensions of the jejunum.
17. Reservoir containing saline at room temperature for fluid gastric distension.
18. A steel ring to stabilize the intraoperative situs.
19. Bipolar silver–silver chloride electrodes.
20. Oscilloscope (e.g. DL 1200A, Yokogawa, Tokyo, Japan).
21. Micro 1401 interface (Cambridge Electronic Design).
22. PC running "Spike 2" software version 4.13 (Cambridge Electronic Design).

2.5. Esophagus of Ferret and Mouse In Vitro (see Fig. 3)

1. Mice weighing about 20–30 g (e.g. male C57BL/6 mice from Charles River) and ferrets weighing about 0.4–1.0 kg (e.g. Charles River, Yokohama, Japan).
2. An organ bath containing of two chambers (5):
   (a) An *organ ch*amber with dimensions about 13.0 cm × 4.0 cm × 1.0 cm for the ferret and 6.0 × 2.5 × 1.2 cm for the mouse.

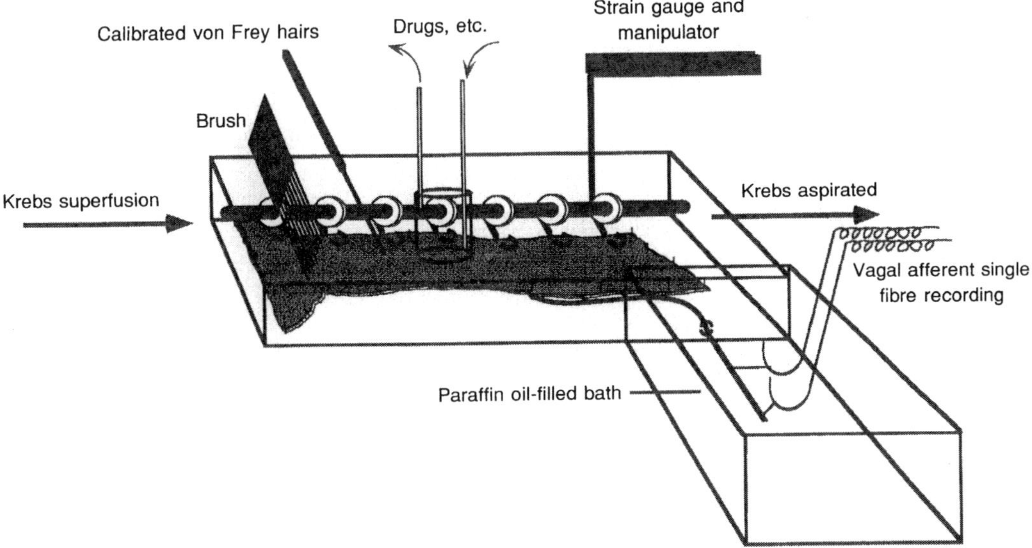

Fig. 3. Schematic diagram of the apparatus used for recording single gastro-esophageal afferent fibres in vitro. This comprises a Perspex chamber in which the esophagus and part of the stomach is pinned mucosa uppermost. The vagus nerve is drawn into a second chamber where fibres are teased back onto a recording electrode. Drugs are applied to the afferent fibre receptive field using a small cylinder. Circular tension is applied to the tissue via a pulley system connected to a balance. The pulley system is also used in conjunction with a force transducer to measure muscular activity. The pulley system is always hooked to the edge of the esophagus adjacent to the receptive field

(b) An isolated *recording chamber* with dimensions about 5.0 cm × 5.0 cm × 1.0 cm for the ferret and 3.7 cm × 3.7 × 1.2 cm for the mouse.

3. Modified Kreb's solution: 118.1 mM NaCl, 4.7 mM KCl, 25.1 mM $NaHCO_3$, 1.3 mM Na_2PO_4, 1.2 mM MgCl, 1.5 mM $CaCl_2$, 1.0 mM citric acid, 11.1 mM glucose; with 95% O_2/5% CO_2.
4. Pentobarbitone sodium (Abbott GmbH & Co KG) for intraperitoneal (i.p.) injection to produce anaesthesia in rats. The injectable product should be stored at room temperature.
5. Heavy liquid paraffin (BDH) prewarmed to a temperature of 37°C for electrical isolation within the nerve dissection area.
6. Pair of platinum wire recording electrodes, about 0.25 mm diameter (Conatex).
7. Fine watchmakers forceps and iris scissors (Fine Science Tools GmbH).
8. Dissection microscope (e.g. model M900) (D.F. Vasconcellos S.A.).
9. Fibre-optic light source (e.g. KL 2500 LCD) (Schott) for illumination during nerve preparation.
10. Biological amplifier (BA1, JRAK).

11. Scaling amplifier (SA1, JRAK).
12. Filter (F1 filter, JRAK).
13. Oscilloscope (e.g. DL 1200A, Yokogawa, Tokyo, Japan).
14. PC running "Spike 2" software version 4.13 (Cambridge Electronic Design).
15. Blunt glass rods/brushes.
16. 1,000 mg von Frey probes.
17. A pulley and cantilever system.
18. A small cylindrical chamber (1 cm diameter) for introducing agents to receptive fields.

2.6. Pancreas of the Rat In Vitro

1. Rats weighing 200–300 g (e.g. male Sprague–Dawley rats from Harlan Industries) (see Note 34).
2. Pentobarbitone sodium (e.g. Nembutal Sodium®, Abbott GmbH & Co KG) for intraperitoneal (i.p.) injection to produce anaesthesia in rats. The injectable product should be stored at room temperature.
3. Modified Kreb's solution: 151 mM Na^+, 4.7 MK^+, 2.8 M Ca^{2+}, 0.6 mM Mg^{2+}, 143,7 mM Cl^-, 1.3 mM $H_2PO_4^-$, 16.3 mM HCO_3^-, 0.6 mM SO_4^{2-}, 7.7 mM glucose; pH maintained at 7.4 with 95% O_2/5% CO_2.
4. Dex–Kreb's solution (see Note 37): modified Kreb's solution is supplemented with Dextran (MW 64,000–76,000; Sigma-Aldrich) at 1.5% w/v, protease inhibitor cocktail at 0.2 ml/L (Sigma-Aldrich) and soybean trypsin–chymotrypsin inhibitor at 2 mg/L (Sigma-Aldrich). The Dex–Kreb's is maintained at 4°C until just prior to the commencement of the stabilization period when it is warmed via a heat exchanger to achieve and maintain a bath temperature of 32–33°C.
5. Peristaltic pump (Watson-Marlow, Falmouth, Cornwall, UK) for perfusion of the organ bath.
6. Dissection dish lined with Sylgard (Dow Corning).
7. A 24G Optiva® i.v. catheter (Smiths Medical, Carlsbad, CA) for cannulation of the hepatic termination of the common bile duct (CBD).
8. A polyvinyl catheter (0.5 mm OD, 0.2 mm ID, 10 cm in length) for perfusion of the CBD.
9. A manometer for measuring the concurrent distension of the CBD and pancreatic duct (PD).
10. Vaseline.
11. Pair of platinum wire recording electrodes, about 0.25 mm diameter (Conatex).
12. Fine watchmakers forceps and iris scissors (e.g. Fine Science Tools GmbH).

13. Dissection microscope (e.g. model M900) (D.F. Vasconcellos S.A.).
14. Fibre-optic light source (e.g. KL 2500 LCD) (Schott), for illumination during nerve preparation.
15. DAM50 differential amplifier (World Precision Instruments, Sarasota, FL).
16. BPF-932 band-pass filter (CWE Inc., Ardmore, PA).
17. Audio mixer, e.g. Stereo Sound Mixer CE (Jaycar Pty Ltd., Adelaide, SA, Australia).
18. PowerLab recording system using Chart v5.1 (ADInstruments, Castle Hill, NSW, Australia) for monitoring and recording of nerve discharges.
19. A Grass S48 stimulator (Grass Medical Instruments Company, Quincy, MA).
20. Custom-designed search probe allowing focal electrical stimulation at 20 V, 0.5 ms duration via a Grass S48 stimulator (see Note 38) to search for receptive fields. This probe consists of a custom-built concentric electrode (1.2 mm OD) with an adapted blunt end (tip radius ~ 2 mm) which permits simultaneous mechanical probing of the tissue surface.
21. Stainless steel well (1 cm OD) for drug application.

2.7. Gall Bladder of the Possum In Vivo

1. Australian Brush-tailed possums (*Trichosurus vulpecula*), body weight about 1.5 kg, from Harlan Industries (San Diego, CA) (see Note 41).
2. Xylazine (Rompun®, Bayer) and ketamine (Ketalar®, Park Davis) for intraperitoneal (i.p.) injection to produce anaesthesia in mice.for anaesthesia.
3. Thiopentone (Pentothal®, Abbott).
4. Lethabarb® (Virbac Pty, Ltd., Baronia, Vic, Australia).
5. Heavy liquid paraffin (BDH) prewarmed to a temperature of 37°C for electrical isolation within the nerve dissection area.
6. Gelfoam (Upjohn, Pty Ltd., Rydalmere, NSW, Australia) to prevent the exposed nerve trunk from drying out.
7. Polyvinyl catheters (1.5 mm OD, 0.9 mm ID) to cannulate the left femoral artery (for maintaining anaesthesia) and to cannulate the right femoral vein (for maintaining hydration).
8. Balloon catheters (catheter 2.4 mm OD, 1 mm ID, 40 mm balloon length) for insertion into the *gall bladder* or the *duodenum*.
9. A 22 g and 24 g indwelling catheter (Optiva, Medex Medical Ltd., Rossendale, Lancashire, UK) for insertion into the proximal *common bile duct (CBD)* and *pancreatic duct (PD)*.

10. A polyvinyl catheter (4.8 mm OD, 2.9 mm ID) for insertion into the *duodenum* during vagal nerve recording.
11. A Foley balloon catheter (4.7 mm, CR Baird Inc.) for insertion into the *stomach* to achieve gastric balloon distension.
12. Animal ventilator (Phipps and Bird Inc., Richmond, VA).
13. Fluid manometers.
14. Homeothermic heating blanket (Harvard Apparatus).
15. Pressure transducer (Transpac IV, Abbot Ireland) to measure blood pressure.
16. PowerLab recording system (ADInstruments) using Chart (5.1) software to constantly monitor blood pressure.
17. 10 cm diameter copper ring (2.2 mm OD) to provide good earthing for *splanchnic* nerve recordings. For *vagal* nerve recordings, a 5 cm diameter copper ring (1 mm OD) is used (see Note 42).
18. A water-heated perspex box to maintain animal body temperature.
19. A purpose-built acrylic recording chamber with glass base (about 2 × 3 cm).
20. Pair of platinum wire recording electrodes, about 0.25 mm diameter (Conatex).
21. Fine watchmakers forceps and iris scissors (e.g. Fine Science Tools GmbH).
22. Dissection microscope (e.g. model M900) (D.F. Vasconcellos S.A.).
23. Fibre-optic light source (e.g. KL 2500 LCD) (Schott) for illumination during nerve preparation.
24. DAM50 differential amplifier (World Precision Instruments).
25. BPF-932 band-pass filter (CWE Inc.).
26. Audio mixer, e.g. Stereo Sound Mixer CE (Jaycar Pty Ltd.).
27. PowerLab recording system using Chart v5.1 (ADInstruments) for monitoring and recording of nerve discharges.

2.8. Urinary Bladder of the Mouse In Vitro

1. Mice weighing about 25–30 g (e.g. male C57BL/6 mice from Charles River).
2. Kreb's solution: 120 mM NaCl 120, 5.9 mM KCl, 1.2 mM NaH_2PO_4, 1.2 mM $MgSO_4$, 15.4 mM $NaHCO_3$, 2.5 mM $CaCl_2$, 11.5 mM glucose; maintained at 7.4 with 95% O_2/5% CO_2.
3. Fine metal rod, e.g. 25 G needle (Becton–Dickinson) for insertion into the lumen of the urinary bladder.

4. Syringe-type infusion pump (e.g. sp210iw, World Precision Instruments) for infusion in and withdrawal from the urinary bladder at a constant rate.
5. A 100 ml Hamilton syringe for intravesical injection of drugs into the urinary bladder.
6. Pressure transducer (NL108T2, Digitimer) for recording of intraluminal pressure in the urinary bladder.
7. A suction glass electrode (tip diameter, 50–100 mm) for recording the nerve activity.
8. Fine watchmakers forceps and iris scissors (e.g. Fine Science Tools GmbH).
9. Dissection microscope (e.g. model M900) (D.F. Vasconcellos S.A.).
10. Fibre-optic light source (e.g. KL 2500 LCD) (Schott) for illumination during nerve preparation.
11. Neurolog headstage NL100 (Cambridge Electronic Design).
12. Neurolog preamplifier NL104 (Cambridge Electronic Design).
13. Neurolog filter NL125 (Cambridge Electronic Design).
14. Spike processor (e.g. Digitimer D130, Digitimer).
15. Oscilloscope (e.g. Tektronix TDS 210, Telektronix GmbH).
16. Micro 1401 interface (Cambridge Electronic Design).
17. PC running "Spike 2" software version 4.13 (Cambridge Electronic Design).

2.9. Ureter of the Guinea-Pig In Vitro

1. Guinea pigs weighing 300–400 g (e.g. from Harlan Industries).
2. An organ bath (outer dimensions about 108 × 80 × 25 mm) consisting of two parts was especially designed (6) for this experimental setup (see Fig. 4).
   (a) an *oxygenating chamber* (volume ~20 ml) and a *main chamber* (~35 ml) including a 5 mm high rubber platform for the mounting of the ureter. Heating coils controlled by a feed-back electronic device and a thermistor fixed close to a heating coil near the platform are used to maintain the bath temperature at 37 ± 1°C. The main chamber is continuously perfused with synthetic interstitial fluid (SIF) via the oxygenating chamber at a flow rate of 3–4 ml/min. The bath level should be kept at 2–3 mm above the platform by an adjustable suction tube. The ureter is fixed onto the rubber platform and cannulated through both ends (cannula outer diameter 0.75–1.00 mm, or, if the kidney pelvis is included 1.34 mm).

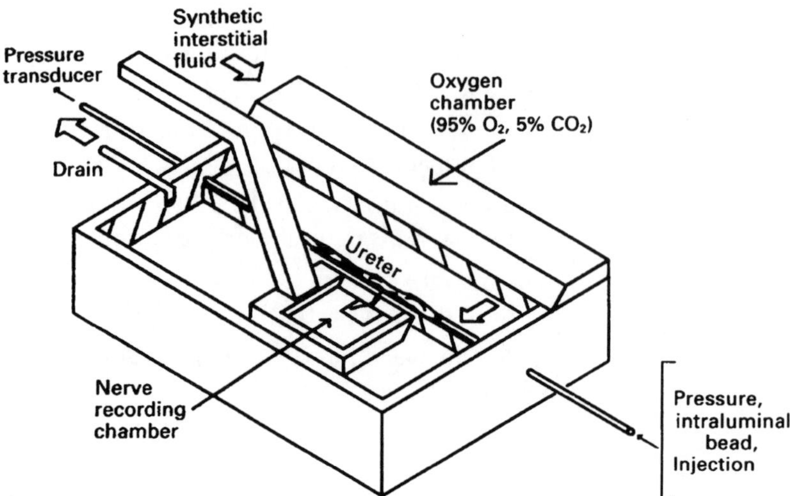

Fig. 4. Schematic diagram of the organ bath used for the recording of single units from the guinea pig ureter. The organ bath is continuously perfused (3–4 ml/main) with synthetic interstitial fluid (SIF) which is oxygenated in a oxygenation chamber. The bath temperature is kept at 37°C and the intraluminal pressure is continuously monitored. The ureter is cannulated and mounted on a rubber platform. Recordings of afferent nerve activity are made from fine ureteric nerves in a movable nerve recording chamber. Increases in intraluminal pressure, insertion of intraluminal glass beads and probing of the ureteric wall can be used as mechanical stimuli

(b) a movable *recording chamber* (outer dimensions about 40 mm × 30 mm × 5 mm) filled with warm heavy liquid paraffin. Between both chambers, there is a small slot (0.5 mm) through which the nerves can be passed. A small sponge in the slot between both chambers prevents leakage between both chambers.

3. Synthetic interstitial fluid (SIF): 107.7 mM NaCl, 3.48 mM KCl, 1.53 mM $CaCl_2$, 20.2 mM $MgSO_4$, 26.2 mM $NaHCO_3$, 1.67 mM NaH_2PO_4, 9.64 mM sodium gluconate, 5.55 mM glucose, and 7.6 mM sucrose; pH maintained at 7.4 with 95% O_2/5% CO_2.
4. Pressure transducer (NL108T2, Digitimer) for recording of intraluminal pressure.
5. A fine platinum wire about 0.25 mm diameter (Conatex), which is attached to a small manipulator mounted directly onto the recording chamber (not shown in Fig. 10.4) to perform monopolar recordings of electrical activity and a silver–silver chloride pellet as the indifferent electrode.
6. Fine watchmakers forceps and iris scissors (e.g. Fine Science Tools GmbH).
7. Dissection microscope (e.g. model M900) (D.F. Vasconcellos S.A.).
8. Fibre-optic light source (e.g. KL 2500 LCD) (Schott) for illumination during nerve preparation.

9. Biological amplifier (BA1, JRAK).
10. Scaling amplifier (SA1, JRAK).
11. Filter (F1 filter, JRAK).
12. Micro 1401 interface (Cambridge Electronic Design).
13. PC running "Spike 2" software version 4.13 (Cambridge Electronic Design).
14. Small blunt glass probes (diameter 0.5 mm)

2.10. Testis of the Dog In Vitro

1. Male mongrel dogs.
2. Pentobarbitone sodium (e.g. Nembutal Sodium®, Abbott Gmbh) for intraperitoneal (i.p.) injection or intravenous infusion to produce anaesthesia in rats. The injectable product should be stored at room temperature.
3. Homeothermic heating blanket (Harvard Apparatus).
4. Modified Kreb's solution: 110.9 mM NaCl, 4.8 mM KCl, 2.5 mM $CaCl_2$, 1.2 mM $MgSO_4$, 1.2 mM KH_2PO_4, 24.4 mM $NaHCO_3$, 20 mM glucose; pH maintained at 7.4 with 95% O_2/5% CO_2.
5. Heavy liquid paraffin (BDH) prewarmed to a temperature of 37°C for electrical isolation within the nerve dissection area.
6. Vaseline.
7. A copper-constantan thermocouple.
8. Glass rods with a small rounded tip.
9. Calibrated von Frey-type nylon hairs with a tip of 0.4 mm in diameter.
10. Fine watchmakers forceps tip and iris scissors (e.g. Fine Science Tools).
11. Dissection microscope (e.g. model M900) (D.F. Vasconcellos S.A.).
12. Fibre-optic light source (e.g. KL 2500 LCD) (Schott) for illumination during nerve preparation.
13. Biological amplifier (BA1, JRAK).
14. Scaling amplifier (SA1, JRAK).
15. Filter (F1 filter, JRAK).
16. Oscilloscope (e.g. DL 1200A, Yokogawa).
17. PC running "Spike 2" software version 4.13 (Cambridge Electronic Design).

2.11. Uterine Cervix of the Rat In Vivo

1. Adult virgin female rats weighing 200–300 g (e.g. female Sprague–Dawley rats from Harlan Industries) (see Note 61).
2. Halothane, pentobarbital and alpha-chloralose for anaesthesia.

3. Heavy liquid paraffin (BDH) prewarmed to a temperature of 37°C for electrical isolation within the nerve dissection area.
4. Dash 8u recorder (Astromed, West Warwick, RI) for monitoring of arterial blood pressure and heart rate.
5. Homeothermic heating blanket (Harvard Apparatus).
6. Heat lamps for maintaining body temperature in the range of 37–38°C.
7. Fine metal rods, e.g. 23G needles (Becton–Dickinson) for inserting both uterine cervical osses.
8. Force transducer (e.g. FT 03, Grass Instruments).
9. A bipolar stainless electrode.
10. Fine watchmakers forceps and iris scissors (e.g. Fine Science Tools GmbH).
11. Dissection microscope (e.g. model M900) (D.F. Vasconcellos S.A.).
12. Fibre-optic light source (e.g. KL 2500 LCD) (Schott) for illumination during nerve preparation.
13. Audioamplifier (e.g. model AM8, Grass Instruments).
14. Oscilloscope (e.g. model 450, Gould, Cleveland, OH).
15. Thermal-sensitive recorder (e.g. model K2G, Astro-Med GmbH, Rodgau, Germany) for recording the neurogram.
16. Micro 1401 interface (Cambridge Electronic Design).
17. PC running "Spike 2" software version 4.13 (Cambridge Electronic Design).
18. A stimulating electrode connected to a Grass stimulator (Grass Medical Instruments).
19. Uninsulated needle electrodes for insertion in the rectus abdominis muscle.

3. Methods

3.1. Small Bowel of Rat and Mouse In Vivo

1. General anaesthesia is induced with an intraperitoneal injection of the appropriate anesthetic:
   (a) For rats (7), general anaesthesia is produced with an intraperitoneal (i.p.) injection of pentobarbitone sodium (60 mg/kg, see Note 3).
   (b) For mice (8), general anaesthesia is induced with an intraperitoneal injection of ketamine, xylazine and acepromazine (80, 50 and 1 mg/kg respectively).

2. The level of anaesthesia is maintained over the course of the experiment by infusing the required substances intravenously (i.v.). For this purpose, the right external jugular vein is cannulated with a catheter (see Note 4).

   (a) For rats, the appropriate level of anaesthesia (see Note 3) is maintained over the course of the experiment by infusing pentobarbitone sodium (0.5–1 mg/kg/min) intravenously.

   (b) For mice, the appropriate level of anaesthesia is sustained by intravenous (i.v.) infusion of ketamine at a rate of 0.7–1.4 mg/kg per min.

3. The left carotid artery is exposed, separated from the vagus nerve, and cannulated with a heparinized catheter to facilitate arterial pressure recording with a Neurolog NL108 (see Note 5).

4. Body temperature is monitored with a rectal thermometer and maintained at around 37°C by means of a heating blanket.

5. An incision is made in the neck, and the trachea is cannulated to maintain a patent airway.

6. A midline laparotomy is performed and the cecum is excised to create space in the abdominal cavity. A 10 cm (rat) or 5 cm (mouse) length of proximal jejunum is identified (typically 1–5 cm distal of the ligament of Trietz). This is ligated, and incisions are made on the antimesenteric border at each end. The loop is flushed through with saline.

7. A 3.5 cm balloon (diameter 0.8 cm) is passed into the jejunum and secured in place at the aboral end of the 10 cm loop. The balloon is then connected to a barostat to enable distensions of the jejunum.

8. The small abdominal wall incisions are sutured, the muscle and skin of the large abdominal incision are sewn to a steel ring and the resulting well is filled with prewarmed (37°C) liquid paraffin.

9. There are typically two mesenteric nerve bundles, which run alongside the two blood vessels located in the mesenteric arcade supplying the jejunum. The connective tissue spanning this arcade is dissected to leave a piece of connective tissue attached to the right side of the arcade. The arcade is then placed on a black perspex platform.

10. With the use of a dissection microscope and illumination from a fibre-optic light source, a single paravascular nerve bundle (approximately 1 cm in length) is exposed by dissection of the overlaying fat and connective tissue. The nerve bundle is severed about 5–10 mm distal from the wall of the jejunum (see Note 6) and cleared of fat and connective tissue.

11. The nerve bundle is then attached to one of a pair of platinum recording electrodes, with a sliver of connective tissue wrapped around the other to act as a reference.
12. The electrodes are connected to a single channel 1902 amplifier, and the signal is differentially amplified and filtered. The afferent nerve signal, together with the blood-pressure recording and the pressure/volume read-out from the barostat, are passed into a micro 1401 amplifier, viewed online and captured by a PC running "Spike 2" software.
13. The viability of the preparation should now be assessed, e.g. with a bolus dose of 2-m-5-HT (30 μg/kg i.v. for the rat) or a slight distension held for 5 s of the jejunum (see Note 7). If there is no afferent response to these test stimuli, a different mesenteric nerve bundle should be dissected and tested.
14. *Ramp* and *phasic* distensions can be produced using a computer-driven barostat with Protocol PlusTM Deluxe software.
    (a) During *ramp* distensions, the balloon is inflated so that the pressure in the jejunum rises by 2 mmHg every 4 s (0–60 mmHg over 120 s).
    (b) *Phasic* distensions can be performed by rapidly inflating the balloon to a preset pressure and holding the pressure for some time (e.g. 25 s), after which the balloon is rapidly deflated (see Note 8).
15. Animals are killed at the end of an experiment by an anesthetic overdose.

3.2. Small Bowel of the Rat and Mouse In Vitro

1. Rats are anesthetized with pentobarbitone sodium at a dose of 60 mg/kg i.p. For the mouse, ketamine, xylazine and acepromazine are injected i.p. at doses of 80, 50 and 1 mg/kg, respectively.
2. A midline laparotomy is performed and the terminal jejunum and its arterial supply are identified. A branching section of artery with a clear projection to a segment of the jejunum (see Note 9) is chosen, and any side branches are ligated.
3. The jejunal segment with its attached mesenteric arcade is quickly removed, immersed in ice-cold Kreb's buffer, and rats and mice are then killed by anesthetic overdose.
4. The lumen of the gut is washed through with ice-cold Kreb's solution and the segment is dissected from the surrounding tissue.
5. The gut is placed in the *organ chamber* of the organ bath (see Subheading 2.1 and Fig. 1), and perfused serosally with Kreb's solution (see Note 10) at a rate of 5–10 ml/min.
6. The gut "tube" in the organ chamber is cannulated at both ends by glass cannulas. Throughout the experiment, the gut

segment is constantly perfused intraluminally with Kreb's solution (see Note 10) at a rate of 5–10 ml/h against a distal pressure head of 2 cmH_2O.

7. The mesenteric arcade is pulled through the aperture between *organ* and *recording chambers*.
8. Now, the mesenteric artery is cannulated using a fine polyethylene cannula to permit intravascular perfusion or drug administration. The cannula is passed into the cut end of the arteriole and tied in place with a fine silk suture. The system is connected to a pressure transducer to allow monitoring of VPP (see Note 11). The artery is perfused with modified Kreb's solution (see Note 10) using a peristaltic pump (see Note 12).
9. The slot between the two chambers is now sealed with vaseline, and the recording compartment is filled with heavy liquid paraffin for electrical isolation. The preparation is then allowed to warm slowly, reaching a working temperature of 32–34°C before mesenteric nerve recording is obtained (see Note 10).
10. The mesenteric nerves are dissected on a piece of black Perspex inserted into the base of the recording chamber using fine watchmakers forceps and iris scissors under a dissecting microscope (20× to 40× magnification) and with fibre optic illumination. The dissection starts by removing the fat surrounding the neurovascular bundle to expose the arteriole and vein that supply the segment (see Note 13). When nerves are identified, 1–3 mm lengths of these nerves are gently peeled away from fat and connective tissue for recording.
11. Fine filaments supplying the segment are wrapped around one arm of a bipolar platinum recording electrode with an adequate length of connective tissue attached to the second electrode.
12. The electrodes are connected to a neurology headstage (NL100), and the signal is amplified (NL104, 20,000×) and filtered (NL125, band width 100–3,000 Hz). Then, the signal is relayed to a spike processor (Digitimer D130) to allow discrimination of action potentials from noise using a manually set amplitude and polarity window. The whole nerve recording is displayed on a storage oscilloscope (e.g. Tektronix TDS 210). The nerve signal is recorded (20 kHz sampling rate) through a Micro 1401 interface to a computer running "Spike 2" software. Whole nerve activity is continually monitored as spike discharge (impulses (imp)/s) and intraluminal pressure is sampled at 100 Hz.
13. The preparation is left to stabilize for up to 60 min, at least 10–15 min (see Note 14).
14. To distend the intestine, a three-way tap on the intraluminal outlet cannula is closed while perfusion with Kreb's solution

continues. In this manner, the gut segment can be distended up to 60 mmHg in approximately 120 s, before the three-way tap is opened to return intraluminal pressure to baseline.

15. To test the effect of chemical substances, different ways of drug administration are possible (see Note 15):
    (a) The perfusate can be switched from pure Kreb's solution to a specific test solution diluted in Kreb's solution.
    (b) Direct application of the substance to the serosa of the gut using a syringe or pipette.
    (c) Intraluminal injection of the drug.
    (d) Injection into the arteriole supplying the segment of jejunum.

3.3. Colon of the Rat In Vitro

1. Rats are anesthetized with Nembutal (60 mg/kg i.p.).
2. After a midline laparotomy, 4–5 cm of distal colon lying oral to the rim of the pelvis are removed, along with the lumbar colonic nerves (LCNs) and the neurovascular bundle containing the inferior mesenteric ganglion (IMG), the intermesenteric nerve and the lumbar splanchnic nerves (see Note 18).
3. The tissue is transferred into ice-cold, modified Kreb's solution (saturated with 95% O_2/5% CO_2) for dissection and animals are then killed by severance of the abdominal aorta.
4. The distal colon is opened longitudinally off-centre to the antimesenteric border in order to orientate LCN insertions along the edge of the opened preparation. The fecal pellets are removed.
5. The colon is mounted mucosa side up into the colonic compartment of the organ bath (*mucosal chamber*), so that the serosal surface lies directly over the lower basement *serosal chamber*. In this position, the insertion points of the lumbar colonic nerves (LCN) should lie along the edge of the tissue abutting the wall that separating the two compartments of the bath. Approximately 1 cm of colon should lie below the insertion point most closely related to the IMG and 4 cm should lie above this point. Both surfaces of the tissue are now superfused with appropriate Kreb's solutions (see Subheading 2) at a rate of 15 ml/min.
6. Connective tissue is dissected away from the neurovascular bundle (see Note 19). The neurovascular bundle is tied and cut at the level of insertion of the artery into the abdominal aorta.
7. The neurovascular bundle is pulled through a hole into the paraffin-filled compartment. The bundle lies now over a mirror in a small blister of Kreb's solution that is continuous with the solution in the colonic compartment.

8. Under a dissecting microscope, afferent strands are teased away from the neurovascular bundle (which comprises lumbar splanchnic nerves and intermesenteric nerves) and placed on a platinum wire recording electrode. A reference electrode is positioned in the blister of solution in which the neurovascular bundle lies.
9. Neural activity is differentially amplified (BA 1, SA 1), filtered (F1), and displayed on an oscilloscope (e.g. Tektronix TDS 210). Amplified neural recordings are recorded onto hard disk, along with amplified length and/or tension recordings from muscle via a micro 1401 interface. Single fibre activity is discriminated off-line for analysis using "Spike 2" software. Action potentials are discriminated as single units on the basis of distinguishable waveform, amplitude, and duration (see Note 20).
10. Search stimuli for the receptive fields of afferent fibres should now be applied. They include three mechanical stimuli (see Note 21):
    (a) Ungraded *circumferential stretch* is applied to tissue via the pulley system.
    (b) The mucosal surface is firmly *probed* with the blunt end of a glass rod (tip contact area 6 mm^2 with a transmural pressure of approximately 50 kPa).
    (c) The mucosal surface is lightly *stroked* with the end of a fine paint brush.
11. After a receptive field has been identified, the temperature of the bath is increased to 32°C and routine tests begin.
12. Mechanical stimuli that can be applied manually to the identified receptive field include e.g. the change of circumferential length (0–10 mm from tissue resting length) or probing with calibrated von Frey hairs.
13. Chemical stimuli are applied to the site of the receptive field on the mucosal surface by adding into a 1 cm diameter ring that is placed directly around the receptive field (see Note 22). The ring is then lifted and the area of tissue is superfused with Krebs solution for washout (see Note 23).

3.4. Stomach of the Rat In Vivo

1. Rats are anesthetized initially with an intraperitoneal injection of pentobarbital sodium (45–50 mg/kg) and anaesthesia is subsequently maintained with a constant intravenous infusion of pentobarbital (5–10 mg/kg/h).
2. The right femoral vein is cannulated for infusion of fluid and anesthetic.
3. The right femoral artery is cannulated and connected to a pressure transducer (Transpac IV) for monitoring blood

pressure and heart rate. The mean arterial pressure is maintained at 80 mmHg with supplemental intravenous injection of 5% dextrose in saline administered in a bolus of 1–1.5 ml as required.

4. The trachea is intubated to permit artificial ventilation with room air.
5. The rat is paralyzed with pancuronium bromide at a dose of 0.2–0.3 mg/kg i.v. (see Note 25) and mechanically ventilated with room air (70 strokes/min, 2.0–2.5 ml stroke volume).
6. Core body temperature is maintained at 36°C by a hot water circulating heating pad placed under the rat and an overhead feedback-controlled heat lamp (thermoprobe inserted into the rectum).
7. The abdomen is opened by a transverse epigastric incision 4–5 cm in length.
8. The right vagus nerve is isolated from the esophagus, and a pair of Teflon-coated, 40-gauge stainless steel wires stripped at the tips are placed around the nerve and sealed with non-reactive Wacker gel.
9. For phasic balloon gastric distension (9), a flexible latex balloon is placed surgically in the stomach through the fundus (see Note 26). The balloon catheter is connected to a distension control device (Barostat) via a low-volume pressure transducer (NL108T2).
10. For fluid gastric distension, the stomach is intubated with flexible plastic tubing via the mouth, esophagus, and cardia. The catheter is secured by a ligature around the esophageal-gastric junction. A second piece of flexible plastic tubing is introduced distally through the pylorus and is secured by a ligature placed caudal to the pyloric sphincter; the duodenum is ligated close to the pyloric ring. For GD, the oral catheter is connected to a reservoir containing saline at room temperature. Constant pressure distension is controlled by the distension control device (Barostat) with the distal catheter clamped. Intragastric pressure is monitored by connecting the distal catheter via a three-way stopcock to a low-volume pressure transducer (NL108T2).
11. The left gastric artery is now freed from connective tissue under a microscope and cannulated for infusion of drugs.
12. The abdomen is closed with silk sutures.
13. The right vagus nerve is exposed by a ventral midline incision in the neck. The sternocleidomastoid, sternohyoid, and omohyoid muscles are removed.
14. The skin is reflected laterally and tied to a frame to make a pool for warm heavy liquid paraffin (37°C).

15. The nerve is dissected away from the carotid tissue sheath, decentralized close to its entry to the nodose ganglion, and placed over a black micro-base plate. The perineural sheath is removed in the pool of warm liquid paraffin (37°C), the nerve is split into thin bundles, and fine filaments are teased from the bundle to obtain a single unit.
16. Electrical activity of the single unit is recorded by placing the fibre over one arm of a bipolar silver-silver chloride electrode. A fine strand of connective tissue is placed over the other pole of the electrode for differential recording.
17. Action potentials are monitored continuously by analogue delay and are displayed on a storage oscilloscope (e.g. DL 1200A) after low noise AC differential amplification. Action potentials are processed through a window discriminator and counted (1-s binwidth) online using "Spike 2" software.
18. Mechanosensitive gastric muscle afferents in the vagus nerve should now be identified by response to a test stimulus of gastric distension, e.g. 40 mmHg for 5 s (see Note 27).
19. At the end of experiment, rats are killed with an overdose of pentobarbital.

3.5. Esophagus of Ferret and Mouse In Vitro

1. (a) Mice are killed by CO_2 inhalation followed by cervical dislocation and the thorax is opened by a midline incision.
   (b) Ferrets are deeply anesthetized with sodium pentobarbitone (50 mg/kg i.p.) and the thorax is opened as described for the mouse. The ferrets are then killed by exsanguination.
2. In both animal species, the stomach, esophagus with attached vagal nerves, heart and lungs are removed and placed in a modified ice-cold Kreb's solution (see Note 28), saturated with 95% O_2/5% CO_2.
3. The heart, lungs and major blood vessels are removed and the vagus nerve is cleared of connective tissue. The diaphragm is also cleared from around the lower esophageal sphincter. The temperature is maintained at 4°C during dissection (see Note 28).
4. (a) In the ferret, the preparation is then opened out longitudinally along the esophagus and the greater curve of the stomach (2 cm length of stomach). Then it is pinned out flat, mucosa side up, in the *organ chamber*.
   (b) For the mouse, the dorsal aspect of the stomach is removed completely to pin the tissue flat in the *organ chamber* with a straight edge.
5. The *organ chamber* (both, for ferret and mouse respectively) is perfused now at a rate of 11–12 ml per min with Kreb's solution, temperature maintained at 34°C.

6. The vagus nerve (free length 3.0 cm in the ferret) is drawn through a small hole into an isolated *recording chamber*. There the nerve is laid on a mirror and bathed in heavy liquid paraffin.
7. Under a dissecting microscope, the nerve sheath is gently peeled back to expose the nerve trunk. Using fine forceps, nerve fibres are teased apart into 8–12 bundles. Then one by one, the small nerve bundles are placed onto a platinum recording electrode. A reference electrode rests on the mirror in a small pool of Krebs' solution. Figure 3 illustrates the in vitro preparation described.
8. Afferent neural activity is amplified with a biological amplifier (BA1) and scaling amplifier (SA1), filtered (F1) and monitored using an oscilloscope (e.g. DL 1200A). Single units are discriminated on the basis of action potential shape, duration, and amplitude using "Spike 2" software (see Note 29).
9. The location of receptive fields along the esophagus should now be determined by mechanical stimulation with either a blunt glass rod or a brush. The size of the receptive field is determined by gently probing the receptive field using a 1,000 mg von Frey probe and measuring the area where a response is elicited. Mechanical thresholds are determined using calibrated von Frey hairs.
10. Tension can be applied via a claw made from bent dissection pins attached with thread to the pulley and cantilever system (see Fig. 3). To balance the cantilever, weights are placed on the opposite side (see Notes 30 and 31).
11. Chemosensitivity of esophageal vagal afferents should be determined after mechanical thresholds have been established (see Note 32). The chemosensitivity of esophageal fibres is examined by applying directly onto the mucosal surface overlying the receptive field (see Note 33); agents are introduced to the receptive field by means of a small cylindrical chamber placed around the area of the receptive field (see Fig. 3).

3.6. Pancreas of the Rat In Vitro

1. After anaesthesia with Nembutal® (60 mg/kg i.p.), the abdomen and thoracic cavity are opened via a large midline incision.
2. Following suitable careful gross dissection of connective tissue and removal of visceral fat, the entire viscera including the aorta, vena cava, esophagus, stomach, duodenum and kidneys is harvested en bloc and rinsed several times in ice-cold modified Kreb's solution (10). The tissue is transferred to a dissection dish lined with Sylgard which contains ice-cold modified Kreb's solution (superfused with 95% O_2/5% CO_2) and is immersed in ice. The tissue is rinsed several times with

fresh ice-cold modified Kreb's solution prior to and during the subsequent tissue dissection.

3. The distal colon is detached from the pancreas and removed together with the small bowel not connected to the pancreas.
4. The hepatic artery and portal vein are identified and ligated, all other liver attachments are sectioned and the liver is removed. The hepatic end of the common bile duct (CBD) is tied off with suture ligatures.
5. With the aid of a dissection microscope, the complex consisting of the celiac and superior mesenteric ganglia is located and the left splanchnic nerve identified. The nerve is carefully dissected away from the surrounding tissue and a 2–3 cm length cephalad to the celiac/superior mesenteric ganglia complex is freed.
6. To complete the dissection, the vena cava is separated from the aorta by blunt dissection and removed along with the renal and portal veins.
7. The kidneys are removed and all remaining fatty tissue is cleared (see Note 35).
8. The gastric artery and attachments between the stomach and the spleen are cut, and the stomach and duodenum are removed by sharp dissection.
9. The hepatic termination of the common bile duct (CBD) is identified and cannulated with a 24G Optiva® i.v. catheter and secured with a silk ligature. The duodenal end of the CBD is either ligated with a silk suture to permit subsequent duct distension, or cannulated with a polyvinyl catheter and secured with a silk suture for duct perfusion with chemical mediators.
10. The duodenum is cut caudad to the pancreatic attachments and the small bowel distal to this point is removed.
11. Each lobe of the liver is carefully removed leaving the major hepatic vessels, ducts and common hepatic branch of the vagus nerve intact. The cut ends of duct branches leading to the common bile duct (CBD) are tied with silk sutures.
12. The heart and lungs are removed by sharp dissection and the diaphragm is cleared from around the lower esophageal sphincter.
13. The vagal nerves are identified along the thoracic esophagus and (using sharp dissection) isolated from the connective tissue up to a point 2–3 cm proximal to the junction of the celiac and hepatic branches.
14. The kidneys and surrounding fatty tissue are removed while leaving the celiac/superior mesenteric ganglia complex intact.

15. To complete the dissection, the stomach is opened along the greater curvature and flushed several times with ice-cold modified Kreb's solution.
16. The duodenal end of the CBD is ligated with a silk suture for duct distension experiments (see Note 36).
17. Each preparation is tautly pinned out in the organ bath (see Figs. 5 and 6) for the spinal and vagal afferent preparations respectively.
18. The common bile duct (CBD) catheter is connected to a manometer for the concurrent distension of the common bile duct (CBD) and pancreatic duct (PD).
19. The bath is superfused with Dex–Kreb's solution (saturated with 95% O_2/5% CO_2) at a rate of 6–7 ml/min via a peristaltic pump.
20. The splanchnic or vagal nerve trunks are positioned in the adjacent paraffin-filled recording chamber through a small hole in a sliding plexiglass "gate" which is sealed with vaseline to prevent Dex–Kreb's from entering the paraffin bath (see Figs. 5 and 6).
21. With the aid of fine forceps and a dissection microscope, each nerve trunk is desheathed and teased into fine nerve bundles.

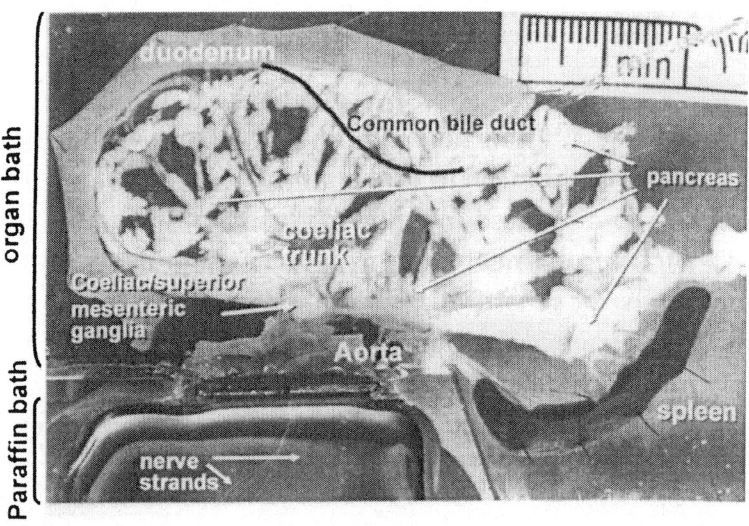

Fig. 5. A representative image of the rat pancreatic spinal afferent preparation. The tissue is pinned in the organ bath such that the aorta is located adjacent to the plexiglass "gate" which isolates the paraffin bath. This facilitates the positioning of the splanchnic nerve in the paraffin bath. The course of the common bile duct is shown by the overlaid black line. The catheter placed in the proximal common bile duct is visible in the top right hand part of the image. Note that the duodenal segment is not part of the preparation but is included in the image to aid orientation. The scale in the top right hand corner of the bath illustrated the dimension of the preparation. Teased nerve bundles (strands) from the left splanchnic nerve are visible in the paraffin bath (bottom left side)

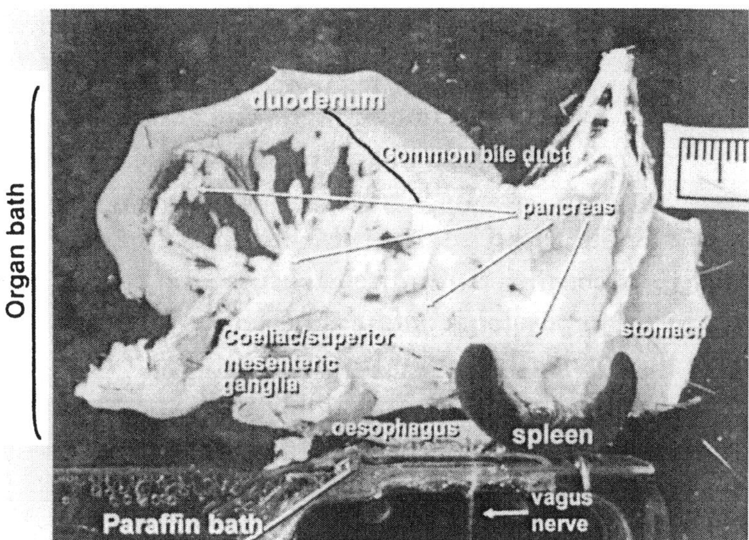

Fig. 6. Representative image of the rat pancreatic vagal afferent preparation. The tissue is pinned with the esophagus adjacent to the plexiglass "gate" to allow the isolated vagal nerves to be passed into the paraffin bath. The stomach and duodenum are pinned out to allow access to the pancreas in a similar arrangement to the isolated spinal afferent preparation (see Fig. 5). The course of the common bile duct is shown by the overlaid black line. The spleen is left unpinned to allow manipulation of the preparation to gain access to pancreatic tissue, as required. The scale on the right hand side of the bath illustrates the dimension of the preparation

Teased nerve bundles are subsequently positioned individually on a platinum recording electrode which is connected to a DAM50 differential amplifier, a BPF-932 band-pass filter, a Stereo Sound Mixer CE and a PowerLab recording system for extra-cellular nerve recording. Nerve discharges are monitored and recorded on a PowerLab recording system using Chart v5.1.

22. During recording from each individual nerve bundle, an initial search of the preparation for receptive fields should be conducted via a search probe.
23. Distension of the CBD/PD can be achieved by applying a distension pressure with warm Dex–Kreb's solution (up to 44 mmHg) via a manometer connected to a syringe (see Note 39).
24. Chemosensitivity of the identified unit can be assessed by application of chemicals (e.g. 0.1 ml) directly to the receptive field in a stainless steel well placed over the site or via injection (0.3 ml for vascular or duct administration followed by a flush with 0.5 ml Dex–Krebs) into the CBD/PD system or the gastric artery (see Note 40).

3.7. Gallbladder of Opossum In Vivo

1. Anaesthesia is induced with intramuscular xylazine (10 mg/kg Rompun®) and ketamine (20 mg/kg Ketalar®).

2. The left femoral vein is cannulated with a catheter to maintain anaesthesia for the duration of the experiment with a constant infusion of sodium thiopentone (5–10 mg/kg/h Pentothal®).
3. To measure blood pressure, the left femoral artery is cannulated with a polyvinyl catheter, connected to a pressure transducer (Transpac IV) and constantly monitored on a PowerLab recording system. The right femoral vein is also cannulated with a polyvinyl catheter, here for continuous infusion of saline at 6 ml/h throughout the entire experiment to maintain hydration.
4. All animals are artificially ventilated with a small animal ventilator via a tracheostomy.
5. Body temperature is maintained at 37°C with a homeothermic heating blanket.
6. Following a midline incision, the gut is gently mobilized to provide access to the gallbladder, common bile duct, sphincter of Oddi, pancreas and duodenum (11). The majority of the gut is not manipulated during the experiment and placed in a plastic bag on the warming blanket or platform. Other exposed tissues are covered with wet gauze and food wrap to maintain moisture content. A copper ring is sewn to the edge of the abdominal incision to provide good earthing for the nerve recordings (see Note 42).
7. In order to activate mechanosensitive afferents, balloon or fluid distension of the gallbladder, duodenum, common bile duct (CBD), and pancreatic duct (PD) is performed (see Fig. 7).
   (a) In the *gallbladder*, a balloon catheter is inserted, secured with a purse string suture and subsequently distended with saline (2–7 ml).
   (b) To achieve distension of the *duodenum*, a balloon catheter is inserted (see Subheading 3.8) and positioned in the duodenum (2 cm proximal to the sphincter of Oddi-duodenal junction), secured with a purse string suture and subsequently distended with saline (2–7).
   (c) A 22 g and 24 g indwelling catheter (Optiva, see Subheading 3.9) is inserted through the sphincter of Oddi and positioned in the proximal *common bile duct (CBD)* and *pancreatic duct (PD)*, respectively. These catheters are connected to fluid manometers, and the fluid level in each manometer is varied to impose known distension pressures (0–20 mmHg) in the biliary and pancreatic ducts.
8. For vagal afferent recordings, fluid distension of the *duodenum* (5–30 ml) can be used.
   (a) Following ligation of the pylorus, a polyvinyl catheter (see Subheading 3.10) is inserted into the *duodenum* via

a stab incision and secured 4 cm anal to the sphincter of Oddi-duodenal junction with a ligature. Saline is introduced through this catheter via a syringe (see Note 43).

(b) In addition, a Foley balloon catheter (see Subheading 3.11) may be inserted through the animal's mouth and esophagus and positioned in the *stomach* in order to achieve gastric balloon distension (5–30 ml).

9. *Splanchnic* nerve isolation: The left splanchnic nerve is isolated and carefully exposed at the level of the diaphragm. The nerve is then followed to its junction with the sympathetic chain. A segment of sympathetic chain approximately 1 cm in length in the cephalic direction is cleared of connective tissue and then cut at the cephalic end of this segment (see Fig. 7).

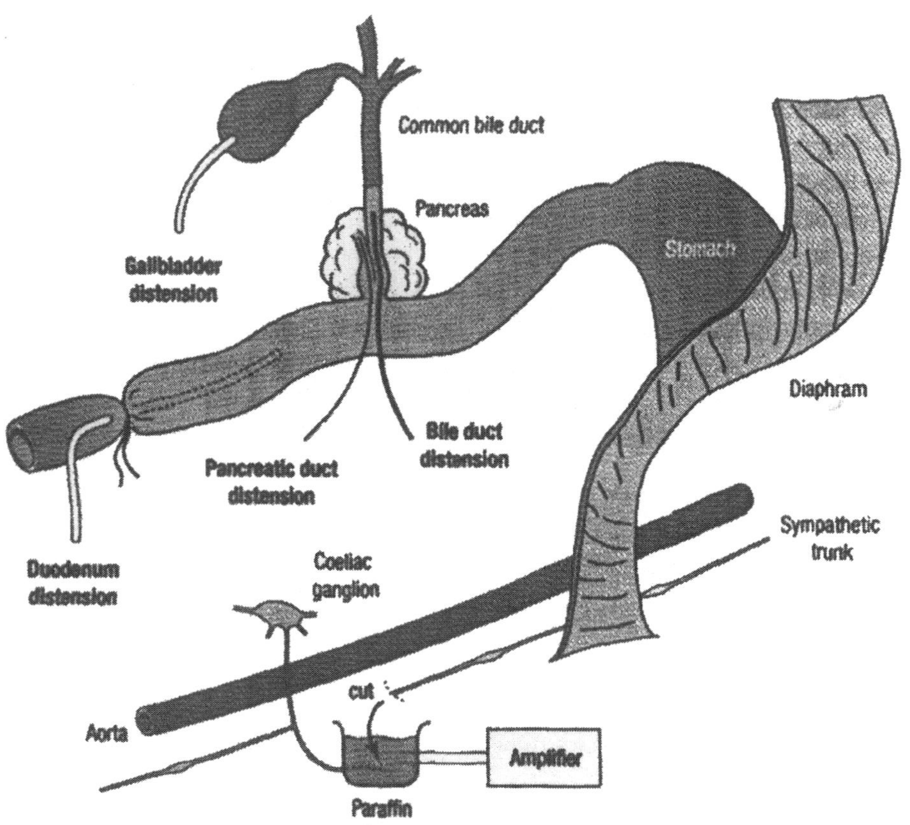

Fig. 7. Splanchnic nerve/sympathetic chain preparation. Schematic diagram illustrating key features of the preparation. The left splanchnic nerves close to the coeliac ganglion are dissected, followed up to the sympathetic chain which is then cut and the free end mounted in a paraffin-filled bath to record action potentials. In separate animals the cervical vagus nerve is dissected to record action potentials (not shown). In both preparations, balloons are placed in the gallbladder and duodenum. The common bile duct and the pancreatic duct are cannulated via the sphincter of Oddi for separate distension of the biliary or pancreatic systems. A foley catheter is inserted into the stomach (not shown) for gastric distension (vagal nerve recordings only)

The exposed nerve trunk is covered with gauze soaked with saline until it is subsequently desheathed (see below).

10. *Vagal* nerve isolation: The left cervical vagus nerve is exposed by blunt dissection and retraction of the thyroid gland, trachea, carotid artery and jugular vein. The nerve is cleared of adhering tissue and then transected at the cephalad end of this cleared segment to produce a sufficient length of free nerve to position in the recording chamber. The exposed nerve trunk is covered with gauze soaked with saline until it is subsequently desheathed (see below).
11. Following surgical preparation, the animals are relocated to a Faraday cage and positioned on a water-heated perspex box to maintain animal body temperature at 37°C.
12. The free *sympathetic* chain or *vagal* nerve trunk is manoeuvred into an acrylic recording chamber, which is secured immediately adjacent to the nerve trunk and filled with heavy liquid paraffin. The remainder of the exposed nerve trunk is covered with gelfoam to prevent it from drying out. With the aid of a dissecting microscope, the nerve trunk is desheathed and nerve fibres are teased free.
13. Individual fibres are placed on the platinum recording electrode. The platinum reference electrode is positioned against the glass base within a drop of saline in the recording chamber. The platinum electrode is connected to a differential amplifier (DAM 59), a bandpass filter (BPF-932), an audio mixer (e.g. Stereo Sound Mixer CE), and a PowerLab recording system.
14. Experimental manipulations should commence following a stabilization period of about 60 min. For each nerve fibre, spontaneous and evoked discharges are monitored and recorded on a PowerLab recording system (see Note 44).
15. At the completion of the experiment, all animals are euthanised with a bolus intravenous dose of Lethabarb®.

3.8. Urinary Bladder of the Mouse In Vitro

1. Mice are killed by exposure to rising concentrations of CO_2 gas.
2. The whole urinary tract attached to the lower vertebrae and surrounding tissues is quickly isolated *en bloc* (12) and placed in a chamber, where it is continuously superfused with Kreb's solution saturated with 5% CO_2 and 95% O_2 (see Note 45).
3. A 25 gauge needle is inserted into the lumen of the urinary bladder and is connected to a syringe-type infusion pump (sp210iw), a pressure transducer (NL108T2), and a 100 ml Hamilton syringe via an Omnifit-adapter. This enables infusion and withdrawal of medium (Kreb's solution) at a constant rate (0.1 ml/min), recording of intraluminal pressure and intravesical injection of drugs.

4. The preparation is allowed to stabilize for about 60 min while the mouse urinary tract is perfused as stated above.
5. With the aid of a dissecting microscope, a branch of the pelvic nerve arising from the urinary bladder is dissected.
6. The nerve activity is recorded with a suction glass electrode connected to a Neurolog headstage (NL100) and a preamplifier (NL104). Signals are amplified (NL104, 10.000x), filtered (NL125, band-pass 200–4,000 Hz), and relayed to a spike processor (D310) that discriminates neural impulses from noise with a manually set amplitude and polarity window. The nerve activity and the intraluminal pressure are recorded on tape and on a computer with a micro 1401 interface and "Spike 2" software.

3.9. Ureter of the Guinea-Pig In Vitro

1. Animals are killed by cervical dislocation.
2. The part of the urinary system containing the bladder, both ureters and both kidneys must be quickly removed within 2–3 min of death and should be washed twice (5 min) at room temperature in synthetic interstitial fluid (SIF).
3. One whole ureter (ureter length 40–50 mm) cut close to the bladder (if possible including part of the renal pelvis) and the corresponding ureteric nerves, is carefully dissected and transferred into an organ bath at 37°C (see Note 46).
4. The ureter is fixed onto the rubber platform of the organ bath and is cannulated through both ends for intraluminal perfusion with oxygenated SIF at low rates of 0.02–0.05 ml/min (see Note 47).
5. Perfusion pressure is continuously monitored using a pressure transducer (NL108T2, see Note 48).
6. Before starting the electrophysiological recordings (see Note 49), the ability of the preparation to produce contractions should be tested (see Note 50).
7. Small branches (diameter 10–40 μm, length 3–6 mm) of the hypogastric nerve or small nerves arising from the inferior mesenteric ganglion or from the pelvic plexus are carefully dissected from the connective tissue and fat using fine watchmaker forceps and iris scissors under a dissecting microscope.
8. Then, the small nerves are passed through a small slot (0.5 mm) into the movable *recording chamber* filled with warm heavy liquid paraffin. A small sponge is used to prevent leakage between both chambers.
9. Monopolar recordings of electrical activity are performed using a fine platinum wire which is attached to a small manipulator mounted directly onto the recording chamber (not shown in Fig. 1). A silver-silver chloride pellet is used as the

indifferent electrode (see Note 51). The electrical signals are amplified (BA1, SA), filtered (F1, band pass 10 Hz–15 kHz) and recorded on tape and on a computer with a micro 1401 interface and "Spike 2" software.

10. Single units are discriminated according to their size and shape (see Note 52).
11. The mechanosensitivity of single units and their receptive field size can be determined by their responses to probing of the ureter with small blunt glass probes (see Note 53).
12. Distension produced by an increase in intraluminal hydrostatic pressure can be used to quantify the responses of the units. Pressure–response curves of mechanosensitive fibres can be obtained by a series of intraluminal distensions with duration of 30 s starting e.g. from pressures of 5 mmHg up to 90 mmHg (see Note 54).

3.10. Testis of the Dog In Vitro

1. Animals are anesthetized with pentobarbital sodium administered intravenously (~30 mg/kg). Thereafter, the cephalic vein of one side is cannulated for supplemental administration of the anesthetics in all animals (see Note 55).
2. The testis and epididymis of both sides are carefully exposed at the tunica vaginalis visceralis and excised from animals (13) with spermatic cord attached (see Notes 56 and 57).
3. The testis and epididymis are held in a modified Kreb's solution (saturated with 5% CO_2–95% O_2).
4. The spermatic cord is held in a pool of heavy liquid paraffin (*oil pool*), separated from a pool of Kreb's solution (*test pool*) by vaseline.
5. The temperature of the *test pool* is measured by a copper-constantan thermocouple and is adjusted by controlling the temperature of the water circulating in the outer trough. The base temperature of the *test pool* is usually set at 34 ± 0.2°C.
6. Afferent neural activity is amplified with a biological amplifier (BA1) and scaling amplifier (SA1), filtered (F1) and monitored using an oscilloscope (e.g. DL 1200A). Single units are discriminated on the basis of action potential shape, duration, and amplitude using "Spike 2" software (see Note 58).
7. Receptive fields of a unit are sought by probing with a glass rod with a small rounded tip. The mechanical threshold of a unit can be measured by means of calibrated von Frey-type nylon hairs with a tip of 0.4 mm in diameter, which are applied at exactly the receptive site under direct visual observation with a binocular microscope.
8. Chemical stimulation can be applied by replacing the Kreb's solution in the test pool with a stimulus solution of the same

temperature, and the test pool is then rinsed several times with Kreb's solution (see Note 59).

9. Heat stimulation can be carried out by raising the temperature of the Kreb's solution from 34 to 50°C (see Note 60). Response to cold stimulation can be tested by replacing the Kreb's solution of 34°C by another with a temperature of <20°C.

3.11. Uterine Cervix of the Rat In Vivo

1. Under halothane anaesthesia, the carotid artery is catheterized for continuous monitoring of arterial blood pressure and heart rate, the jugular vein is cannulated for i.v. application of drugs, and the trachea is cannulated for artificial ventilation.
2. Halothane is then discontinued and anaesthesia maintained with pentobarbital (10 mg/kg i.v.) and alpha-chloralose (40–50 mg/kg i.v.). Body temperature is maintained in the range of 37–38°C with a circulating water heating pad and heat lamps throughout the experiment.
3. Through a small midline laparotomy incision, fine metal rods are inserted through both uterine cervical osses. The rods enter from the uterus and leave through the vaginal wall, both as near as possible to the cervix. Uterine cervical distension (UCD) is applied to the cervix by pulling one of the rods manually (see Fig. 8), while the other rod is fixed to a force transducer (FT 03).
4. A midline laparotomy is now performed, the intestines are wrapped in plastic and retracted to the side, and the hypogastric nerve is identified in the right retroperitoneal space.

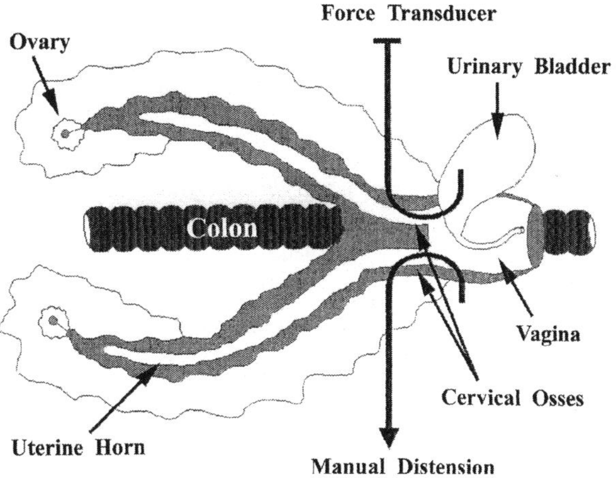

Fig. 8. Diagram illustrating the experimental setting to study the effects of EMG responses to UCD. After a small midline laparotomy incision, two metal rods are inserted into the osses of the uterine cervix and separated manually. A force transducer fixed at one rod detectes the distension. Single-unit EMG activity from the rectus abdominis muscle is transformed into digital signals

5. The distal cut end of the nerve is draped on a platform and covered with heavy liquid paraffin. Small nerve filaments are teased gently under operating microscopy. Single-unit afferent nerve activity is recorded with a bipolar stainless electrode. The nerve filaments are dissected gradually until single-unit activity of afferents is isolated.
6. The action potential of the afferent is amplified and processed through an audioamplifier (model AM8) and an oscilloscope (model 450). The neurogram is recorded on a thermal-sensitive recorder (model K2G) and the single unit is identified initially by examining the waveform and the spike amplitude on the oscilloscope at a rapid sweep speed as well as by checking the recorded sound frequency related to each spike activity. Furthermore, the signals are digitized at a sampling rate of 20 kHz and recorded into a computer through a micro 1401 interface for subsequent off-line analysis (see Note 62). An amplitude threshold is set for the recorded action potential of nerve fibres. When an event is detected, the associated waveform (6 ms) is extracted and displayed continuously in a separate software oscilloscope window. Discharge frequency can be quantified by using analysis software "Spike 2".
7. Afferents innervating the cervix are now searched using gentle mechanical stimulation of the visceral surface of the cervix. Receptive fields of afferents are verified with a stimulating electrode connected to a Grass stimulator (10–30 V, 0.3 ms, 0.2–0.5 Hz). First, the threshold of afferents to cervical distension is determined, produced by manual distraction (through the fine metal rods inserted into both cervical osses) while measuring the force on a force transducer (FT 03, see Note 63).
8. After determining basal activity and threshold to mechanical stimulation, chemical substances (e.g. bradykinin) can be topically applied to the receptive field of afferents using a cotton-tipped applicator. The response of the afferent unit should immediately be recorded. Afferent response to mechanical stimulation (e.g. 20, 40, and 80 g for 5 s at 2 min intervals) can be determined as well.
9. To examine reflex responses induced by uterine cervical distension (UCD), uninsulated needle electrodes are inserted in the rectus abdominis in its right inguinal part, never changed in its position, and EMG activity is monitored. Processing is similar to single unit afferent nerve activity as described above.
10. At the end of the experiments, rats are killed by an overdose of intravenous (i.v.) pentobarbital.

4. Notes

1. Animals are allowed free access to both regular solid food and water.
2. Changes in intraluminal pressure reflect intestinal motor activity.
3. Each segment of jejunum should be about 30 mm long (for both, rat and mouse tissue) and should contain one single straight neurovascular bundle. Keeping to these demands, nerve preparation will show reproducible results.
4. The preparation is allowed to warm slowly, reaching a working temperature of 32–34°C before mesenteric nerve recording is obtained. Warming up should only begin after sealing the slot between the two chambers with vaseline and filling the recording compartment with heavy liquid paraffin, i.e. immediately before nerve preparation starts. This procedure helps to maintain the viability of the tissue.
5. Vascular perfusion pressure (VPP) can be used as an index of vascular tone/blood flow.
6. Pulsatile flow in the artery can be avoided by passing the vascular fluid through a bubble trap. To prevent fluid build-up in the recording chamber, the venous effluent should be allowed to drain into the gut chamber by puncturing the small veins draining the segment.
7. In most preparations, two nerve fascicles are found running between the artery and vein. If preparation of the first nerve does not show appropriate results, the second nerve can be used for experiment.
8. Experiments should only be performed on preparations, which show continous baseline afferent discharge and robust responses to a priming exposure of a testing substance (e.g. 5-HT).
9. A minimum interval of 15–20 min should be left between each stimulus.
10. Here, particular consideration is given to maintaining the viability of the mucosa. For this reason, several features should be considered:
    (a) A mixture of short chain fatty acids (butyrate, 2 mM and acetate, 20 mM) replaces glucose in the mucosal superfusate.
    (b) The prostaglandin synthesis inhibitor indomethacin (3 μM) is added to Kreb's solutions to reduce prostaglandin synthesis and suppress potential inhibitory actions of endogenous prostaglandins.

(c) The L-type calcium channel antagonist nifedipine (1 mM) is added as well to suppress smooth muscle activity that might otherwise give rise to indirect responses secondary to contractile effects of administrated substances (e.g. 5-HT). Nifedipine is also used to inhibit degranulation of mast cells and enterochromaffin cells that could similarly give rise to secondary effects. Both surfaces of the tissue are superfused with Kreb's solution at a rate of 15 ml/min.

(d) Bath temperature should be maintained at 21°C prior to the commencement of the experimental protocol and raised to 32°C only following identification of a viable fibre. This procedure should be followed to reduce the rate of deterioration of the mucosa.

11. During baseline conditions, the tissue should be maintained at approximately in situ longitudinal and circumferential length.

12. The pelvic and hypogastric nerves are not included in the preparation.

13. To add support to the preparation, blood vessels are not dissected away from the nerve.

14. Strands of nerve should be discarded or separated into smaller bundles if spontaneous activity of more than three different action potential profiles is observed. Data should be excluded if the shape and character of two units merge together, such that they can't be discriminated confidently by visual inspection.

15. The criteria used for classification of afferents are based on their responses to the three distinct mechanical stimuli described here:

(a) Afferents that respond to probing of the colon but not to stretch or mucosal stroking are classed as serosal receptors.

(b) Afferents that respond to ≥5 mm circular stretch and probing but not to mucosal stroking are classed as muscular receptors.

(c) Afferents that respond to mucosal stroking with a 0.1 mN von Frey hair and probing but not to circumferential stretch are classed as mucosal receptors.

16. Chemical stimuli should be applied usually for 2 min before being aspirated from the ring.

17. The tissue should be superfused for at least 3 min before reapplication of the ring for administration of another stimulus. Chemicals should be administered in a special order, so that noxious stimuli (e.g. 50 mM HCl or 100 μM capsaicin) are

given later in the order to avoid damage or desensitization earlier on in the protocol. In order to exclude the possibility that chemically induced responses are secondary to induced muscular activity, sensitive strain gauge recordings of muscular activity should be routinely made concurrently with neural recordings.

18. Food, but not water, is withheld for 24 h before surgery.
19. Supplemental doses of pancuronium bromide (0.2–0.3 mg/kg/h) are given when necessary to maintain paralysis during the experiment.
20. The balloon should occupy approximately two-thirds of the proximal stomach. The pylorus mustn't be obstructed, so that no blockage of gastric emptying may occur. The outside diameter of the balloon when inflated is greater than the intraluminal diameter of the stomach of the rat. Therefore, the pressure measured during GD reflects actual intragastric pressure.
21. At the end of the protocol for each fibre, the abdomen should be opened, and the mechanosensitive receptive field can be located by probing the stomach with a fine, blunt glass rod.
22. This temperature should be maintained during dissection to preserve the tissue and prevent metabolic degradation.
23. Usually, it is very rare with the described size of the strands used to have more than three units / nerve strands; however, when this occurs, the strand can be split further to reduce the number of units. If this can't be managed, this preparation should be discarded.
24. The claw should always be hooked to the edge of the stomach or esophagus adjacent to the receptive field under investigation.
25. All tension-sensitive afferents respond to stretch in both the *longitudinal* and *circular* direction, while no afferents exist that respond only to *longitudinal* stretch. For this reason and also to provide optimum control, stretch is applied in a *circular* direction.

    Tension response curves should be obtained for each receptive field because they can be used in combination with von Frey thresholds to determine whether the receptive fields are located in the mucosa or the muscle layer of the esophageal wall, or both.
26. In all experiments, the mechanical sensitivity of receptive fields should be checked between each drug application to ensure continued viability of the unit under investigation. Further application of other drugs should not be undertaken if a certain drug desensitizes the receptive field to mechanical stimulation.

27. It is important to note that chemosensitivity of *one* fibre only per experiment is evaluated to avoid bias due to sensitization or desensitization. After removal of the drug from around the receptive field, the afferent fibres must be allowed to return to a normal baseline level of activity (at least 5 min of normal baseline activity should be maintained before the addition of another drug).
28. Rats should be fasted overnight.
29. The area near the celiac/superior mesenteric ganglia complex should be avoided.
30. In a few preparations, the vagal trunks should be cleared as described and the gastric vagal branches should be cut caudad to the celiac and hepatic branches. The esophagus and stomach should then be removed. This may improve the recording of pancreatic afferent signals by eliminating afferent signals of gastric and esophageal origin.
31. Dex–Kreb's solution is superior to modified Kreb's solution in maintaining pancreatic tissue integrity over the experimental period (4–6 h).
32. Experimental manipulations should only commence following a stabilization period of about 1 h.
33. During each period of duct distension, the region of the CBD-duodenal junction should be viewed via the dissection microscope to confirm that PD duct distension is achieved and no leakage of fluid into the duodenum occurs.
34. Washout periods should be performed over a period of 10–20 min.
35. Animals should be fasted for 18 h.
36. The smaller copper ring (1 mm OD) used here is due to the smaller abdominal incision required for the surgery.
37. This catheter also serves as a drain for this segment of the duodenum.
38. The Chart module (5.1) and Spike Histogram v2.2 software can be used for nerve spike discrimination and analysis of spike discharge rate.
39. The chamber temperature should be kept at ~26°C.
40. The other ureter can be prepared similarly, should then be mounted onto a piece of rubber and can be kept in oxygenated SIF at 4°C, if necessary overnight (it can be used for an experiment the next day).
41. This flow rate is within the physiological range of urine flow in the guinea-pig.
42. Contractions of the ureter are indicated by short (1–3 s) increases in intraluminal pressure (10–30 mmHg).

43. Recordings can be made between half an hour and 9 h after the cannulation of the ureter.
44. This can be tested either by electrical stimulation or by direct mechanical stimulation of the smooth muscle.
45. Using this technique, small nerves as short as 2 mm can be utilized for recording.
46. If the discrimination of single units is not possible, attempts can be made to reduce the number of units by cutting/fibre teasing, or (if impossible) the nerve must be discarded.
47. The ureter should be initially touched and about 3 s later be pressed for about 1 s. In addition, small glass beads (diameter 0.5–0.9 mm) fixed onto a fine tungsten wire or an adljustable umbrella-like distension device can be used for intraluminal stroking or for a local (1–2 mm) distension of the ureteric wall, respectively.
48. The interval between these stimuli should be at least 3 min and ought to be extended according to the stimulus intensity and the responses of the unit.
49. The corneal and flexion reflexes are checked every 30 min, and the animals are maintained in an areflexic state by administering supplemental doses (about one-tenth of initial dosage) of pentobarbital sodium via a venous cannula when necessary.
50. In most cases, the preparations from both sides can be used.
51. Until the second testis is excised, the body temperature should be maintained in the physiological range using a heat pad.
52. Usually, it is very rare with the described size of the strands used to have more than three units/nerve strands; however, when this occurs, the strand can be split further to reduce the number of units. If this can't be managed, this preparation should be discarded.
53. The interval between tests should be ~10 min.
54. This can be achieved by raising the temperature of the water circulating in the outer trough to 65 or 70°C.
55. The rats have free access to standard food and tap water and are allowed to habituate to the housing facilities for at least one week before the day of the experiment.
56. Single-unit recording should now be ensured by checking the constancy of the shape and polarity of the displayed spike waveform on PC.
57. Units are classified as *low threshold* if they respond to distension <20 g and as *high threshold* if they responded to distension >40 g.

References

1. Mueller MH, Glatzle J, Kampitoglou D, Kasparek MS, Grundy D, Kreis ME (2008) Differential sensitization of afferent neuronal pathways during postoperative ileus in the mouse jejunum. Ann Surg 247:791–802
2. Brunsden AM, Jacob S, Bardhan KD, Grundy D (2002) Mesenteric afferent nerves are sensitive to vascular perfusion in a novel preparation of rat ileum in vitro. Am J Physiol Gastrointest Liver Physiol 283:G656–G665
3. Rong W, Winchester WJ, Grundy D (2007) Spontaneous hypersensitivity in mesenteric afferent nerves of mice deficient in the sst2 subtype of somatostatin receptor. J Physiol 581:779–786
4. Lynn PA, Blackshaw LA (1999) In vitro recordings of afferent fibres with receptive fields in the serosa, muscle and mucosa of rat colon. J Physiol 518(Pt 1):271–282
5. Page AJ, Blackshaw LA (1998) An in vitro study of the properties of vagal afferent fibres innervating the ferret oesophagus and stomach. J Physiol 512(Pt 3):907–916
6. Cervero F, Sann H (1989) Mechanically evoked responses of afferent fibres innervating the guinea-pig's ureter: an in vitro study. J Physiol 412:245–266
7. Grundy D, Booth CE, Winchester W, Hicks GA (2004) Peripheral opiate action on afferent fibres supplying the rat intestine. Neurogastroenterol Motil 16(Suppl. 2):29–37
8. Hillsley K, McCaul C, Aerssens J, Peeters PJ, Gijsen H, Moechars D, Coulie B, Grundy D, Stead RH (2007) Activation of the cannabinoid 2 (CB2) receptor inhibits murine mesenteric afferent nerve activity. Neurogastroenterol Motil 19:769–777
9. Ozaki N, Sengupta JN, Gebhart GF (1999) Mechanosensitive properties of gastric vagal afferent fibers in the rat. J Neurophysiol 82: 2210–2220
10. Schloithe AC, Sutherland K, Woods CM, Blackshaw LA, Davison JS, Toouli J, Saccone GT (2008) A novel preparation to study rat pancreatic spinal and vagal mechanosensitive afferents in vitro. Neurogastroenterol Motil 20:1060–1069
11. Schloithe AC, Woods CM, Davison JS, Blackshaw LA, Toouli J, Saccone GT (2006) Pancreatobiliary afferent recordings in the anaesthetised Australian possum. Auton Neurosci 126–127:292–298
12. Vlaskovska M, Kasakov L, Rong W, Bodin P, Bardini M, Cockayne DA, Ford AP, Burnstock G (2001) P2X3 knock-out mice reveal a major sensory role for urothelially released ATP. J Neurosci 21:5670–5677
13. Kumazawa T, Mizumura K (1980) Chemical responses of polymodal receptors of the scrotal contents in dogs. J Physiol 299: 219–231

Chapter 11

Human Correlates of Animal Models of Chronic Pain

Arpad Szallasi

Abstract

Neuropathic pain is defined by International Association for the Study of Pain as "pain initiated or caused by a primary lesion or dysfunction in the nervous system which can persist long after the initial injury has healed". Given the complexity of neuropathic pain ("lesion or dysfunction" encompasses a wide variety of disease states, ranging from trauma through neurotoxins and infections to metabolic disturbances), it is hardly surprising that an array of models has been developed for this pain condition, many of which are described in this volume. This chapter addresses the clinical correlates of these pain models.

Key words: Neuropathic pain, Animal models, Clinical correlates

1. Definition of Chronic Pain

Chronic pain is commonly defined as pain lasting longer than 3 months though some experts advocate 6 months as diagnostic criterion (1). Chronic pain can be subdivided into four major categories, namely neuropathic pain, nociceptive pain, mixed pain, and idiopathic pain (2).

Neuropathic pain is defined by the International Association for the Study of Pain (IASP) as "pain initiated or caused by a primary lesion or dysfunction in the nervous system which can persist long after the initial injury has healed" (3). An alternative definition of neuropathic pain was recently suggested by Treede and colleagues as pain arising as a direct consequence of a lesion or disease affecting the somatosensory system (4). Prime examples of neuropathic pain include pain secondary to nerve injury or multiple sclerosis as well as trigeminal neuralgia. Neuropathic pain is characterized by spontaneous pain, hyperalgesia (increased pain response to painful stimuli), and allodynia

Arpad Szallasi (ed.), *Analgesia: Methods and Protocols*, Methods in Molecular Biology, vol. 617,
DOI 10.1007/978-1-60327-323-7_11, © Springer Science+Business Media, LLC 2010

(pain evoked by stimuli that are normally not painful). Of note, these symptoms are also present in other forms of chronic pain. Indeed, sensory loss (this is a neurological sign, "numbness" is the corresponding symptom) is probably the only sign which is somewhat unique to neuropathic pain (it can also be detected in mixed pain). Examples of nociceptive and idiopathic pain are postoperative pain and fibromyalgia, respectively. Cancer and low back pain are considered to be mixed in etiology.

2. Types of Chronic Pain

As detailed in the chapters by Drs. Modir and Wallace, several good human models are available to study the effect of analgesic drugs on acute nociceptive pain. To investigate chronic pain, a number of animal models have been developed over the last two decades. Murine models of osteoarthritis and canine bone cancer may be used to study human nociceptive and mixed pain, respectively. Idiopathic pain is hard to model for obvious reasons.

Neuropathic pain is of special interest because it is also a major contributor to mixed pain conditions like the common low back pain. Given the complexity of neuropathic pain ("lesion or dysfunction" encompasses a wide variety of disease states, ranging from trauma through neurotoxins and infections to metabolic disturbances), it is hardly surprising that an array of models (mostly rodent) has been developed for this pain condition. The clinical correlates of these animal models are not always clear that hinders drug development. Somewhat arbitrarily, neuropathic pain can be further subdivided as peripheral and central. Most patients are believed to have peripheral neuropathic pain.

3. Clinical Correlates of Some Commonly Used Rodent Pain Models

Commonly used animal models of neuropathic pain are described in details in the subsequent chapters. Here, I deal only with the clinical correlates.

1. Unilateral ligation of the L5/L6 (or L5 only) spinal nerves in rats mimics the effects of nerve plexus injury in man (5).
2. Chronic compression by stainless steel rods of L4 and L5 dorsal root ganglia (DRG) in rats is a model of nerve root pain secondary to herniated disk or spinal stenosis in man (6).
3. Crush by forceps of the sciatic nerve in rats is a model of sciatic nerve contusion (7).

4. Partial (30–50%) and unilateral ligation of the rat sciatic nerve is believed to mimic complex regional pain syndrome (CRPS) in man (though essentially this is also nerve injury pain model). A recent CRPS model (post-ischemia) was developed by Gary Bennett and colleagues (8).
5. The so-called "spared nerve injury" (the tibial and common peroneal branches of the sciatic nerve are ligated, whereas the sural nerve remains intact) model was suggested to correspond to various peripheral neuropathies in man (9).
6. The chronic constriction injury model (also known as the Bennett model) utilizes loose ligatures placed at the sciatic nerve at mid-thigh level. This was suggested to mimic such diverse human pain conditions as sciatica secondary to lumbar disk herniation or nerve entrapment, heavy metal poisoning, anoxia, and metabolic disorders such as painful diabetic polyneuropathy (10).
7. Neuroma generation by severing the saphenous nerve is a model for human neuromas (a sequel to traumatic injury of peripheral nerves) (11).

Clinical pain is, of course, a subjective experience that hinders the extrapolation of animal experiments to pain patients.

References

1. http://www.vachronicpain.org
2. McMahon S, Koltzenburg M (eds) (2005) Wall and Melzack's textbook of pain, 5th edn. Churchill Livingston
3. http://www.iasp-pain.org
4. Treede RD, Jensen TS, Campbell JN, Cruccu G, Dostrovsky JO, Griffin JW, Hansson P, Hughes R, Nurmikko T, Serra J (2008) Neuropathic pain: redefinition and a grading system for clinical and research purposes. Neurology 47:1630–1635
5. Kim SH, Chung JM (1992) An experimental model for peripheral neuropathy produced by segmental spinal nerve ligation in the rat. Pain 50:355–363
6. Hu SJ, Xing JL (1998) An experimental model for chronic compression of dorsal root ganglion produced by intervertebral foramen stenosis in the rat. Pain 77:15–23
7. Bester H, Beggs S, Woolf CJ (2000) Changes in tactile stimuli-induced behavior and c-fos expression in the superficial dorsal horn and in parabrachial nuclei after sciatic nerve crush. J Comp Neurol 428:45–61
8. Coderre TJ, Xanthos DN, Francis L, Bennett GJ (2004) Chronic post-ischemia pain (CPIP): a novel animal model of complex regional pain syndrome-type I (CRPS-I; reflex sympathetic dystrophy) produced by prolonged hindpaw ischemia and reperfusion in the rat. Pain 112:94–105
9. Decosterd I, Woolf CJ (2000) Spared nerve injury: an animal model of persistent peripheral neuropathic pain. Pain 87:149–158
10. Bennett GJ, Xie YK (1988) A peripheral mononeuropathy in rat produces disorders of pain sensation like those seen in man. Pain 33:87–107
11. Rivera L, Gallar J, Pozzo MA, Belmonte C (2000) Responses of nerve fibres of the rar saphenous nerve neuroma to mechanical and chemical stimulation. J Physiol 527:305–313

Chapter 12

Human Experimental Pain Models 1: The Ultraviolet Light UV-B Pain Model

James G. Modir and Mark S. Wallace

Abstract

The UV-B pain model utilizes ultraviolet light to induce a small area of inflammation allowing assessment of mechanical and thermal thresholds. Pharmacologic testing has mainly focused on reduction of primary hyperalgesia, although the effect of analgesics on secondary hyperalgesia has also been investigated. The model requires an instrument to precisely generate controlled UV-B tissue hyperalgesia. Initially, a minimum dose to induce tissue hyperalgesia is determined; subsequently, dosages are delivered in set quantities. Tissue is then assessed for inflammation using color Doppler imaging or flare measurements. Heat pain thresholds and pain tolerance are often evaluated using a commercially available thermal sensory testing device. Analgesics can be administered to determine the influence on these clinical endpoints.

Key words: Ultraviolet radiation (UV-B), Inflammation, Pain model, Hyperalgesia, Analgesics, Human experimental pain

1. Introduction

Ultraviolet radiation (UV-B) is utilized to induce a controlled area of inflammation without causing continuous pain (1). This permits assessment of mechanical and thermal pain thresholds. Studies have focused on using this model to assess the effect of peripherally acting analgesic medications on primary hyperalgesia. Gustorff et al. have proposed that the model may promote a brief secondary hyperalgesia, which appears to respond to opioids (2). Similar to the electrical pain model, Koppert et al have demonstrated that UV light may signal silent nociceptors contributing to hyperalgesia (3).

Pharmacological analysis using the UV-B pain model has shown variable results. Morphine significantly increased pain

Arpad Szallasi (ed.), *Analgesia: Methods and Protocols*, Methods in Molecular Biology, vol. 617,
DOI 10.1007/978-1-60327-323-7_12, © Springer Science+Business Media, LLC 2010

thresholds to UV-B treated areas, but not to mechanical pain thresholds (4). Gabapentin has been shown to lack antihyperalgesic effect and was not shown to have an opioid-enhancing effect. On the other hand, the study also showed that remifentanil increased the heat pain tolerance threshold significantly, but showed a minimal reduction in the area of secondary hyperalgesia (5). In addition, the selective COX-2 inhibitor, rofecoxib, increased the heat pain tolerance threshold and diminished the area of secondary hyperalgesia (6). Furthermore, the nonsteroidal anti-inflammatory ibuprofen was also shown to decrease the area of secondary hyperalgesia to mechanical stimuli (7).

2. Materials

2.1. Determining Minimum Erythema Dose (MED)

1. Calibrated UVB-source (Sellasol, Sellas Medizinische Gerate GMBH, Gevelsberg-Vogelsand, Germany), wavelength 290–320.
2. Saalmann multitester SBB LT 400TM (Saalmann Medizintechnik, Herford, Germany).
3. Chromameter CR-400 (Konica Minolta, Japan).

2.2. Assessing UVB Induced Inflammation

1. Laser Doppler Imager LDI-2 (Moor Instruments, Devon, UK).

2.3. Measuring Heat Pain Threshold and Tolerance

1. Thermal sensory testing device TSAII-2001 (Medoc, Ramat Yishai, Israel).

3. Methods

3.1. Determining Minimum Erythema Dose (MED)

1. Protective eye glasses are required prior to switching on the multitester and worn throughout testing. The MED must be determined prior to initiating the experimentally induced hyperalgesia to control for interindividual variations in UV-B skin sensitivity.
2. Prior to testing, the skin should be cleaned with hydrex solution to remove any cosmetics.
3. Five distinct spots are irradiated with UV-B using the multitester (see Note 1). It is important to align the multitester, so that no light escapes (Fig. 1).

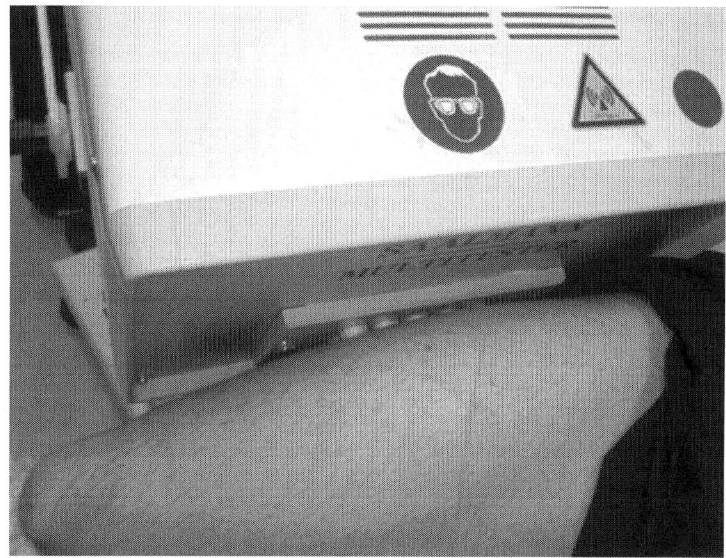

Fig. 1. Example of proper placement of Saalmann Multitester on the thigh. Photo courtesy of Boris A. Chizh, MD PhD

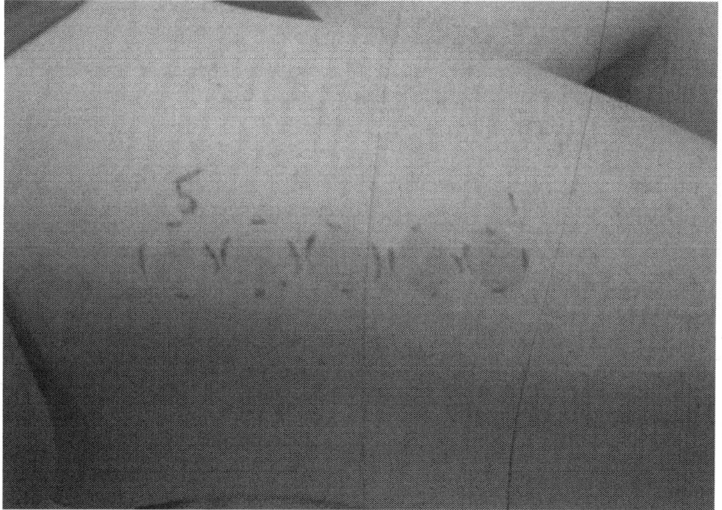

Fig. 2. Example of responses to graded UB-V irradiation. Photo courtesy of Boris A. Chizh, MD PhD

4. Start with 100–40 mJ/cm^2 of UV-B irradiation. This is accomplished using the 5 hole template. The dose is set to 100 mJ/cm^2 and the 5 sites are irradiated simultaneously. The template is graded out at different levels, with the highest dose being clear and the lowest dose graded down by 60% (Fig. 2). Exposure time is usually under 60 s. Utilizing the same machine for each patient may reduce any variation in emission intensity (see Note 2) (8).

5. The MED is ascertained using a colorimetric analysis, which is either perceived visually or by a chromameter (see Note 3).
6. Erythema and eschar formation is scored in a scale of 0–4 (see Note 4).
7. Colorimetry can also be used to assess skin color change, especially if discrepancies in the score arise. The area measured is 8 mm and a change of 3 units on red scale equates to approximately a grade 1 MED, as compared to the visual scale.

3.2. Assessing UV-B-induced Inflammation

1. Diminishing interindividual variability is important for reliable results when performing algesimetric testing. Typically, the site is irradiated with 3× MED and assessed for inflammation with color Doppler and heat pain thresholds and tolerance are also performed (see Note 5).
2. Inflammation is assessed using color Doppler imaging. After UV-B irradiation is performed, the subjects return for a baseline assessment of inflammation. This is usually performed 24 h postirradiation since this normally corresponds to the plateau phase of inflammation and hyperalgesia (see Note 6).
3. Flare measurements are typically performed with a laser Doppler. These measurements are taken 24 h postirradiation and then repeated approximately 6 h after treatment with the experimental medication.
4. Flare area is estimated by analyzing an area of 16 × 8 cm around the stimulation site with a resolution of 22,400 pixels. The flare area is then calculated from all pixels around this site in which values exceeded the 95 percentile of the baseline distribution.

3.3. Measuring Heat Pain Thresholds and Tolerance

1. Heat pain thresholds and tolerance are assessed using a commercially available thermal sensory testing device. After UV-B irradiation is performed, the subjects return for a baseline assessment for heat pain threshold and tolerance measurements, which are usually performed 24 h postirradiation corresponding to the plateau of inflammation and hyperalgesia (see Note 6).
2. A computer-assisted 3 × 3 cm Peltier device is positioned on the upper-inner thigh corresponding to the test site for UV-B irradiation (see Note 7). To determine the heat threshold, the probe is set to 32°C and increased incrementally by 1 degree per second until the subject first senses heat. This measurement is then repeated three times to generate a mean threshold measurement.
3. Heat pain tolerance test is performed in a similar manner, except that the subject stops the test when the heat stimulus is intolerable. A maximum temperature is set to 50°C to avoid burn injury.

4. Notes

1. Patients are usually asked to avoid sun exposure to these test sites prior to testing in order to avoid external UV interference. The areas tested should be distinct and documented each session to avoid accumulating UV exposure and confounding results (7). The inner thigh is often used since it is less exposed to natural light. Performing these sessions during the winter months can also reduce exogenous exposure to UV-B (2).
2. Some studies have excluded patients who fail to develop erythema after UV-B is applied since such patients may not provide adequate results during algesimetric testing (9).
3. To perform this visually, the OECD Guideline for Testing of Chemicals No. 404, adopted on 24th April 2002: "Acute Dermal Irritation/Corrosion" scale is utilized (8, 10).
4. Erythema and eschar formation scale:
   (a) No erythema
   (b) Very slight erythema (barely perceptible)
   (c) Well-defined erythema
   (d) Moderate to severe erythema
   (e) Severe erythema (beet redness) to eschar formation
5. Hoffmann et al. demonstrated that irradiating a 5 cm diameter circular spot with 3× MED on the ventral-medial side of the upper leg induced reproducible erythema (11). Subsequently, the new test spot can receive fixed units of MED, such as 1× MED or 3× MED (personal communication).
6. The time course is well described by Hoffman and Schmelz (11). In their study, UV-B treatment increased blood flow by up to eight-fold, but peaked at 12 h after irradiation and normalized by 96 h. On the other hand, the development of mechanical and thermal hyperalgesia was delayed in comparison to changes in blood flow, reaching a plateau at 24 h and peaking at 48 h postirradiation (11). Thus, laser Doppler imaging and psychometric testing should occur 24 h after irradiation, so that both inflammation and mechanical or thermal hyperalgesia can be assessed.
7. The size of the peltier probe varies. Both 3×3 cm and 1.8×1.8 cm probes have been utilized with success (2, 9). Also, when securing the probe to the skin, consider using elastic wrap to insure close contact of probe to skin. The curvilinear shape of the thigh should also be considered (2). The interstimulus time is 15 s for heat perception and 60 s for heat tolerance (2). Standardized training and measurements of thresholds were performed prior to UVB irradiation of subjects to avoid first-time bias (12).

References

1. Harrison GI, Young AR, Mcmahon SB (2004) Ultraviolet radiation-induced inflammation as a model for cutaneous hyperalgesia. J Invest Dermatol 122:183–189
2. Gustorff B, Anzenhofer S, Sycha T, Lehr S, Kress HG (2004) The sunburn pain model: the stability of primary and secondary hyperalgesia over 10 hours in a crossover setting. Anesth Analg 98:173–177
3. Koppert W, Brueckl V, Weidner C, Schmelz M (2004) Mechanically induced axon reflex and hyperalgesia in human UV-B burn are reduced by systemic lidocaine. Eur J Pain 8(3): 237–244
4. Koppert W, Likar R, Geisslinger G, Zeck S, Schmelz M, Sittl R (1999) Peripheral antihyperalgesic effect of morphine to heat, but not mechanical, stimulation in healthy volunteers after ultraviolet-B irradiation. Anesth Analg 88:117–122
5. Gustorff B, Hoechtl K, Sycha T, Felouzis E, Lehr S, Kress HG (2004) The effects of Remifentanil and Gabapentin on hyperalgesia in a new extended inflammatory skin pain model in healthy volunteers. Anesth Analg 98:401–407
6. Sycha T, Anzenhofer S, Lehr S, Schmetterer L, Chizh B, Eichler HG, Gustorff B (2005) Rofecoxib attenuates both primary and secondary inflammatory hyperalgesia: a randomized, double blinded, placebo controlled crossover trial in the UV-B pain model. Pain 113(3): 316–322
7. Bickel A, Dorfs S, Schmelz M, Forster C, Uhl W, Handwerker HO (1998) Effects of antihyperalgesic drugs on experimentally induced hyperalgesia in main. Pain 76(3):317–325
8. Chizh BA (2008) Personal Communication
9. Chizh B, O'Donnell M, Napolitano A, Wang J, Brooke A, Aylott M, Bullman J, Gray EJ, Lai RY, Williams PM, Appleby JM (2007) The effects of the TRPV1 antagonist SB-705498 on TRPV1 receptor-mediated activity and inflammatory hyperalgesia in humans. Pain 132(1):132–141
10. OECD (Organisation for Economic Cooperation and Development) (2002) OECD guideline for testing of chemicals No. 404: acute dermal irritation/corrosion. Organisation for Economic Cooperation and Development, Paris, pp 1–13
11. Hoffmann RT, Schmelz M (1999) Time course of UVA- and UVB-induced inflammation and hyperalgesia in human skin. Eur J Pain 3(2):131–139
12. Yarnitsky D, Sprecher E, Zaslansky R, Hemli JA (1996) Multiple session experimental pain measurement. Pain 67:327–333

Chapter 13

Human Experimental Pain Models 2: The Cold Pressor Model

James G. Modir and Mark S. Wallace

Abstract

The cold pressor test is a reliable pain model in which subjects submerge their hands and forearms into ice water while onset to pain, pain intensity, and tolerance are assessed. Although originally developed as a model for hypertension, the paradigm leads to development of reproducible pain responses allowing assessment to analgesic medications. However, analgesic variability to various medications has been observed. A recent study suggests that methodological discrepancies may contribute to such inconsistencies. The model may be more reproducible by utilizing consistent protocols.

Key words: Cold pressor test, Analgesia, Human experimental pain, Hyperalgesia, Nociceptors

1. Introduction

The Cold Pressor (CP) test is a well-established pain model in which subjects are asked to submerge their hands and forearms into ice water. The three primary outcomes typically measured include time to onset of pain, pain intensity (VAS), and pain tolerance (time to hand withdrawal). Subjects report two temporally separated pain responses. Immediately, they may experience a pure cold sensation, often followed by a radiating deep, dull aching pain in clinical quality and intensity, which tends to dominate other sensations (1, 2). The freezing water causes an acute and tonic noxious cold pain stimulus by activating peripheral nociceptors and central pain systems, which is often accompanied by an autonomic response. In fact, the model was originally developed to test antihypertensive medications (2). Nevertheless, the pain response is often reproducible making the model ideal for measuring reduction of pain to various pharmaceuticals.

Arpad Szallasi (ed.), *Analgesia: Methods and Protocols*, Methods in Molecular Biology, vol. 617,
DOI 10.1007/978-1-60327-323-7_13, © Springer Science+Business Media, LLC 2010

However, variability in analgesia to different classes of drugs has been observed (3). For instance, the model is reliable in demonstrating reduction in pain following administration of opioids (4). In addition, the analgesic effects of acupuncture and transcutaneous nerve stimulation in a trial of 46 subjects have been documented (5). On the other hand, the efficacy of nonsteroidal anti-inflammatory drugs (NSAIDS) has produced conflicting results. The effect of acetaminophen has shown to provide a modest reduction in pain from the CP model (3). Oral venlafaxine, amitriptyline, and imipramine showed no effect (6, 7). Finally, Gabapentin improved the acute analgesic effect of morphine when used in the CP model (8).

In an attempt to understand these conflicting outcomes, Mitchell et al. performed a study that showed how inconsistencies in methodology of the cold pressor test affect clinical endpoints. Their study demonstrated that variations in water temperature as small as 2°C can result in significant differences in both pain intensity levels and tolerance times (9). Furthermore, in line with previous studies of human experimental pain, gender differences in CP test have been observed (2, 9).

Subject safety is prioritized by avoiding the cold pressor test in certain subpopulations. Contraindications to the test include cardiac or vascular disease, especially Raynaud's Syndrome, blood pressure problems, diabetes, epilepsy, pregnancy, and recent serious injuries (9).

2. Materials

1. Circulating and cooling water bath (Jeiotech model VTRC 620, Seoul, Republic of Korea)
2. Water cooler

3. Methods

General Screening Criteria: Subjects are chosen and those patients with contraindications are excluded. In addition, subjects who can tolerate the ice bath for the maximal period of time are also generally eliminated. Other considerations include excluding subjects with neurologic or psychiatric illness, patients who are taking the medication to be tested, and patients who fulfill the DSM-IV criteria for substance dependence. Some studies even perform breathalyzer and drug screening prior to testing.

1. The subjects are tested in a quiet, comfortable room with no audible or visual distractions.
2. Their dominant arm and hand temperature are normalized by submersion into a warm bath at 35°C for 2 min (see Note 1).
3. Subjects are asked to submerge their dominant hands into the cold water tank, which is continuously circulating to provide a constant temperature around the appendage. The temperature of the cold water tank should be maintained at 1.0°C ±0.3°C (see Note 2). The volunteers are instructed to keep their hands submerged until it proves to be intolerable. Testing is usually stopped at 120 s. The subjects are asked to provide continuous VAS scores and tolerance time is measured in seconds with a stopwatch.
4. Pharmaceutical testing is employed in the same manner, administering the medication according to its pharmacokinetics. The same endpoints are measured and compared.

4. Notes

1. Studies from Mitchel et al. demonstrated that a difference as little as 2°C can alter pain intensity levels and tolerance (9). Thus, every effort should be made to insure adequate circulation of water temperature with frequent temperature measurements. Some experiments have used an aquarium pump instead of the aforementioned unit from Jeiotech. Tank sizes vary from 6 to 14 L (6, 7, 9).
2. Variation in insertion depth is common in most protocols, but consistency is most important. At least 16 cm of submersion should provide adequate testing conditions. In addition, studies vary as to whether they standardize the extremity to a specific temperature prior to submersion into cold water. The temperature of the cold water bath also varies in the literature with a range of 0–2°C. Generally speaking, the extremity temperature should be measured prior to submersion into cold water to control for variability in baseline extremity temperature. Most studies also provide multiple training sessions to both eliminate patients who are tolerant to the effect of cold and familiarize volunteers with the study session procedure (4).

References

1. Fruhstorfer H, Lindblom U (1983) Vascular participation in deep cold pain. Pain 17(3): 235–241
2. Compton P, Charuvastra VC, Ling W (2003) Effect of oral ketorolac and gender on human cold pressor pain tolerance. Clin Exp Pharmacol Physiol 30(10):759–763
3. Yuan CS, Karrison T, Wu JA, Lowell JP, Lynch JP, Foss JF (1998) Dose-related effects of oral acetaminophen on cold-induced pain: a double-blind, randomized, placebo-controlled trial. Clin Pharmacol Ther 63(3): 379–383
4. Jones SF, McQuay HJ, Moore RA, Hand CW (1988) Morphine and Ibuprofen compared using the cold pressor test. Pain 34(2): 117–122
5. Ashton H, Ebenezer I, Golding JF, Thompson JW (1984) Effects of acupuncture and transcutaneous electrical nerve stimulation on cold-induced pain in normal subjects. J Psychosom Res 28:301–308
6. Enggard TP, Klitgaard NA, Gram LF, Arendt-Nielsen L, Sindrup SH (2001) Specific effect of venlafaxine on single and repetitive experimental painful stimuli in humans. Clin Pharmcol Ther 69(4):245–251
7. Enggard TP, Poulsen L, Arendt-Nielsen L, Hansen SH, Bjornsdottir I, Gram LF, Sindrup SH (2001) The analgesic effect of codeine as compared to imipramine in different human experimental pain models. Pain 92(1–2): 277–282
8. Eckhardt K, Ammon S, Hofmann U, Riebe A, Gugeler N, Mikus G (2000) Gabapentin enhances the analgesic effect of morphine in healthy volunteers. Anesth Analg 91(1):185–191
9. Mitchell LA, MacDonald RA, Brodie EE (2004) Temperature and the cold pressor test. J Pain 5(4):233–237

Chapter 14

Human Experimental Pain Models 3: Heat/Capsaicin Sensitization and Intradermal Capsaicin Models

James G. Modir and Mark S. Wallace

Abstract

The heat/capsaicin sensitization and intradermal capsaicin injection models are safe and noninvasive paradigms to generate stable, long-lasting, and reproducible injury capable of producing an area of both primary and secondary hyperalgesia. Risk of skin injury is substantially reduced since lower levels of thermal and chemical irritation produce long-lasting cutaneous hyperalgesia. Rekindling sustains central sensitization by providing peripheral nociceptive input. The intradermal capsaicin model has been widely used to test analgesic efficacy for a wide range of analgesics. Unlike the heat/capsaicin sensitization model, intradermal capsaicin results in a brief painful stimulus followed by a long lasting area of secondary hyperalgesia. The intradermal injection of capsaicin results in a transient, intense stinging sensation at the site of injection (e.g. heat allodynia) followed by a persistent area of secondary tactile allodynia.

Key words: Heat/capsaicin sensitization, Hyperalgesia, Rekindling, Central sensitization, von Frey hair, Intradermal capsaicin

1. Introduction

1.1. The Heat/Capsaicin Sensitization Model

The heat/capsaicin sensitization model was developed as a safe, noninvasive paradigm to generate stable, long-lasting, and reproducible injury capable of producing an area of both primary and secondary hyperalgesia. Lower levels of thermal and chemical irritation produce long-lasting cutaneous hyperalgesia without skin injury sufficient to test oral analgesic pharmaceuticals. This model also avoids the extreme pain associated with intradermal capsaicin injection and the potential for tissue injury associated with the burn injury model (1–4).

Arpad Szallasi (ed.), *Analgesia: Methods and Protocols*, Methods in Molecular Biology, vol. 617,
DOI 10.1007/978-1-60327-323-7_14,

One theory that arose to explain the stability and duration of cutaneous sensitization was that the effect of heat and capsaicin was synergistic. A recent study by Dahl et al. tested that assertion. They found that the combination of heat and capsaicin were neither additive nor synergistic when compared with each stimulus alone. In fact, the study demonstrated that the rekindling procedure produced the stability and reproducibility. Rekindling is accomplished by reheating the skin to 40°C for 5 min at 40 min intervals during the study day. The process of rekindling is thought to sustain central sensitization by maintaining a peripheral nociceptive input. Finally, the study demonstrated that the area of secondary hyperalgesia to von Frey hair stimulation is more reproducible than to brush (2).

One study showed that oral lamotrigine administered 90 min before initiation of the heat/capsaicin model did not significantly prevent sensitization of the nociceptive system. In addition, lamotrigine administered at induction did not suppress established secondary hyperalgesia. Lamotrigine had no analgesic effect on acute thermal nociception. In contrast, both intravenous remifentanil and oral hydromorphone significantly suppressed established secondary hyperalgesia and acute thermal nociception (2). In a different study, the analgesic effect of a single oral dose of the combination of 30 mg morphine and 30 mg of dextromethorphan was not superior to that of morphine alone when measured on acute thermal pain and experimental cutaneous sensitization in healthy volunteers (3).

1.2. The Intradermal Capsaicin Model

The intradermal capsaicin model is a safe method of producing an area of both primary and secondary hyperalgesia. It has been widely used to test analgesic efficacy of a wide range of analgesics and routes of administration including oral, intravenous, and intrathecal. Unlike the heat/capsaicin sensitization model, intradermal capsaicin results in a brief painful stimulus followed by a long lasting area of secondary hyperalgesia (5, 6).

The intradermal injection of capsaicin results in a transient report of an intense stinging sensation at the site of injection followed by a persisting tactile hypersensitivity in the area immediately surrounding the injection site (e.g. a secondary tactile allodynia) (5, 6). The pharmacology of this model of human experimental pain has been addressed with different classes of agents that include: opioids, NMDA antagonists, cannabis, sodium channel antagonists, and tricyclic antidepressants (7–10). The opioids, NMDA antagonists, and cannabis, significantly decrease pain and allodynia in this model of human experimental pain. In contrast, other nonopioids (intravenous lidocaine and tricyclic antidepressants) have minimal effect.

2. Materials

2.1. The Heat/ Capsaicin Sensitization Model

1. Capzaisin-HP cream (Chattem Inc., Chattanooga, TN).
2. 0.075% capsaicin solution (Clay-Park Labs, Bronx, NY).
3. 1-inch foam paintbrush.
4. Touch-Test Sensory Filament 5.46 (North Coast Medical, Morgan Hill, CA).
5. 26-g von Frey hair (Semmes–Weinstein monofilaments, Stoelting, IL).
6. Computer-controlled Peltier device (Medoc TSA 2001, Ramat Yishai, Israel).

2.2. Intradermal Capsaicin Model

1. Capsaicin is dissolved at 10 mg/ml in 20% cyclodextrin or 15% Tween-80.
2. 1-inch foam paintbrush.
3. Touch-Test Sensory Filament 5.46 (North Coast Medical).
4. 26-g von Frey hair (Semmes–Weinstein monofilaments).
5. Medoc TSA 2001 (Medoc).

3. Methods

3.1. Heat/Capsaicin Sensitization

1. The stimulation site (22.8 cm^2) is outlined by tracing the outside of the thermode with a felt-tip pen on the volar side of the dominant forearm.
2. Sensitization is initiated by heating the skin to 45°C for 5 min with the thermode.
3. Topical capsaicin cream is applied to the skin site for 30 min.
4. The sensitization is maintained throughout the study day by heating the skin with a lower temperature (40°C) for 5 min at 50-min intervals with the thermode (see Note 1).
5. The area of secondary hyperalgesia is quantified using a 1-inch foam paintbrush and a 26-g von Frey hair (a mildly noxious pin-like sensation,) by stimulating along 4 linear paths arranged vertically and horizontally around the stimulation site in 5-mm steps at 1-s intervals (see Note 2). Stimulation along each path is initiated well outside the hyperalgesic area and continued toward the treated skin area until the subject reports a definite change in sensation (burning, tenderness, more intense pricking). The border is marked on the skin with a felt-tip pen, and the rostral–caudal and lateral–medial dimensions are measured for surface area calculations (see Note 3).

3.2. Injection of Intradermal Capsaicin and Pain Assessments

1. Using a 27 g or 30 g hypodermic needle, 10–25 µl of the capsaicin solution is injected intradermally on the forearm or anterior thigh (see Note 4).
2. Spontaneous pain intensity is assessed using the VAS at the time of injection (time 0) and every 5 min up to 20 min (see Note 5).
3. Elicited pain intensity can also be assessed to von Frey hair stimulation, stroking and a 40°C stimulus at the injection site every 5 min. The Area under the time versus pain intensity curve can be used as the Primary Endpoint (Fig. 1).
4. The area of secondary hyperalgesia is quantified using a 1-inch foam paintbrush and a 26-g von Frey hair (a mildly noxious pin-like sensation,) by stimulating along 4–8 linear paths arranged vertically, horizontally, and diagonally around the stimulation site in 5-mm steps at 1-s intervals. Stimulation along each path is initiated well outside the hyperalgesic area and continued toward the treated skin area until the subject reports a definite change in sensation (burning, tenderness, more intense pricking). The border is marked on the skin with a felt-tip pen, and the rostral–caudal and lateral–medial dimensions are measured for surface area calculations (Fig. 2).

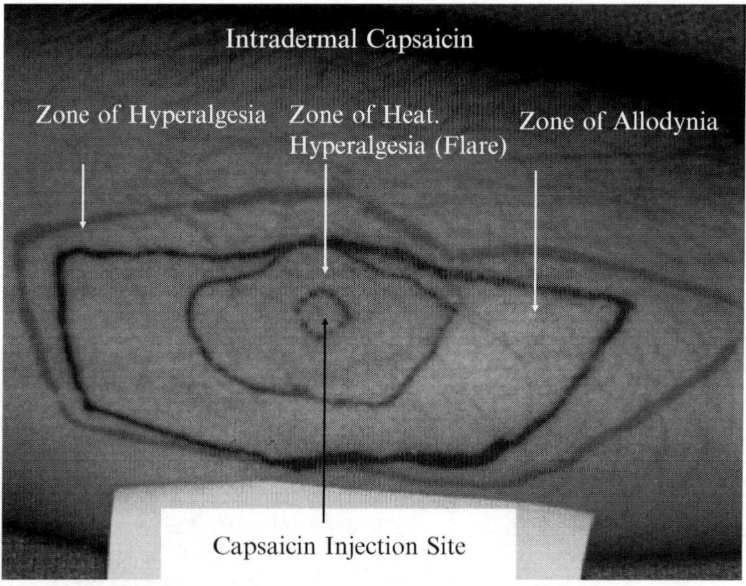

Fig. 1. Example of spontaneous pain over time after intradermal capsaicin

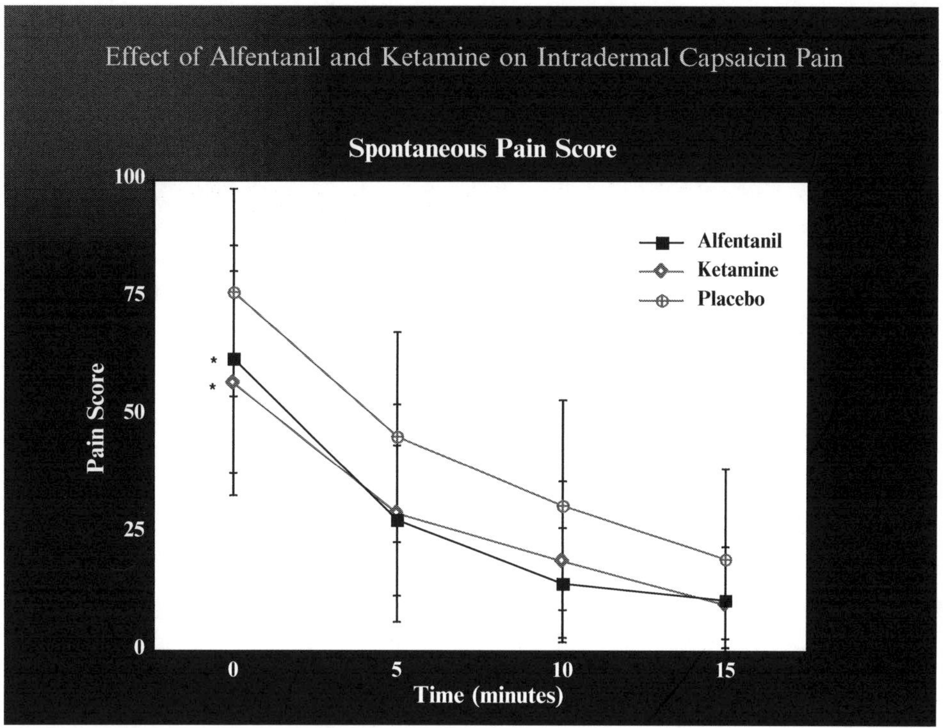

Fig. 2. Zones of hyperalgesia and allodynia after intradermal capsaicin

4. Notes

1. Rekindling is typically performed 4 times during the study day. Areas of secondary hyperalgesia to brush and von Frey hair stimulation are measured after each rekindling (1).
2. To improve reproducibility, it is recommended that a separate training day for the subjects to educate them on methods. The ability to discriminate between normal and hyperalgesic skin is critical. Measurements should be performed by only one investigator; when a crossover design is employed, the same investigator should perform the testing. Testing days must be close enough together to allow the same reference point when performing experiments using 2 or more evaluation days; however, they must also be distant enough to allow the skin to return to baseline thresholds (2).
3. Vital signs (heart rate, blood pressure, and respiratory rate) are assessed every 30 min during the study day. There are minimal safety concerns. The pain is not as severe as the intradermal capsaicin. If the patients cannot tolerate the pain of the capsaicin, it can be wiped off using a soap cleanser and ice applied.

4. If the subjects cannot tolerate the pain of the injection, ice can be applied. If this is ineffective, the site can be infiltrated with local anesthetic.
5. To improve reproducibility, it is recommended that a separate training day for the subjects to educate them on methods. The ability to discriminate between normal and hyperalgesic skin is critical. Measurements should be performed by only one investigator; when a crossover design is employed, the same investigator should perform the testing. Testing days must be close enough together to allow the same reference point when performing experiments using 2 or more evaluation days; however, they must also be distant enough to allow the skin to return to baseline thresholds. Typically, at least 4 days is sufficient between testing. It has been suggested that keeping the skin temperature constant will decrease variability between subjects.

References

1. Petersen KL, Jones B, Segredo V, Dahl J, Rowbotham MC (2001) Effect of remifentanil on pain and secondary hyperalgesia associated with the heat–capsaicin sensitization model in healthy volunteers. Anesthesiology 94(1): 15–20
2. Dirks J, Petersen KL, Dahl JB (2003) The heat/capsaicin sensitization model: a methodologic study. J Pain 4(3):122–128
3. Petersen KL, Maloney A, Hoke F, Dahl JB, Rowbotham MC (2003) A randomized study of the effect of oral lamotrigine and hydromorphone on pain and hyperalgesia following heat/capsaicin sensitization. J Pain 4(7):400–406
4. Frymoyera AR, Rowbothama MC, Petersen KL (2006) Placebo-controlled comparison of a morphine/dextromethorphan combination with morphine on experimental pain and hyperalgesia in healthy volunteers. J Pain 8(1):19–25
5. LaMotte RH et al (1991) Neurogenic hyperalgesia: psychophysical studies of underlying mechanisms. J Neurophysiol 66:190–211
6. LaMotte RH, Lundberg LE, Torebjork E (1992) Pain, hyperalgesia and activity in nociceptive C units in humans after intradermal injection of capsaicin. J Physiol 448: 749–764
7. Wallace MS et al (2002) Concentration-effect relationships for intravenous alfentanil and ketamine infusions in human volunteers: effects upon acute thresholds and capsaicin-evoked hyperpathia. J Clin Pharmacol 42:70–80
8. Wallace MS et al (1997) Concentration-effect relations for intravenous lidocaine infusions in human volunteers: effect on acute sensory thresholds and capsaicin-evoked hyperpathia. Anesthesiology 86:1262–1272
9. Wallace MS, Grubbs D (2002) Effects of oral desipramine on capsaicin induced hyperalgesia. Anesth Analg 95:973–978
10. Ando K et al (2000) Neurosensory finding after oral mexiletine in healthy volunteers. Reg Anesth Pain Med 25:468–474

Chapter 15

The Value of the Dental Impaction Pain Model in Drug Development

Stephen A. Cooper and Paul J. Desjardins

Abstract

The modern version of the Dental Impaction Pain Model (DIPM) was developed in the mid-1970s. Since that time, several hundred studies have been conducted by numerous investigators. Today it is arguably the most utilized of all the acute pain models. Its popularity is due to the success rate of the studies, fast subject entry, and cost effectiveness. The surgical procedure is extremely standardized, and the surgery requires either minimal or no use of CNS depressant anesthetics. The methodology is similar to that utilized in other acute pain models; however, the DIPM is much more versatile than most other models. The model can be easily adapted to perform multiple-dose studies, pharmacokinetics/pharmacodynamics (PK/PD) correlations, preemptive interventions, and sleep–pain studies. A few investigators have even developed microdialysis techniques, wherein they insert probes into extraction sockets to collect exudates for measuring biochemical mediators of pain or drug levels at the site of injury. In many instances, an accomplished site can complete a study of several hundred subjects in approximately 3 months. There are studies in the literature that have incorporated up to six treatment arms in one study and clearly separated the drugs from each other. The exquisite assay sensitivity is due to the homogeneity of the study population, the predictable level and appropriate intensity of the postsurgical pain, and the minimizing of variability by using only one or two study centers. The DIPM has been employed to evaluate NSAIDs (both nonselective and selective Cox inhibitors), opioids and combination analgesics, as well as some investigational drugs with unique mechanisms of action. The model is particularly useful for proof-of-concept studies that require dose-ranging and profiling the time–effect curve for efficacy including onset, peak effect, and duration of analgesic activity.

Key words: Acute pain, Dental impaction pain, First perceptible relief, Meaningful relief, Visual analog pain score

1. Introduction

During my training in dental school, I became curious as to why almost every patient with a traumatic procedure received the same analgesic prescription. Even in this early stage of my career,

Arpad Szallasi (ed.), *Analgesia: Methods and Protocols*, Methods in Molecular Biology, vol. 617,
DOI 10.1007/978-1-60327-323-7_15, © Springer Science+Business Media, LLC 2010

I suspected that treating pain was far more complex and more deserving than this simplistic approach. This led to my interest in pharmacology and eventual pursuit of an NIDR fellowship under the mentorship of Dr. William T. Beaver. Dr. Beaver, Emeritus Professor at Georgetown University, Department of Pharmacology, is one of the world's leading experts in analgesic methodology and the conduct of clinical trials in cancer and postsurgical pain. In 1971, with my background in dentistry and his expertise in Analgesiology, we embarked on the development of the Dental Impaction Pain Model. Today, there are literally hundreds of published studies utilizing this model, and it still remains one of the most widely used models for studying acute pain drugs.

Since the initial studies published in the mid-1970s, Paul Desjardins, Raymond Dionne, Kenneth Hargreaves, Elliot Hersh, Abraham Sunshine, and several other investigators have contributed to the growth and development of this model. This paper covers the following topics:

- Characteristics of the Dental Impaction Pain Model (DIPM)
- Early studies that established the DIPM
- Studies that demonstrate the versatility of the DIPM
- Methodology
- Extrapolating the results from the DIPM to other pain conditions
- Debunking some myths about the DIPM

2. Characteristics of the Dental Impaction Pain Model

How does a symptom like pain from a dental surgical procedure become transformed into a validated, standardized pain model? To be considered a representative model for acute pain, the experimental model should have assay sensitivity to discriminate against placebo as well to explore the full range of dosages for the control and experimental drugs. The ability to demonstrate efficacy across a broad spectrum of prototype analgesics determines the overall utility of the model. In addition, the model must have reproducible results, a low placebo response, and results that can be generalized across a variety of pain states. The ideal acute pain model characterizes the onset, peak effect, and duration of effect of the experimental drug across a range of dosages. As we will see, the DIPM meets all these criteria and the results from studies have clearly predicted the ultimate treatment regimens for many experimental drugs that were eventually approved for treating acute pain by the FDA and other international regulatory bodies.

It is also important to define the limitations of any acute pain model. They do not predict long-term toxicity, rare adverse events, or efficacy beyond the scope of acute pain. The efficacy results from acute pain studies are just one key aspect in assembling the puzzle of a full analgesic development program.

There are several demographic factors that make the DIPM an ideal model. The study subjects are young, healthy adults with impacted third molars commonly called wisdom teeth. The population of subjects is large in number and very homogeneous. Usually, the subjects are not even aware of their condition until a dentist makes the diagnosis from a radiographic exam. Given this demographic profile, the population rarely has any preexisting pain or complicating medical illnesses involving confounding medications. The surgical procedure is elective, relatively short (less than 30 min), and very standardized. Unlike many other surgical interventions, the procedure requires minimal sedation or anesthesia and is often performed with just a local anesthetic. Avoiding the carry-over effects of general anesthesia is an important advantage in that subjects are alert and ambulatory with no memory impairment or drug-induced nausea. Most important, the surgical procedure results in an intensity level of postoperative pain that optimizes assay sensitivity. The pain is sufficiently intense that placebo is virtually ineffective; while drugs like aspirin, ibuprofen, and codeine-like opioids have only modest analgesic activity. This results in the ideal situation of both optimal "downside" and "upside" assay sensitivity (Fig. 1).

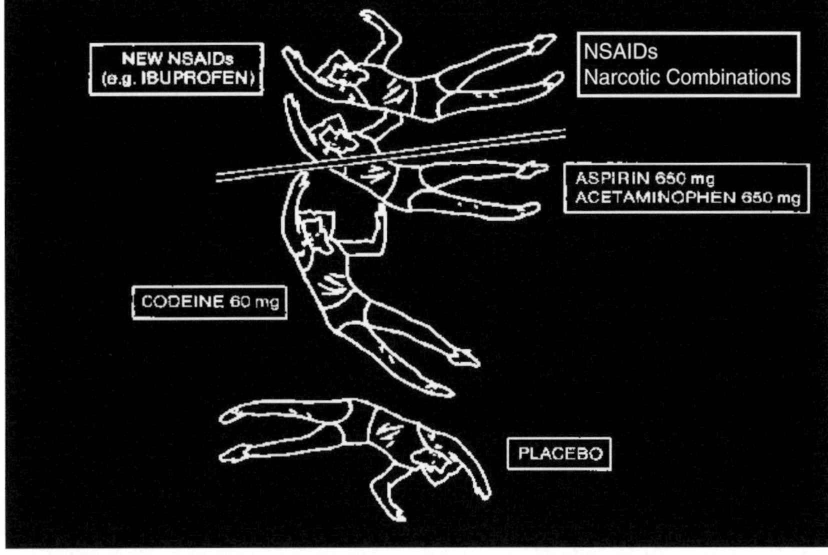

Fig. 1. Assay sensitivity – the model must be able to separate active drug from placebo as well as more efficacious drugs from less efficacious drugs

3. Versatility of the Dental Impaction Pain Model

There were several seminal studies performed in the late 1970s and early 1980s that defined the sensitivity, reproducibility, and versatility of the DIPM. One of the first published studies demonstrated that ibuprofen was a superior analgesic to aspirin (1). At the time, this was a major breakthrough and opened the door to the development of many new NSAID analgesics. One of these new NSAIDs was indoprofen. Although the drug was never approved in the US, its development program offered the opportunity to replicate studies using the same study site and research coordinator. This happened because in the original study, the aspirin control treatment failed stability testing and the pivotal study had to be repeated using the identical treatment arms. As shown in Fig. 2, the results were remarkably reproducible (2). The development program for zomepirac sodium (Zomax[R]) offered an opportunity to utilize the DIPM for early dose ranging in humans. Based on animal data, two dosages (50 mg and 100 mg) were chosen and compared to aspirin 650 mg using a sequential design which was an early form of the "Adaptive Design" that has recently gained popularity. With a sample size of just ten per group, there was a clear-cut separation of active drugs from placebo and both dosages of zomepirac were superior to aspirin. By protocol design, in the second sequence, a third

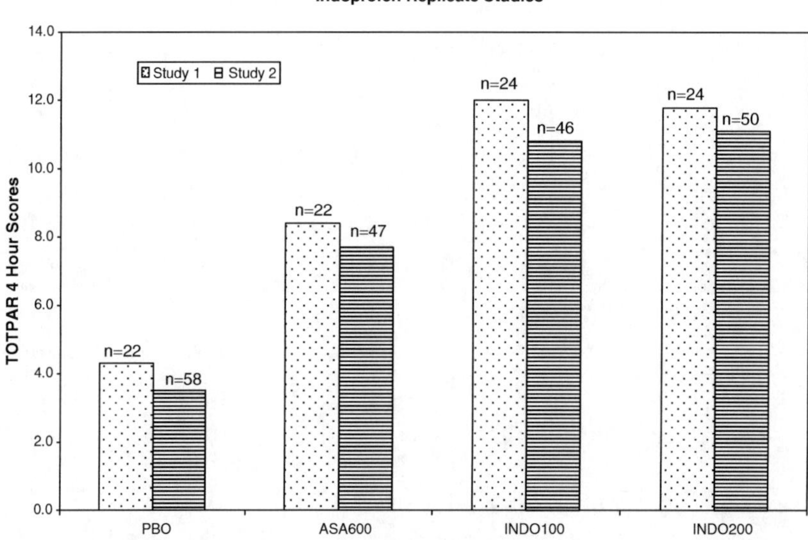

Fig. 2. Replicate studies evaluating the NSAID indoprofen demonstrating the reproducibility of the DIPM. Mean Total Pain Relief Scores over 4 h (TOTPAR4) are plotted for each treatment group in the replicate studies. Reproduced from ref. 2

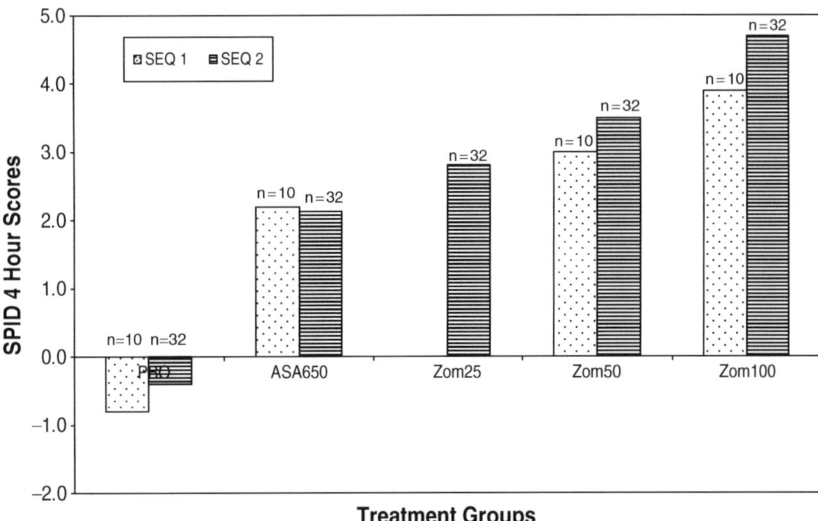

Fig. 3. Dose ranging study that used a sequential design evaluating an investigational NSAID, zomepirac. This design demonstrated that with as few as ten subjects per group, the DIPM has exquisite assay sensitivity. Mean Sum Pain Intensity Difference Scores over 4 h (SPID4) are plotted for each treatment group and for each sequence. Reproduced from ref. 3

dosage of 25 mg was added and this fell right in line on the linear part of the log dose–effect curve (Fig. 3) (3). To this day, we do not believe that any pain model can duplicate this level of assay sensitivity. Equally as impressive, this pilot dose ranging study accurately predicted the analgesic dose–effect of zomepirac across a wide array of acute pain models. Unfortunately, because of the short exposure time to drug, what the DIPM will not predict is long-term toxicity, which eventually led to the demise of both indoprofen and zomepirac.

As the DIPM became more widely utilized, investigators and pharmaceutical sponsors began to recognize its versatility. The following representative studies from the archival literature depict a variety of study designs that demonstrate durability of the surgical pain over time, the ability to quantify onset of effect, opportunities to correlate pharmacodynamics to pharmacokinetics (PK/PD modeling), and pretreatment to prevent or reduce postsurgical pain.

The surgical pain resulting from impaction surgery is most intense within a few hours after surgery intensifying as the local anesthetic effect dissipates. The intensity of the pain generally remains relatively constant for at least 12 h and then tapers off over the next 1–2 days. Figure 4 shows that the DIPM can easily accommodate single-dose evaluations lasting 12 h and even extending to 24 h. In these two studies, three doses of regular release ibuprofen (200 mg in Study 1 and 400 mg in Study 2) were compared to three doses of codeine or a single dose of a

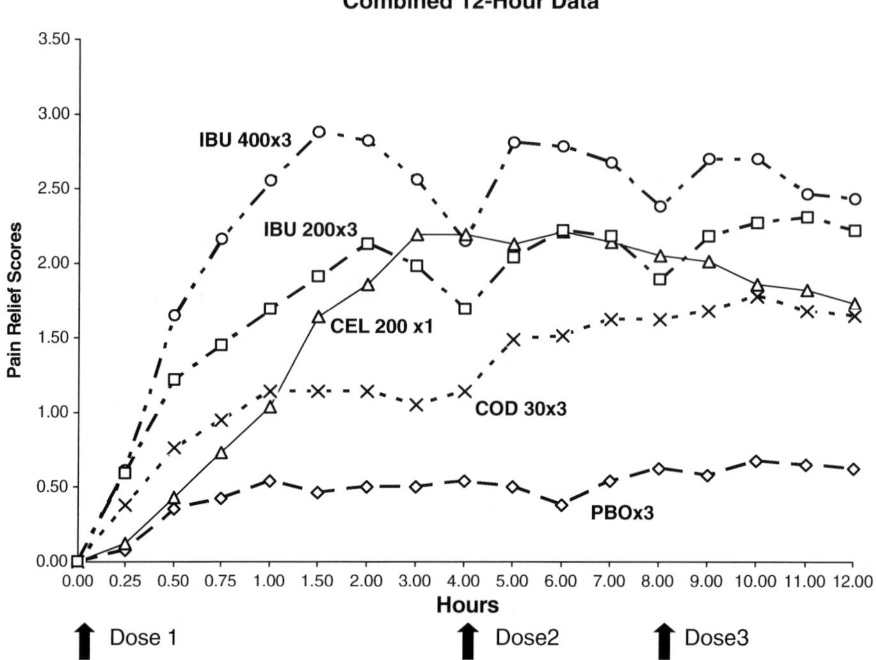

Fig. 4. Two studies with 12-h observations demonstrate reproducibility, durability, and assay sensitivity of the model. Mean Pain Relief Scores are plotted against time in hours. Reprinted with permission of Oral Surgery, Oral Medicine, Oral Pathology, Elsevier, Inc. (4), and reprinted with permission of the American College of Clinical Pharmacology (5)

controlled release ibuprofen in Study 1 and three doses of placebo or a single dose of celecoxib in Study 2. The two studies are combined into a single graph to further demonstrate the durability, reproducibility, and assay sensitivity of the DIPM (4, 5). Note the dose–effect of the 200 mg and 400 mg ibuprofen as well as the consistent peak and trough time-effect of the three doses of ibuprofen over the 12-h studies. Interestingly, these studies were performed at different sites, using independent research coordinators and separated by 10 years of time. In another multiple dose study that extended for 7 days, over 70% of subjects continued their pain medication for 3 days (Fig. 5) (6). Thus, it is quite feasible to evaluate a single dose of analgesic hourly for 12 h and extend daily observations for multiple doses for up to 3 days.

The DIPM is probably the most efficient acute pain model for assessing onset of analgesia. The two-stopwatch method measuring both First Perceptible Relief and Meaningful Relief was developed by Paul Desjardins using this model (7). After ingesting the study medication, the subject is given a stopwatch and asked to depress the button when first perceiving any relief (First Perceptible Relief). If and when this stopwatch is depressed, the subject is then given a second stopwatch and asked to depress the button when the relief is perceived as meaningful (Meaningful Relief). Using this method, onset to First Perceptible and

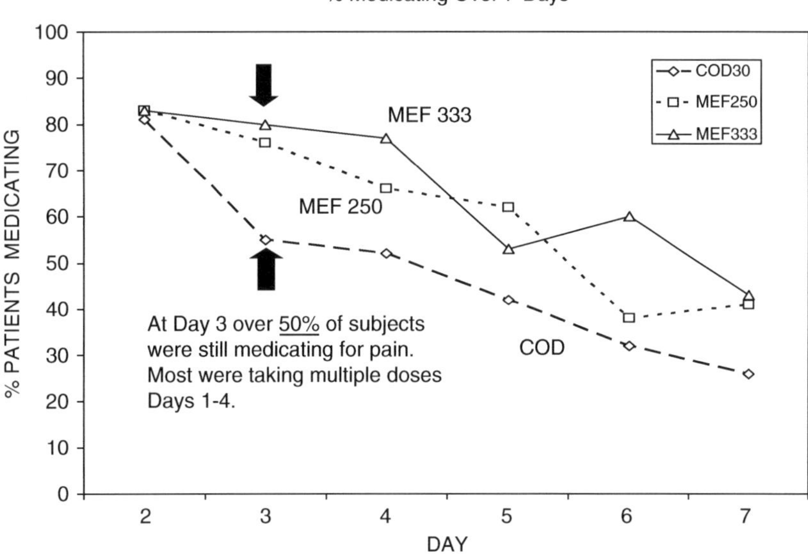

Fig. 5. Multidose study evaluating mefanamic acid demonstrates that there is sufficient postsurgical pain to dose over a 3-day period. The percentage of patients taking medication for each treatment group is plotted against days. Reproduced from ref. 6

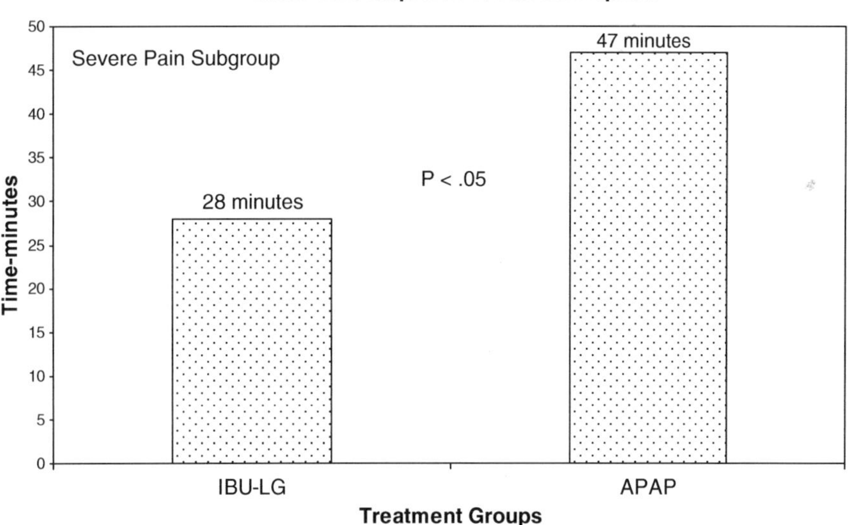

Fig. 6. Two Stopwatch data for ibuprofen liquigels demonstrates that the DIPM is ideal for assessing onset of effect of acute pain medications. Mean time in minutes to achieving Meaningful Relief is plotted for ibuprofen 400 mg and acetaminophen 1,000 mg. Reproduced from ref. 8

Meaningful Relief can be quantified to the nearest minute. The studies evaluating the benefits of the liquigel formulation of ibuprofen clearly demonstrated the power of this technique in comparing the relative onset of pain relief between ibuprofen and acetaminophen (Fig. 6) (8).

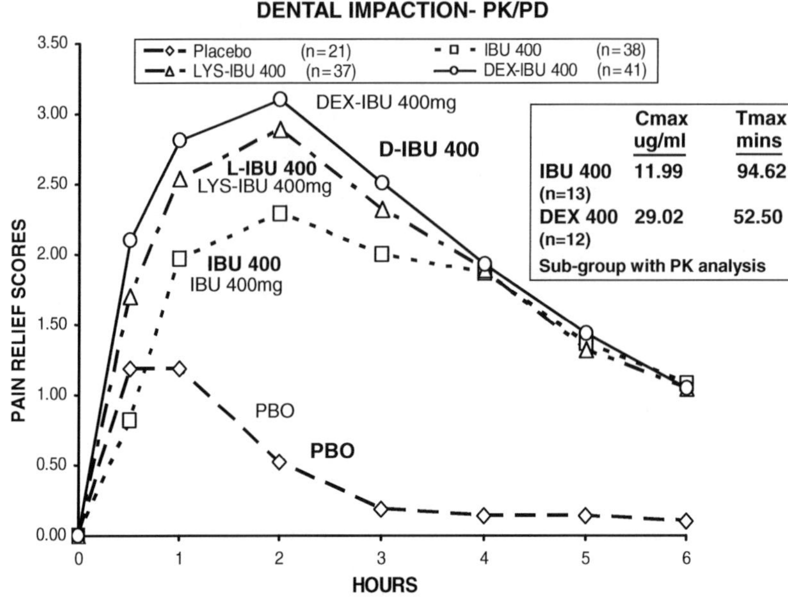

Fig. 7. PK/PD data for ibuprofen enantiomers demonstrates that the DIPM can be adapted to collect plasma and correlate plasma levels of drug to efficacy measurements. Mean Pain Relief Scores are plotted against time in hours with the inset showing the mean C_{max} and T_{max} values for a subset of subjects treated with racemic and S+ ibuprofen treatments. Reproduced from ref. 9

The DIPM is particularly well suited for PK/PD modeling. An indwelling catheter can be placed just prior to surgery, and the predictability of the onset of postsurgical pain within 2–4 h facilitates the collection of blood samples. The study depicted in Fig. 7 is based on a subset of subjects having blood draws that received either racemic ibuprofen or just the S+ isomer of ibuprofen. The PK profile for the S+ isomer clearly showed a higher C_{max} and shorter time for T_{max} and this nicely correlated with the clinically faster onset for the S+ version of ibuprofen (9).

The DIPM also is ideally suited for evaluating pretreatment prior to the onset of the pain. The experimental drugs or placebo can be administered either just prior to surgery or immediately after surgery, but prior to the local anesthetic wearing off. The primary endpoint of the study can either be measuring the time to onset of moderate pain (≥50 mm on a VAS scale) or measuring the area under the curve (AUC) for pain intensity over the entire course of the postoperative treatment. A study by Dionne et al. showed an initial pretreatment dose with the NSAID ibuprofen significantly delayed the onset as well as reduced the level of postoperative pain when compared to pretreatment with placebo (Table 1) (10). In another study by Dionne et al., ibuprofen was effective, while neither acetaminophen nor an acetaminophen–codeine combination was effective as a pretreatment therapy (11). This makes clinical sense in that neither acetaminophen nor codeine

Table 1
Onset and severity of postoperative pain after pretreatment with either placebo or ibuprofen 400 mg following surgical removal of impacted wisdom teeth

Treatment	Time to postoperative medication in minutes	Initial postoperative pain – # subjects		
		Severe	Moderate	None
Pre-placebo Post-Asa 650 mg	133.0 ± 11.8[a]	6	15	0
Pre-placebo Post-Ibu 400 mg	140.6 ± 11.1	10	14	0
Pre-Ibu 400 mg Post-Asa 650 mg	236.3 ± 30.8	5	17	1
Pre-Ibu 400 mg Post-Ibu 400 mg	241.2 ± 24.9	3	17	2
All placebo pre	137.1 ± 8.0	16	29	0
All ibuprofen pre	238.5 ± 19.9	8	34	3

[a]Standard error of mean

directly inhibits the local mediators of pain and inflammation. These studies demonstrate that the anti-inflammatory component is critical for a drug to be effective as pretreatment therapy.

4. Methods

The methods for assessing analgesia used in the DIPM are very similar to those for other acute pain models (1). The surgical procedure itself can involve 1–4 impacted third molars, but the mandibular teeth are of most importance. This is because the mandibular bone is much denser than the cancellous maxillary bone, thus resulting in greater trauma in a more confined tissue space (see Note 1). The impacted teeth are classified as either tissue, partial bony or full bony impactions. The amount of bone removal appears to be correlated to the level of postsurgical pain; therefore, full bony mandibular impactions result in the greatest level of postsurgical pain. The upside sensitivity of the model is actually enhanced as the level of postsurgical pain increases. The Bunionectomy Pain Model has many similarities to the DIPM and this bony surgical procedure creates even more severe and enduring pain. Some investigators believe that this model has equal or greater assay sensitivity to the DIPM (12).

Most study centers use only local anesthetics with a vasoconstrictor for the surgical procedure. If additional pain control is required during surgery, inhalation nitrous oxide can be administered (see Note 2). Once surgery is completed, the subject is moved to a quiet evaluation room and kept isolated from other study subjects. Research coordinators continually monitor subjects and wait for the postsurgical pain to reach at least a moderate intensity. Many sites record both a categorical score (moderate or severe) and confirm this with a Visual Analog score of at least 50 mm on the 100 mm VAS scale (see Note 3). Once the baseline score is established, study medication is administered and the subject is now questioned by the research coordinator at the designated observation times using validated patient reporting scales. The number of observations depends on the drug being studied and the need to capture early onset values. Most commonly, evaluations are done at 0.25, 0.50, 0.75, 1, 1.5, 2 h and extending hourly for as many hours as desired. At each observation, subjects are asked a series of questions related to efficacy and side effects. Typical questions are as follows:

1. What is your pain intensity level at this time?

   None (0), Slight (1), Moderate (2), or Severe (3)

   (A 100-mm VAS scale or a 0–10 numerical scale could be substituted for the Likert scale.)

2. How much relief do you have from your starting pain?

   None (0), A Little (1), Some (2), A Lot (3), or Complete (4)

   (A 100-mm VAS scale or a 0–10 numerical scale could be substituted for the Likert scale.)

3. Have you noticed any other effects from the study medication?

This is a nonleading question aimed at eliciting any possible adverse effects from the study medication.

If onset of effect is a key parameter being investigated, then the two stopwatch method also can be employed. The subject is given a stopwatch approximately 5 min after receiving the study medication. The subject is instructed to press the stopwatch as soon as any perceptible relief is felt. At this point, the subject receives a second stopwatch and is instructed to press this one when the relief becomes meaningful (see Note 4).

At the completion of the evaluation period or at the time the subject takes a rescue analgesic, whichever comes first, a Global Evaluation question is asked:

How would you rate the study medication you received?

Poor (0), Fair (1), Good (2), Very Good (3), or Excellent (4)

From these analgesic scales, a variety of endpoints can be quantified to generate a comprehensive profile of the study medications. For time-action, areas-under-the-curve (AUCs) can be generated for changes in pain intensity (SPID – Sum of Pain Intensity Differences) and relief (TOTPAR – Total Pain Relief). Peak effect would be the highest level for either pain reduction (PPID – Peak Pain Intensity Difference) or pain relief (PREL – Peak Pain Relief). Onset can be quantified in a variety of ways including the stopwatch measures of First Perceptible and Meaningful Relief in minutes or calculating the median time that the study population took to achieve a certain level of pain relief, e.g. "some relief". Duration of analgesia can be assessed by calculating the mean or median time to taking the first dose of rescue analgesic.

One critical aspect to the success of the study is employing a trained research coordinator. Some coordinators are much more adept at understanding when it is appropriate to administer the study medication and, equally as important, when it is appropriate to administer any rescue medication. It cannot be overemphasized how much of an impact this can have on the sensitivity of any individual pain study (see Note 5).

5. Discussion

Few researchers argue about the sensitivity and versatility of the DIPM, but some skeptics question whether the data from this model are representative across various pain states. To address this question, we searched the archival literature for studies in other pain models that included the same treatment groups that were used in dental impaction studies. Our goal was simply to compare apples to apples. Three studies representative of the data (Figs. 8–10) that clearly demonstrate the results from the DIPM are almost identical to those from general surgery, OB–GYN surgery, and bunionectomy. In Fig. 8, a factorial study evaluating an ibuprofen–codeine combination produced almost identical results in both the DIPM and general surgery models (13, 14). Figure 9 compares the narcotic combination ibuprofen–oxycodone and again the results for the DIPM, and OB–GYN models are comparable with the noteworthy exception that the DIPM required far less subjects to achieve the same result (15, 16). Figure 10 compares a Cox-2 Selective Inhibitor valdecoxib in DIPM and Bunioectomy Model and again the results are remarkably similar (17). We are not aware of any general analgesic drug, NSAID or opioid, used for acute pain that was ineffective in the DIPM while effective in other acute pain models.

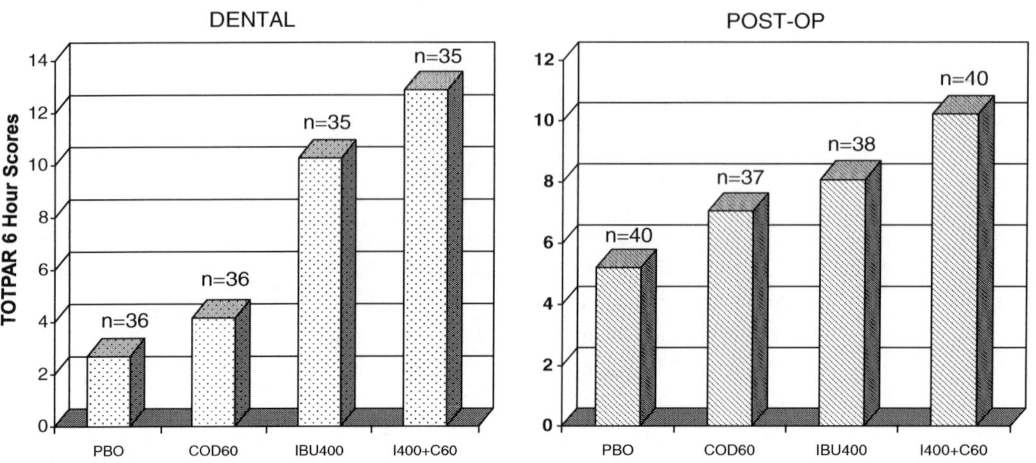

Fig. 8. Comparability of acute pain models – Postsurgical vs. DIPM. Mean Total Pain Relief Scores over 6 h (TOTPAR6) are plotted for both the Postsurgical Pain Study and the DIPM. Reproduced from refs. 13, 14

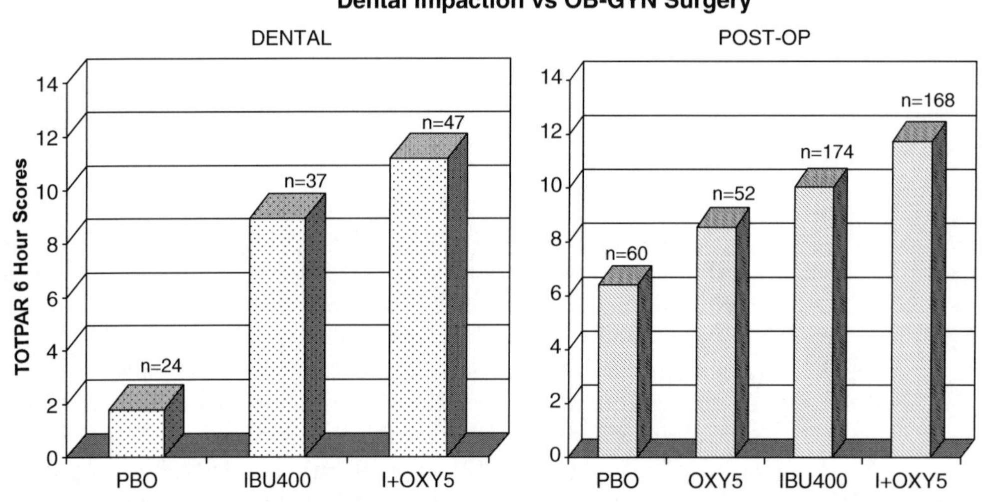

Fig. 9. Comparability of acute pain models – Postsurgical OB–GYN vs. DIPM. Mean Total Pain Relief Scores over 6 h (TOTPAR6) are plotted for both the Postsurgical Pain Study and the DIPM. Reproduced from refs. 15, 16

It is valid to conclude that the DIPM is particularly amenable to evaluating the NSAID-class of drugs. There are a plethora of DIPM articles in the archival literature that describe the efficacy of just about every NSAID and selective Cox-2 inhibitor. Also, it is fair to conclude that the DIPM is sensitive to opioid drugs when therapeutic levels of these drugs are tested. Unfortunately, many studies utilizing the DIPM were evaluating very low dosages

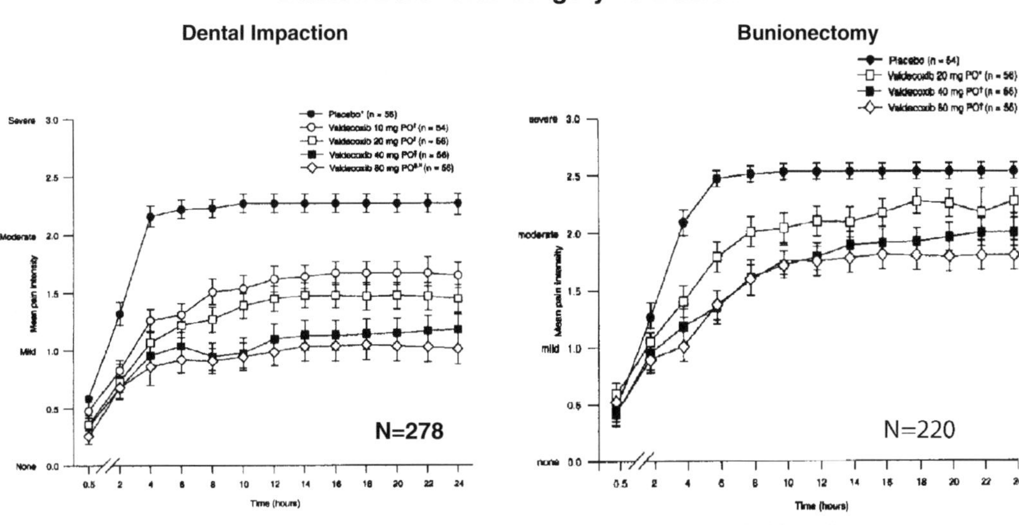

Fig. 10. Comparability of acute pain models – Bunionectomy vs. DIPM. Mean Pain Intensity Scores are plotted against hours for both the Bunionectomy Model and DIPM. Reprinted with permission of Anesthesiology (17)

of drugs like codeine 30–60 mg and oxycodone 2.5–5 mg. By the oral route, these dosages are equivalent to only 1.25–2.5 mg of intramuscular morphine, so it is not surprising that at these dosages, codeine and oxycodone had only mediocre efficacy. When higher dosages of opioids are evaluated in the DIPM, they clearly demonstrate a dose–effect relationship that is seen in other acute pain models (18–20).

There are situations where the DIPM, or any other acute pain model, are inappropriate. In many instances, drug development teams correctly choose the DIPM for the proof-of-concept studies based on its proven assay sensitivity, fast subject recruitment, and cost effectiveness. On occasion, they make this choice without carefully assessing whether the mechanism of action and projected efficacy profile of their experimental drug is well suited for an acute pain model whose underlying nociceptive pain is predominantly caused by inflammatory mediators. Prodrugs, drugs with slow onset of action, and some drugs with unique mechanism of actions also may not be appropriate for this model. In some cases, adapting the traditional model and using a pretreatment strategy might be a viable alternative. This often can be predicted by the profile established in the preclinical animal models.

We believe that a critical review of the DPIM trials clearly documents and establishes the DIPM as one of the premiere acute pain models. However, it is not the best model for long-term studies extending 3 or more days or for predicting long-term safety. For proof-of-concept, dose-ranging and comparing relative efficacies of acute analgesics to known standards, no other model has been as widely utilized, demonstrates more versatility or has better predictability than the DIPM.

6. Notes

1. The degree of difficulty for the surgical removal of impacted teeth is best judged by the oral surgeon. From the panographic X-ray, the teeth are classified as tissue, partial, or full bony impactions. Mandibular full bony impactions generally result in the most intense postsurgical pain. The experience and skill of the surgeon are also key factors in the postoperative pain experience. Four bony impactions surgically removed by an inexperienced oral surgery resident can lead to postoperative pain during the first 12–24 h that would rival a kidney stone. In contrast, a very experienced surgeon can remove four impactions in less than 10 min with much less surgical trauma.
2. Most experienced study sites perform the surgery under short-acting local anesthetics. Lidocaine and mepivacaine with or without a vasoconstrictor are most commonly used. In addition, nitrous oxide can be administered as an adjunct to pain control. Ideally, the local anesthetic should last for 45–90 min into the postsurgical period so that subjects can be moved to the recovery area and have sufficient time to stabilize. Some protocols allow the use of conscious sedation during surgery. In this scenario, short-acting intravenous drugs such as midazolam and fentanyl are most appropriate. Long-acting sedatives and narcotics should be avoided.
3. Investigators and the FDA enjoy debating over which efficacy scales are most sensitive. The fact is that no scale makes up for an insensitive model or inexperienced investigators. Visual Analog, Likert, and Numerical scales have all been used successfully in the DIPM. One official at the FDA has commented in a presentation that the VAS is probably the most difficult for subjects to comprehend. All of these scales relate to questions on pain intensity and relief from the starting pain and are asked repeatedly over the observation period. These scales are used to generate the time–effect curves for pain intensity, pain intensity difference (PID), and pain relief (REL). In addition, a Global Evaluation scale is often utilized to assess the subject's overall experience. More comprehensive Quality of Life (QOL) scales are not appropriate for these short-term studies.

4. The two-stopwatch method is a relatively new addition to the armamentarium of efficacy measures. It is designed to capture onset of analgesic effect in a systematic and reproducible manner. Subjects are carefully instructed to push the first stopwatch after taking the study medication when they first perceive "any" pain relief. Often, this is a false positive (or placebo effect) and can be a misleading measure. Thus, most investigators rely on giving a second stopwatch to the subjects after the first one is pushed. The subjects are instructed to push this stopwatch only when their pain relief becomes "meaningful" to them and this time is used as a surrogate for onset time. What is "meaningful relief"? It is whatever that particular subject believes it to be. The question is simply put: "press the stopwatch when you feel that your pain relief is meaningful to you". This method is quite sensitive for quantifying onset of effect. If subjects do not push both of the stopwatches within 2 h after medicating, then it is appropriate to censor the data at that point. These data are best analyzed using a responder analysis. Some investigators use the First Perceptible time for onset, but include only those subjects in the analysis that confirm the First Perceptible with a Meaningful Relief response. Those not confirming are censored with the maximum time to onset.
5. It is worth making a special note related to the research coordinators. No acute pain study will be successful without well trained research coordinators. The coordinator is the person most influential in determining when to administer the study medication and when it is appropriate to rescue the subject. Medicating too soon or too late and rescuing too soon are all recipes for a failed study. Above and beyond recording data with the measuring scales, the conduct of the study is as much an art as a science. Unfortunately, some coordinators never make the grade. Before allowing a research coordinator to participate in a sponsored study, it is a very good idea to set up a double-blinded dress rehearsal using standard drugs such as placebo, acetaminophen, and acetaminophen + hydrocodone. Most good sites have new coordinators work for several weeks with a research coordinator experienced in the conduct of acute analgesic studies.

References

1. Cooper SA, Needle SE, Kruger GO (1977) An analgesic relative potency assay comparing aspirin, ibuprofen and placebo. J Oral Surg 35:898–903
2. Cooper SA, Breen JF, Giuliani RL (1979) Replicate studies comparing the relative efficacies of aspirin and indoprofen in oral surgery outpatients. J Clin Pharmacol 19:151–159
3. Cooper SA, Reynolds DC, Kruger GO, Gottlieb S (1980) An analgesic relative potency assay comparing zomepirac sodium and aspirin. J Clin Pharmacol 20:98–106

4. Cooper SA, Quinn PD, MacAfee K, Hersh EV, Sullivan D, Lamp C (1993) Ibuprofen controlled release formulation – a clinical trial in dental impaction pain. Oral Surg Oral Med Oral Path 75:677–683
5. Doyle G, Jayawardena S, Ashraf E, Cooper SA (2002) Efficacy and tolerability of nonprescription ibuprofen versus celecoxib for dental pain. J Clin Pharmacol 42:912–919
6. Cooper SA, Hersh EV, Betts NJ, Wedell D, Quinn P, Lamp C, Herman D, Reynolds D, Gallegos LT, Reynolds B (1994) Multidose analgesic study of two mefanamic acid formulations in a postsurgical dental pain model. Analgesia 1:65–71
7. Desjardins PJ, Black P, Papageorge M, Norwood T, Shen DD, Norris L, Ardia A (2002) Ibuprofen arginate provides effective relief from postoperative dental pain with more rapid onset of action than ibuprofen. Eur J Clin Pharmacol 58(6):387–394
8. Hersh EV, Levin L, Cooper SA, Doyle G, Waksman J, Wedell D, Hong D, Secreto SA (2000) Ibuprofen liquigel for oral surgery pain. Clin Ther 22:1306–1318
9. Cooper SA et al (1994) Pharmacokinetic/pharmacodynamic study of ibuprofen formulations. Clin Pharmacol Ther 55:126
10. Dionne RA, Cooper SA (1978) Evaluation of preoperative ibuprofen for postoperative pain after removal of third molars. Oral Surg Oral Med Oral Path 45:851–856
11. Dionne RA, Campbell RA, Cooper SA, Hall DL, Buckingham B (1983) Suppression of post-operative pain by preoperative administration of ibuprofen in comparison to placebo, acetaminophen, and acetaminophen plus codeine. J Clin Pharmacol 23:37–43
12. Desjardins PJ, Shu VS, Recker DP, Verburg KM, Woolf CJ (2002) A single preoperative oral dose of valdecoxib, a new cyclooxygenase-2 specific inhibitor, relieves post-oral surgery or bunionectomy pain. Anesthesiology 97:565–573
13. Cooper SA, Engel J, Ladov M, Precheur H, Rosenheck A, Rauch D (1982) Analgesic efficacy of an ibuprofen–codeine combination. Pharmacotherapy 2:162–167
14. Sunshine A, Roure C, Olson N, Laska EM, Zorrilla C, Rivera J (1987) Analgesic efficacy of two ibuprofen–codeine combinations for the treatment of postepisiotomy and postoperative pain. Clin Pharmacol Ther 42:374–380
15. Cooper SA (1993) Analgesic efficacy of an ibuprofen–oxycodone combination. Clin Pharmacol Ther 53:148
16. Singla N, Pong A, Newman K, MD-10 Study Group (2005) Combination oxycodone 5 mg/ibuprofen 400 mg for the treatment of pain after abdominal or pelvic surgery in women: a randomized, double-blind, placebo- and active-controlled parallel-group study. Clin Ther 27:45–57
17. Daniels SE, Desjardins PJ, Talwalker S, Recker DP, Verburg KM (2002) The analgesic efficacy of valdecoxib vs. oxycodone/acetaminophen after oral surgery. J Am Dent Assoc 133:611–621
18. Desjardins PJ, Norris LH, Cooper SA, Reynolds DC (2000) Analgesic efficacy of intranasal butorphanol (Stadol NS) in the treatment of pain after dental impaction surgery. J Oral Maxillofac Surg 58(Suppl. 2):19–26
19. Daniels S, Casson E, Stegmann JU, Oh C, Okamoto A, Rauschkolb C, Upmalis D (2009) A randomized, double-blind, placebo-controlled phase 3 study of the relative efficacy and tolerability of tapentadol IR and oxycodone IR for acute pain. Curr Med Res Opin 25:1555–61
20. Kleinert R, Lange C, Steup A, Black P, Goldberg J, and Desjardins, P (2008) Single dose analgesic efficacy of tapentadol in postsurgical dental pain: results of a randomized, double-blind, placebo-controlled study. Anesth Analg 107:2048–55

Chapter 16

Live Cell Imaging for Studying G Protein-Coupled Receptor Activation in Single Cells

Deepak Kumar Saini and Narasimhan Gautam

Abstract

G protein-coupled receptors (GPCRs) constitute the single largest family of target proteins for drugs of pain and anesthesia. Non-invasive assays based on the activity of G protein-based sensors in living cells allow the identification of potentially novel compounds for anesthesia and pain management with high specificity. Quantitative information about the efficacy of any molecule or drug compound that acts through a GPCR can be obtained through this approach. Furthermore, live cell assays provide spatio temporal information that is valuable in high content screening of compounds. Here, we describe the use of various fluorescently tagged G protein subunits and methods for using translocation and FRET-based G protein sensors in studying GPCR activation in living cells.

Key words: Live cell imaging, GPCR, G protein, Translocation, FRET, Fluorescence microscopy

1. Introduction

G protein-coupled receptors (GPCRs) constitute the largest family of cellular proteins which regulate almost all cellular responses mediated by an extracellular stimulus. This ability to regulate GPCR activation and deactivation externally has made them the most attractive target for therapeutic drug discovery. The human genome encodes for approximately 750 GPCRs, of which 30% are non-odorant GPCRs, which are potential targets for developing therapeutic interventions (1). Less than half of these receptors have known ligands, leaving a large number of orphan GPCRs, for which no known ligand exists.

Approximately 45% of drugs in the market today are targeted against GPCRs, which include those involved in pain and anesthesia (2). A number of GPCRs including opioid, cannabinoid, metabotropic

Arpad Szallasi (ed.), *Analgesia: Methods and Protocols*, Methods in Molecular Biology, vol. 617,
DOI 10.1007/978-1-60327-323-7_16, © Springer Science+Business Media, LLC 2010

glutamate, and cytokine receptors have been suggested to play a role in pain perception and anesthesia (3–7). Although existing anesthetics targeting some of these GPCRs have worked well in pain management, they suffer from undesirable psychoactive side effects because they activate GPCRs in the central nervous system. To facilitate the development of new drugs, which can potentially overcome these side effects, specific agonists to the non-CNS-associated GPCRs such as CB2 cannabinoid receptors or cytokine receptors need to be identified (3, 8).

In order to prevent the side effects of anesthesia such as the slowing down of respiration and gastric inconsistency, a deeper understanding of the effects of existing anesthetics on different GPCRs is critical (3). It is known that these side effects are due to the cross reactivity of the anesthetics with other GPCRs. The existing system to study this cross reactivity relies on monitoring Ca^{+2}-dependent Cl^- currents and works only for Gq-coupled receptors. Hence, this necessitates a system which can detect effects of various anesthetics on Gi/o coupled receptors in intact cells (7, 9).

Using live cell imaging techniques, we describe two distinct "sensors" involving protein translocation (10, 11) and FRET (12), for monitoring the activation of GPCRs in living cells. The translocation technique is effective in detecting GPCR activation with all α subunit types whereas the FRET methodology can specifically detect the activation of αo/αi-coupled receptors. The techniques are non-invasive, use intact cells for analysis and most importantly monitor G protein activation, which is the first step of GPCR activation. Targeting the primary step in a GPCR activation pathway allows the identification of molecules that directly act on GPCRs rather than for a downstream component of the pathway.

We make use of fluorescently tagged G protein subunits to detect spatio-temporal changes in response to receptor activation in living cells. We have previously shown translocation of a family of G protein βγ subunits from plasma membrane to intracellular membranes on GPCR activation (11). Detailed characterization of translocation properties of βγ subunits has indicated it to be a very potent sensor for detecting GPCR activation in a living cell. Here, we describe the translocation technique as a tool for studying GPCRs as well as G protein activation. Similarly, we report the methodology to use the FRET sensor which we had previously devised to detect G protein activation in response to GPCR activation in living mammalian cells. The sensor comprises αo-CFP and YFP-βγ subunits which provide a FRET signal in basal cells due to the formation of the G protein αβγ heterotrimer. On receptor activation, the G protein heterotrimer dissociates into αo-CFP and YFP-βγ complex. This dissociation leads to the spatial separation of the G protein subunits thus abrogating the FRET signal. This loss of FRET is monitored as an indicator of GPCR activation in living cells (12).

2. Materials

2.1. Plasmids and Constructs

All cDNAs were cloned in the mammalian expression vector pCDNA3.1 (Invitrogen, Carlsbad, CA). The expression of cloned cDNAs was driven from a CMV promoter. The fluorescent proteins used were obtained from R. Tsien (UCSD, CA) and cloned either at N- or C-terminus of the cDNAs.

1. Fluorescently tagged G protein subunits
   - αo-CFP – CFP was fused to the internal region of αo subunit (12).
   - YFP-γ subunit. YFP was fused to the N-terminal of the cDNA.
2. Untagged G protein alpha subunits – αo and αq

2.2. Cell Culture and Transfection

1. CHO wild type cells – From ATCC.
2. CHO cells stably expressing M2 or M3 receptor were originally obtained from Dr. Peralta (13).
3. Dialyzed fetal bovine serum (Atlanta Biologicals, Lawrenceville, GA) (See Note 1). Stored in aliquots at –20°C after decomplementation. The final concentration of dFBS in media is 10%.
4. Penicillin, 10^6 U/ml in water. Stored as 0.5 ml aliquots at –20°C. Final concentration 100 U/ml. Cell culture grade.
5. Gentamicin, 50 mg/ml in water. Stored as 0.5 ml aliquots at –20°C. Final concentration 50 µg/ml. Cell culture grade.
6. Streptomycin, 100 mg/ml stock solution in water. Final concentration 100 µg/ml. Cell culture grade.
7. Methotrexate: 5 mM solution prepared in 0.1 M Sodium carbonate, pH 5.2. The solution was prepared in the dark and stored in aliquots in amber colored tubes at –20°C. The solution was diluted in media before use. (See Note 2.)
8. CHO-IIIa growth media (Invitrogen) supplemented with 10% dialyzed fetal bovine serum (Atlanta Biologicals), penicillin, streptomycin, gentamicin, and amphotericin B. The media was supplemented with methotrexate for maintaining stable cell lines. All the components were mixed and filter sterilized before use. The prepared media was stored at 4°C upto 4 weeks and prewarmed at 37°C before use.
9. 20 mM sterile EDTA solution, cell culture grade.
10. Optimem low serum media (Invitrogen). Stored as sterile aliquots at 4°C.
11. Lipofectamine 2000 (Invitrogen). Stored at 4°C.

12. No. 1.5 glass cover slips (15 × 40 mm), sterilized by soaking in 95% ethanol and then flaming them inside a hood. Sterile coverslips were stored in a sterile tissue culture dish.
13. 60 mm sterile tissue culture dishes.

2.3. Cell Stimulation

1. Hank's balanced salt solution (HBSS) free of Mg and Ca salts (Mediatech, Manassas, VA) was supplemented with 10 mM HEPES, pH 7.0 and 1 g/L glucose. The buffer was stored at 4°C and warmed at 37°C before use.
2. Carbachol – Muscarinic receptor agonist. 0.1 M solution was prepared in HBSS buffer (mentioned above) and aliquots were stored at –80°C. The solution was diluted in HBSS buffer before use to provide a final concentration of 100 μM.
3. Atropine – Muscarinic receptor antagonist.0.1 M solution in ethanol, prepared fresh in dark tubes. Diluted to 100 μM in HBSS before use.

2.4. Live Cell Imaging

1. Perfusion ready imaging chamber for 15 × 40 mm coverslips (Model No. RC30; Warner Instruments, Hamden, CT).
2. 15 × 30 mm cover glass (#1.5)
3. 250 μm thick channel gasket (Warner Instruments) which has a total imaging volume of 25 μl.
4. Automated perfusion/fluid delivery system, 8 or 4 – valve (Automate Scientific, Berkeley, CA). The Teflon valves in the device are controlled by a digital controller, where the opening and closing of valves can be either programmed or controlled manually. The system will also require syringe reservoirs for holding solutions, silicone tubing, perfusion manifold for linking multiple inputs to one output port, a flow rate controller, and waste collection reservoir.
5. Wide field fluorescence microscope equipped for live cell imaging. The setup of microscope and other components for live cell imaging is shown in Fig. 1. Please note that the components listed are named with their generic terminologies and may have different company names. We use Nikon TE2000E inverted microscope with 63× Plan Apo oil immersion objective for our imaging experiments. (See Note 3.)
6. Immersion oil for objective lens, type DF (Cargille Labs, Cedar Grove, NJ). (See Note 4.)
7. Computer software for image capturing and analysis. We use Metamoprh 6.7 (Molecular Devices Inc., Sunnyvale, CA) to control the image acquisition process and for data analysis.

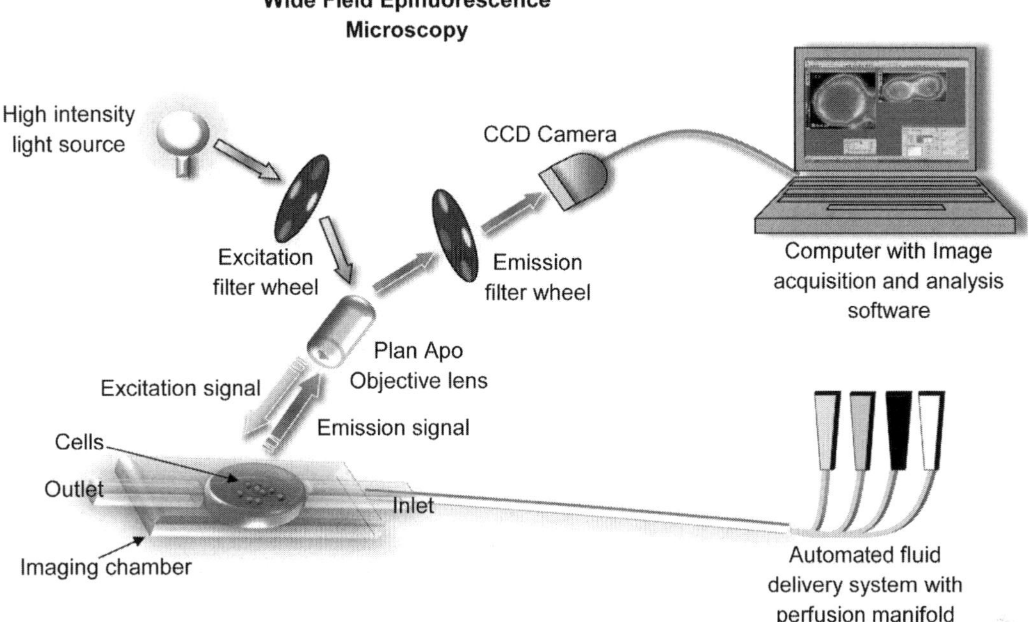

Fig. 1. *Wide-field epifluorescence microscopy based live cell imaging system.* Nikon TE2000E inverted microscope with 60× oil immersion objective lens was equipped with the components listed below. High intensity *white light* was generated using a 103 W Hg Arc lamp (Sylvania) housed in an isolated lamp housing which delivered the light through a liquid light guide (Exfo-Xcite fluorescence illumination). Excitation and emission filter wheels and excitation shutter were from Sutter Instruments (Lambda 10-2). Image registered sub-pixel resolution filter sets for specific excitation and emission wavelengths (Chroma Technology) were used in the filter wheels. The fluorescence signal was detected using a 12-bit Hamamatsu Orca ER CCD camera (Hamamatsu Photonics). All the devices were connected to a computer and were controlled by Metamorph imaging software (Molecular Imaging Inc.). Automated fluid delivery system was a standalone system with a controller (Automate Scientific) to regulate the valves for timed delivery of various solutions

3. Methods

3.1. Cell Culture and Transfection

1. Maintain the CHO cells stably expressing M2 or M3 receptor (as required) in 100 mm dishes in CHO-IIIa media containing 10% dialyzed fetal bovine serum, penicillin (100 U/ml), streptomycin (100 μg/ml), and Amphotericin B (25 ng/ml). Add methotrexate to the media based on the receptor present in the cells, for M2 cells use 0.5 μM of methotrexate and 0.25 μM for M3 cells.
2. For imaging experiments, use cells grown to 70–80% confluency in 100 mm dishes. Aspirate the spent media from the dishes and add 4 ml EDTA solution to the dishes. Incubate the dishes at 37°C, 5% CO_2 for 2–5 min to dislodge the adherent cells. Remove adherent cells by repeatedly pipetting the EDTA solution up and down in the dish. Collect the detached cells in a 15-ml tube and count using a hemocytometer. Pellet the cells by centrifugation (1,000×g, 3–4 min) and remove

EDTA by aspiration. Resuspend the cells to a final concentration of one million cells/ml. For seeding for imaging applications, place 15 × 40 mm (No. 1.5) sterile coverslips in 60 mm sterile dishes. Spread 200 μl of cell suspension containing 200,000 cells on the coverslips and add 4 ml fresh CHO-IIIa media. Grow the cells for another 16 h at 37°C, 5% CO_2 before transfection. (See Note 5.)

3. Transfect the cells using lipofectamine 2000 as per the manufacturer's instructions. For each transfection reaction, add 8 μl of lipofectamine 2000 to a 1.5-ml microfuge tube containing 100 μl of cold Optimem and incubate at RT for 5 min. Meanwhile, add various DNAs to be transfected to 100 μl of warm Optimem in a 1.5 ml microfuge tube. We use 1 μg DNA for YFP tagged constructs, 1.5 μg for CFP tagged constructs and 1 μg for untagged constructs per transfection. Add the DNA mix to the tube containing the lipofectamine–Optimem mix. Gently flick to mix the two solutions. Do not mix the solution by repeat pipetting as lipofectamine is hydrophobic and sticks to pipette tips, and this can change the effective concentration. Incubate the mix at RT for 30 min. Remove growth media from the 60 mm dishes in which transfection needs to be done and replace it with 4 ml of warm Optimem. Gently add 200 μl of the DNA–lipofectamine mix per dish. The mix is added in a gentle stream, without generating droplets as they roll to the edge of the dish. Gently mix the transfection solution by swirling the dishes. Incubate the cells for 5 h at 37°C, 5% CO_2. After incubation, remove optimem from the dishes and replace with 4 ml of pre warmed CHO-IIIa media. Further, incubate the cells for 16 h (overnight) at 37°C, 5% CO_2. (See Note 6.)

3.2. Translocation Assay: Imaging Translocation of G Protein βγ Subunit in Response to Receptor Activation

Based on the classical model, activation of a GPCR in a cell leads to activation and dissociation of the G protein αβγ heterotrimer in α and βγ subunits when the γ subunit associated is capable of translocation away from the plasma membrane (14, 15). Six of the γ subunits, γ1, γ5, γ9, γ10, γ11, and γ13 translocate, whereas the other six, γ2, γ3, γ4, γ7, γ8, and γ12 do not. Of the six subunits capable of translocating, four of them, viz. γ1, γ9, γ11, and γ13 translocate rapidly with $t_{1/2}$ less than 20 s on activation of a GPCR (10, 11). This rapid translocation is reversible and the βγ subunits revert back to the plasma membrane with similar kinetics on receptor inactivation. Here, we use YFP-tagged G protein γ11 subunit to visualize reversible βγ complex translocation mediated through muscaranic receptors in living CHO cells. The translocation is measured by monitoring intensity changes of YFP-βγ in the Golgi as a function of GPCR activation status. The assay indicates the potency of βγ translocation as a sensor for GPCR activation and deactivation.

1. Pre-warm HBSS buffer containing 10 mM HEPES, pH 7.0 and 1 g/L glucose in a 37°C water bath.
2. Prepare the GPCR (muscaranic receptor) agonist (carbachol) and antagonist (atropine) 30 min before imaging. Dilute 100 mM stock of both agonist and antagonist 100 μM in pre-warmed HBSS buffer. We generally prepare 20–30 ml of the solutions for imaging.
3. Prepare the perfusion system before the imaging experiment. Valves number 1, 2, and 3 are used. Position 1, HBSS buffer; 2, agonist and 3, antagonist. Set up the tubing from the valves to the perfusion manifold and then connect it to the flow controller. Check the flow rate by checking the amount of HBSS buffer which flows through the system in a minute and then accordingly adjust the flow rate to 0.5–1 ml/min. We generally use 0.5 ml/min for our experiments. (See Note 7.)
4. Prepare the imaging chamber for mounting the cover slip as per the manufacturer's guidelines. We use an RC30 imaging chamber with 250 μm gaskets for our imaging. Apply vacuum grease on the mounts to prevent leaking between the cover slips and the mount. (See Note 8.)
5. For imaging the cells, use fine tipped forceps to remove the cover slip containing the transfected cells from the dish and quickly rinse the cover slip in a dish containing HBSS buffer. Gently wipe the bottom of the cover slip and place it on the imaging chamber. Quickly add a small volume of the buffer to prevent drying (~0.5 ml). Close the chamber gently making sure that no air bubbles are trapped inside. Attach the perfusion manifold outlet to one of the inlets of the imaging chamber and attach the other end of the chamber (outlet) to a tube which directs the solution coming out of the imaging chamber to a collection container.
6. Place the assembled imaging chamber on the microscope stage with cover slip containing the cells facing towards the objective lens. Keep the HBSS buffer perfusing continuously through the cells.
7. To image, choose the excitation and emission filters based on the type of fluorophore present in the cells. For imaging YFP-γ subunits. excitation filter 500/20 is used. (See Notes 9 and 10.) Visually select the cells which have good YFP expression on the plasma membrane along with a small amount in the intracellular membranes. After selecting the cells, image the cells using the live imaging mode through the camera. To rapidly acquire and focus the images without bleaching the fluorophores, image them with short acquisition duration (0.1–0.2 s) using 10% neutral density filter. We perform acquisition in autoscale mode of the Metamorph software

which adjusts the brightness and contract of the images automatically to provide best image. (See Note 11). Acquire images for YFP at higher excitation duration (0.5–1 s) to obtain images with better signal (generally a PM signal between 600 and 1,400 is optimal for experiments).

8. Once acquisition conditions are finalized, acquire images at 10 or 20 s interval using a time lapse imaging mode (lambda stack) of the software. This mode generates a temporal stack of the images while recording elapsed time. Such temporal stacks can be streamed to generate a movie or they can be used for intensity plot measurements.
9. While acquiring images in the temporal mode, change solutions in the imaging chamber at set time intervals using perfusion controller. Our set intervals for solution perfusion are, 0–40 s, HBSS buffer; 40 s to 2′ 40 s, agonist (100 μM carbachol in HBSS buffer) and 2′ 40 s to 4 min antagonist (100 μM atropine in HBSS buffer). During solution perfusion and switching, acquire images continuously to the temporal stack for a total of 4 min duration.
10. Plot the YFP intensity changes on the PM and Golgi of single cells to monitor the translocation of G protein βγ complex. (Fig. 2a, b). Before selecting the region for intensity measurements, ascertain that the cells under observation do not change focus or shape or move. These alterations can interfere with the intensity measurements.
11. Plot the intensity changes as a function of time to relate the changes in GPCR activation or inactivation (Marked by arrows in Fig. 2b).

3.3. FRET Assay: Imaging GPCR Activation Through Monitoring Dissociation of G Protein Heterotrimer in Living Cells

G protein heterotrimer consisting of αβγ subunits undergoes GPCR activation dependent dissociation into free G protein α subunit and βγ subunits. We have used this dissociation of α and βγ subunits to generate a FRET sensor (12, 16). FRET or Forster resonance energy transfer takes place between two fluorescent proteins or molecules when they are in close physical proximity (~10–100 Å) provided that excitation spectra of one fluorophore overlaps with the emission spectra of other fluorophore (17, 18). The amount of resonance or non-radiative energy transfer decreases by a factor of 6 with respect to distance between the two fluorophores. Such energy transfer or FRET can be measured by monitoring the intensity changes in emission of the energy donor molecule. Also, FRET can be effectively measured by monitoring the emission of acceptor molecule by exciting the donor molecules only. The emission in this situation will originate only from the transferred energy or FRET.

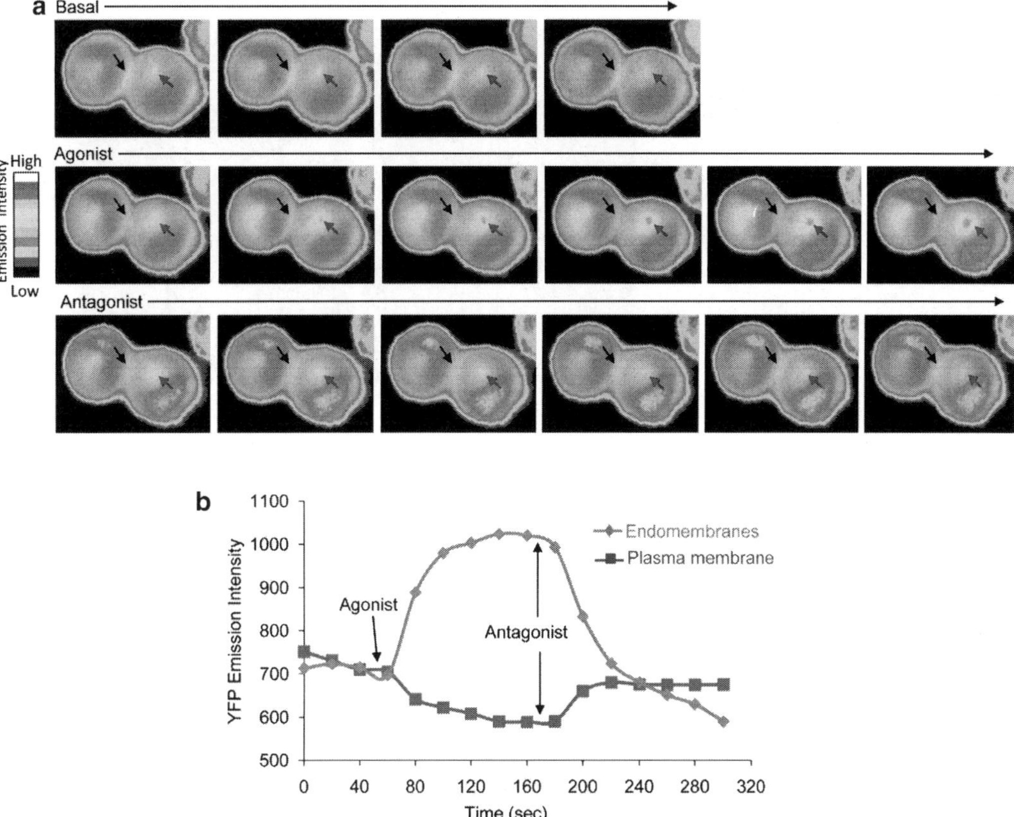

Fig. 2. *Translocation of G protein YFP-γ11 subunit on activation of M2 receptor*. CHO-M2 cells expressing YFP-γ11 were used. The cells were mounted on an imaging chamber and imaged as described. (**a**) Images of cells taken at 20 s intervals showing the translocation of YFP-γ11 from plasma membrane to the intracellular region on receptor activation. The βγ complex reverse translocates back to plasma membrane on receptor deactivation. *Arrows* indicate the regions where changes in the cell are observed and plotted as under (*Black*, plasma membrane; *Red*, endomembranes). (**b**) Plots showing the change in the YFP emission intensity in the endomembrane region (Golgi) and the plasma membrane of the cell as a result of translocation of G protein βγ complex. Agonist (100 μM carbachol) addition after 40 s and antagonist (100 μM atropine) after 2′40 s is indicated by arrows on the plot

It is important to choose FRET pairs carefully to obtain the best signal to noise ratio. Amongst fluorescent proteins, CFP and YFP proteins are the most widely used FRET pair. Here, we use the same pair as a sensor for monitoring GPCR activation dependent dissociation of αo-CFP and YFP-βγ subunits. In basal state, FRET signal is obtained due to energy transfer from αo-CFP to YFP-βγ subunits. On receptor activation, the heterotrimer dissociation leads to abrogation of FRET, thus generating an effective imaging sensor for GPCR activation measurement (Fig. 3). The sensor is based only on αo subunit and is not dependent on the type of γ subunit type used. Here, we used CHO-M2 cells transfected with αo-CFP and YFP-γ11. We have obtained similar results using other γ subunits or using YFP-tagged β1 subunit instead of γ subunit (12).

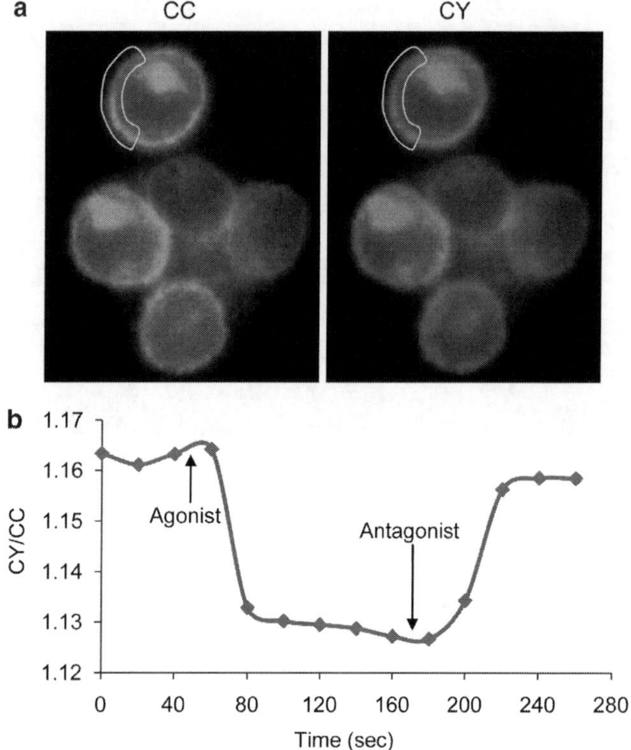

Fig. 3. *Change in FRET by G protein dissocation through activation of a GPCR.* M2 CHO cells expressing αo-CFP and YFP-γ11 were used. Cells expressing almost equal intensities of both CFP and YFP were used for the assay. The cells were imaged as described with images captured at 20 s interval in CC and CY channel only. YY channel was not imaged to prevent its bleaching which can change the FRET measurements. (**a**) Images of cells captured using CC and CY channels. CC showing expression of αo-CFP and CY, FRET from CFP to YFP (See Subheading 3.4). The plasma membrane region selected for measuring changes in the emission intensity is indicated. (**b**) Ratiometric plot of changes in emission intensities of CC and CY channels at the plasma membrane region on receptor activation and deactivation. The time of addition of agonist and antagonist is indicated by arrows

1. Process and mount the cover slip containing CHO-M2 cells expressing the fusion constructs as mentioned in subheading 3.2 on the imaging chamber.
2. Select cells expressing similar levels of CFP and YFP for imaging.
3. Capture temporal stack for the cells by imaging them in CC and CY excitation and emission filter combinations. (CC, *CFP* excitation filter and *CFP* emission filter; CY, *CFP* excitation filter and *YFP* emission filter).
4. Treat the cells with agonist and antagonist while capturing images at 20 s intervals as described in subheading 3.2.
5. Separate the temporal stack into sequential CC and CY images.

6. Select a region from the plasma membrane for CC and CY emission intensity measurements. Mark the region in the CC image sets and transfer the region to CY to facilitate identical positioning of the selected region.
7. Measure the intensity changes as a function of time.
8. Plot CY/CC changes as a function of time with agonist and antagonist addition time points marked.

3.4. FRET Assay: Monitoring Protein–Protein Interaction in Living Cells by Acceptor Photobleaching

The FRET measurement obtained by continuously measuring donor and FRET emission is a reliable tool to study dynamic changes in interaction of two proteins such as the ones described above. However, direct measurement of FRET by monitoring acceptor emission on donor excitation suffers from limitations arising from acceptor cross-excitation and donor bleed through. Cross excitation of acceptor refers to the emission obtained from acceptor when it is cross excited by donor excitation wavelength. For example, YFP emission observed through YFP filter set when excited by CFP excitation wavelength corresponds to cross excitation. This is estimated by measuring CY emission from cells expressing YFP alone. Donor bleed through refers to the amount of emission obtained in acceptor channel on excitation of the donor, i.e., CFP emission detected in the YFP filter set through CFP excitation. This is measured by measuring CY emission from cells expressing CFP alone (Fig. 4). The FRET signal contamination by acceptor cross-excitation and donor bleed through reduces the significance of the actual FRET signal.

To overcome these problems, dynamic FRET changes are measured using ratiometric calculation based on independent CC and CY reading to generate CY/CC ratio. Besides ratiometric plotting, acceptor photobleaching, is also used to confirm FRET. In acceptor photobleaching, the acceptor molecules (YFP) are photobleached by exposing them to high intensity light. The bleached acceptor is incapable of accepting FRET energy from the donor molecule leading to gain in emission intensity of donor which was previously lost because of FRET. Thus on acceptor photobleaching a gain in donor emission is observed if there is FRET because of physical proximity of partner proteins, as in the case of inactive heterotrimer. In case there is no proximity and FRET is absent, no gain in donor emission is observed on pbotobleaching as in the case of the activated heterotrimer, where αo-CFP and YFP-γ subunits are physically separated (Fig. 5). Here, we use CHO-M2 cells stably expressing αo-CFP and YFP-γ11 subunits to study FRET by studying acceptor photobleaching.

1. Grow cells in CHO-IIIa media containing methotrexate and G418 (500 μg/ml) on 35-mm glass-bottom petri dishes for 16 h before the experiment.

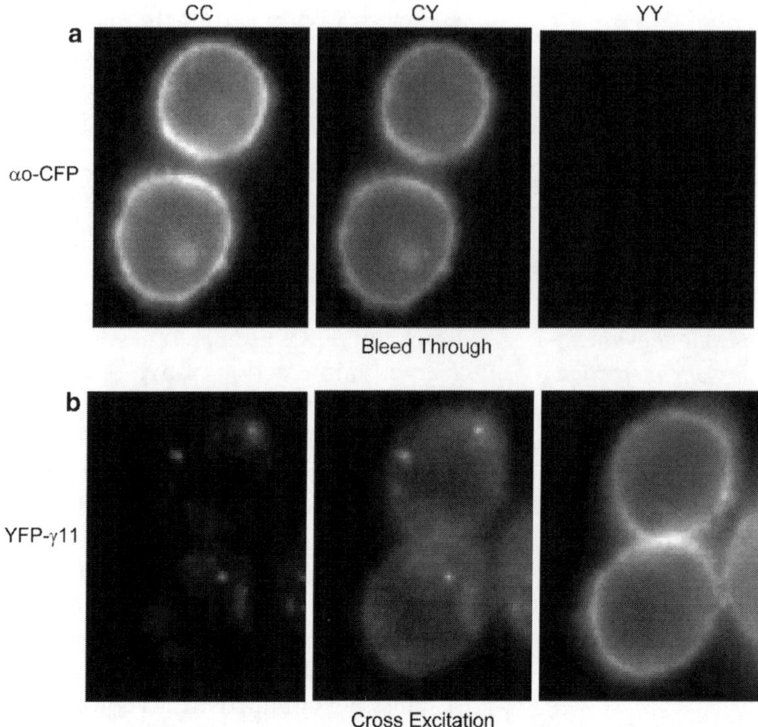

Fig. 4. *Cross excitation and bleed through analysis.* CHO-M2 cells independently expressing αo-CFP and YFP-γ11 were imaged in CC, CY, and YY channel. (**a**) CFP and (**b**) YFP. The amount of CFP fluorescence observed by CFP excitation and YFP emission corresponds to bleed through of CFP in YFP channel. The YFP fluorescence observed by CFP excitation and YFP emission channel corresponds to cross excitation of YFP by CFP excitation light

2. Replace media with 2 ml of pre-warmed HBSS buffer containing 10 mM HEPES, pH 7.0 and 1 g/L d-glucose before imaging.
3. Image the cells in an open dish on an inverted microscope. Select the cells with relatively equal levels of expression of CFP and YFP for the experiments. Capture two images with CC settings as pre-bleaching images.
4. Switch to live view mode for detecting YFP emission. Completely remove the neutral density filter, allowing 100% YFP excitation light to illuminate the sample. Continue imaging the cells without engaging the auto balance setting to allow the observation of the gradual loss of YFP fluorescence. After bleaching of YFP, switch back the neutral density filter to imaging setting as it was before. (See Note 12.)
5. Capture images in CC channel for CFP emission.
6. Select a specific plasma membrane region of the cell and compare the CFP intensity before and after the YFP photobleaching experiment.

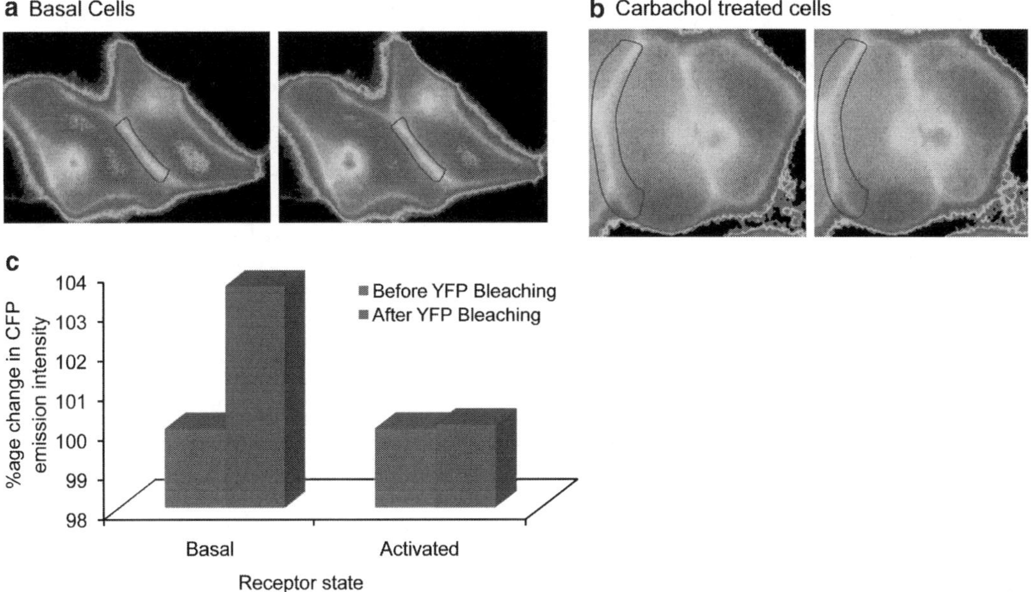

Fig. 5. *Acceptor photobleaching showing presence of FRET between αo-CFP and YFP-βγ*. CHO-M2 cells expressing αo-CFP and YFP-γ11 were used. Cells with almost equal emission intensities of CFP and YFP were used for the experiment. Images for the cells were captured in CC and YY channel in the resting and agonist stimulated state before photobleaching. YFP was then bleached with maximum excitation illumination. Another set of images in CC and YY channel was captured to record the changes in emission intensities. (**a**) Images of CFP expression in basal cells before and after photobleaching. Small increase in intensity of CFP observed after photobleaching indicates FRET. This shows that in resting cells, αo-CFP and YFP-γ11 are physically close and are interacting with each other. (**b**) Images for CFP in agonist stimulated cells before and after photobleaching. No increase in intensity of CFP observed after photobleaching indicates absence of FRET. The absence of FRET shows the loss of interaction as well as physical proximity between αo-CFP and YFP-γ11 on receptor activation. (**c**) Plots showing the changes in CFP emission after YFP photobleaching in basal and agonist treated conditions. The gain in CFP emission is due to loss of YFP emission due to FRET between αo-CFP and YFP-γ11 in basal state

7. Since G protein heterotrimer has tightly associated alpha and beta gamma subunits in its basal state, acceptor photobleaching leads to an increase in CFP emission. The gain in CFP emission corresponds to the resonance energy which was transferred from CFP to the YFP molecules.
8. To evaluate the loss of FRET, treat the cells with muscarinic receptor agonist (carbachol) which leads to activation and dissociation of G protein heterotrimer. This dissociation consists of separation of αo-CFP and YFP-βγ. This spatial separation prevents transfer of resonance energy from CFP to YFP.
9. Photobleaching in this situation does not show any significant increase in CFP emission as there is no FRET.
10. The plasma membrane intensity measurements in cells before and after treatment with agonist will reflect the presence and absence of FRET respectively (Fig. 3).

3.5. Dynamic FRET: Translocation Assay for Monitoring Activation of GPCR in Living Cells

The methods described above are very sensitive for detecting GPCR and G protein activation in living cells using imaging technology. The sensitivity of the assays is dependent on the choice of plasma membrane or intracellular region selected for measuring the changes in intensities of the fluorescent sensors. Even minor changes in cell shape during the experiment can limit the choice of regions for intensity analysis. We overcame this limitation by devising an assay which uses the main features of both translocation and the FRET assay. The assay effectively monitors dynamic FRET changes in G protein heterotrimer association and dissociation. Using YFP- tagged translocation proficient γ-subunits, activation of GPCRs lead to dissociation of the heterotrimer followed by translocation of βγ complex. (See Note 13). Translocation ascertains the complete dissociation which leads to a robust FRET change detected as FRET loss in the assay. The assay is adaptable to whole image analysis avoiding the need for selecting specific regions for measuring intensity changes. Here, we use αo-CFP and YFP-γ11 to detect the FRET changes mediated by translocation of YFP-11. Measurement of CC and CY emission intensities before and after receptor stimulation shows clear changes in the FRET.

1. Process and mount the cover slip containing CHO-M2 cells expressing the fusion constructs as mentioned in subheading 3.2 on the imaging chamber.
2. Select cells expressing similar levels of CFP and YFP for imaging.
3. Capture images every 20 s for cells in CC and CY excitation and emission filter combinations. (CC, *C*FP excitation filter and *C*FP emission filter; CY, *C*FP excitation filter and *Y*FP emission filter) in temporal stacks.
4. Treat the cells with agonist and antagonist while capturing images at 20 s intervals as described in subheading 3.2.
5. Separate the temporal stack into sequential CC and CY images.
6. Measure the intensity of the whole image for both CC and CY channels.
7. Plot CY/CC changes as a function of time with agonist and antagonist addition time points marked.

4. Notes

1. Undialyzed serum contains small agonist molecules which can stimulate GPCRs to induce basal level of activation. It is therefore important to use dialyzed serum which provides minimal background.

2. Methotrexate degrades rapidly when exposed to light. Store very small aliquots at –20°C and do not reuse the stocks once thawed.

3. Plan Apo lenses are corrected for various aberrations such as spherical aberration in four wavelengths (dark blue, blue, green, and red), chromatic aberrations and for flatness of field. These corrections allow for better alignment of images obtained using various excitation and emission lights. Other lenses such as Fluar or Apochromat lenses yield poorly aligned images.

4. Only oil formulated for fluorescence microscopy is used to avoid background fluorescence. Fluorescence arising from the oil can lead to interference with the actual fluorescence signals from the fluorophores.

5. We generally grow 0.2 million cells for 16 h before transfection for our experiments. When the transfection needs to be performed the same day, we seed 0.4 million cells per cover slip. The cells are then allowed to adhere for a minimum 2 h before transfection.

6. To test the transfection efficiency of the cells, we generally grow cells in a glass bottom dish (In vitro Scientific or Mattek) and directly visualize the cells after transfection without setting up the perfusion system. This allows us to estimate the transfection efficiency for the entire transfected population.

7. Perfusion manifolds (Harvard apparatus) have multiple inputs and one output. They allow delivery of various solutions with minimum dead volume and without mixing them. While connecting tubings to the manifold and subsequently to the flow rate controller, we ensure that no air bubbles are trapped in the delivery lines. Presence of bubbles in the imaging chamber ruins an imaging experiment. We run the buffer and solutions through the tubing for a short time to remove the bubbles adhering to the dry wall of the tubing. Bubbles are removed by tapping them with fingertips while draining the solution. We drain the tubing and other components with HBSS buffer alone if the agonist and antagonists are limiting.

8. We apply grease through a fine tipped syringe. This allows us to apply minimum grease on the imaging assembly. Avoid applying excessive grease as it can block the fluid delivery outlets on the imaging chamber.

9. We use the following filter combinations for our experiments. All the filters are image registered sub-pixel resolution quality. For CFP, 436/20 excitation filter, 470/30 emission filter and for YFP, 500/20 excitation filter, 535/30 emission filters were used.

10. The designation of the filters is based on the wavelength it allows to pass through followed by total bandwidth range, e.g. 500/20 stands for main wavelength as 500 nm and band width is 20 nm, which means it allows light from 490 to 510 nm range.
11. The auto adjust features of the software provide the best signal to noise ratio using the brightest pixel of the focused plane as a reference. Though it is incapable of distinguishing the signal arising from the actual expression versus background debris, the auto balance feature is very useful in observing cells with different expression levels without adjusting any other control while selecting the cells for experiment.
12. Setting up this experiment without the software control is an issue, as the locations of the neutral density filters in the microscope might have access problems. We try and position the neutral density filters in our microscope out of the way of other devices attached to the microscope. In the Nikon microscope, we have placed the filter wheels, light source, and stage controllers on the opposite side of neutral density filters to allow unhindered access to them. Since imaging is performed in a room with almost negligible light, executing this task in dark may become a little complicated. We use a remote controlled low intensity lamp close to the microscope (facing away from the microscope) while moving the neutral density filters. This helps unnecessary movements of the sample which is very critical for FRET analysis.
13. The FRET assay works with all γ subunit types, whereas the translocation assay works with only 6 of the 12γ subunit types. Of the six translocation proficient γ subunits, only four translocate rapidly, γ1, γ9, γ11, and γ13s. Thus, only these four subunits are useful for rapid monitoring of GPCR activation in the translocation assay. Due to the translocation, the FRET assay is also more sensitive when these translocating γ subunits are used. This feature has been used to develop the FRET – translocation assay.

Acknowledgments

The authors would like to thank Vani Kalyanaraman, Mariangela Chisari, and Joonho Cho for their technical help and discussions. This research was supported by National Institutes of Health grants GM 69027 and GM080558 (N.G.) and AHA postdoctoral fellowship (DKS).

References

1. Vassilatis DK, Hohmann JG, Zeng H, Li F, Ranchalis JE, Mortrud MT, Brown A, Rodriguez SS, Weller JR, Wright AC, Bergmann JE, Gaitanaris GA (2003) The G protein-coupled receptor repertoires of human and mouse. Proc Natl Acad Sci U S A. 100:4903–4908
2. Bleicher KH, Bohm HJ, Muller K, Alanine AI (2003) Hit and lead generation: beyond high-throughput screening. Nat Rev Drug Discov 2:369–378
3. Ahmad S, Dray A (2004) Novel G protein-coupled receptors as pain targets. Curr Opin Investig Drugs 5:67–70
4. Stein C, Schafer M, Machelska H (2003) Attacking pain at its source: new perspectives on opioids. Nat Med 9:1003–1008
5. Dray A (2003) Novel molecular targets in pain control. Curr Opin Anaesthesiol 16:521–525
6. Hruby VJ, Porreca F, Yamamura HI, Tollin G, Agnes RS, Lee YS, Cai M, Alves I, Cowell S, Varga E, Davis P, Salamon Z, Roeske W, Vanderah T, Lai J (2006) New paradigms and tools in drug design for pain and addiction. AAPS J 8:E450–E460
7. Minami K, Uezono Y (2006) Gq protein-coupled receptors as targets for anesthetics. Curr Pharm Des 12:1931–1937
8. Malan TP Jr, Ibrahim MM, Lai J, Vanderah TW, Makriyannis A, Porreca F (2003) CB2 cannabinoid receptor agonists: pain relief without psychoactive effects? Curr Opin Pharmacol 3:62–67
9. Minami K, Uezono Y (2005) The effects of anesthetics on G-protein-coupled receptors. Masui 54:118–125
10. Akgoz M, Kalyanaraman V, Gautam N (2004) Receptor-mediated reversible translocation of the G protein betagamma complex from the plasma membrane to the Golgi complex. J Biol Chem 279:51541–51544
11. Saini DK, Kalyanaraman V, Chisari M, Gautam N (2007) A family of G protein betagamma subunits translocate reversibly from the plasma membrane to endomembranes on receptor activation. J Biol Chem 282:24099–24108
12. Azpiazu I, Gautam N (2004) A fluorescence resonance energy transfer-based sensor indicates that receptor access to a G protein is unrestricted in a living mammalian cell. J Biol Chem 279:27709–27718
13. Peralta EG, Winslow JW, Peterson GL, Smith DH, Ashkenazi A, Ramachandran J, Schimerlik MI, Capon DJ (1987) Primary structure and biochemical properties of an M2 muscarinic receptor. Science 236:600–605
14. Gilman AG (1987) G proteins: transducers of receptor-generated signals. Annu Rev Biochem 56:615–649
15. Cabrera-Vera TM, Vanhauwe J, Thomas TO, Medkova M, Preininger A, Mazzoni MR, Hamm HE (2003) Insights into G protein structure, function, and regulation. Endocr Rev 24:765–781
16. Janetopoulos C, Jin T, Devreotes P (2001) Receptor-mediated activation of heterotrimeric G-proteins in living cells. Science 291:2408–2411
17. Kenworthy AK (2001) Imaging protein-protein interactions using fluorescence resonance energy transfer microscopy. Methods 24:289–296
18. Sekar RB, Periasamy A (2003) Fluorescence resonance energy transfer (FRET) microscopy imaging of live cell protein localizations. J Cell Biol 160:629–633

Chapter 17

Recombinant Cell Lines Stably Expressing Functional Ion Channels

Florian Steiner, Sraboni Ghose, and Urs Thomet

Abstract

Ion channels are membrane proteins that gate the flow of ions into and out of a cell. They are present in the membranes of human, animal, plant, and bacterial cells. They are profoundly involved in diverse tasks ranging from neuronal functions to hormonal secretion and cell division. Biophysical characterization and modulation of ion channel targets are important approaches in modern drug discovery. With the heterologous expression of the nicotinic acetylcholine receptor alpha7 (nAChRα7) in a host cell, we show a way to construct and use such a stable cell-based expression system for electrophysiological assays.

Key words: Ion Channels, Stable cell line, Patch-clamp, Membrane localization, Ligand-gated, nAChRα7

1. Introduction

Ion channels are integral membrane proteins that allow the flow of ions across membranes in all living cells. They have an important role in many diverse physiological processes such as nervous transmission, muscle contraction, learning and memory, secretion, cell proliferation, regulation of blood pressure, fertilization, and cell death (1). Ion channel dysfunction results in pathophysiology, they are therefore a major target class for therapeutic intervention. The number of genes expressing ion channels again underlines their biological importance. More than 400 genes encode potential ion channels representing 1–2% of our genetic endowment (2).

Ion channels have proven to be a difficult class for rational drug discovery efforts. Earlier, ion channel-targeted drugs were discovered and optimized using animal models with the molecular target remaining unknown for decades in some cases (3).

Arpad Szallasi (ed.), *Analgesia: Methods and Protocols*, Methods in Molecular Biology, vol. 617,
DOI 10.1007/978-1-60327-323-7_17, © Springer Science+Business Media, LLC 2010

Technological advances such as patch clamping made the analysis of ion channels possible at the single molecule level (4). Although it is considered the gold standard of ion channel analysis, patch clamping is laborious and requires technically skilled operators and is not conducive to the screening of chemical libraries. Systematic high throughput screening was not possible until recently. Ion channels are thus considered an underexploited target class.

Besides being drug discovery targets per se, ion channels are increasingly important in safety studies in the preclinical stages of drug development. Off-target drug-ion channel interactions can have major consequences. For example, the cardiac potassium channel hERG (human ether a-go-go related gene) is an important regulator of the duration of the plateau phase of the cardiac action potential (1). Susceptibility to the potentially lethal arrhythmia torsade de pointes could be correlated in certain individuals with hERG block by various pharmacological agents (5). Therefore, safety studies of unwanted drug interactions with the hERG channel have significantly increased the volume of ion channel assays carried out during drug development. It is now a regulatory requirement to test all new drug candidates in an hERG channel assay and provide proof of noninterference with hERG channel activity (FDA Document S7B Nonclinical Evaluation of the Potential for Delayed Ventricular Repolarization (QT Interval Prolongation)). It is thus increasingly important to develop the capability to carry out large-scale ion channel assays. Indirect assays such as ion-sensitive dyes or radioactive flux and binding assays lack sensitivity and have a higher potential for false positives (6). The major technological advance in recent years has been the advent of parallel planar patch-clamp electrophysiology (7). These automated systems now allow direct electrophysiology-based medium throughput screening campaigns (8). These systems work well for voltage-gated ion channels. For assays with ligand-gated ion channels, the manual patch-clamp system still produces best data if high throughput is not the major concern.

Well defined assays require a stable biological preparation on which chemical libraries can be tested. Primary cultures of tissue-dissociated cells are not an option, the only viable alternative being the heterologous expression of the given ion channel. Transient transfection of ion channel encoding cDNA is possible (9) and has been used, but batch variability remains a concern. The generation of stable cell lines may be one way to minimize variability of the reference biological signal.

Ion channels are not just isolated proteins, they form part of complex structural and signalling entities in cells. Their associated accessory subunits are not only important for the functionality of the native channel but also ensure correct assembly, trafficking, insertion, and retrieval (10). This multiple subunit structure gives rise to a large number of structural variants. Analysis of the genomic sequence from different individuals provides variants for ion channel genes adding a further level of complexity to channel structure with implications for the biophysical behaviour of the channel. The potassium channel family is the biggest and most diverse of the ion channel classes with 75 distinct mammalian genes identified and sequenced so far (11). Alternate splicing during mRNA processing adds another source of diversity. In case of the SK1 subtype of SKCa channels for example, as many as 32 splice variants are predicted and mRNA for 20 of these have already been detected in the mouse brain.

To demonstrate the generation of stable ion channel cell lines, we have selected the nicotinic acetylcholine receptor alpha7 (nAChRα7). This ligand-gated neuronal isoform has been implicated in neuropathic pain (12). The rapid desensitation of this receptor requires fast application of the ligand (13). This is why we chose a manual patch-clamp rig for experiments with this particular ion channel. We chose rat neuronal GH4C1 cells for host cell because this cell line endogenously expresses the chaperone RIC-3, which is required for proper processing and sorting of acetylcholine receptors (14).

2. Materials

2.1. Cloning

1. pcDNA3 vector (5,446 bp, Invitrogen, Carlsbad, CA).
2. Ampicillin is dissolved at 100 mg/mL in dH_2O and then stored at –20°C until used.
3. 10 cm Petri dishes for bacterial plates (Greiner Bio-One GmbH, Germany).
4. Proofread polymerase kit, e.g. Finnzymes Phusion™ polymerase (New England Biolabs Inc, Ipswich, MA).
5. *Bam*HI and *Xho*I restriction enzyme kits (New England Biolabs).
6. T4 DNA Ligase (New England Biolabs).
7. 50×TAE Buffer Stock solution: 242 g Tris base, 57.1 ml glacial acetic acid 37.2 g $Na2EDTA{\cdot}2H_2O$, dH_2O to 1 L.
8. 10× loading buffer: 20% (w/v) Ficoll 400, 0.1 M disodium EDTA, pH 8.0, 1% (w/v) SDS, 0.25% (w/v) bromophenol blue.
9. QiaexII Gel extraction Kit (Qiagen, Valencia, CA).
10. QIAprep Spin Miniprep kit (Qiagen).

11. SeaKem LE Agarose (BioConcept, Allschwil, Switzerland), for gels use 0.7% (w/v) in 1× TAE and 2 μl of 10 mg/ml ethidium bromide stock solution.
12. Chemically competent DH5α cells (Invitrogen).
13. LB agar ampicillin plates (100 μg/mL ampicillin, used from stock).

Glycerol 50% (v/v) in dH_2O, autoclaved.

2.2. Cell Culture

1. GH4C1 cells (Health Protection Agency Culture Collections, Salisbury, UK).
2. Lipofectamine 2000 (Gibco/BRL, Bethesda, MD).
3. Optimem (Gibco/BRL).
4. Dulbecco's Modified Eagle's Medium (DMEM+Glutamax) (Gibco/BRL) supplemented with 10% foetal calf serum (FCS).
5. Trypsin/EDTA (Gibco/BRL).
6. Neomycin (Sigma, St-Louis, MO), 50 mg/mL stock solution, store at –20°C
7. Phosphate buffered saline (PBS) (Gibco/BRL).

2.3. Electrophysiology

1. Acetylcholine chloride (Sigma), 1 mM working concentration (15).
2. Bath solution: 120 Mm NaCl, 3 mM KCl, 2 mM $CaCl_2$, 2 mM $MgCl_2$, 10 mM glucose10, 10 mM HEPES; adjust pH to 7.3 with NaOH.
3. Pipette solution: 60 mM CsCl, 60 mM CsF 60, 10 mM EGTA, 10 mM HEPES; pH (CsOH) 7.30.
4. Inverted microscope (Zeiss), WPC-100 patch-clamp amplifier (Abimek, Germany), ISO-2 recording software (MFK, Frankfurt, Germany), micromanipulator (Märzheuser), rapid solution changer (RSC-200, BioLogic Science Instruments, Knoxville, TN), integrated into a PC computer. Borosilicate micropipettes are prepared from capillary tubes (Warner Instruments) on a pipette puller (PC-10, Narishige) shortly before experimentation. Our patch-clamp setup is isolated from vibration using a TMC anti-vibration table.

3. Methods

Choosing the appropriate coding sequence(s) for expression of the desired ion channel protein(s) is the most important decision in such a project. Some ion channels are functional as homomultimers, others only as heteromultimers. Sometimes, the beta subunits in heteromultimers can be recruited if one chooses a host cell that endogenously expresses the required protein cofactors. In addition, for several ion channels, several sequence variants are known. In the case of the Cystic Fibrosis Receptor (CFTR), these exceed 1,500 variants (according to the CFTR mutation database), but in most cases there are about a dozen described variants. Some of these variants have been functionally characterized; most have not. It is thus imperative to do literature research on which experiments have been done and what sequences have been used for the particular experiments. NCBI lists most published sequences in the "Nucleotide" database (http://www.ncbi.nlm.nih.gov/sites/entrez).

The second important decision is choosing the right expression system, the host cell. Human embryonic kidney cells (HEK-293) cells or Chinese hamster ovary cells (CHO) are most commonly used due to their unproblematic handling in cell culture and a high expression rate of proteins. In some cases, a specific ion channel is described to require a specific host cell in order to be functionally active. The endogenous expression of specific membrane proteins that interact with the ion channel as mentioned above can be critical. For this project, the neuronal subtype nAChRα7 ion channel, rat pituitary-derived GH4C1 host cells are required. The fact that that only one full coding sequence has been described so far (16), and published as Locus NM_000746, facilitates the selection of the coding sequence. Since this CDS is commercially available, we will not go into details of doing RT-PCR on tissue to obtain the cDNA. This method would also imply that the cDNA obtained may be a different allele of the gene and might contain sequence variations from the published sequence.

This article also assumes basic cloning and cell handling experience. It also assumes basic handling of a manual patch-clamp rig that features a fast perfusion system for the application of the ligand.

3.1. Cloning

1. The nAChRα7 alpha subunit coding sequence (CDS) can be obtained by RT-PCR (or from companies that offer this service, e.g. OriGene, Rockville, MD). Another method is to have the entire sequence synthesized, e.g. from GENEART (Regensburg, Germany). Having it synthesized has the advantage of directly adding the appropriate cutting sites 5′ and 3′ of the coding sequence and thus being able to directly proceed to cloning into an expression vector. For this, common noncutting sites that are compatible with the pcDNA3 vector multi cloning site (MCS) are required (see Note 1). For the nAChRα7 CDS, the cutters *Bam*HI and *Xho*I are suitable 5′ and 3′ cutters.

They also share similar reaction conditions as outlined by the vendor (New England Biolabs Inc, Ipswich, MA).

2. If the DNA is synthesized, the *Bam*HI (GGATCC) cutting site should be inserted in 5′ to the Kozak sequence and the start ATG (bold) of the CDS (CTCAACATG). Similarly, 3′ to the stop codon (bold), the *Xho*I cutting site (TAACTCGAG) should be inserted.
3. 1 μg of the synthesized plasmid can be processed in a double digest with 1 μl each of *Bam*HI and *Xho*I enzyme. 4 μl of 10× NEB Buffer 3 and 4μl of 10× bovine serum albumin (BSA, included as 100× stock solution along with the restriction enzymes) are added as well with a volume of dH_2O that brings the reaction volume to 40 μl. The reaction mix is then incubated at 37°C for 1 h.
4. Following the reaction, add 4 μl of 10× loading buffer and purify the fragments on a 0.7% 1× TAE agarose gel.
5. Excise the 1.6 kb band with a scalpel and recover the DNA fragment with the QiaexII kit according to the manufacturer's instructions.
6. To obtain the nAchRα7 CDS by PCR, dilute the cDNA template to a concentration of ~50 μg/μl. Use the sense and the antisense primer shown in Table 1 for PCR.
7. For a PCR reaction mix, we recommend a volume of 50 μl. Sense and antisene primers are detailed in Table 1. 1 μl template DNA, 1 μl of each sense and antisense primers (10 mM), 1 μl of dNTPs (200 μM each), 10 μl 10×HF Buffer and 0,5 μl polymerase.

   For PCR, you can use the following cycling conditions: an initial denaturation phase of 30 s at 98° that is shortened to 20 s during the cycles. The annealing temperature is 64°C for 30 s, extension at 72°C for 1 min for 35 cycles. A final extension of 5 min at 72°C completes the program.
8. Purify the 1.6 kb DNA fragment on a 0.7% 1×TAE agarose gel. Make sure that you use reduced brightness on the UV transilluminator and proceed quickly when cutting out the band, as UV is extremely mutagenizing to DNA. Recover the DNA by using the QiaexII kit as instructed in the manual.

Table 1
PCR Primers

PCR primer 1	5′-CGGGATCCCTCAACATGCGCTGCTCGCCGGGA-3′
PCR primer 2	5′-CCGCTCGAGTTACGCAAAGTCTTTGGACACGGCCT-3′

9. The PCR fragment can then be processed with a double digest of *Bam*HI and *Xho*I. Use the total volume of the eluted DNA from step 9 of this section and add 4 μl of 10× NEB Buffer 3 and 4 μl of 10× BSA. 4 μl of each *Bam*HI and *Xho*I are added last. Incubate 1 h at 37°C.
10. Digest 1 μg of pcDNA3 vector with a similar double digest of *Bam*HI and *Xho*I in a 40 μl volume. Incubate 1 h at 37°C. Both fragments, vector (5.4 kb) and insert (1.6 kb), can be gel-purified as described above. After recovery, they now possess compatible 5′ and 3′ overhangs for ligation of the insert.
11. For ligation, a molar ratio of 3:1 insert vs. vector is recommended for optimal results. 50–400 ng of linear vector DNA and the corresponding amount of insert should be used. Sometimes, ligation efficiency can be increased when it is performed at 16°C overnight instead of 20 min at room temperature.
12. The ligation product can then be transformed into chemically competent DH5α cells and plated on an ampicillin containing LB agar plate. As negative control, an equal amount of linearized pcDNA vector can be transformed in a similar fashion in DH5α cells and plated. Incubate the plates at 37°C overnight. The ligation product should yield many more colonies than the negative control. If that is not the case, the ligation should be repeated, as the chance of successful insertions is very low.
13. If there is a higher number of colonies on the ligation sample, pick 12 to 24 colonies and grow them in 5 ml LB medium (100 mg/ml ampicillin) at 37°C on a shaker. Shake vigorously (250 rpm or more).
14. The next day, from each culture, take 70 μl of bacteria and transfer in an Eppendorf tube. 15. Add 30 μl of 50% glycerol and mix gently. These glycerol stocks should be stored at −70°C, although for a short time (days), −20°C is adequate.
15. Use the Miniprep kit to obtain plasmid DNA from the bacteria to be used in a restriction digest. Any enzyme that you keep in stock and that cuts within the insert as well as in the vector and produces an easily recognizable band pattern can be used. For example, *Afl*III produces 4 bands (3,783 bp, 2,044 bp, 743 bp, 333 bp) with the correct sequence that contains the insert, whereas the empty vector yields only two bands (3,402 bp, 2,044 bp).

    Clones that yield a correct restriction digest pattern should be sequenced. The primers listed in Table 2 can be used to sequence the sense strand.

Table 2
Sequencing Primers

Sequencing primer[a]	5′-CGTATTAGTCATCGCTATTA-3′
Sequencing primer 2	5′-TCCAGAGGAAGCTTTACAAG-3′
Sequencing primer 3	5′-CCTTTGATGTGCAGCACTGC-3′
Sequencing primer 4	5′-GATAGCCCAGTACTTCGCCA-3′
Sequencing primer 5	5′-ACGATGAGCACCTCCTGCAC-3′

[a]Primer 1 primes on the vector sequence 5′ of the insertion

16. When the sequence is confirmed to be correct, this pcDNA3 construct can be tested by transient transfection into GH4C1 cells (see Note 2.).
17. To create a stable cell line, the circular plasmid DNA has to be linearized. This will decrease the likelihood of the vector integrating into the genome in a way that disrupts the gene of interest or other elements required for protein expression. Suitable enzymes for linearization are for example: *Bgl*II, *Pvu*I, *Mlu*I.

3.2. Transfection and Cell Culture

1. For a functional assay using only transiently expressing cells, use a 35 mm dish of GH4C1 cells grown to ~90% confluence.
2. Transfect 2 μg of circular pcDNA3 nAChRα7 plasmid and 2 μg of a GFP-expressing plasmid using 10 μl of Lipofectamine2000 according to manufacturer's instructions. Following the transfection, cells are incubated in DMEM containing 10% FCS.
3. 16 h posttransfection, cell can be analyzed under the fluorescence microscope of the manual patch-clamp rig. Bright green cells are expected to coexpress the ion channel and can be tested for nAChRα7 activity.
4. When the proper functioning of the cloned plasmid is confirmed, a stable cell line can be created from this plasmid DNA:
   Linearize the cloned pcDNA3 plasmid with either *Bgl*II, *Pvu*I,or *Mlu*I
   Transfect GH4C1 cells (grown to ~90% confluence in a 25 ml flask) with 0.2 μg of linear DNA in 5 μl Lipofectamine2000 according to the manufacturer's protocol. Although higher amounts of DNA can be used, for creation of stable cell lines, less material is usually more efficient.
5. After transfection, incubate the cells in DMEM supplemented with 10% FCS.

6. About 16 h posttransfection, detach the cells by removing the old medium and carefully washing the cells with 10 ml 1×PBS. Add 1 ml 1× trypsin/EDTA and tilt the flask such that the entire surface is covered by the liquid. Carefully aspirate the trypsin and incubate the cells for 1 min at 37°C. The cells should then start to detach from the bottom of the flask. Add fresh DMEM (10% FCS, 0.5 mg/ml neomycin) and resuspend cells. Make sure that there are no clumps, then transfer them to a 75 ml flask
7. 24 h later, change the medium to 10% FCS in DMEM supplemented with 0.5 mg/ml neomycin.
8. Incubate the cells for 7–14 days and leave them untouched at least for 7 days (see Note 3.). Count the number of colonies that have formed after 1 week.
9. Once the colonies are visible to the eye and are about 3 mm in diameter, detach the cells.
10. Transfer this pool in a new 75 ml flask.
11. Passage the cells three times in neomycin selection medium once they attain ~90% confluence.
12. After this first round of selection, proceed with cloning the cells. For this, wash and detach the cells as detailed in step 11 of this section. Take half of those cells and freeze them in liquid nitrogen as the original first round of selection.
13. Prepare a 96 well plate with 80 μl of fresh DMEM (10% FCS, 0.5 mg/ml neomycin) per well.
14. Count the other half of the cells with a cytometer.
15. Dilute a fraction of this pool to a cell density of 0.5 per 20 μl volume. For this, use serial dilutions (e.g. one in ten) and make sure that you work rapidly and constantly shake the cells in the medium. Otherwise, cells will decant rather fast and tend to aggregate as clumps.
16. Add 20 μl of the diluted cells in suspension to each well. With this dilution, you expect a single colony in every second well. This means if you counted 20 individual colonies in the first selection, a 96 well plate should do and there is no need for expanding more clones. Up to 30 initial colonies can be distributed in a single 96 well plate.
17. Incubate this 96 well plate at 37°C.
18. After a few days, you should be able to see single colonies emerging from a singe cell in the wells. Mark those wells with a pen and let the cells grow for about 2 weeks.
19. Once big colonies have formed (about 1/5 of the well diameter), the medium colour will also start to change due to a shift in the pH level.

20. Prepare a 24 well plate with 400 μl DMEM (10% FCS, 0.5 mg/ml neomycin) per well. For each promising colony in the 96 well plate, one well in (a) 24 well plate(s) has to be prepared.
21. At this point, choose the successful single colonies for further passaging. Aspirate the medium of those wells, wash them carefully with 100 μl PBS, then add 40 μl trypsin. Trypsin is rather aggressive to the cells; process no more than 5 cell clones at a time, otherwise the procedure will take too long and the cells will start to suffer in the trypsin medium. Once the cells are detached, add 80 μl of medium, resuspend the cells by gently pipetting up and down and transfer them in different wells of the prepared 24 well plate(s).
22. Let the cells grow and passage them twice. After the first passage, the cell clones can be expanded in 6 well plates. The cell number of a 6 well plate is sufficient for both freezing cells and for manual patch clamp assays. From this second passage, cell clones can be functionally analyzed. Discard the clones that fail electrophysiological validation at this point.

3.3. Functional Assay

1. Cells are finally plated into 35 mm Petri dishes at a density low enough to record single cells (17).
2. Place the Petri dish on the stage of the inverted microscope and perfuse them continuously with the standard bath solution (1 ml/min). All solutions are to be maintained at room temperature (unless otherwise required).
3. After formation of a giga-Ohm seal between the patch electrode (pipette resistance range 2–6 MΩ) and the cell, the cell membrane across the pipette tip is ruptured by suction to assure electrical access to the cell interior (whole-cell patch-clamp configuration). Seal resistance should be over 1 GΩ without using leak current compensation. Access resistance below 10 MΩ is acceptable. The series resistance should be compensated to at least 80%.
   As soon as a stable seal is established, acetylcholine-induced inward currents are measured upon brief applications of ligand to the patch-clamped cell. A two-barreled application system is used to achieve drug exchange within milliseconds (required to record the full amplitude of channel response before desensitisation, Fig. 1).
4. Once the control response is established, it is recommended to repeat the ligand application 2–3 times before further recording (dose-response curves, modulation experiments).

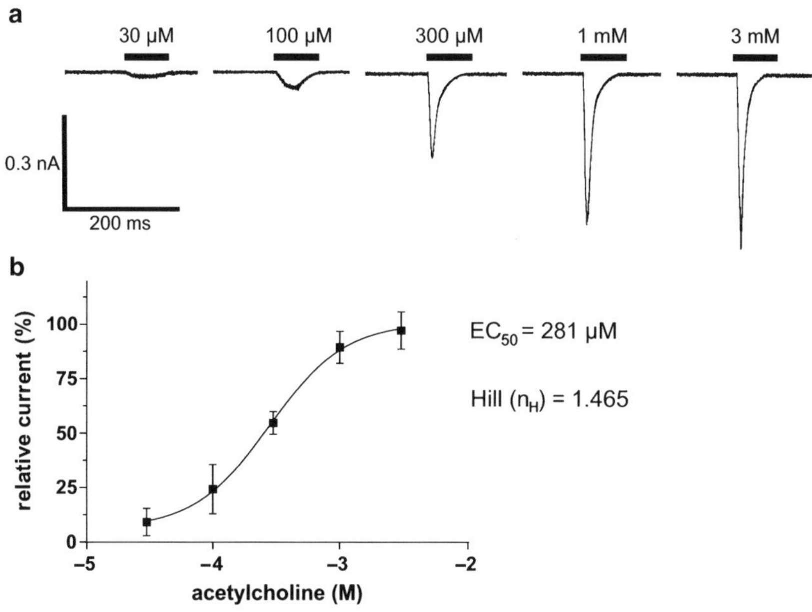

Fig. 1. Acetylcholine-induced responses of the α7 nicotinic acetylcholine receptors in GH4C1 cells. Panel A shows representative current traces of five applications of acetylcholine. 30 μM, 100 μM, 300 μM, 1 mM, and 3 mM acetylcholine were applied during the time indicated by the *black horizontal bar* on top of the traces. Any employed perfusion system must apply the desired ligand concentration around the cell in a time less than 2 ms. Otherwise, the channel will desensitize before the desired ligand concentration is reached and the response will reflect a lower ligand concentration. Saturation of the acetylcholine response is reached around 3 mM concentration. Panel B illustrates the normalized response of the ion channel. The half maximal effective concentration (EC_{50}) of this channel is at 281 μM acetylcholine. Corresponding data points are mean ±SEM of $n=3$ cells. The Hill coefficient (n_H) is 1.46 and thus shows the positive cooperativity of the nAChRα7 channel in opening the conductance

4. Notes

1. There are of course many other possible cloning vectors and systems currently available, most notably from Invitrogen, Inc. These site-directed integration strategies have the drawback of being dependent on a specific host cell. As we want to stress the flexibility of choosing different host cell lines for individual ion channels, this protocol is limited to the traditional way of creating a stable cell line. For efficient expression of the nAChRα7 receptor, GH4C1 cells (or other RIC-3 expressing host cells) are required. These cells as such are not compatible with current directed DNA integration protocols.
2. It is recommended that functional validation of the construct be carried out before one does all the work for the creation of the stable cell line. Transient expression together with a GFP reporter gene will allow the discrimination of ion channel-expressing cells. For this, a plasmid that encodes for free green

fluorescent protein (GFP) can be cotransfected in equal amount as the cloned pcDNA3-derived vector. Transfection with Lipofectamine2000 (or calcium phosphate) introduces many copies of a plasmid into a cell. Proper mixing of the GFP plasmid and the nAChRα7 plasmid ensures that most transfected cells express both proteins. GFP-expressing cells should be patched 24–48 h after transfection.

3. During the first selection round, it is stated that you should not touch the cells for at least a week. We recommend not touching the flask to reduce the formation of satellite colonies. This way, you will be able to see by eye the individual colonies that are forming in the flask. Count the number of visible clones. The colonies that form are all unique clones. This number of clones gives an idea of how many clones should be created by limiting dilution. For example if you count 10 colonies, there will be no point in creating more than a dozen limiting dilutions of the total cells in this flask, as there are only 10 different clones to be expected. This can be taken into consideration when you decide how many clones you want to produce by limiting dilution.

Acknowledgments

The authors thank Céline Wimmersberger for technical assistance.

References

1. Ashcroft F (2000) Ion Channels and Disease. Academic Press, San Diego, CA, p 481
2. Venter JC, Adams MD, Myers EW, Li PW et al (2001) The sequence of the human genome. Science 291:1304–1351
3. Li S, Gosling M, Poll CT, Westwick J, Cox B (2005) Therapeutic scope of modulation of non-voltage-gated cation channels. Drug Discov Today 10:129–137
4. Hamill OP, Marty A, Neher E, Sakmann B, Sigworth FJ (1981) Improved patch-clamp techniques for high-resolution current recording from cells and cell-free membrane patches. Pflugers Arch 391:85–100
5. Fermini B, Fossa AA (2003) The impact of drug-induced QT interval prolongation on drug discovery and development. Nat Rev Drug Discov 2:439–447
6. Xu J, Wang X, Ensign B, Li M, Wu L, Guia A, Xu J (2001) Ion-channel assay technologies: quo vadis? Drug Discov Today 6:1278–1287
7. Wang X, Li M (2003) Automated electrophysiology: high throughput of art. Assay Drug Dev Technol 1:695–708
8. Dunlop J, Bowlby M, Peri R, Vasilyev D, Arias R (2008) High-throughput electrophysiology: an emerging paradigm for ion-channel screening and physiology. Nat Rev Drug Discov 7:358–368
9. Bianchi BR, Moreland RB, Faltynek CR, Chen J (2007) Application of large-scale transiently transfected cells to functional assays of ion channels: different targets and assay formats. Assay Drug Dev Technol 5:417–424
10. Deutsch C (2003) The birth of a channel. Neuron 40:265–276
11. Jenkinson DH (2006) Potassium channels–multiplicity and challenges. Br J Pharmacol 147(Suppl 1):63–71

12. Feuerbach D, Lingenhoehl K, Olpe HR, Vassout A, Gentsch C, Chaperon F, Nozulak J, Enz A, Bilbe G, McAllister K, Hoyer D (2009) The selective nicotinic acetylcholine receptor alpha7 agonist JN403 is active in animal models of cognition, sensory gating, epilepsy and pain. Neuropharmacology 56:254–256
13. Lyford LK, Rosenberg RL (1999) Cell-free expression and functional reconstitution of homo-oligomeric alpha7 nicotinic acetylcholine receptors into planar lipid bilayers. J Biol Chem 274:25675–25681
14. Treinin M (2008) RIC-3 and nicotinic acetylcholine receptors: biogenesis, properties, and diversity. Biotechnol J 3:1539–1547
15. Zwart R, Vijverberg HP (1997) Potentiation and inhibition of neuronal nicotinic receptors by atropine: competitive and noncompetitive effects. Mol Pharmacol 52:886–895
16. Gault J, Robinson M, Berger R, Drebing C et al (1998) Genomic organization and partial duplication of the human alpha7 neuronal nicotinic acetylcholine receptor gene (CHRNA7). Genomics 52:173–185
17. Verdoorn TA, Draguhn A, Ymer S, Seeburg PH, Sakmann B (1990) Functional properties of recombinant rat GABAA receptors depend upon subunit composition. Neuron 4:919–928

Chapter 18

Ion Channels in Analgesia Research

Tamara Rosenbaum, Sidney A. Simon, and Leon D. Islas

Abstract

Several recent techniques have allowed us to pinpoint the receptors responsible for the detection of nociceptive stimuli. Among these receptors, ion channels play a fundamental role in the recognition and transduction of stimuli that can cause pain. During the last decade, compelling evidence has been gathered on the role of the TRPV1 channel in inflammatory and neuropathic states. Activation of TRPV1 in nociceptive neurons results in the release of neuropeptides and transmitters, leading to the generation of action potentials that will be sent to higher CNS areas, where they will often be perceived as pain. Its activation will also evoke the peripheral release of pro-inflammatory compounds that may sensitize other neurons to physical, thermal, or chemical stimuli. For these reasons, and because its continuous activation causes analgesia, TRPV1 is now considered a viable drug target for clinical use in the management of pain. Using the TRPV1 channel as an example, here we describe some basic biophysical approaches used to study the properties of ion channels involved in pain and in analgesia.

Key words: TRPV1, Pain, Nociceptors, Nonstationary noise analysis, Open probability, Transient transfection

1. Introduction

The capsaicin receptor, TRPV1, has been implicated in physiological processes such as the detection of noxious physical and chemical stimuli, making it a promising target for pain-relieving drugs. TRPV1-containing neurons can be rendered insensitive to further painful stimuli through receptor desensitization in response to some agonists, which can result in a generalized lack of responsiveness of this protein to further noxious stimuli. Moreover, some local anaesthetics are able to permeate through the TRPV1 channel and block neuronal sodium channels from the intracellular side, providing a means for controlling the activity of these cells containing nociceptors and thus, pain itself (1).

Arpad Szallasi (ed.), *Analgesia: Methods and Protocols*, Methods in Molecular Biology, vol. 617, DOI 10.1007/978-1-60327-323-7_18, © Springer Science+Business Media, LLC 2010

Some reagents such as certain classes of antibiotics, fatty acids, and anaesthetics induce analgesia. Until recently, the underlying mechanism for the analgesic effects of these agents was unknown. It has now been shown that they act as potent blockers of TRPV1 by lowering the open channel probability.

The use of a combination of techniques has allowed us to better understand how this channel works and elucidate how molecules with analgesic effects regulate the perception of pain. These techniques include transient transfection of the ion channel into a nonnative cellular system, where its properties can be studied in isolation, using classical approaches of cellular biophysics, such as patch-clamp recording, which permit the study of how the channel's biophysical properties are affected using open probability and nonstationary noise analysis.

2. Materials

2.1. Cell Culture and Transient Transfection

1. Human embryonic kidney cells (HEK 293) (American type culture collection, Manassas, VA).
2. Complete growth medium; Dulbecco's Modified Eagle's Medium (DMEM) (Gibco/BRL, Bethesda, MD) supplemented with 10% fetal bovine serum (Gibco/BRL), 1% L-glutamine (Invitrogen, Carlsbad, CA) and 0.5% penicillin–streptomycin (Invitrogen). Cells must be grown in an atmosphere of 95% air and 5% CO_2.
3. Trypsin-EDTA 0.05% (Gibco/BRL)
4. Lipofectamine reagent (Invitrogen)
5. pRES-Green fluorescent protein (GFP) and TRPV1 cDNA's in mammalian-cell expression vectors
6. 35 and 100 mm dishes (Corning, Corning, NY)
7. Sterilized cover glass pieces cut to no more than 2 × 2 cm

2.2. Electrophysiological Recording

1. Axopatch 200B (Axon Instruments, Foster City, CA) or EPC-10 (Heka Elektronik, Mahone Bay, NS, Canada) with an external Bessel filter (Frequency Devices, Ottawa, IL).
2. RSC-100 rapid solution changer (Bio-Logic Science Instruments, France) or VC-77SP (Warner Instruments, Hamden, CT).
3. Picospitzer apparatus (Intracel, Herts, UK).
4. Igor Pro software (Wave Metrics, Lake Oswego, OR) and Matlab software (The Mathworks, Natick, MA).

2.2.1. Low Divalent Recording Solution for Inside-Out Patch-Clamp Experiments

To avoid acute desensitization and tachyphlaxis and facilitate the interpretation of the results, low divalent recording solutions are used, prepared with deionized water (pH to 7.2 with NaOH).

1. 130 mM NaCl
2. HEPES-free acid, 3 mM
3. EDTA, 200 μM

2.2.2. Intracellular and Extracellular Recording Solutions for Whole-Cell Patch-Clamp Experiments

1. Extracellular solution: 140 mM NaCl, 3 mM KCl, 2 mM $MgCl_2$, 2 mM $CaCl_2$ and 5 mM HEPES and the pH adjusted to 7.3 with NaOH.
2. Intracellular pipette solution: 140 mM KCl, 0.5 mM EGTA, 5 mM HEPES, 3 mM Mg-ATP and 10 mM glucose, and the pH is adjusted to 7.3 with KOH.

2.3. Capsaicin Stock and Dilutions

1. 4 mM Capsaicin (Sigma, St. Louis, MO) stock in absolute ethanol.
2. Capsaicin dilutions to 10 nM, 25 nM, 50 nM, 100 nM, 250 nM, 500 nM, 1 μM and 4 μM prepared in low divalent recording solution.

2.4. Glass Pipette Fabrication

1. P-97 horizontal micropipette puller (Sutter Instrument Co., Novato, CA).
2. Borosilicate glass (Sutter Instrument).
3. MF-830 microforge (Narishige, Japan).
4. Sylgard polymer coating (Dow Corning Corp., Midland, MI) which is cured under a heated filament or Q-dope (GC Electronics).

3. Methods

HEK cells constitute a very useful model in the study of ion channel properties outside their native expression systems. These cells are not electrically excitable and therefore, "contamination" from introduced ion channels is readily attained. The use of reagents such as Lipofectamine renders cells more viable for experiments, where cell membranes must be in good conditions for lengthy recordings. Cotransfection with GFP cDNA permits the identification of those cells that were successfully transfected without having to attach a fluorescent molecule to the ion channel, which may produce a protein that might not express or function as well.

3.1. HEK293 Cell Transient Transfection

From a 100 mm culture dish where cells have grown to 70–80% confluency:

1. Prepare 35 mm culture dishes by placing side by side as many cut cover glass pieces as possible in a sterile environment. Cut cover slips with a diamond pen into 0.5 × 0.5 cm squares.
2. Remove and discard culture medium.
3. Add 0.5–1 ml of Trypsin-EDTA solution to dish and place dish in a 37°C incubator.
4. Add 5 ml of complete growth medium and aspirate cells by gently pipetting.
5. Add appropriate aliquots (300–400 μl) of the cell suspension to 35 mm culture dishes with cover glasses.
6. Incubate cultures at 37°C for 24 h prior transfection.
7. To transfect one 35 mm dish prepare:
8. Tube 1: 0.5 μg of TRPV1 cDNA; 0.5 μg of pRES-GFP cDNA; 99 μl serum-free DMEM.
9. Tube 2: 5 μl Lipofectamine; 95 μl serum-free DMEM.
10. Mix both tubes and incubate at room temperature for 45 min.
11. While incubating the DNA and Lipofectamine solution, use a serological or Pasteur pipette attached to a vacuum to remove all existing media from the 35 mm culture dishes and replace it with 800 μl serum free DMEM (no L-glutamine or antibiotic should be included) and incubate at 37°C for 45 min.
12. After 45 min, add the transfection solution to the cells by pipetting and gently mix the media.
13. Incubate for 6 h at 37°C before removing and replacing transfection solution with complete growth media.
14. Incubate cells in complete growth media for at least 12–24 h before performing an experiment.

3.2. Protocol for Current Recording of TRPV1 Channels in HEK Cell Excised Membrane Patches

Single channel or macroscopic currents can be recorded in HEK cells shortly after TRPV1 transfection. Both types of data can be obtained with the use of cell attached or detached patch clamp recording. The cells are used for experiments one or two days after transfection. Using the transfection protocol in Subheading 3.1, the density of channels in the membrane is high enough to allow recordings of macroscopic currents (several nanoamperes (nA) of current). The use of smaller DNA quantities (1–2 μg) for transfection allows for recordings of single-channels.

1. Pull and polish pipettes to have a resistance of 10–15 MΩ and coat with Sylgard or Q-Dope (see Note 1). Backfill the pipette with the low divalent solution and form a very high resistance (>10 GΩ) seal between the tip of the glass pipette and the membrane cell.

2. The membrane patch is excised in order to obtain a seal in the inside-out patch-clamp configuration. This is accomplished by lifting the pipette slowly which is usually not a problem if the cells are well attached to the substrate. The bath solution should be the low divalent solution.
3. Currents are low-pass filtered at 2 kHz with the built-in filter of the patch-clamp amplifier (Axopatch 200B or EPC-10) or with an external Bessel filter and sampled at 10 kHz.
4. Place the tip of the patch pipette near the perfusion tube that contains a saturating solution of capsaicin (4 μM). Activation of channels can be attained by the following voltage step protocol. Hold the membrane at 0 mV for 100 ms and step the voltage from –120 mV to 100 mV for 300 ms in 20 mV increments and return the voltage to 0 mV for 100 ms. This protocol should elicit macroscopic current activation.
5. If single channel recording is performed, then the presence of a single channel in the patch can be assessed by the absence of overlapping channel openings under conditions of high open probability (see Note 2). For steady-state measurements, the patch is moved in front of the perfusion tube of an RSC-100 rapid solution changer that contains a saturating solution of capsaicin (4 μM). Membrane patches should be held at the voltage of interest and recordings performed for a long period of time, typically several seconds to minutes.
6. For single-channel level studies of the activation in response to voltage steps, one may measure for example, the first latency to opening, for which a large number of sweeps (200–300) are needed and leak subtraction should be applied. The voltage steps can be shorter (100–200 ms) and leak subtraction is performed as follows: all the sweeps without openings (null sweeps) are averaged together to produce an ensemble null sweep. This is then subtracted from each of the sweeps that contain active channels. The use of a rapid solution changer makes it possible to apply different solutions directly to the patch, without changing the whole bath solution, minimizing changes in the solution level that in turn reduces changes in the pipette capacitance and reduces subtraction artefacts.

3.3. Protocol for Whole-Cell Current Recording of TRPV1 Channels in HEK Cells

Macroscopic currents can also be recorded in the whole-cell configuration of the patch clamp in order to keep the integrity of the cell compartments as well as some of the intracellular signalling elements.

1. Pull pipettes to have a resistance of 3–5 MΩ and coat with Sylgard or Q-Dope (see Note 1). Backfill the pipette with the intracellular recording solution (low divalent solution). The bath solution should be the extracellular solution. Next, form a high resistance (>2–3 GΩ) seal between the tip of the glass

pipette and the cell membrane and compensate for the fast capacitative transient, which arises mostly from the pipette itself.

2. Apply gentle suction to rupture the membrane patch underneath the patch pipette tip using either a syringe or a mouthpiece. A sign that the membrane has been ruptured is the sudden increase in the leak and capacitative currents. At this point, suction may have to be continuously applied in order to avoid resealing of the membrane. The slow component of the capacitative transient, which arises mainly from the cell membrane, should be compensated at this time. Series resistance may be compensated by observing a speeding up of the remaining capacitative transient in the oscilloscope screen.
3. Currents are low-pass filtered at 2 kHz with the built-in filter of the patch-clamp amplifier or with an external Bessel filter. Currents are sampled at 5 kHz, which satisfies the Nyquist criterion (2).
4. Hold the voltage at around 70 mV and step the voltage from −120 mV to 100 mV for 100–200 ms in 10–20 mV increments and return to the holding potential. This protocol should elicit macroscopic current activation.
5. Agonists such as capsaicin or other substances can be applied by changing all the solution in the bath chamber (particularly in the case of a chamber with small volume) or by using the picospritzer apparatus which supplies reproducible pressure pulses for rapid ejections of picoliter to nanoliter volumes of chemical solutions of interest through a glass pipette positioned near the cell.

3.4. Protocol for Non-Stationary Noise Analysis of TRPV1 Currents in HEK Cells

Noise analysis is a technique by which one can determine the single-channel current (i), the number of channels in the patch (N), and the open probability (p) from macroscopic current recordings. Even though better estimates of these parameters can be measured directly by single-channel recording, noise measurements allow for a faster and less analysis-intensive determination, also, some channels may have an immeasurably small single-channel conductance, precluding single-channel analysis. The term non-stationary refers to the fact that the measurement is carried out when the current is changing in time (3). The two main quantities needed are the mean current, $\hat{I}$ and the time-dependent variance, $\sigma^2(t)$. Noise analysis of TRPV1 can be carried out with the use of macroscopic currents recorded in cell-attached or inside-out patches or in whole-cell configuration. In the protocol presented below, the purpose is to determine the maximum value of p and the corresponding values of i and N. Many pharmacological agents exert their effects either by changing the open probability or the single channel current. By using this technique, these can be rapidly estimated.

1. For non-stationary noise analysis, good quality recordings are needed and this is accomplished when pipette-membrane seals are of high resistance > 1 GΩ. Pipettes need to be coated with either Q-Dope or Sylgard to reduce stray capacitance and extraneous noise (see Note 1). Recording solutions are the same as in subheading 3.2. This protocol can be carried out with macroscopic recordings obtained either in the inside-out patch or whole-cell configurations (see Note 3).
2. Once a current recording is stable, many records can be taken (between 100 and 200 sweeps), under the same experimental conditions. The duration of the voltage pulse should be long enough to reach a current level that does not change with time (steady-state activation) and the magnitude of the applied voltage should be one that produces saturation of the conductance-voltage relationship. For example, at a capsaicin concentration of 4 μM, a pulse of 100 ms duration is sufficient to reach steady-state activation and the conductance–voltage relationship saturates near 100 mV (open probability ~0.9).
3. A number of different algorithms have been developed to obtain the mean current and the variance, but the method that is least likely to introduce errors because of drift in the base line current is the algorithm developed by Conti et al. (4) or Conti et al. (5). The analysis of records is carried out as follows. A difference record, δs, is calculated by subtracting pairs of continuous sweeps, $(s_i - s_{i+1})$. An example is shown in Fig. 1a. Note that these sweeps need not be leak-subtracted. The variance, σ^2 is calculated as the ensemble-average of the quantity, δs^2 as (Fig. 1b):

$$\sigma^2 = \left\langle \frac{\delta s^2}{2} \right\rangle \tag{1}$$

4. The mean current, $\hat{I}$, can be obtained as the ensemble-average of the n leak-subtracted (see Note 4) sweeps as: $\hat{I} = \frac{1}{n}\sum_i^n s_i$, (Fig. 1c).
5. Once the variance and mean are calculated, these two quantities are plotted in a variance vs. mean graph (Fig. 1d). If the records come from N channels with an open-state single-channel current i, and open probability p, the mean current, $\hat{I}(t)$ can be expressed as: $\hat{I}(t) = iNp(t)$ and the variance is given by:

$$\sigma^2 = i^2 Np(t)(1 - p(t)) \tag{2}$$

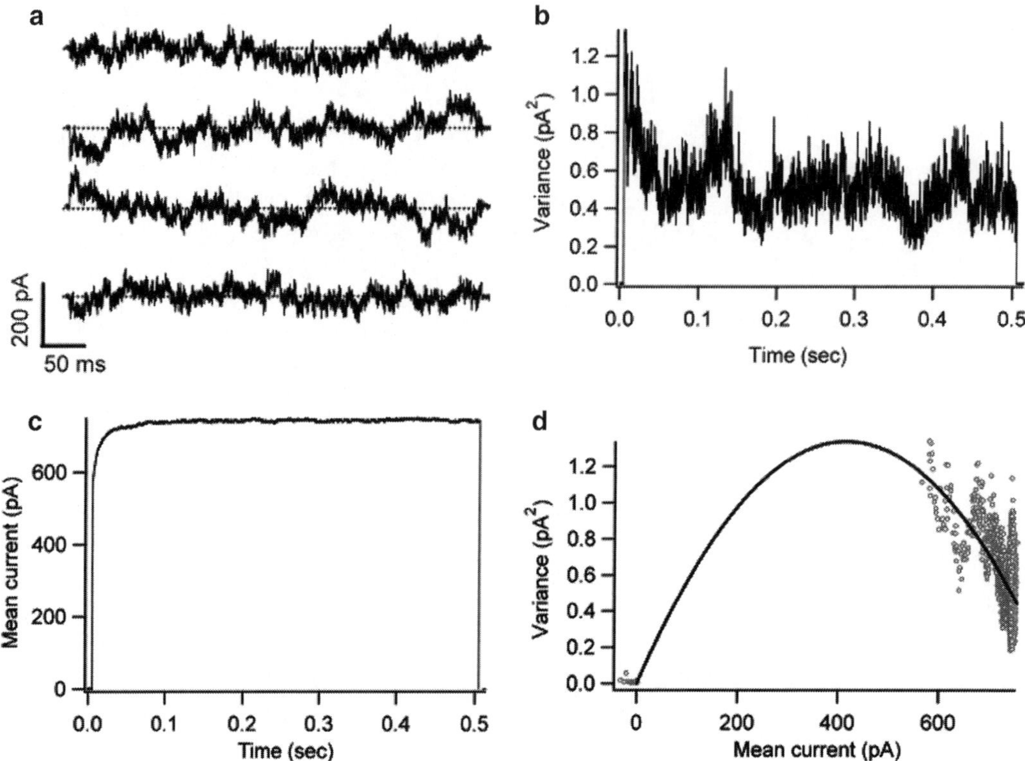

Fig. 1. *Nonstationary noise analysis of capsaicin-activated currents through TRPV1 channels.* (**a**) Four difference records, δs obtained from eight consecutive current traces. Currents were recorded in the inside-out configuration at 100 mV in the presence of 4 μM capsaicin. The dotted lines represent the zero current levels. (**b**) The time-dependent variance obtained from records such as in **a**. (**c**) The mean time-dependent current obtained as the ensemble-average of all 120 records obtained in this experiment. (**d**) Mean-variance plot is obtained by graphing the data in **b** as a function of the data in **c** for each time point. The continuous curve is a fit of Eq. 18.3 with parameters: i = 6.46 pA, N = 128 and p = 0.90

6. Combining these two equations, we obtain an expression for the variance vs. mean relationship:

$$\sigma^2(\hat{I}) = i\hat{I} - \frac{\hat{I}^2}{N} \tag{3}$$

7. This is a parabolic function and can be fitted to the data to give estimates of N and i (Fig. 1d). The open probability at the maximum value of $\hat{I}(t)$ can then be calculated from the equation: $\hat{I}(t) = iN\, p(t)$.
8. The data manipulation described here can be readily implemented into data analysis programs such as Igor Pro.

3.5. Protocol for Determination of the Channel Open Probability

The estimation of the open probability, p, of ion channels is a common experimental procedure. For example, the interaction between drugs that produce current block and the channel is frequently state-dependent and consequently, the open probability is a function of both the capsaicin and blocker concentrations. In order to correctly measure these state-dependent interactions, one may need to measure p over a large range of agonist concentrations. The measurement of p is typically carried out using either single-channel or macroscopic current recordings. In single-channel experiments, the open probability, p, can be estimated directly by measuring the total open time and dividing it by the total recording time (6). This measurement can be reliably carried out to a lower limit of around 0.1 (7, 8), because at lower open probabilities, recording times need to be very long. On the other hand, by carefully measuring the amplitude of tail currents (see Note 5) , macroscopic current recordings can provide estimates of p to around 0.001, but the measured conductance-voltage relationship has to be calibrated in order to obtain estimates of the number of channels contributing to the recording (N) and the maximum value of p_{max} (9–11).

Here, we will discuss a less commonly used method that combines macroscopic and single-channel recordings in the same patch and allows estimates of the open probability as a function of capsaicin concentration down to arbitrarily low values (9, 12). However, for this method very stable recordings are required.

1. To reduce capacitative transients and noise, patches with high seal resistances (>5 GΩ) should be obtained with pipettes coated with Sylgard or Q-Dope. Inside-out patches generated in this way tend to allow stable recordings for more than an hour.
2. Macroscopic currents at a saturating capsaicin concentration and a voltage of interest are recorded in the same way as explained in subheading 3.2. Following the methods explained in the previous section, under these experimental conditions, the number of channels N, the single channel current i, and the maximum open probability p_{max} are estimated by nonstationary noise analysis.
3. Macroscopic current recordings are then obtained at decreasing capsaicin concentrations (Fig. 2a). The value of open probability as a function of capsaicin concentration, p(caps) can be estimated from the ionic current as:

$$p(\text{caps}) = \hat{\text{I}}(\text{caps}) / i\text{N}.$$

4. At sufficiently low capsaicin concentrations, the open probability is very small and macroscopic currents are no longer elicited by the voltage pulse. At this point, the gain of the recording amplifier is increased to 50–100 pA/mV, and openings from a single channel or a few channels, out of the many present in the patch, should be visible (Fig. 2b) although the

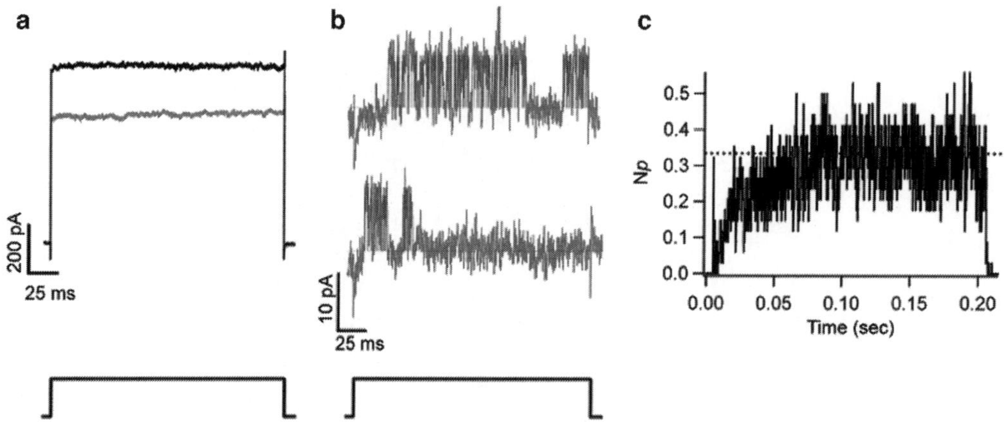

Fig. 2. *Measurement of the open probability from macroscopic and single openings in the same patch.* (**a**) Macroscopic currents from a patch with TRPV1 channels at 4 μM (*black trace*) and 0.25 μM (*grey trace*). The voltage is 60 mV for all recordings. Leak current has been subtracted. Noise analysis indicated that this patch contained 106 channels. (**b**) Two sweeps (*grey trace*) showing single channel openings at 50 nM capsaicin. The black trace is the idealized trace obtained from the 50% threshold crossing criteria. (c) The ensemble average obtained from 96 idealized traces as in **b**. This curve represents the time-dependent N*p* product. The dotted line indicates the value obtained by averaging the last 50 ms of the curve

duration of the voltage pulse may need to be increased due to the low open probability.

5. At this point, a large number (>300) of sweeps at a given low capsaicin concentration are recorded. It is better if the duration of these pulses is larger than the duration used for macroscopic current recording, a good number is 500–1,000 ms. (see Note 6). To estimate the ensemble open probability, most of these sweeps will contain a few or no openings and all are included in the analysis. However, before performing any analysis, each current trace is leak subtracted using a leak template of averaged null sweeps (sweeps that contain no channel openings), (see Note 7).
6. The ensemble open probability can now be calculated from the leak subtracted sweeps. Each sweep is digitally filtered with a Gaussian filter to 1–1.5 kHz and analyzed with the 50% threshold crossing method (6). Since some sweeps will contain overlapping openings from multiple channels, multiple thresholds should be used to allow detection of overlapping channel openings. The closed and open current levels are idealized to values of 0 and 1, respectively (see Note 8). A Gaussian filter is implemented on software packages such as Igor or Matlab or can be programmed from public domain routines (6).

7. The result of step 6 is an idealized record of open and closed events for each sweep (Fig. 2b). The idealizations of all the sweeps (null traces included) are then ensemble averaged. This ensemble average is the time-dependent product of the total number of channels and the open probability, N*p* (Fig. 2c). The value of N*p* from which *p* is calculated is taken as the steady state value of the N*p* trace and is computed as the mean value of the last milliseconds of the averaged idealization (Fig. 2c).
8. The N*p* data thus obtained at each capsaicin concentration can be normalized by N to obtain *p* and combined with the macroscopic estimates of *p*(caps) to be plotted as a dose-response curve.

3.6. Method to Study the Effects of Channel Blockers or Antagonists on TRPV1 Activity

3.6.1. Obtaining the Initial Capsaicin Dose-Response Curves from Macroscopic Recordings

1. Form a very high resistance seal (> 5 GΩ) between the tip of a glass pipette and the membrane cell.
2. Excise the membrane patch in order to obtain a membrane patch in the inside-out configuration. Internal and external solutions same as above.
3. Currents are low pass-filtered at 2 kHz and sampled at 5 kHz.
4. Hold membrane potential at 0 mV and apply voltage pulses ranging from −120 to +120 mV in 10 or 20 mV increments for 100 ms in order to obtain the current to voltage relations in the absence of ligand.
5. The dose-response curve is obtained by repeating the voltage protocol in step 4 at varying capsaicin concentrations ranging from 10 nM to 4 μM. This allows recording of the voltage and state dependence in the same data set.
6. Subtract the currents obtained without agonist (leak currents) from those obtained in the presence of capsaicin.

3.6.2. Blocker Dose-Responses and Calculation of the Fraction of Current Blocked (F_B)

1. To obtain blocker dose-responses, the same voltage protocol as in step 4 of the previous section must be applied and currents must be measured before and after the blocker is added. Note that these same measurements can be used to study the effects of antagonists also.
2. Several blocker concentrations are used in the presence of one single capsaicin concentration in order to calculate the fraction of current blocked.
3. The fraction of current blocked (F_B) is calculated as:

$$F_B = 1 - \frac{I}{I_o};$$

where I is the current in the presence of blocker and I_o is the current in the absence of blocker.

4. The apparent dissociation constant, K_D, which maybe a function of voltage is obtained for the various blocker concentrations [B] by fitting F_B as a function of blocker concentration with the Hill equation:

$$F_B = \frac{[B]^s}{K_D^s + [B]^s},$$

where s is the steepness factor and $[B]$ is the blocker concentration.

5. Once the K_D for the blocker has been obtained, the protocol in the previous section can be used to determine whether the blocker binds better to the open or the closed states of the channel. This is achieved by comparing the initial capsaicin dose-response in the absence of the blocker with a capsaicin dose-response using a concentration near the K_D of the blocker. If the blocker is more effective at blocking the closed states of the channel, then block will be more evident when lower agonist concentrations are used. The same applies for an open state blocker, where the blocking effect will be larger at higher agonist concentrations.

4. Notes

1. Coating with Q-dope is the easier procedure. The pipette is dipped directly into an eppendorf tube containing Q-dope, enough to cover about a cm of the pipette. Q-dope dries on air in about 30 min. The residue that covers the tip of the pipette is burned off in the microforge at the time of fire polishing, without interfering with sealability. Sylgard is less forgiving. Positive pressure should be applied to the back of the pipette with a syringe attached to a small piece of plastic tubing. Sylgard is applied with another pipette, taking care not to touch the tip (this is better done under a microscope). The Sylgard elastomer is cured by heat, which is applied using a blow dryer.
2. There are other statistical methods to estimate the number of channels on a patch (13). In the case of TRPV1 channels, the maximum open probability is very high, in the order 0.9 and the channels remain open for very long periods. If the number of simultaneously open channels in a patch containing n channels is given by the binomial distribution, then the probability of observing only one open level without overlaps is smaller than 0.18 and becomes vanishingly small as n grows. This means that the estimation of the number of

channels by the overlap method is very reliable when the open probability is high.

3. The disadvantage of parameter estimation using noise analysis from macroscopic currents recorded in the whole-cell configuration is that the large cell capacitance and the whole-cell access resistance R_s, act as an RC circuit, effectively filtering the signal and generally producing lower valued estimates of i, N and p. One way around to reduce this problem is to increase the bandwidth of the recording and to use series resistance and capacitance compensation.
4. Leak subtraction can be done by subtracting from each sweep an average of records obtained at the same voltage but in the absence of capsaicin. Care must be taken that the unliganded open probability is low enough to not introduce an error in the subtraction procedure.
5. At the end of a depolarizing pulse, the channels reach a steady-state open probability. If at this moment the voltage is made more negative, this probability will relax to its corresponding steady-state value at negative voltages, reflecting channel closure. Tail currents are the resulting currents from this deactivation process of the channels. Under symmetrical ionic conditions such as the ones discussed here, these can be recorded at negative potentials using a voltage protocol that includes step depolarisations and a repolarization to a negative voltage. The magnitude of the peak tail current is proportional to the channel open probability at the end of the depolarizing voltage pulse.
6. Longer pulses are needed because at low open probabilities, the latency to first opening is longer (this effect is more relevant in voltage-gated channels with larger voltage dependences). If the duration of pulses is short, the steady-state may not be reached in the ensemble averaged Np trace.
7. Leak subtraction using a leak template is preferred over p/n methods because a smaller number of sweeps are needed to form a low noise leak average (14). The variance of the leak-subtracted trace will be increased by: $(1+1/m)$, where m is the number of averaged sweeps used to form the leak template. This increase in noise becomes negligible if more than 10 null sweeps are averaged to form the leak template. If a p/n type protocol is used, the increase in variance due to leak subtraction is $(1+n^2/m)$, where n is the scaling factor of the p/n leak subtraction trace.
8. Idealizing the closed channel level to 0 and the open channel level to 1 is only valid if there is a single open current level. This idealization method allows us to ignore the absolute value of the single channel current, which would

be a variable, for example if this protocol is used to study the voltage dependence of p. If the channel under study presents multiple open states, the idealization has to take into account this fact. An intermediate threshold corresponding to the intermediate conductance level has to be included in the idealization routine.

Acknowledgments

TR is supported by grant CONACyT No. 58038 and DGAPA–UNAM IN200308. SAS is supported in part by grants NIH Grants GM27278, DC-01065 and by grants from Philip Morris USA and Philip Morris International Inc. LDI is supported by CONACyT grant No. 48990 and DGAPA–UNAM grant IN202006-3.

References

1. Binshtok AM, Bean BP, Woolf CJ (2007) Inhibition of nociceptors by TRPV1-mediated entry of impermeant sodium channel blockers. Nature 449:607–10
2. Colquhoun D, Sigworth F (1995) Fitting and statistical analysis of single-channel records. In: Sakmann B, Neher E (eds) Single-channel recording. Plenum, NY, pp 191–263
3. Sigworth FJ (1980) The variance of sodium current fluctuations at the node of Ranvier. J Physiol 307:97–129
4. Conti F, Hille B, Neumcke B, Nonner W, Stampfli R (1976) Conductance of the sodium channel in myelinated nerve fibres with modified sodium inactivation. J Physiol 262:729–742
5. Conti F, Hille B, Neumcke B, Nonner W, Stampfli R (1976) Measurement of the conductance of the sodium channel from current fluctuations at the node of Ranvier. J Physiol 262:699–727
6. Aldrich RW, Yellen G (1983) Analysis of nonstationary chanel kinetics. In: Sakmann B, Neher E (eds) Single-channel recording. Plenum, NY, pp 287–299
7. Hoshi T, Zagotta WN, Aldrich RW (1994) Shaker potassium channel gating. I: Transitions near the open state. J Gen Physiol 103:249–78
8. Moczydlowski E, Latorre R (1983) Gating kinetics of Ca^{2+}-activated K^{+} channels from rat muscle incorporated into planar lipid bilayers. Evidence for two voltage-dependent Ca^{2+} binding reactions. J Gen Physiol 82:511–42
9. Islas LD, Sigworth FJ (1999) Voltage sensitivity and gating charge in Shaker and Shab family potassium channels. J Gen Physiol 114:723–42
10. Schoppa NE, Sigworth FJ (1998) Activation of shaker potassium channels. I. Characterization of voltage-dependent transitions. J Gen Physiol 111:271–94
11. Zagotta WN, Hoshi T, Dittman J, Aldrich RW (1994) Shaker potassium channel gating. II: Transitions in the activation pathway. J Gen Physiol 103:279–319
12. Hirschberg B, Rovner A, Lieberman M, Patlak J (1995) Transfer of twelve charges is needed to open skeletal muscle Na^{+} channels. J Gen Physiol 106:1053–68
13. Horn R (1991) Diffusion of nystatin in plasma membrane is inhibited by a glass-membrane seal. Biophys J 60:433–39
14. Oseguera AJ, Islas LD, Garcia-Villegas R, Rosenbaum T (2007) On the mechanism of TBA block of the TRPV1 channel. Biophys J 92:3901–3914

Chapter 19

Electrophysiological and Neurochemical Techniques to Investigate Sensory Neurons in Analgesia Research

Alexandru Babes, Michael J.M. Fischer, Gordon Reid, Susanne K. Sauer, Katharina Zimmermann, and Peter W. Reeh

Abstract

The primary afferent nociceptive neuron has recently attracted major research interest because of the cloning of very selectively expressed and well-conserved ion channel genes. All parts of the neuron, sensory terminals, axon and cell body, are accessible to validated research techniques in vitro using various isolated tissues or cells taken from laboratory animals. Single-unit recording and measuring stimulated calcitonin gene-related peptide (CGRP) release as well as patch-clamping and calcium imaging of cultured sensory neurons provide different kinds of information, and no model alone answers all questions. In combination, however, consistent results and complementary evidence form a solid basis for translational research to follow.

Key words: Patch clamp, Calcium imaging, Neuropeptide release, CGRP, Single fibre recording, Dorsal root ganglion, Trigeminal ganglion, Primary culture, Ion channels

1. Introduction

The focus of analgesia/antinociception research has moved away from the CNS including the spinal dorsal horn towards the primary sensory, i.e. nociceptive, neuron in the peripheral nervous system. This reorientation was stimulated by the cloning of the first nociceptor-specific transduction proteins, the ATP receptor-channel P_2X_3 and the heat and proton-activated capsaicin receptor TRPV1, and by the cloning of an essential action potential generator, $Na_V1.8$, in these neurons (1–3). It is obviously the hope of more specific and less unwanted actions that fosters this research direction. Strong support for this vision has recently come from the discovery of a human loss-of-function mutation (in $Na_V1.7$ of the sensory neurons) that results in

Arpad Szallasi (ed.), *Analgesia: Methods and Protocols*, Methods in Molecular Biology, vol. 617, DOI 10.1007/978-1-60327-323-7_19,

complete inability to perceive pain combined with no other neurological deficits (4).

The primary nociceptive neuron is accessible to a number of well-established research techniques that provide insight into cellular and molecular functions of single neurons and/or of defined neuronal subpopulations. The actual nociceptive nerve ending in the peripheral tissue and its unmyelinated or thinly myelinated nerve fibre can be examined by recording the propagated action potentials evoked by defined stimuli, or by measuring the stimulated release of calcitonin gene-related peptide (CGRP) as a lump index of activation of the peptidergic nociceptor subpopulation. Both techniques are applicable to in vivo or ex vivo research on intact animal preparations, and related methods such as microneurography and microdialysis are established in human pain research, which allow for translation of the findings (5, 6).

Nociceptors were studied for the first time in 1969 by Burgess and Pearl in the skin (7). In intact animals, however, it is impossible to achieve control over all experimental variables affecting the skin. There is no method to control the effective concentration of applied chemicals at the receptive site, and some routes of administration (injection, pricking, and blister induction) result in skin damage that may alter nociceptor sensitivity. Even close arterial injection of agents depends on distribution of blood flow, and many substances are highly vasoactive (bradykinin, histamine, and acetylcholine) and thus influence their own distribution. Intact isolated superfused tissue preparations were therefore developed in the 1980s (8)

A versatile model for studying the responsiveness of the primary sensory neurons in the isolated mouse skin is the saphenous skin-nerve preparation (9). It enables extracellular recording of propagated action potentials from the receptive fields of single sensory nerve endings in the skin. The sensory properties are comparable to those obtained in vivo in the same species (10, 11). The skin-nerve preparation is fast to isolate and can be kept viable for more than 12 h under superfusion. Compounds are applied directly to the corium, which avoids diffusion barriers and allows tight control of the concentration of chemicals. Therefore, this preparation has been used for a wide variety of pharmacological studies of a wide variety of pro- and antinociceptive compounds on nociceptive nerve endings (12–21) Taking advantage of the uniform genetic background of inbred mice, and genetically modified mice, it is possible to evaluate the influence of single genes or gene products on the sensory transduction process, and on action potential electrogenesis and propagation (16, 22, 23). The basic setup can also be used to investigate the effects of in vivo induced inflammatory conditions (24) and primary afferent aspects of neuropathic pain (25).

Sharing the advantage of employing isolated tissue, the measurement of spontaneous and stimulated CGRP release does not require an intact nerve in continuity with the preparation and, thus, extends the spectrum of investigational tissue. A wide variety of different tissue sections such as skin flaps, segments of colon or oesophagus, desheathed peripheral nerves, or nerve sheaths, or whole isolated organs such as the heart, trachea, or dura mater of the skull have been used in such experiments on rats and mice. Stimuli to induce the neurosecretion include noxious heat, mechanical distension, and antidromic electrical stimulation – through an intact nerve in this exceptional case – as well as a plethora of chemicals activating G protein-coupled or ionotropic receptors in the nerve endings and axons. An obvious limitation to this approach is the restriction to CGRP-expressing neurons, which, however, play an essential role in inflammatory sensitization to heat and hyperalgesia (16). Drug effects evaluated have been those of calcium channel blockers, cholinergics, COX inhibitors, triptans, cannabinoids, opiates, local and general anaesthetics, whereby not only inhibitory but, concentration-dependently, also excitatory actions were encountered in certain cases (26–28). Although specific for nociceptors, observed drug effects on stimulated CGRP release do not necessarily reflect interference with the mechanisms of sensory transduction or activation because the stimulus response additionally depends on a whole cascade of events leading to vesicular exocytosis of CGRP. Control experiments, using unspecific activation by external KCl (inducing depolarization and calcium influx), are therefore required to delineate the mechanism of drug action. On the other hand, CGRP release measurements are potentially more sensitive (to stimulation as well as drug effects) than action potential recordings because they do not depend on depolarization exceeding action potential threshold (26). In fact, neuropeptide release does not depend on depolarization at all but just on calcium influx (29). In this respect, CGRP release findings are expected to correlate well with results from calcium imaging of cultured sensory neurons.

Cell bodies of sensory neurons in primary culture, taken from the dorsal root (DRG), trigeminal, or nodose/jugular ganglia, are established as a surrogate model of their former, axotomized, peripheral nerve endings (Subheading 3.1). They are accessible to patch-clamping (Subheading 3.2) and calcium microfluorimetry (Subheading 3.3), high-resolution techniques that allow for the fine dissection and analysis of mechanisms related to activation, sensitization and inhibition. The same techniques are applied to heterologous expression systems that provide further reduction of the biological complexity. Immortal cell lines, such as HEK 293 or CHO, are transiently or stably transfected so as to express ion channels, G-protein-coupled receptors, or combinations of them.

Heterologous expression systems combined with fully automated calcium imaging or patch-clamping are also the basis of high-throughput screening that allows pharmaceutical companies to search within days for functional agonists or antagonists among millions of compounds.

However, the reductionistic approach obviously conveys the problem of increasing the distance to "real life". The enzymatic dissociation of the ganglia alters the neurons; various different culture conditions cause more or less uncontrolled de- and re-differentiations, and, in consequence, the composition of functional membrane proteins changes (30, 31). For example, cultured DRG neurons show hardly any heat-activated currents if isolated from TRPV1 null mutant mice; in contrast, polymodal nociceptors from the skin of those animals respond almost normally to noxious heat, as do the whole animals (23, 32). In recent studies, cultured DRG neurons from Nav1.8$^{-/-}$ mice became unexcitable when cooled to 10°C, while the excitability of cutaneous nerve endings appeared similar to wildtype animals (33). Thus, radically different conclusions could be drawn from intact animals or skin-nerve preparations on one side and the cellular model on the other.

2. Materials

2.1. Culture of Primary Sensory Neurons

1. Dulbecco's Modified Eagle Medium (DMEM) (Sigma, St. Louis, MO) supplemented with gentamicin at 50 μg/ml and stored in aliquots at –20°C.
2. Poly-D-lysine is dissolved in distilled water at 0.1 mg/mL and stored in 5 ml aliquots at –20°C.
3. Incubation solution for the enzymatic treatment of DRG: 155 mM NaCl, 1.5 mM K_2HPO_4, 5.6 mM HEPES 5.6, 4.8 mM NaHEPES, 5 mM glucose, supplemented by gentamicin 50 μg/ml. This solution is stored in 10 ml aliquots at –20°C.
4. Nerve growth factor NGF 7S (Sigma) is dissolved in serum-containing medium to form a stock solution at 10 μg/mL. The stock solution is stored in 0.4 ml aliquots at –20°C. The final concentration is 100 ng/mL (see Note 1).
5. Dissection instruments: large, medium and very fine scissors, fine forceps (Dumont no. 5), scalpel with no. 11 blade.
6. Syringes, needles for handling medium and solutions: 10 ml and 30 ml syringes with 18-gauge needles.
7. Syringe filters for sterilizing solutions: 25 or 30 mm diameter for medium, 13 mm diameter for poly-lysine, and the incubation

solution for the enzymatic treatment (Millipore filters type GVWP02500 and GVWP01300; see Note 2). These disposable membranes fit into holders (Millipore SX0002500 or SX0001300) and are sterilized by dry heat (110°C for 1 h).

8. Glass Pasteur pipettes, short type (15 cm long), with teats. These are heat-sterilized before use.
9. Sterile 35 mm culture dishes: these should have ventilated lids.
10. Cover slips, round, borosilicate, 15 or 25 mm diameter, no. 1½ thickness (see Note 3).
11. Collagenase (Sigma) and dispase (Gibco/BRL, Bethesda, MD). Store desiccated at –20°C (collagenase) or 4°C (dispase). For convenience, these are stored in aliquots of ~3 mg (collagenase) and ~10 mg at –20°C in 1.5 ml microcentrifuge tubes.
12. Binocular dissecting microscope with cold light source. Ideally, this should be sited in a laminar flow hood; if it is on an open bench, it should be in a quiet corner of the laboratory without draughts or through traffic.
13. Medium for growing dissociated neuronal cells (TNB100, Biochrom, Berlin, Germany) (see Note 4).
14. Dye and membrane permeablizer (e.g. Fura2-AM and Pluronic F127, Invitrogen, Carlsbad, CA).

2.2. Setup for Patch-Clamping and Calcium Imaging

1. An inverted fluorescence microscope (e.g. IX-70 from Olympus or Eclipse 200 from Nikon) for carrying out simultaneous patch-clamp and calcium microfluorimetry measurements. (See Note 5). If cells are pre-selected with Ca^{2+} imaging (see Note 6), the microscope for imaging and patch-clamping will be identical. Inverted microscopes allow good access to the cells in a culture dish or recording chamber.
2. Vibration isolation tables, required to damp microscopic movements and vibrations present to various degrees in all buildings (63-500 series, Technical Manufacturing Corporation, Peabody, MA) (see Note 7).
3. Superfusion application system allowing application of different solutions during the experiment. Commonly, gravity-driven fluid application is used. Solutions are led through tubing to a manifold with a single outlet (e.g. Warner ML or MP series) positioned close to the cell under study. A system with electronically controlled valves adds to ease and precision of the experiment.
4. For constant temperature, an in-line solution heater (e.g. Warner SF-28, Warner Instruments, Hamden, CT) and a

device to hold the recording dish (PDMI-2, Digitimer, Welwyn Garden City, UK) can be used. For full temperature control, a few laboratory-made Peltier-controlled devices are available. Most can heat, some can additionally cool (34–36). Usually the temperature controlling element is placed in the final common pathway, after the manifold.

5. External solution for whole cell recording: 140 mM NaCl, 5 mM KCl, 2 mM $CaCl_2$ (or 1 mM $MgCl_2$ 1), 10 mM HEPES, 4.55 mM NaOH, 5 mM glucose, pH 7.4 at 25°C. For calcium imaging, some attention should be given to the calcium concentration. Calcium influx upon increase of calcium conductance correlates to the extracellular calcium concentration; for a slow rise of the intracellular calcium, the physiological free calcium level of 1.25 mM can be reduced to as low as 0.05 mM.
6. Pipette solution: 135 mM KCl, 1.6 mM $MgCl_2$, 2 mM EGTA, 2.5 mM Mg-ATP, 10 mM HEPES. This is filtered and stored in 1 ml aliquots at –20°C. The pH is adjusted to 7.3 with NaOH. For special purposes (for instance to block particular current components), solutions can be altered, e.g. to block K^+ channels intracellular CsCl replaces KCl allowing to study Na^+ and Ca^{2+} channels.
7. Faraday cages: made of wire mesh (e.g. aluminium) for isolating the patch-clamp headstage (pre-amplifier) from electrical interference. All equipment is sited inside the Faraday cage.
8. Amplifiers: Axopatch 200B (Molecular Devices, Union City, CA) and the EPC series (HEKA, Bellmore, NY). Amplifiers are delivered with headstage and pipette holder.
9. Digitizer and data-recording device to acquire data with at least 20 kHz.
10. Basic two-channel storage oscilloscope.
11. Micromanipulator (mechanical, hydraulic, motorized, or piezoelectric) for positioning the patch pipette. The amplifier headstage is mounted directly on the micromanipulator. The manipulator must be fixed very securely to the microscope to prevent transmission of mechanical disturbances to the patch pipette.
12. Pipette puller is used to thin capillary glass with one or more initial pulls, then broken into two pipettes with the final pull; e.g. P-97 Flaming/Brown (Sutter Instrument Company, Novato, CA) or Narishige PC-10 (Narishige International Limited, London, UK).
13. Pipette microforge. This device is used for heat-polishing the patch pipettes, usually just before using the pipette for

recording. This ensures a very clean and smooth tip, essential for achieving high-resistance seals to cell membranes. A commercially available device can be used (e.g. Narishige MF-830).

14. Borosilicate glass capillaries for standard whole-cell patch recording (e.g. GC150TF-10, Harvard Apparatus), with 1.5 mm outer diameter and 1.17 mm inner diameter.
15. Silver wire coated with silver chloride serves as reference electrode (or bath electrode) and is mounted inside a short (2 cm) polythene tube (1.5 mm O.D.) filled with 4% agar (see Subheading 3.2).
16. U-tube to apply positive pressure to the pipette while approaching the cell. The U-tube is filled with water, and pressure of about 10–20 cm of water is applied continuously via a side port to the pipette holder by way of flexible tubing.
17. Optical recording (see Note 8).

2.3. Neurochemical Studies

1. CGRP double-antibody sandwich enzyme immunoassay (EIA) kit (SPIbio, Montigny-le-Bretonneux, France). Detection range = 2–1,000 pg/mL.
2. Temperature controlled water bath
3. Microplate washer.
4. Microplate wells pre-coated with CGRP monoclonal antibody (SPIbio) (see Note 9).
5. Spectrometer plate reader (Dynex Opsys MR Microplate Reader, Dynex Technologies Inc., Chantilly, VA) with the appropriate software.
6. EIA buffer (supplied with the kit) is dissolved in distilled water to achieve two different concentrations; a 5× concentration is added to the samples and 1× concentration to dissolve the tracer. EIA buffer is stable for 1 month at 4°C. The concentrated EIA buffer contains 1 M sodium phosphate, 1% BSA, 4 M NaCl, 10 mM EDTA, 0.1% hydrochloric acid and a composition of peptidase inhibitors.
7. Anti-CGRP-AChE tracer (supplied with the kit) is dissolved in 10 ml 1× EIA buffer. Allow to rest for 5 min until it is completely dissolved and then mix gently. The tracer is stable for 1 month at 4°C. The tracer is a acetylcholine esterase (AChE) – Fab' conjugate that binds selectively to separate epitope of the CGRP molecule and by that builds up the double-antibody-CGRP sandwich (see Note 10).
8. Wash buffer (supplied with the kit): 1 mL of the concentrate is dissolved in 400 mL distilled water together with 200 μL

Tween-20. After mixing, it is stored in aliquots at 4°C and used at room temperature.

9. Ellmann's reagent (SPIbio) is dissolved in 49 mL distilled water and 1 mL wash buffer. Ellmann's reagent is freshly prepared and contains 5,5′-dithio-bis-[2-nitrobenzoic acid] (DTNB) for thiol colorimetric measurement of the AChE activity (37).
10. CGRP Standard: 1,000 pg/mL lyophilized CGRP, which is diluted to concentrations fitting the expected CGRP range.
11. Synthetic interstitial fluid (SIF) (38): 107.8 mM NaCl, 26.2 mM $NaHCO_3$, 9.64 mM Na-gluconate, 7.6 mM sucrose, 5.05 mM glucose, 3.48 mM KCl, 1.67 mM NaH_2PO_4, 1.53 mM $CaCl_2$ and 0.69 mM $MgSO_4$, gassed with 95% oxygen and 5% carbon dioxide creating pH 7.4.

2.4. Skin-Nerve Preparation

The technique is described in details elsewhere (39). Briefly,

1. Recording chamber with two compartments: (a) an organ bath for superfusion and oxygenation of the skin-nerve flap, and (b) an adjacent recording chamber where single-fibre activity is recorded from nerve filaments.
2. Tubing and connectors to establish a fluid superfusion. Fluid flow is regulated via a drop chamber of an infusion system (i.v. extension set; dial-a-flo®, Abbott); a cylinder with compressed carbogen gas (5% CO_2, 95% O_2) is necessary to gas the physiologic buffer solution, and a thermostatically perfused glass heat exchanger is used to pre-warm the solution before it enters the organ bath.
3. Two-stage amplifier for single-fibre recording. (a) Low noise AC-coupled differential amplifier (World Precision Instruments, Sarasota, FL). (b) A second stage amplifier equipped with high- and low- pass filters, Vernier adjustment, a Noise Cut (anti-noise-filter that cuts out inevitable resistive noise), and a notch filter (a band-pass filter centred on 50/60 Hz that eliminates AC cycles).
4. Two channel storage oscilloscope
5. Amplified loudspeaker
6. Digital thermometer
7. Data acquisition system for extracellular recordings using Dapsys (Johns Hopkins University, Baltimore, MD), requiring a DAP5400a board from Microstar Labs (Bellevue, WA), or Spike 2 requiring an AD converter
8. SD9 Square Pulse Stimulator (Grass Telefactor, Warwick, RI)
9. Metal microelectrodes
10. von Frey hair

3. Methods

3.1. Sensory Neuronal Cell Culture

1. To minimize bacterial contamination, use skin disinfectant before opening the skin and work under laminar airflow conditions. Sterilize dissecting instruments in 70% ethanol. Remove frozen solutions (poly-lysine and culture medium) from the freezer.
2. If using cover slips, clean and sterilize these in 70% ethanol. Dip cover slips briefly in 99% ethanol and leave to dry in a sterile environment.
3. Remove the spine from the sacrificed animal by cutting along both sides through the ribs and back muscles. Place the spine into a sterile container filled with DMEM (e.g. plastic culture dish). Open the spine by cutting along the dorsal and ventral surfaces with fine, strong scissors.
4. Remove the spinal cord. The DRGs will now be visible between the vertebrae (see Note 11). Under the dissecting microscope gently grip the spinal roots with fine forceps, lift very gently to avoid snapping the fragile spinal root and use fine scissors to cut around the dura holding the DRG in position (see Note 11). Transfer each ganglion into the culture dish with DMEM. Remove attached dura to reduce non-cellular parts.
5. Transfer the ganglia into a reaction tube with MEM and the enzymes for digestion. Digestion time is essential and can vary for different enzymes, e.g. incubate for 1 h at 37°C for 1 mg/ml collagenase and 3 mg/ml dispase. This should be done conveniently in the CO_2 incubator, when the enzymes were diluted in a CO_2-buffered solution.
6. Previously or during the incubation, coat the cover slips or culture dishes with poly-lysine. Add poly-lysine solution to the centre area of each cover slip or dish; the amount defines the coated area, which should reflect the needs for later recording. Allow the solution to stand on the cover slips for 30 min then remove by suction, and wash distilled water before drying in a sterile environment.
7. Add NGF if desired (see Note 1) and then warm the culture medium in a 37°C water bath. Stop digestion by diluting the enzymes with about 8 ml of MEM, let the tissue sink down and remove the supernatant. Repeat this once and then reconstitute the neurons in about 0.5 ml of medium.
8. Triturate the neurons by sucking them into a heat-polished Pasteur pipette and expelling them back for around 15 times. This produces a cloudy suspension of single DRG cells; if a few clumps remain, do not triturate further to avoid damage to the DRG neurons.

9. Place the dried cover slips in culture dishes or appropriate-sized well plates. Centrifuge the tube again with the 800 g for 2 min to produce a loose pellet of cells. Remove the supernatant and add culture medium. The amount of culture medium should slightly exceed the volume needed for plating. Use a low concentration for a low cell density suitable for patch-clamp experiments; a higher density is desirable for calcium imaging, use around 10–100 μL per dish. Let the cells settle for 6–10 min, then very gently add culture medium (1–2 mL depending on culture dish) to avoid drying. Then, place into the CO_2 incubator until use.

3.2. Patch-Clamp Recordings on Single Cells

1. Patch pipettes are normally pulled in a batch of 20 or more pipettes at the beginning of the recording day. Before pulling, gently flame polish the ends of the capillary tubes to avoid damage to the rubber O-ring in the pipette holder. Pull pipettes at a resistance of 2–4 MΩ and store them in a clean box until use.
2. Chloride coating of silver wires electrolytically: immerse wires in 150 mM NaCl, connect first to the cathode of a 9 V battery to clean them briefly, then for several minutes to the anode of a 1.5 V battery to coat them; use a carbon rod (from an old battery) as the reference electrode. The chloride coating becomes visible as smooth and dark grey lining. Coated are the wires of the pipette holder and the bath electrode. Chloride coating is usually done on a weekly basis.
3. Assembly of bath electrode: mount the silver wire inside a short (2 cm) polyethylene tube (1.5 mm outer diameter) filled with 4% agar, dissolved in extracellular recording solution. When dissolved, the hot solution is sucked into the polyethylene tube using a syringe, left to solidify, and the tubing cut into 2 cm lengths. The assembly is placed in the recording chamber such that the lower, agar-filled end of the plastic tube is in contact with the bath solution.
4. Preparation of recording solutions: extracellular solutions should be drawn into syringes and 0.22 μm filters placed on the ends. An aliquot of the pipette solution is thawed and drawn into a 1 ml syringe; if it contains ATP, it should be kept on ice for the whole day.
5. Preparation of superfusion application system: extracellular solutions to be used during recordings are filled into the syringes and the manifold outlet is positioned near its final position.
6. Preparation of recording dish: recordings may be made in the plastic culture dish in which the cells were grown (or in a cover slip chamber if they were grown on cover slips). Medium will be replaced by extracellular solution.

7. Apply positive pressure to the pipette using the U-tube and lower the pipette into the recording dish. The pipette is moved with the coarse manual micromanipulator under microscopic observation using a low-power (4×) objective.
8. When the pipette is within less than 10 μm of the cell, it should be moved with the fine movement of the manipulator. At this point, a pulse of about 1–5 mV and about 50 ms duration should be applied through the pipette tip at about 1 Hz, and the current visualized on the oscilloscope or monitor of the acquisition system. When the current in response to the voltage pulse starts to decline in amplitude, it is assumed that the pipette is touching the cell and the positive pressure should be turned off. Gentle negative pressure is then applied and the current pulse should decline rapidly and then become invisible, indicating that the resistance between pipette and membrane has risen to an extremely high value (see Note 12). It can be measured by most data acquisition systems, and should be at least 4 GΩ for good-quality recordings. At this point, the "cell-attached" configuration has been reached, and openings of single ion channels may become visible if the recording gain is increased.
9. Currents across the whole cell membrane are measured in the whole-cell configuration (see Note 13). The voltage-clamp mode of the amplifier is chosen and a potential of –60 mV to –80 mV should be applied. From the "cell-attached" configuration, going into the conventional "whole-cell" configuration requires rupturing of the membrane fragment at the tip of the pipette, either by increased suction, or by a brief high voltage pulse (e.g. 800 mV for 500 μs) provided by the patch clamp amplifier (the Zap function, available on only some amplifiers). As this happens, the almost flat current line obtained upon Giga-seal formation changes suddenly and transient currents due to the cell capacitance will be seen on the display at the beginning and end of the test voltage pulse. This transient current can be cancelled using the RC-circuitry (C-slow and R-series) on the patch clamp amplifier. The capacitive transients enable the investigator to measure the cell capacitance, which can be used to determine cell size, as well as the access resistance and the membrane resistance of the cell.
10. Study of single channels can be done in excised membrane patches. There are two excised patch modes: inside-out and outside-out. For more details, guidance can be sought in a number of published sources in relation to specific experimental situations (40, 41).
11. Current-clamp recording allows the effect of a stimulus or algogen on the cell's membrane potential or action potential

activity to be studied, and may be an important guide to the health of a cell that is being recorded; if the resting membrane potential is more positive than about –40 mV, the cell is unlikely to be healthy and the experimenter may want to proceed to another cell. In current-clamp recording, the membrane current is kept at zero and variations in membrane potential are followed, thus imitating the natural situation wherein any changes in membrane current will either depolarize or hyperpolarize the cell.

12. Voltage-clamp recording uses a preset desired membrane potential (the "holding potential"). The ion currents active at that particular potential are recorded. To record voltage-gated currents, voltage pulses are applied, usually generated by the data acquisition software and applied through the computer interface into the amplifier. If these are fast currents, such as those mediated by sodium channels of the Na_v family, a good cancellation of the capacitive transients is absolutely required for a high-quality artefact-free recording (see Note 14).

3.3. Calcium-Imaging Using Single Cells

1. Prepare staining solution: dilute the Fura2-AM dye in medium at 3–10 μM, and let it warm in the incubator before adding Pluronic (0.02–0.1%) to permeabilize the membranes.
2. Incubate the neurons for about 30 min with the dye at 37°C. In an appropriate-sized multi-well plate, about 250 μl of staining solution is sufficient to submerge the 15 mm diameter cover slip. The incubation time and concentration should be adapted individually according to success defined by recording a sufficient fluorescence signal compared to a cell-free area (see Note 15). Wash cells once to remove the dye, wait about 15 min to allow deesterification of the acetoxymethylester dye (see Note 16).
3. Place cover slip in recording chamber, mount it on the microscope, place and start the perfusion (see Note 17) and the suction system to equilibrate fluid levels
4. After selecting a suitable region with a sufficient number of individual cells, acquire a bright field image (e.g. for measuring cell diameter later). Acquire a fluorescence image and compare with the bright field image to select regions of interest (CCD camera-based setups allow offline analysis if all images are stored, online monitoring based on at least some regions of interest is recommended).
5. Start recording fluorescence and the application of substances according to your protocol. For Fura2-AM alternating illumination at 340 and 380 nm and a ~450 nm long-pass filter are a standard choice. Select the acquisition rate.

Available exposure times and acquisition rates a highly dependent on the system, the chosen parameters should reflect the investigated process.

6. For offline analysis, select regions of interest. Subtract recorded background intensity at a cell free spot. For ratio imaging with Fura2-AM, do this for illumination at 340 and 380 nm and calculate the ratio (F340/F380). The resulting time-course is analysed, the extracted features should reflect the process under investigation but also limitations of the method (see Note 18).

3.4. Neuropeptide Release Measurement

1. Samples of different tissues or organs from mouse or rat are harvested from animals freshly sacrificed in pure CO_2 atmospheres (see Note 19). Tissues may include skin, trachea, dura, nerve, colon, heart, and kidney slices. DRG, trigeminal or nodose and jugular ganglia can be used intact or as cultured sensory neurons. In some cases, the preparations, e.g. skin flaps, are mounted on arylic glass sticks with fine threads with the corium side exposed to improve the contact of the innervated tissue to the stimulation solution. After preparation, tissues are incubated in SIF for about 30 min inside a thermostatic shaking water bath. Depending on the preparation, the organ bath is set to the appropriate temperature, e.g. for skin preparations 32°C and for preparations of internal organs, such as the trachea, 37 or 38°C (see Note 19).
2. The preparations are passed through a series of incubation steps; the duration of incubation is adjusted with respect to the organ and the expected density of peptidergic innervation, which determines the measurable amount of neuropeptides released from the tissue at rest and in response to stimulation. Glass or plastic reaction tubes can be used to expose the tissue to stimulation and to collect the neuropeptide containing eluate. The size of the used reaction tubes should be adjusted to the size of the preparation. Incubation volume should be minimized, but for CGRP detection by means of EIA, at least 100 μl are required. Usually two individual values for basal (i.e. control) release (see Note 20), one for stimulated release (see Note 21) and two final values to demonstrate recovery are acquired. This protocol is adapted for each means of stimulation such as heat, cold, distension or electrical stimulation. If available, bilateral preparations from one animal allow for a matched-pairs comparison, usually decreasing variability and thus the total number of experiments required to achieve a meaningful result.
3. Acquisition of neuropeptide containing fluid: samples of fluid are collected and transferred to tubes after each incubation step, i.e. when the tissue sample is transferred to the consecutive

tube. 100 µl of incubation fluid is collected in a tube, mixed with 25 µl EIA buffer (5×), and stored on crushed ice. If required, samples can be stored at −20°C and accumulated, until final processing.

4. Wash the pre-coated EIA plates (96 wells or fractions of a whole plate) four times with 300 µl prepared wash buffer, and then carefully empty the plate (invert and shake). Allow all samples and solutions to reach room temperature before use.
5. Transfer 100 µl of each sample to a separate well of the EIA plate. On each EIA plate, one or two blank values (unused samples of the incubation and stimulation solutions) and a quality control, supplied with the kit, need to be determined (internal controls). In addition, two series of progressively diluted CGRP standards are required on each plate (see Note 22). To this end, the commercial kit contains a vial with 1,000 pg/ml lyophilized CGRP. The standards should cover a broad range of concentrations in order to calibrate the measurements, e.g. 250, 125, 62.5, 31.3, 15.6, 7.8 and 0 pg/mL. Controls are also set up (see Note 23).
6. Add 100 µl of the prepared tracer to each well, cover the plate by a foil to avoid drying and store overnight (16–20 h) at 4°C for incubation.
7. Wash four times with 300 µl wash buffer, and then empty the plate by turning it over and shaking it. Then, add 200 µl of prepared Ellmann's reagent. Incubate in the dark for about 1 h, and then the plate is placed in the shaker (3 s, 9 Hz, 30 nm) and read with the microplate reader at 405 and at 490 nm. Data gained from the 490 nm measurement are subtracted from the 405 nm data during the data analysis to account for light absorption in the plastic bottom. The signal increases linearly with time as long as the acetylcholine esterase is saturated with Ellman's reagent. Make sure to measure in this linear range; the duration of this depends on the incubation temperature and the highest concentration on the plate (should be part of the standard curve). The reader is a filter photometer that measures the optical density (OD) of each well. The concentration of the neuropeptide in the standard or sample is determined by the Beer–Lambert law.
8. Draw the standard concentration/OD data points and fit them with an appropriate function. The resulting curve is then used to convert the measured OD of each sample into a concentration of neuropeptide. The standard CGRP concentration curve is usually not linear in the lowest concentration range; the Akima fit, a special cubic spline function, which constructs a smooth locally fitted curve through all data points, can be used to fit the curve. This eliminates the systematic overestimation of very low sample concentrations produced

by high standard curve values. Concentrations are compiled and analysed in a spreadsheet program, such as Excel.

3.5. Single Fibre Recordings

1. The skin of the lower leg of a mouse or rat is subcutaneously excised using surgical dissection tools. The saphenous nerve is dissected over its entire length up to the inguinal ligament and separated from connective tissue and detached from the vessels running side by side with the nerve. The whole skin flap in continuity with the saphenous nerve is then placed in a pre-gassed SIF-filled beaker. The preparation can so be kept for several hours at refrigerator temperature (up to 8 h).
2. The preparation is mounted in the organ bath chamber by piercing with insect pins through the very edges of the skin into the silicon rubber. The epidermis faces the bottom of the chamber, exposing the corium (dermis) to superfusion with extracellular solution and allowing access to receptive fields. The end of the nerve is threaded through the hole into the adjacent recording chamber and immersed in paraffin oil, which is applied on top of the aqueous solution in the recording chamber.
3. A single-fibre terminal/single-fibre receptive field is identified by teasing the saphenous nerve in filaments of smaller and smaller size. Filaments are placed on the monopolar electrode and recorded from. Subdivision of filaments should lead to increased signal-to-noise ratio of the action potentials and a reduction in the required amplifier gain.
4. Verification of single C-units within a strand of several fibres by using the marking protocol: The "marking phenomenon" is employed to identify the particular electrically evoked spike within a train of others or within a compound waveform (consisting of two or more spikes of similar latency). Spikes evoked by natural stimulation of the receptive field under investigation cause a latency shift (to the right) of the electrical response.
5. Characterization of identified single receptive fields by classification of fibre type. Single-fibres are classified according to conduction velocity. The mechanical threshold is tested by using calibrated von Frey monofilaments with uniform tips. Thermosensitivity is assessed for each single-fibre using controlled heat and cold stimulation.
6. Experimental design. The most convenient way of applying drugs to isolated receptive fields is the use of an application system that allows to simultaneously control the temperature. This bears the advantage that potential sensitizing effects of compounds can be tested by superfusion (e.g. heat sensitizing effect of capsaicin or cold sensitizing effect of menthol).

4. Notes

1. Addition of growth factors and time in culture should be given a careful thought. Growth factors are not necessary to cultivate the neurons, however they change expression rates. The latter is also true for the culture duration and differentiation state (age of the animal) at the time of recording. Some peripherally transported receptors are barely expressed in acutely dissociated cell bodies, which are usually analysed as a model of their former nerve endings. Cell survival decreases with time in culture. At least a screen of recording at different culture durations is recommended. For patch-clamp recordings in whole-cell configuration, the so-called 'space clamp' problem results from large pipette-distant cell membrane surfaces, a culture duration not much longer than 24–48 h is favoured by most experimenters to avoid growth of processes.
2. *Sterile filters for cell cultures*: the pore size should be 0.22 μm and the membrane material should have good biocompatibility. We use hydrophilic PVDF filters from Millipore; of all commonly used filter membranes, hydrophilic PVDF has the lowest protein binding and the lowest concentration of water-extractable material. Filters with higher levels of extractables have been shown to damage cultured cells (42). The same PVDF filters are used to filter patch-clamp recording solutions; here they do not need to be sterile.
3. *Glassware for Ca-imaging*: The material has to pass ultraviolet excitation light; therefore, the cell culture plastic ware is not suited. Glass bottom dishes, even precoated, can be bought but are rather expensive. A cover slip holder allows growing neurons on custom coated cover slips with little expenses.
4. Serum-free medium can avoid the presence of undefined constituents in serum that may alter the growth or properties of cells. Defined serum replacements suitable for neurons should be preferred (43, 44). In our hands, neurons grown in serum-free medium are a little more fragile and it is more difficult to maintain stable patch-clamp recordings; a possible advantage is that the growth of other cell types in the culture (Schwann and satellite cells, fibroblasts) is inhibited.
5. *Grounding the setup*: Removal of electrical interference (or pick-up), in particular the 50- or 60-cycle line frequency noise (also known as "hum") coming from the electrical network of the building, is essential for high-resolution, low-noise recording of membrane currents, especially in the single-channel configurations. For this purpose, one has to connect all metallic objects near the preparation to one reliable ground point.

Make all connections with copper braid or multi-stranded wire and not with single-core wires: multi-strand wire is better at carrying high-frequency signals. We connect large items further from the preparation (anti-vibration table and Faraday cage) to the amplifier's chassis ground (this point is available on most amplifiers as a 4 mm socket on the case). Smaller metal items close to the headstage (microscope, micromanipulator and application system), as well as the bath electrode, are connected to the ground terminal on the headstage. These two ground points are connected by a single connection within the amplifier. It is essential that they are *only* connected at that point, because an additional connection outside the amplifier will create a ground loop (45); for this reason, the microscope is insulated from the antivibration table. It will be necessary to make a tour of the microscope with an ohmmeter and measure resistances between its parts; these may be high if metal parts have been painted or otherwise treated. All parts of the microscope should be connected with resistances of a small fraction of an ohm; it will probably be necessary to attach copper braid to parts that are not well connected, making small tapped holes in the microscope body if necessary to attach the braid. Make sure any holes are away from optically critical parts of the microscope. The perfusion system may also act as an antenna and, depending on the resistance of the bath electrode, may generate hum, in which case it may be necessary to shield the tubing with aluminium foil.

6. *Choice of microscope objective*: For patch-clamping, good visualization of the cells is crucial. We find phase contrast objectives to be the best, although other systems such as Nomarski and Hoffmann optics are also used. The magnification of the objective should be 40×. If working with plastic dishes (which bottoms are about 1 mm thick), a long working distance objective is essential. With DRG neurones, being a heterogeneous population, it is very useful to pre-select neurons for a given response using Ca^{2+} imaging (Subheading 3.3). This has been widely used in sensory physiology (34, 46–48) Here, a high numerical aperture (N.A.) is essential; if a 40× objective is used, the N.A. should be at least 0.95. A suitable alternative is a 20× objective with N.A. at least 0.7. If thermal stimuli are to be used, choose a dry objective (47) because an oil-immersion objective may distort the thermal stimulus due to its high thermal mass and good thermal contact with the cell under study.

7. *Layout of the laboratory*: Advice on setting up a cell culture laboratory and on finding the most suitable spot with least electrical and vibration interference for a patch-clamp setup can be found in the comprehensive book by (49).

8. A variety of setups is possible, depending on the means of illumination by laser or by a light source, from which a single wavelength is selected by filters or by a prism-based method. Fluorescence acquisition is possible via a photomultiplier or a CCD camera setup, the latter allows tracking responses of multiple individual cells, resulting in a manifold higher output compared to patch-clamping. This is a main reason to prefer calcium imaging vs. patch-clamping when possible.
9. Measurement of intracellular calcium is the most common target, Fura2 the preferred dye. The membrane permeable Fura2-AM (e.g. Invitrogen) and a membrane permeabilizer to enhance dye loading (e.g. pluronic F127, Invitrogen) are recommended.
10. Assay specification: The antibody against human CGRP is 100% cross-reactive with rat and human CGRP-α/β but does not cross-react with the CGRP fragments (23–37) and (28–37) (SPIbio, commercial information). In our hands, the minimum detection limit is 2 pg/ml for CGRP. The intra- and interassay coefficients of variation with repeated measurements was determined 15–20% for the low basal release values and 10–15% for the higher values of stimulated release.
11. Instead of an AChE-coupled secondary antibody, a radioactive labelling and detection (RIA) can be used, the resulting sensitivity is similar (50).
12. *Spinal levels of DRGs*: If DRGs from defined spinal levels are to be used; these can be identified by looking for the stumps of the ribs attaching to the spine. These define the thoracic levels (T1–T13). Each DRG is located immediately *caudal* to the corresponding vertebra. We normally use L1–L6 and S1 DRGs.
13. *Series-resistance compensation*: The series resistance describes the quality of the access between the pipette and the inside of the cell, and its name is derived from the fact that it is "in series" with the membrane resistance. Series resistance is typically about five times higher than pipette resistance. A high series resistance may seriously affect the control of membrane voltage, especially when large ion currents are involved, as the voltage that is applied through the pipette electrode is divided between the two resistances in series (membrane resistance and series resistance): for a 10 MΩ series resistance, an ion current of 1 nA will result in a voltage error of 10 mV, which is quite substantial. If the current under study is activated by depolarization, currents near threshold will be distorted to an extreme degree. Accurate compensation of the series resistance is thus essential.

14. Perforated-patch whole-cell recording: Instead of rupturing the membrane to go into the whole-cell configuration, it is possible to use a pore-forming agent in the pipette, which will allow electrical access by passing monovalent ions while preventing larger cytoplasmic components from leaving the cell. This is essential if one is studying a process that is thought to involve cytoplasmic modulation of an ion channel. Suitable pore-forming agents are amphotericin (51), which is the most reliable in our hands; nystatin gramicidin (52) which has the advantage of being impermeable to chloride ions; and ATP (53). We dip the pipette into amphotericin-free solution before back-filling with amphotericin-containing solution (240 μg/ml). For this to work well, it is essential to use pipette glass *without* a capillary. The tip resistance should be low and the pipettes blunt, to allow good access resistances, and the time of dipping should be carefully controlled to keep the amount of amphotericin-free solution in the tip constant. If this is carefully done, the method works consistently and low-resistance access (sufficient for currents below 1 nA) is gained after as little as 5 min.
15. *Combined patch-clamp and Ca^{2+} imaging*: The perforated-patch whole-cell recording configuration (previous note) makes it possible to combine patch-clamping with Ca^{2+} imaging (Subheading 3.3). Here, the cells are loaded with the Ca^{2+}-sensitive dye, and a preliminary recording may be made in order to pre-select a cell for patch clamp recording. Patch clamping a cell without disrupting the Ca^{2+} recording requires care. Firstly, it is necessary to work at very low light to avoid photobleaching of the dye; red light will largely avoid photobleaching. Secondly, formation of the amphotericin pores in current-clamp mode is inadvisable because the cell may depolarize; for this reason, the cell should be kept in voltage-clamp mode with a holding potential of –60 mV to –80 mV until adequate access has been achieved. This combined approach has been very useful in gaining insight into the ionic currents and membrane electrical activity that underlie the cell's Ca^{2+} signals (54).
16. Procedures are focussed on Fura2-AM because of the widespread use of this method, but apply for other dyes in a similar fashion. Staining: Many labs stain for 30 min with 5 μM Fura-AM and 0.02% pluronic. The authors have experimented with periods of 15–60 min, Fura2-AM 3–30 μM and 0.01–0.2% pluronic. It should be noted that the fluorescence intensity is not in a linear relationship with these parameters. The absolute fluorescence signal (background subtracted) determines the signal–noise ratio. The three above parameters can be reduced as long as the signal–noise ratio at the desired acquisition parameters is good.

17. Often periods of time are given to allow deesterification. The AM ester has an absorption similar to the not calcium-bound Fura2. Too short periods for deesterification will therefore dampen the observed ratio, and too long periods lead to reduction of the fluorescence. We would recommend 10–30 min.
18. A capillary-based perfusion system with a large outlet, covering the complete cell area with a laminar flow and providing defined substance concentrations is desirable. From the capillary tip a laminar flow should reach all cells in the area of view, this can be verified with stained solutions. A capillary-based perfusion allows for fast solution changes, an electronic control of valves is favourable for reproducibility of short applications, and for co-registration of events with the fluorescence signal. Bath applications allow only long application periods. Using syringes mounted on a height-adjustable holder and gravitation as the driving force allows easy adjustment and fail-safe flow rates.
19. *Regarding calcium measurements*: Integrals of the fluorescence or ratio over the application time or full time till recovery are often analysed. Given a fast acquisition compared to the investigated process calcium influx rates can also be analysed. Strong stimuli often reach the cellular calcium limit, which does not code for the applied concentration but is rather determined by an inhibition of further calcium influx by intracellular calcium levels. If this happens fast, a reduction in exposure concentration and time or an analysis method reflecting the increase rather than the maximum should be favoured.
20. *Choice of preparation and animal species*: Expression of different receptors and coexpression with CGRP is variable amongst different tissues and therefore preparation and animal species should be chosen according to the receptor and ion channels under study. Transient receptor potential A1 receptor-channel, for example, is highly expressed in tissues innervated by the vagal nerve (55, 56) and coexpression of TRPV1 with CGRP varies between rat and mouse and even between different inbred mouse strains (16, 57).
21. *Basal release of CGRP*: Apparent basal release (in the absence of stimulation) is high immediately following surgical procedures prior to the release experiment. Therefore, an initial 30 min washout period prior to the experiment is indispensable and helps in establishing stable and reproducible values for actual basal CGRP release. Basal release depends on the temperature and therefore the temperature during initial washout and experiment should not be different.

22. *Calcium-dependence of neuropeptide release*: Depolarization-induced release of neuropeptides from primary afferents dependents on the activation of voltage-gated calcium channels, namely N- and L-type calcium channels (26). These are not involved, if receptor-channels of high calcium conductance such as TRPV1 or TRPA1 are activated (26). In any case, the concentration of extracellular calcium is essential and using calcium-free (and buffered) extracellular solution constitutes an important control experiment establishing whether or not a stimulated CGRP release is mediated by physiological, Ca^{++}-dependent mechanism of vesicular exocytosis or due to an unspecific membrane damage.
23. *Interference with the CGRP assay*: Chemical used for stimulation of CGRP release or its modulation may interfere with steps of the enzyme-immuno assay. Therefore, all solutions used during the experiment should be run as CGRP-spiked controls on the assay.
24. *Control experiments*: Introducing a new preparation or stimulations usually requires some control experiments to validate the CGRP release. High external potassium leads to general depolarization of the neurons causing concentration-dependent (15–60 mM KCl) (26, 58) KCl-induced CGRP release correlated well with the total CGRP content of a tissue, but it represents only a small fraction (1% in 5 min) of it (16). High potassium can be added as final step within one experiment to achieve a maximal response that can be used to normalize preceding responses to other stimuli. High potassium control is essential to discriminate between modulatory influences (of a drug etc.) on sensory transduction and those on the release mechanisms as such (see Subheading 1).

References

1. Novakovic SD, Tzoumaka E, McGivern JG, Haraguchi M, Sangameswaran L, Gogas KR, Eglen RM, Hunter JC (1998) Distribution of the tetrodotoxin-resistant sodium channel PN3 in rat sensory neurons in normal and neuropathic conditions. J Neurosci 18: 2174–2187
2. Caterina MJ, Schumacher MA, Tominaga M, Rosen TA, Levine JD, Julius D (1997) The capsaicin receptor: a heat-activated ion channel in the pain pathway. Nature 389: 816–824
3. Chen CC, Akopian AN, Sivilotti L, Colquhoun D, Burnstock G, Wood JN (1995) A P2X purinoceptor expressed by a subset of sensory neurons. Nature 377:428–431
4. Dib-Hajj SD, Cummins TR, Black JA, Waxman SG (2007) From genes to pain: Na v 1.7 and human pain disorders. Trends Neurosci 30:555–563
5. Namer B, Barta B, Orstavik K, Schmidt R, Carr R, Schmelz M, Handwerker HO (2009) Microneurographic assessment of C-fibre function in aged healthy subjects. J Physiol 587:419–428
6. Orstavik K, Namer B, Schmidt R, Schmelz M, Hilliges M, Weidner C, Carr RW, Handwerker H, Jorum E, Torebjork HE (2006) Abnormal function of C-fibers in patients with diabetic neuropathy. J Neurosci 26:11287–11294
7. Bessou P, Perl ER (1969) Response of cutaneous sensory units with unmyelinated

fibers to noxious stimuli. J Neurophysiol 32:1025–1943

8. Kumazawa T, Mizumura K, Sato J (1987) Response properties of polymodal receptors studied using in vitro testis superior spermatic nerve preparation of dogs. J Neurophysiol 57:702–711
9. Reeh PW (1986) Sensory receptors in mammalian skin in an in vitro preparation. Neurosci Lett 66:141–147
10. Cain DM, Khasabov SG, Simone DA (2001) Response properties of mechanoreceptors and nociceptors in mouse glabrous skin: an in vivo study. J Neurophysiol 85:1561–1574
11. Reeh PW (1988) Sensory receptors in a mammalian skin-nerve in vitro preparation. Prog Brain Res 74(271–6):271–276
12. Bernardini N, Roza C, Sauer SK, Gomeza J, Wess J, Reeh PW (2002) Muscarinic M2 receptors on peripheral nerve endings: a molecular target of antinociception. J Neurosci 22:RC229
13. Kress M, Averbeck B (1997) Release of calcitonin gene-related peptide from sensory neurons in culture. Pflügers Archiv – Europ J Physiol 433:360.
14. Kress M, Riedl B, Reeh PW (1995) Effects of oxygen radicals on nociceptive afferents in the rat skin in vitro. Pain 62:87–94
15. Kress M, Rödl J, Reeh PW (1996) Stable analogs of cyclic AMP but not cyclic GMP sensitize unmyelinated primary afferents in the rat skin to mechanical and heat stimuli but not to inflammatory mediators, in vitro. Neuroscience 74:609–617
16. Mogil JS, Miermeister F, Seifert F, Strasburg K, Zimmermann K, Reinold H, Austin JS, Bernardini N, Chesler EJ, Hofmann HA et al (2005) Variable sensitivity to noxious heat is mediated by differential expression of the CGRP gene. Proc Natl Acad Sci U S A 102: 12938–12943
17. Petho G, Derow A, Reeh PW (2001) Bradykinin-induced nociceptor sensitization to heat is mediated by cyclooxygenase products in isolated rat skin. Eur J NeuroSci 14: 210–218
18. Reeh PW, Petho G (2000) Nociceptor excitation by thermal sensitization – a hypothesis. Prog Brain Res 129:39–50
19. Ringkamp M, Schmelz M, Kress M, Allwang M, Ogilvie A, Reeh PW (1994) Activated human platelets in plasma excite nociceptors in rat skin, in vitro. Neurosci Lett 170:103–106
20. Steen KH, Wegner H, Reeh PW (1999) The pH response of rat cutaneous nociceptors correlates with extracellular [Na+] and is increased under amiloride. Eur J NeuroSci 11:2783–2792
21. Steen KH, Reeh PW, Kreysel HW (1995) Topical acetylsalicylic, salicylic acid and indomethacin supress pain from experimental tissue acidosis in human skin. Pain 62: 339–347
22. Alloui A, Zimmermann K, Mamet J, Duprat F, Noel J, Chemin J, Guy N, Blondeau N, Voilley N, Rubat-Coudert C et al (2006) TREK-1, a K^+ channel involved in polymodal pain perception. EMBO J 25:2368–2376
23. Zimmermann K, Leffler A, Fischer MM, Messlinger K, Nau C, Reeh PW (2005) The TRPV1/2/3 activator 2-aminoethoxydiphenyl borate sensitizes native nociceptive neurons to heat in wildtype but not TRPV1 deficient mice. Neuroscience 135:1277–1284
24. Kirchhoff C, Jung S, Reeh PW, Handwerker HO (1990) Carrageenan inflammation increases bradykinin sensitivity of rat cutaneous nociceptors. Neurosci Lett 111:206–210
25. Koltzenburg M, Kress M, Reeh PW (1992) The nociceptor sensitization by bradykinin does not depend on sympathetic neurons. Neuroscience 46:465–473
26. Spitzer MJ, Reeh PW, Sauer SK (2008) Mechanisms of potassium- and capsaicin-induced axonal calcitonin gene-related peptide release: involvement of L- and T-type calcium channels and TRPV1 but not sodium channels. Neuroscience 151:836–842
27. Averbeck B, Peisler MIIRPW (2003) Inflammatory mediators do not stimulate CGRP release if prostaglandin synthesis is blocked by S(+)-flurbiprofen in isolated rat skin. Inflamm Res 52(12):519–523
28. Averbeck B, Reeh PW, Michaelis M (2001) Modulation of CGRP and PGE2 release from isolated rat skin by alpha-adrenoceptors and kappa-opioid-receptors. Neuroreport 12:2097–2100
29. Huang YM, Neher E (1996) Ca^{2+}-dependent exocytosis in the somata of dorsal root ganglion neurons. Neuron 17:135–145
30. Safronov BV, Bischoff U, Vogel W (1996) Single voltage-gated K+ channels and their functions in small dorsal root ganglion neurones of rat. J Physiol 493(Pt 2):393–408
31. Scholz A, Gruss M, Vogel W (1998) Properties and functions of calcium-activated K+ channels in small neurones of rat dorsal root ganglion studied in a thin slice preparation. J Physiol 513(Pt 1):55–69
32. Woodbury CJ, Zwick M, Wang S, Lawson JJ, Caterina MJ, Koltzenburg M, Albers KM, Koerber HR, Davis BM (2004) Nociceptors

lacking TRPV1 and TRPV2 have normal heat responses. J Neurosci 24:6410–6415

33. Zimmermann K, Leffler A, Babes A, Cendan CM, Carr RW, Kobayashi J, Nau C, Wood JN, Reeh PW (2007) Sensory neuron sodium channel Nav1.8 is essential for pain at low temperatures. Nature 447:855–858
34. Reid G, Flonta ML (2001) Physiology. Cold current in thermoreceptive neurons. Nature 413:480
35. Dittert I, Vlachova V, Knotkova H, Vitaskova Z, Vyklicky L, Kress M, Reeh PW (1998) A technique for fast application of heated solutions of different composition to cultured neurones. J Neurosci Methods 82:195–201
36. Dittert I, Benedikt J, Vyklicky L, Zimmermann K, Reeh PW, Vlachova V (2006) Improved superfusion technique for rapid cooling or heating of cultured cells under patch-clamp conditions. J Neurosci Methods 151: 178–185
37. Ellman GL, Courtney KD, Andres V Jr, Feather-Stone RM (1961) A new and rapid colorimetric determination of acetylcholinesterase activity. Biochem Pharmacol 7:88–95
38. Bretag AH (1969) Synthetic interstitial fluid for isolated mammalian tissue. Life Science 8:319–329
39. Zimmermann K, Hager UA, Hein A, Kaczmarek JS, Turnquist BP, Clapham DE, Reeh PW (2009) Phenotyping sensory nerve endings in vitro in the mouse. Nature Protocols 4(2):174–196
40. Sakmann B, Neher E (1995) Single-channel recording. Plenum, New York
41. Anonymus (2008) *The axon guide: a guide to electrophysiology and biophysics laboratory techniques.* Molecular Devices, Sunnyvale, CA., USA
42. Knight DE (1990) Disposable filters may damage your cells. Nature 343:218
43. Bottenstein JE, Sato GH (1979) Growth of a rat neuroblastoma cell line in serum-free supplemented medium. Proc Natl Acad Sci U S A 76:514–517
44. Bottenstein JE, Skaper SD, Varon SS, Sato GH (1980) Selective survival of neurons from chick embryo sensory ganglionic dissociates utilizing serum-free supplemented medium. Exp Cell Res 125:183–190
45. Purves RD (1981) Microelectrode methods for intracellular recording and ionophoresis. Academic, London
46. Viana F, de la Peña E, Belmonte C (2002) Specificity of cold thermotransduction is determined by differential ionic channel expression. Nat Neurosci 5:254–260
47. Reid G, Flonta ML (2002) Ion channels activated by cold and menthol in cultured rat dorsal root ganglion neurones. Neurosci Lett 324:164–168
48. McKemy DD, Neuhausser WM, Julius D (2002) Identification of a cold receptor reveals a general role for TRP channels in thermosensation. Nature 416:52–58
49. Freshney RI (2005) Cuture of animal cells: a manual of basic technique. Wiley-Blackwell, Oxford
50. Zaidi M, Girgis SI, MacIntyre I (1988) Development and performance of a highly sensitive carboxyl-terminal-specific radioimmunoassay of calcitonin gene-related peptide. Clin Chem 34:655–660
51. Rae J, Cooper K, Gates P, Watsky M (1991) Low access resistance perforated patch recordings using amphotericin B. J Neurosci Methods 37:15–26
52. Kyrozis A, Reichling DB (1995) Perforated-patch recording with gramicidin avoids artifactual changes in intracellular chloride concentration. J Neurosci Methods 57:27–35
53. Lindau M, Fernandez JM (1986) A patch-clamp study of histamine-secreting cells. J Gen Physiol 88:349–368
54. Reid G, Babes A, Pluteanu F (2002) A cold- and menthol-activated current in rat dorsal root ganglion neurones: properties and role in cold transduction. J Physiol 545:595–614
55. Nassenstein C, Kwong KK, Taylor-Clark TE, Kollarik M, Macglashan DW, Braun A, Undem BJ (2008) TRPA1 expression and function in vagal afferent nerves innervating mouse lungs. J Physiol 586(6):1595–1604
56. Fajardo O, Meseguer V, Belmonte C, Viana F (2008) TRPA1 channels mediate cold temperature sensing in mammalian vagal sensory neurons: pharmacological and genetic evidence. J Neurosci 28:7863–7875
57. Price TJ, Flores CM (2007) Critical evaluation of the colocalization between calcitonin gene-related peptide, substance P, transient receptor potential vanilloid subfamily type 1 immunoreactivities, and isolectin B4 binding in primary afferent neurons of the rat and mouse. J Pain 8:263–272
58. Kress M, Izydorczyk I, Kuhn A (2001) N- and L- but not P/Q-type calcium channels contribute to neuropeptide release from rat skin in vitro. Neuroreport 12:867–870

Chapter 20

The Genetics of Pain and Analgesia in Laboratory Animals

William R. Lariviere and Jeffrey S. Mogil

Abstract

Pain and analgesia traits are heritable in humans and in mice. To better understand the mechanisms of heritability, animal models that provide greater control than is possible in humans over genotype, previous history, environment, and stimulus parameters are available. This chapter will highlight several common methods to study the genetic mechanisms of *heritable* sensitivity to pain and pain-related traits in rodents. Methods to demonstrate and estimate the heritability of a trait are discussed, as are genetic correlation analysis and linkage mapping. Practical concerns are highlighted throughout this chapter. Due to limitations on the use of humans for similarly powered experiments, these and other animal models remain an essential component in the study of heritable mechanisms of pain and analgesia.

Key words: Genetics, Heritability, Genetic correlation, Gene mapping, Linkage, Strain differences

1. Introduction

The study of the genetics of heritable pain sensitivity in rodent models of pain has proven to be a valid and productive endeavor. Novel genetic relationships among types of pain models have been detected (1–3), and novel genes identified via mapping studies have been convincingly demonstrated to be responsible for variability in several pain traits (4–6). Moreover, findings from mouse genetic studies have been translated to humans (5, 7, 8). One can study the role of single genes in pain and analgesia with transgenic knockout mice, or with oligonucleotides or small-interfering RNA (siRNA) that inhibits the function of specific genes. However, these methods do not directly examine heritable variability. This chapter will concentrate on common methods used to study the genetic mechanisms of *heritable* sensitivity to pain and pain-related traits in rodents.

Arpad Szallasi (ed.), *Analgesia: Methods and Protocols*, Methods in Molecular Biology, vol. 617,
DOI 10.1007/978-1-60327-323-7_20,

2. Heritability of Pain Traits

The heritability of a trait is the proportion of the overall variability observed in that trait that is due to inherited genetic factors. Determining the heritability of a trait is the first step in examining the genetic factors that contribute to trait variability. Heritability estimates provide a gauge of the value of subsequent genetic mapping studies. Only if a significant proportion of the variability can be ascribed to genetic factors will it be of value to pursue the identification of those genes. To quantify the heritability of a trait, the "narrow-sense heritability" (h^2) can be calculated by comparing the between-strain (or allelic) variance (V_A) with the total variance comprised of the between-strain variance and the within-strain (or environmental) variance (V_E): $h^2 = V_A/(V_A + V_E)$ (9). Narrow-sense heritability can be easily calculated based on the results of a one-way analysis of variance (ANOVA) of an inbred strain survey as described below. "Broad-sense heritability" can also be estimated, but is significantly more complex especially if little is known about the genetic mechanisms of variability in the trait. Broad-sense heritability includes allelic (or additive) variance in the numerator in addition to other genetic sources of variance including allelic dominance and gene–gene interactions (called epistasis), which are mostly unknown at present.

Several methods and animal models exist that one can use to determine whether a trait is heritable. The careful choice of the appropriate model can maximize the yield and impact of the results. Some models have greater long-term utility of the results, allowing for further comparisons with previous and additional experiments, and justifying their increased costs. In many cases, the matching of short-term and long-term goals and the available and expected budget for the overall research program is critical.

2.1. Selective Breeding

Selective breeding, or artificial selection, of rats or mice is one method to demonstrate that genetic factors contribute to a pain trait. In a population of outbred rodents, trait variability will exist within the strain. If the trait is heritable, successive breeding of highly sensitive members of the strain with other highly sensitive members will result in progeny that are more sensitive overall than progeny of highly resistant members of the strain. With successive generations, the distribution of sensitivity will be forced toward the extremes of the range seen prior to selective breeding due to the additive effects of fixation of alleles (i.e., gene variants) segregating in the population. Successful selection is *prima facie* evidence of heritability. Selective breeding for highly heritable traits largely controlled by one (monogenic) or a few genes (oligogenic) requires fewer generations of breeding to produce progeny with extreme sensitivities when compared with traits that are less heritable or more polygenic. Several examples of selective breeding of pain traits exist in the literature, including programs for neuropathic pain, and drug- and stress-induced analgesia (10–13).

2.2. Inbred Strain Differences

Strain comparisons can also be used to demonstrate and quantify the influence of heritable factors on pain sensitivity. With this method, the type, number, and selection of strains is critical. Numerous comparisons have been performed between two outbred or inbred strains of rats or mice. Comparing outbred strains is problematic because they are not isogenic; trait (phenotypic) differences might be due to genotype and might also be due to chance selection of individuals in the sample. Two-strain comparisons have serious limitations that should dissuade one from picking such a limited comparison to reveal genetic mechanisms. For instance, although the genetic background is known to differ between the Lewis and Fisher 344 inbred rat strains, the two strains also have known differences in hormonal responsivity to stressors and stressor-induced behavioral patterns (14, 15). As such, it becomes exceedingly difficult to ascribe strain differences in a pain trait to any of the numerous alleles that differ between the strains. It is much preferable to use larger panels of inbred strains with known genomic differences (16).

2.3. Genetic Reference Populations: Standard Inbred (SI) and Recombinant Inbred (RI) Strains

SI and RI mouse strains are genetic reference populations in which alleles of genes throughout the genome have been forced into homozygosity by inbreeding for over 20 generations. RI strains are derived by crossing two SI strains and fully inbreeding the F2 progeny (see Fig. 4 for an illustration). For both SI and RI strains, the genotype of each inbred strain is fixed over time. Another way of saying this, of course, is that within-strain, individual SI and RI mice are clones of each other. A panel of SI or RI mouse strains can be used to estimate the narrow-sense heritability (h^2) of a pain trait by comparing the between-strain variance (V_A) with the total variance based on the results of a one-way analysis of variance (ANOVA) by dividing the between-strain sum of squares (SS) term by the sum of the between-strain and within-strain SS terms.

One should be cautious not to over interpret heritability estimates since they are specific to the particular conditions of the experiment. These include the dose or intensity of the pain producing stimulus, the experimenter, the rodent strains chosen, and known and unknown environmental factors. Optimization of these parameters using one or a limited number of outbred strains can greatly increase the heritability obtained in a panel of inbred strains, providing heritability estimates that can be much larger in rodent models than those obtained in human subjects, and in turn, facilitating subsequent studies. The mosaicity of inbred strains is an important factor to consider when selecting strains in order to maximize the genetic diversity among strains being tested. Several articles examining the mosaicity of inbred rodents using a range of methods can be referred to for the phylogenetic placement of inbred strains of mice or rats in their respective evolutionary trees (17–19).

Paying careful heed to environmental factors can also increase heritability estimates. For most pain traits in humans and in many rodent pain models, genetic factors account for a minority (<50%) of the total variability in the trait (20) although a median of approximately ~50% heritability has been demonstrated over numerous pain-related traits in SI mice (1, 3, 21, 22). Thus, to minimize environmental noise, strict control is necessary of environmental factors including experimenter, season, cage density, time of day, humidity, diet, housing, social factors (including proximity to other mice during testing) genetic background of cagemates, habituation to the testing room and apparatus, and state of arousal during testing, all of which can affect pain traits and may interact with genotype (23–29).

3. Genetic Correlations

Once heritability of the trait has been determined and quantified, the same genetic resources can be used to perform a genetic correlation analysis. Genetic correlation analysis is a method that allows for the understanding of the biological basis of a trait prior to determination of the responsible genes (30–32). Given a particular strain distribution pattern (SDP) of means for a trait determined in an inbred strain survey, for example, strong positive correlation with the strain means for a second trait indicates that similar genetic mechanisms underlie heritable variability in both traits (see Fig. 1). If the genetic correlation between the strain means for the two traits is close to zero, it indicates that independent genetic mechanisms underlie variability in each of the traits. If a strong negative correlation exists between two traits, the same genetic mechanisms may increase one trait and decrease the second trait. Note that genetic similarities or dissimilarities suggest biological similarities or dissimilarities, respectively, and this suggestion can be quite heuristic.

Calculation of a genetic correlation is performed with a Pearson correlation coefficient or a Spearman rank correlation coefficient, with the distribution of the strain means determining the most appropriate method (30). Note that the correlation is calculated using strain *mean* values and not using values from individual mice, which would contain environmental variability as well. As a general rule, a minimum of eight strains should be used in order for the correlations to indicate common or distinct mecha-

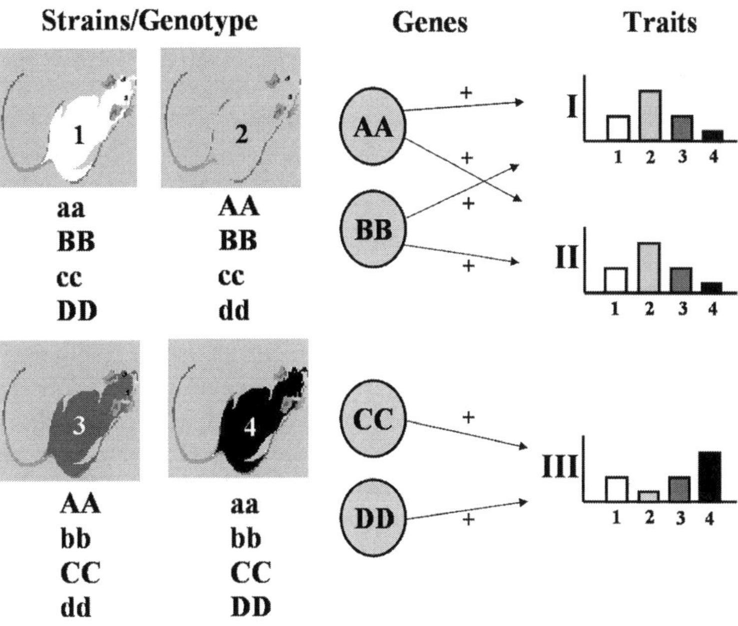

Fig. 1. Genetic correlation analysis. A genetic correlation analysis examines whether the heritable variability in two traits (or phenotypes) is due to the same underlying genetic mechanisms. Inbred strains of mice or rats are tested for their responsiveness or sensitivity to determine the strain distribution pattern (SDP) of means for the traits. Pearson's correlation coefficient or a Spearman rank correlation is then calculated between the means of each trait. If the SDPs are similar and a sufficient number of strains have been tested, the traits are "genetically correlated", and the correlation can be ascribed to common genetic mechanisms. The figure demonstrates the logic behind this inference. Fully inbred strains have alleles forced into homozygosity throughout the genome as demonstrated in the figure (e.g., AA). Pain traits are considered to be polygenic with several genes contributing to increases or decreases of the traits. For this example, we will assume that the capital letter alleles of A and B genes contribute to increases in traits I and II, but not trait III, and C and D genes contribute positively to trait III, but not to traits I and II. Phenotyping the mice produces similar SDPs for traits I and II. Since trait III is mediated by different genes, C and D, the SDP for the same strains is different from those of traits I and II. By adding up the gene effects for each contributing gene, one can see the relationship between genotype of each inbred strain and the phenotype value (e.g., strain 2 has two positively contributing alleles to traits I and II). Therefore, even prior to determining the precise mechanisms of heritability, one can make the inference regarding shared genetic mechanisms based on similar SDPs for two or more traits. Note that use of this method requires a significant number of inbred strains (preferred minimum of 11; absolute minimum of 8) be simultaneously phenotyped, and environmental factors must be strictly controlled throughout the experiment

nisms and to be able to detect statistically significant correlations. It is ideal to have a wide range of strain means that are continuously distributed, as comparisons with or between bimodally distributed traits or traits exhibiting a poor spread of means are not as valid or informative with respect to indicating common genetic mechanisms.

3.1. Genetic Correlations Among Multiple Traits

When a sufficient number of traits have been tested in the same inbred strains, the genetic relationships among the traits can be determined and a genetic framework developed using multivariate statistical methods. A growing literature of SI and RI "strain surveys" exists, with online resources to search these data and to directly compare previous and new strain surveys (e.g., http://www.jax.org/phenome, http://www.genenetwork.org). Provided enough common strains were selected in each strain survey, multivariate analyses can be used to visualize the genetic relationships among a group of pain traits simultaneously (2, 3). Using the multivariate methods of multidimensional scaling (MDS) and principal components analysis (PCA), clustering of genetically similar traits in a two- (or three-) dimensional representation of the genetic correlations can be easily illustrated, as can informative genetic relationships among groups of traits, and even potentially meaningful dimensions or factors that distinguish the traits. One can also determine the relative similarity of inbred strains for a set of related traits to identify outlier strains, for instance (33).

In both MDS and PCA methods, a set of points representing each trait is plotted with the distance between points fitting as closely as possible a matrix of measured similarities between the traits such as correlations. In the two-dimensional MDS plot, points representing highly positively correlated traits will have the smallest distances between them, highly negatively correlated traits will have the largest inter-point distances, and uncorrelated traits will have intermediate distances between their points. In a two-dimensional PCA graph, points at the end of vectors emanating from the center are plotted. Angles between vectors that are close to zero indicate highly positively correlated traits, angles close to 180° indicate highly negatively correlated traits, and angles close to 90° indicate uncorrelated traits. The MDS and PCA plots are usually complementary, each providing additional information. Note that each trait in the multivariate analysis has an influence on the relative position of every other trait. Thus, adding a new trait that is differentially correlated with two positively correlated traits can change the relative position of the two moderately positively correlated traits. Incomplete data sets (with few strains in common between traits) can also have profound effects on the overall 2-D representation, as can bimodally distributed traits or strain means with a small range of values.

These multivariate methods have been used to identify genetically fundamental types of pain (as clusters of assays), and to determine the genetic relationships among hypersensitivity measures and their relation to baseline nociceptive measures (2, 3) (see Fig. 2). We observed, for example, that mechanical hypersensitivity is distinct from thermal hypersensitivity, even when induced in the same nerve injury model, and that thermal hypersensitivity models differ in their genetic relatedness to baseline nociception models.

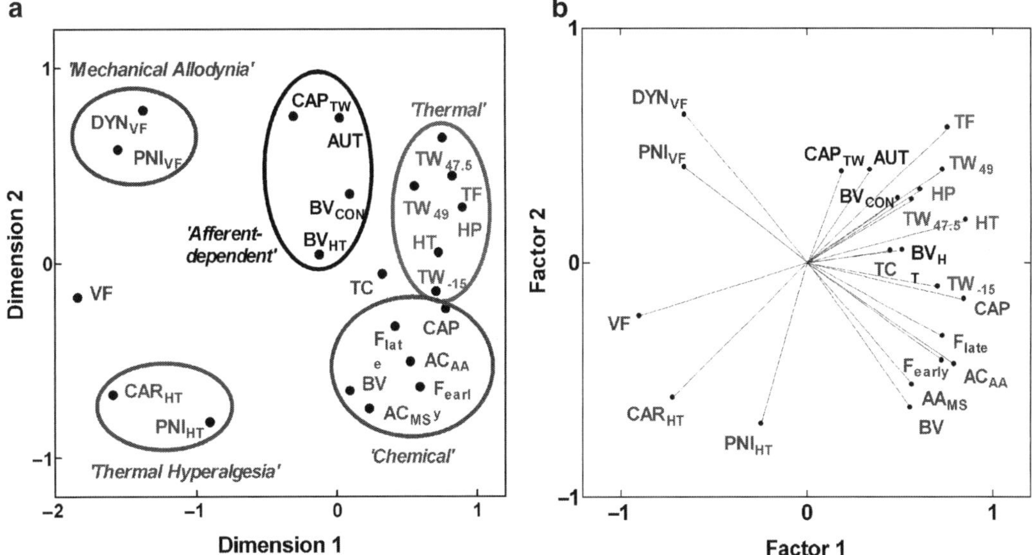

Fig. 2. Multivariate statistics methods for genetic correlation analysis of several traits simultaneously. Multidimensional scaling (MDS) and principal components analysis (PCA) plots facilitate visualization of the genetic relationships among a group of pain traits simultaneously. Clustering of genetically similar traits in a two-dimensional representation of the matrix of pairwise trait correlations can be easily determined, as can informative genetic relationships among groups of traits and meaningful dimensions or factors that distinguish the traits. (**a**) With MDS, points representing highly positively correlated traits will be closest, highly negatively correlated traits will be furthest apart, and uncorrelated traits will have intermediate distances between their points. (**b**) With a PCA, traits are represented as points at the end of vectors. Highly positively correlated traits have angles between their vectors close to zero, highly negatively correlated traits have angles close to 180°, and uncorrelated traits have between-vector angles close to 90°. Each method can provide complementary information. For example, from the PCA plot in (**b**) it is apparent that the "Afferent-dependent" hypersensitivity traits represented with black points and font are genetically related to the "Thermal" nociception traits with red points and font, but this is not obvious from only the MDS plot in (**a**). See refs. 2, 3 for full description of assays represented in the figure. Figure reprinted from (3) with permission from the International Association for the Study of Pain® (IASP®)

The methods can also be effectively used to compare pain traits to traits of another biological domain that are hypothesized to be genetically related (e.g., locomotion, anxiety, neurotransmitter release in specific brain areas, hormone release). Numerous traits from several domains have been examined in SI and RI mouse strains and have been placed in online databases for perusal and analysis by the interested investigator (http://www.jax.org/phenome, http://www.genenetwork.org). These resources should be consulted during selection of strains to include in a new strain survey. Data sets of baseline mRNA transcript expression in specific brain areas and other tissues, obtained by microarray gene expression profiling, are also available online for particular RI strains, permitting direct comparisons of pain traits with transcript expression profiles.

4. Linkage Mapping Studies of Pain and Analgesia

Of course, the main reason to employ genetic animal models is because they allow a relatively inexpensive path to the identification of the responsible genes. Using linkage mapping, one is lead to those genes by their genomic position alone, and thus no prior assumptions are necessary. This allows for the discovery of entirely novel determinants of pain sensitivity.

4.1. Techniques

4.1.1. Theory of Linkage

Linkage mapping, including QTL mapping, exploits the phenomenon of homologous recombination (also called crossing-over) to estimate the distance between genomic loci (34). Recall that during meiosis, DNA strands can physically break, switch places, and reattach to one another such that the resulting haploid chromosome (to be packaged in a gamete) is *recombinant*, containing, for example, paternal alleles proximal to the breakpoint and maternal alleles distally. Homologous recombination occurs quite naturally as a way to produce new genotypic combinations. Because crossing-over occurs commonly (approximately once per 100 Mb per meiosis) and randomly (with the exception of so-called recombination "hot spots" and "dead spots"), the probability of any two loci on a chromosome being separated from each other (i.e., independently assorted) by a cross-over event is directly related to their physical distance on that chromosome. (Note that the independent assortment of loci on *different* chromosomes is assured, and known even by Mendel.) As a practical matter, then, the genetic distance between two loci can be defined as the number of offspring who are recombinant for those two loci (i.e., a cross-over occurred between the loci) out of the total number of offspring; this ratio provides the recombination frequency, θ, which ranges from 0–50%. Loci with $\theta < 50\%$ are thus "linked". In experimental organisms like mice, where matings can be constructed so that the divergent parental genotypes are known and the genotypes and phenotypes of offspring can be easily typed (called "genotyping" and "phenotyping," respectively), calculation of θ is trivial. Somewhat more computationally intensive (and beyond the scope of this chapter) are the inferential statistics used to determine whether linkage at any θ is statistically reliable. These include the logarithm of the odds (LOD) score, the χ^2 statistic, and, increasingly, p-values estimated by iterative permutation of the actual data set.

It is important to understand that linkage can be demonstrated between any two loci on a chromosome, regardless of what those loci are. One can talk about linkage between two genes, between a gene and a genomic "marker", between two markers, or, importantly, between a marker and a phenotype itself (because the phenotype is being affected by a DNA sequence with a particular location). Genomic markers used in linkage mapping have evolved from restriction fragment length polymorphisms (RFLPs) to microsatellites (simple sequence repeat polymorphisms; SSRPs), to single-nucleotide polymorphisms (SNPs), with the more modern markers exhibiting higher frequencies in the genome (thus ensuring fuller coverage). Linkage mapping of a trait is in fact the demonstration of linkage between the phenotype and a genomic marker, followed by an inference of linkage between the genomic marker and the responsible DNA variant. Transitive logic ties the phenotype with the DNA variant, which is of course the point of the exercise. See Fig. 3 for an illustration of the principles underlying linkage mapping.

4.1.2. Implementation of Linkage Mapping in Segregating Populations

The most straightforward way to implement linkage mapping in an experimental organism like the mouse is to create a segregating population (i.e., F2 hybrid or backcross) from inbred parental genotypes displaying a large phenotypic strain difference. By doing this, one maximizes the number of trait-relevant genes that can be found (since only genes with variant alleles in the two parental strains are "visible" to linkage mapping), and guarantees that only two genotypes are possible in the backcross (one homozygous, one heterozygous) and three genotypes are possible in the F2 hybrid (two homozygous, one heterozygous) at the responsible variant and all strongly linked markers. One great advantage of using experimental organisms rather than human pedigrees for linkage mapping is that it is perfectly feasible to create segregating populations numbering the hundreds or even thousands (in lower organisms like *Drosophila* and in plants even much higher numbers are routine), providing as much statistical power as is necessary to detect QTLs, which often account for only a small percentage of the genetic variance. As microsatellite and/or SNP genotyping has become quite affordable, the limiting factor is phenotyping cost and effort. Typically, all subjects of the segregating population are phenotyped, and genomic DNA obtained from any tissue is then genotyped at approximately 100 microsatellites spanning the genome. Interval mapping can then be performed on the data to detect linkage by interpolating between the markers (e.g., ref. 35). It is important to note that due to the large distance of linkage disequilibrium (LD) around microsatellite markers (≈100 kb), QTL mapping typically provides only a very rough estimate of the location of the responsible variant, usually no better than 10 Mb (36) although new and evolving models may significantly increase the resolution (37).

Proceeding from QTL detection to identification of the responsible gene (the quantitative trait gene; QTG) and responsible variant in or near that gene is known as positional cloning, and often proceeds via the construction and testing of congenic

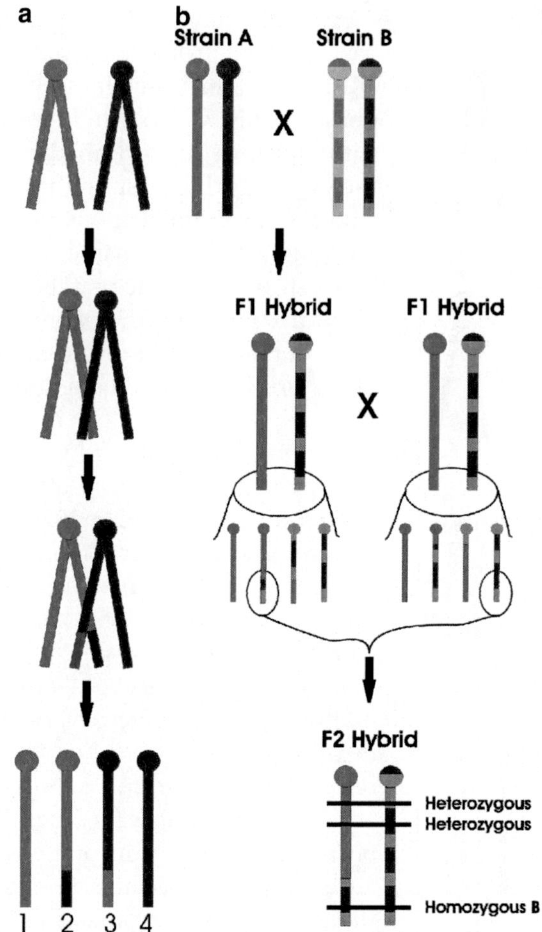

Fig. 3. Linkage mapping theory. Note that murine chromosomes are telocentric, with the centromere (ball) located at the proximal end of the chromosome. Blue and pink colors represent the paternally and maternally derived chromosomes, respectively. For simplicity only one chromosome is illustrated. Graph A shows homologous recombination (crossing-over) in a chromosome during meiosis. During prophase I, the two paired chromosomes (i.e., four chromatids) are found very close to one another, and homologous sites on two chromatids can mesh and exchange places. As a result, four gametes are possible: two nonrecombinant (gametes 1 and 4), inherited unchanged from the parental form, and two recombinant (gametes 2 and 3), in which both paternal and maternal genetic information is represented. Graph B illustrates how homologous recombination produces "linkage" of intra-chromosomal genetic locations in an F2 hybrid mouse. Inbred Strain A (*solid*) and Strain B (*hatched*) when mated will produce identically heterozygous F1 hybrid animals. In the F1 hybrids, however, the effects of homologous recombination can be seen, and both nonrecombinant and recombinant gametes are created. Assuming the highlighted gametes result in the conception of an F2 hybrid, shown, genomic locations (horizontal lines) near each other physically will tend to have the same genotype (in this case, heterozygous), whereas genomic locations far away physically will tend to have a different genotype (in this case, homozygous for Strain B alleles). Thus, physical locations of unknown genetic factors can be estimated (see text)

strains, in which donor genome from one strain is placed ("introgressed") onto the background of another via repeated backcrossing (see ref. 38). The process of congenic strain construction can be speeded up by the use of marker-assisted breeding strategies ("speed congenics") (39), but positional cloning remains laborious and time-consuming (40). Of course, at any point in the process, one is free to entertain and test candidate gene hypotheses of any gene known to reside in the genomic confidence interval containing the QTL.

4.1.3. Advanced Mapping Populations

One weakness of performing linkage mapping using segregating populations is that they are one-shot experiments; the population disappears forever as soon as the subjects are tested and euthanized. More useful might be genetic reference populations, whereby segregation is reinbred so that it is stable, able to be propagated intact through multiple generations so that new phenotypes can be tested at will (see ref. 41). The oldest of these are RI strain sets (42), in which individual members of an F2 hybrid cross are used as progenitors of new inbred strains, each one representing a discrete and unchanging "shuffling" of the progenitor alleles. Other examples of inbred mapping populations include recombinant congenic (RC) strain sets, in which small portions (different in each strain) of "donor" genome are placed on a recipient background (43) and chromosomal substitution strain (CSS; consomic) sets, in which entire donor chromosomes are placed on a recipient background (see ref. 44). See Fig. 4 for an illustration of the construction and use of these models.

The advantage of using stable mapping populations over de novo segregating populations is that the mapping populations have already been genotyped by their developers. To use them, therefore, one only needs to obtain and phenotype the set of strains, and correlate the phenotypic data with databased genotyping data in order to detect linkages. The disadvantage is that for practical reasons, the size of these strain sets is too small to provide statistical power to detect any but the largest linkages; typically, a provisional QTL detection in RI, RC or CSS panels is followed by confirmation in an F2 intercross or backcross (45). In other cases, advanced mapping populations can be used to confirm a linkage and/or reduce the size of the genomic interval containing the QTL (see ref. 41). A new, very powerful (46) advanced mapping population, the Collaborative Cross (37, 47) represents an attempt to combine the advantages of a genetically stable mapping population with the statistical power afforded by the sheer number of strains (500–1,000). The Cross has yet to be completed and used, however, and haplotype mapping of large sets of inbred strains (see below) provides some of the same advantages.

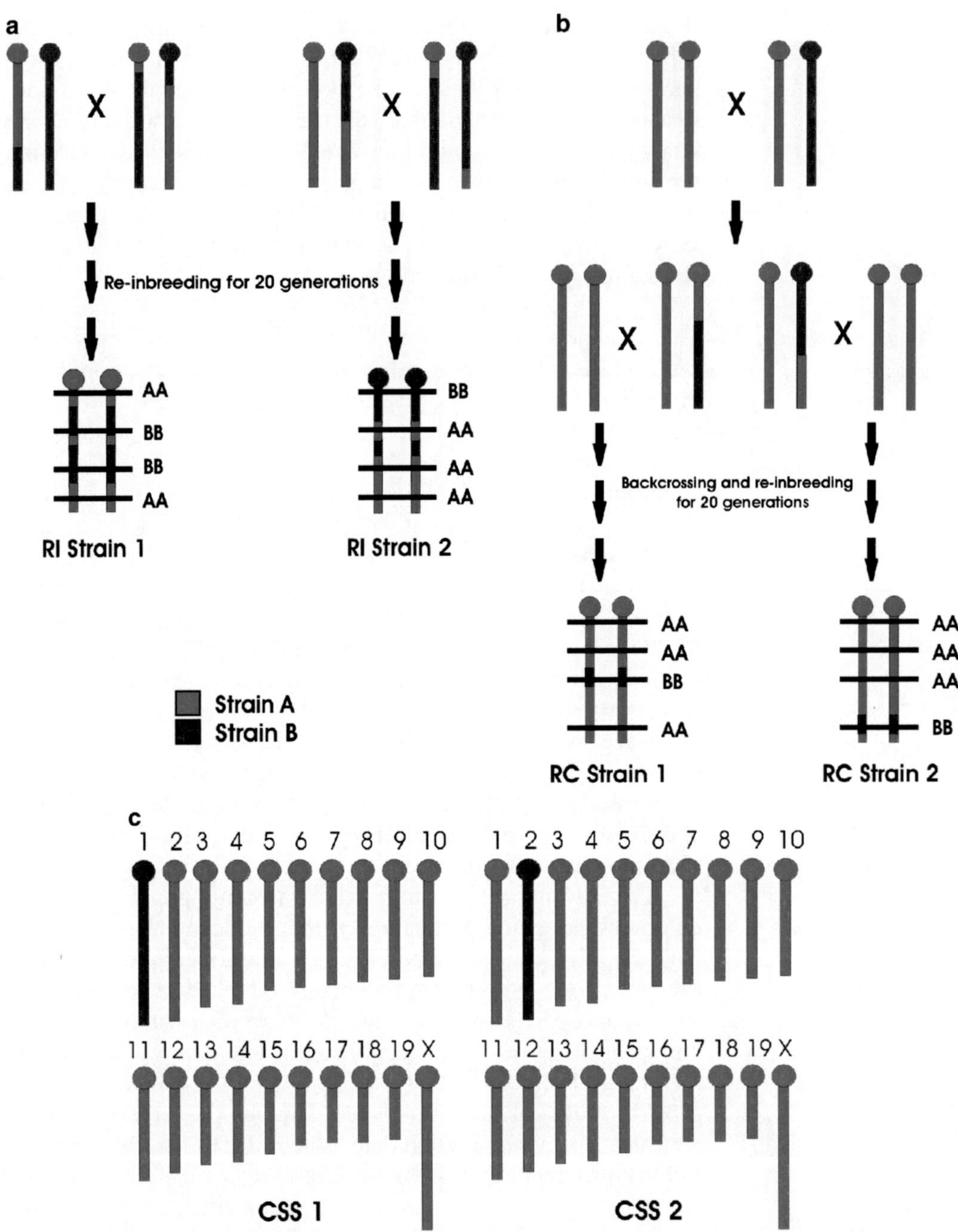

Fig. 4. Advanced QTL mapping populations. Graph A shows the construction of recombinant inbred (RI) strains. Only one chromosome is illustrated for simplicity. F2 hybrids constructed from two strains, Strain A (green) and Strain B (red), are reinbred for 20 generations. Eventually all loci become fixed in a homozygous state, but the pattern of homozygosity differs from one strain (e.g., RI Strain 1) to another (e.g., RI Strain 2). QTL mapping proceeds by identifying a genomic location (horizontal line) in which genotype correlates with the phenotype among a large set of RI strains. Graph B shows the partial construction of recombinant congenic (RC) strains. Again, only one chromosome is illustrated for simplicity. A backcross is first constructed by breeding an F1 hybrid back to one parental strain (in this case, Strain A). The offspring are further backcrossed and then reinbred to homozygosity. Unlike RI strains that are 50% Strain A, 50% Strain B (albeit in different patterns), RC strains are constructed so that they have a minority of "donor" genome (in this case, Strain B)

4.1.4. In silico Haplotype Mapping

A significant disadvantage of both segregating populations and advanced mapping populations derived from them is that only gene variants divergent in the two progenitor strains can be detected; variation contained in the >450 other inbred mouse strains (16), for example, is not brought to bear. A notable exception is the population of mice in the Collaborative Cross, which is derived from an 8-way cross of standard inbred strains (47). Following the sequencing of the (C57BL/6) mouse genome (48) and the re-sequencing of the genomes of many other strains to identify SNPs among them, it has been revealed that variation among inbred laboratory mouse strains is best explained as a mosaic of three founder subspecies: *Mus musculus (M. m.) domesticus*, *M. m. musculus*, and *M. m. molossinus* (18). In fact, SNPs are not inherited independently, but in so-called haplotype blocks (with high LD of SNPs within the block) of varying sizes (but averaging ≈30 kb, approximately the size of a single gene), and only a small number of (typically no more than four) observed haplotypes among large sets of strains. Thus, simply by phenotyping a large (>15) set of strains and comparing the distribution of those phenotypes to the distribution of haplotype blocks across the genome in those same strains (49), one can detect QTLs, and with gene-level (or even subgenic) resolution (see ref. 50). See Fig. 5 for an illustration of haplotype mapping.

Note that haplotype mapping is fundamentally different from standard linkage mapping in that it relies on patterns of LD between strains rather than detecting linkage per se. The limitation of the technique is that its statistical power is limited in the same manner as for advanced mapping populations; only a finite number of strains have been genotyped at SNPs blanketing the genome.

4.2. Findings

Although murine linkage mapping studies of pain and analgesia have been conducted for almost 15 years, the practical challenges surrounding its use have ensured only a small number of published findings. For details of these findings, consult any one of a number of reviews on the topic (20, 51–53). A listing of significant QTLs and the genes possibly (and in some cases, likely) responsible for them is provided in Table 1.

Fig. 4. (continued) placed on a majority "recipient" background (in this case, Strain A). The location of the donor genome differs from one strain (e.g., RC Strain 1) to another (e.g., RC Strain 2). Commonly, a reciprocal RC set is created where the donor and recipient genome is swapped. Again, QTL mapping proceeds by identifying a genomic location (horizontal line) in which genotype correlates with the phenotype among relevant RC strains. Graph C illustrates (the construction process is beyond the scope of this chapter) chromosome substitution strains (CSSs). In these, the donor segment represents an entire chromosome (e.g., chromosome 1 in CSS1 and chromosome 2 in CSS2). The statistically significant phenotypic divergence of a CSS from its background strain is *prima facie* evidence of a QTL on that chromosome

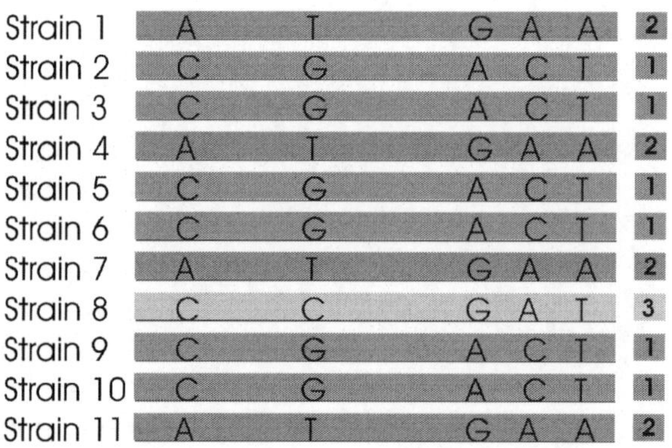

Strain 1 A T G A A 2
Strain 2 C G A C T 1
Strain 3 C G A C T 1
Strain 4 A T G A A 2
Strain 5 C G A C T 1
Strain 6 C G A C T 1
Strain 7 A T G A A 2
Strain 8 C C G A T 3
Strain 9 C G A C T 1
Strain 10 C G A C T 1
Strain 11 A T G A A 2

Fig. 5. Haplotype mapping theory. Along the stretch of DNA illustrated (center), sequencing reveals only five nucleotide bases showing polymorphisms (i.e., single-nucleotide polymorphisms; SNPs) across a set of 11 strains. Although $5^4 = 625$ permutations are possible, in fact only three sequences of these five SNPs (haplotypes) are observed: A-T-G-A-A, C-G-A-C-T, and C-C-G-A-T. This is because these SNPs are inherited together in a haplotype block, and population bottlenecks in the species' history has limited the number of extant haplotypes. We can label the haplotypes in this block in order of their frequency: 1, 2 and 3. QTL mapping proceeds by identifying haplotypes that correlate with the phenotype among a large set of inbred strains

Table 1
Statistically significant QTLs of relevance to pain and analgesia in laboratory mice

Phenotype	Chromosome	LOD[a]	Location[b]	Candidate gene(s)	Reference
Acute/tonic pain					
Capsaicin	2	5.9	30		(55)
	7	4.8	10		(55)
	7	5.8	50		(55)
	8	4.4	30		(55)
Formalin	9	5.2	60	*Atp1b3* (51 cM)	(56)
	10	4.3	70	*Avpr1a* (68 cM)	(56)
Hot-plate	4	3.8 (♂ only)	71	*Oprd1* (65 cM)	(57)
Paw withdrawal	7	6.3	50	*Calca* (54 cM)	(4)
Tail-withdrawal	4	3.6 (♂ only)	56	*Oprd1* (65 cM)	(6)
	7	12.6	33	*Trpv1* (44 cM)	(6)
	11	7.8	46		
Analgesia					
Clonidine	1	4.7	100	*Kcnj9* (94 cM)	(6)

(continued)

Table 1 (continued)

Phenotype	Chromosome	LOD[a]	Location[b]	Candidate gene(s)	Reference
Morphine	1	4.7 (♀ only)	10	*Oprk1* (6 cM)	(58)
	1	3.2	91	*Htr1b* (46 cM)	(6)
	9	5.2 (♀ only)	20	*Oprm1* (8 cM)	(58)
	9	4.5	42		(59)
	10	7.5	9		(60)
Stress-induced	8	6.1 (♀ only)	56	*Mc1r* (68 cm)	(57)
U50,488	8	2.7 (♀ only)	67	*Mc1r* (68 cM)	(5)
WIN55,212-2	1	4.4	100	*Kcnj9* (94 cM)	(6)
	7	4.8	40	*Trpv1* (44 cM)	(6)
Opioid hyperalgesia					
Chronic morphine	5	$p=0.000083$ *	1	*Abcb1b* (1 cM)	(61)
	18	$p=0.00037$ *	34	*Adrb2* (34 cM)	(62)

[a] *LOD* logarithm of the odds score

[b] Location of peak LOD score in centiMorgans (cM), a unit of genetic distance. Note that confidence intervals in QTL mapping projects are generally very large

5. Conclusions

Pain genetics does not need to be conducted in laboratory animals. Genes responsible for monogenic pain disorders like congenital insensitivities to pain and primary erythermalgia can be identified by linkage mapping, and genetic association studies have provisionally implicated a handful of genes in more common pain pathologies (53). The latter technique has suffered from lack of replication (53), however, and so far the powerful methodology of the whole-genome association study (WGAS) remains too expensive to be applied to pain (54). It seems likely, however, that pain genetics in laboratory rodents will continue to play an important role, both in the discovery of novel genes and in the characterization of how their allelic variants produce variable sensitivity to pain and analgesics.

References

1. Mogil JS, Wilson SG, Bon K, Lee SE, Chung K, Raber P, Pieper JO, Hain HS, Belknap JK, Hubert L, Elmer GI, Chung JM, Devor M (1999) Heritability of nociception. I. Responses of eleven inbred mouse strains on twelve measures of nociception. Pain 80:67–82
2. Mogil JS, Wilson SG, Bon K, Lee SE, Chung K, Raber P, Pieper JO, Hain HS, Belknap JK,

Hubert L, Elmer GI, Chung JM, Devor M (1999) Heritability of nociception. II. "Types" of nociception revealed by genetic correlation analysis. Pain 80:83–93

3. Lariviere WR, Wilson SG, Laughlin TM, Kokayeff A, West EE, Adhikari SM, Wan Y, Mogil JS (2002) Heritability of nociception. III. Genetic relationships among commonly used assays of nociception and hypersensitivity. Pain 97:75–86
4. Mogil JS, Meirmeister F, Seifert F, Strasburg K, Zimmermann K, Reinold H, Austin J-S, Bernardini N, Chesler EJ, Hoffman HA, Hordo C, Messlinger K, Nemmani KVS, Rankin AL, Ritchie J, Siegling A, Smith SB, Sotocinal SB, Vater A, Lehto SG, Klussmann S, Quirion R, Michaelis M, Devor M, Reeh PW (2005) Variable sensitivity to noxious heat is mediated by differential expression of the CGRP gene. Proc Natl Acad Sci USA 102:12938–12943
5. Mogil JS, Wilson SG, Chesler EJ, Rankin AL, Nemmani KVS, Lariviere WR, Groce MK, Wallace MR, Kaplan L, Staud R, Ness TJ, Glover TL, Stankova M, Mayorov A, Hruby VJ, Grisel JE, Fillingim RB (2003) The melanocortin-1 receptor gene mediates female-specific mechanisms of analgesia in mice and humans. Proc Natl Acad Sci USA 100: 4867–4872
6. Smith SB, Marker CL, Perry C, Liao G, Sotocinal SG, Austin J-S, Melmed K, Clark JD, Peltz G, Wickman K, Mogil JS (2008) Quantitative trait locus and computational mapping identifies *Kcnj9* (GIRK3) as a candidate gene affecting analgesia from multiple drug classes. Pharmacogenet Genom 18:231–241
7. Mogil JS, Ritchie J, Smith SB, Strasburg K, Kaplan L, Wallace MR, Romberg RR, Bijl H, Sarton EY, Fillingim RB, Dahan A (2005) Melanocortin-1 receptor gene variants affect pain and μ-opioid analgesia in mice and humans. J Med Genet 42:583–587
8. Tegeder I, Costigan M, Griffin RS, Abele A, Belfer I, Schmidt H, Ehnert C, Nejim J, Marian C, Scholz J, Wu T, Allchorne A, Diatchenko L, Binshtok AM, Goldman D, Adolph J, Sama S, Atlas SJ, Carlezon WA, Parsegian A, Lotsch J, Fillingim RB, Maixner W, Geisslinger G, Max MB, Woolf CJ (2006) GTP cyclohydrolase and tetrahydrobiopterin regulate pain sensitivity and persistence. Nature Med 12:1269–1277
9. Falconer DS, Mackay TFC (1996) Introduction to quantitative genetics. Longman, Essex, UK
10. Devor M, del Canho S, Raber P (2005) Heritability of symptoms in the neuroma model of neuropathic pain: replication and complementation analysis. Pain 116:294–301
11. Devor M, Raber P (1990) Heritability of symptoms in an experimental model of neuropathic pain. Pain 42:51–67
12. Panocka I, Marek P, Sadowski B (1986) Inheritance of stress-induced analgesia in mice. Selective breeding study. Brain Res 397:152–155
13. Belknap JK, Haltli NR, Goebel DM, Lamé M (1983) Selective breeding for high and low levels of opiate-induced analgesia in mice. Behav Genet 13:383–396
14. Lariviere WR, Sattar MA, Melzack R (2006) Inflammation-susceptible Lewis rats show less sensitivity than resistant Fischer rats in the formalin inflammatory pain test and with repeated thermal testing. J Neurophysiol 95:2889–2897
15. Sternberg EM, Glowa JR, Smith MA, Calogero AE, Listwak SJ, Aksentijevich S, Chrousos GP, Wilder RL, Gold PW (1992) Corticotropin releasing hormone related behavioral and neuroendocrine responses to stress in Lewis and Fischer rats. Brain Res 570:54–60
16. Beck JA, Lloyd S, Hafezparast M, Lennon-Pierce M, Eppig JT, Festing MFW, Fisher EMC (2000) Genealogies of mouse inbred strains. Nat Genet 24:23–25
17. Petkov PM, Graber JH, Churchill GA, DiPetrillo K, King BL, Paigen K (2005) Evidence of a large-scale functional organization of mammalian chromosomes. PLoS Genet 1:e33
18. Wade CM, Kulbokas EJ III, Kirby AW, Zody MC, Mullikin JC, Lander ES, Lindblad-Toh K, Daly MJ (2002) The mosaic structure of variation in the laboratory mouse genome. Nature 420:574–578
19. Canzian F (1997) Phylogenetics of the laboratory rat *Rattus norvegicus.* Genome Res 7:262–267
20. Mogil JS (1999) The genetic mediation of individual differences in sensitivity to pain and its inhibition. Proc Natl Acad Sci USA 96:7744–7751
21. Wilson SG, Smith SB, Chesler EJ, Melton KA, Haas JJ, Mitton BA, Strasburg K, Hubert L, Rodriguez-Zas SL, Mogil JS (2003) The heritability of antinociception: common pharmacogenetic mediation of five neurochemically distinct analgesics. J Pharmacol Exp Ther 304:547–559
22. Wilson SG, Bryant CD, Lariviere WR, Olsen MS, Giles BE, Chesler EJ, Mogil JS (2003) The heritability of antinociception II: pharmacogenetic mediation of three over-the-counter

analgesics in mice. J Pharmacol Exp Ther 305:755–764

23. Chesler EJ, Wilson SG, Lariviere WR, Rodriguez-Zas SL, Mogil JS (2002) Influences of laboratory environment on behavior. Nature Neurosci 5:1101–1102
24. Chesler EJ, Wilson SG, Lariviere WR, Rodriguez-Zas SL, Mogil JS (2002) Identification and ranking of genetic and laboratory environment factors influencing a behavioral trait, thermal nociception, via computational analysis of a large data archive. Neurosci Biobehav Rev 26:907–923
25. Devor M, Gilad A, Arbilly M, Nissenbaum J, Yakir B, Raber P, Minert A, Pisante A, Darvasi A (2007) Sex-specific variability and a 'cage effect' independently mask a neuropathic pain quantitative trait locus detected in a whole genome scan. Eur J NeuroSci 26:681–688
26. Raber P, Devor M (2002) Social variables affect phenotype in the neuroma model of neuropathic pain. Pain 97:139–150
27. Langford DL, Crager SE, Shehzad Z, Smith SB, Sotocinal SG, Levenstadt JS, Chanda ML, Levitin DJ, Mogil JS (2006) Social modulation of pain as evidence for empathy in mice. Science 312:1967–1970
28. Shir Y, Ratner A, Raja SN, Campbell JN, Seltzer Z (1998) Neuropathic pain following partial nerve injury in rats is suppressed by dietary soy. Neurosci Lett 240:73–76
29. Callahan BL, Gil ASC, Levesque A, Mogil JS (2008) Modulation of mechanical and thermal nociceptive sensitivity in the laboratory mouse by behavioral state. J Pain 9:174–184
30. Crabbe JC, Phillips TJ, Kosobud A, Belknap JK (1990) Estimation of genetic correlation: interpretation of experiments using selectively bred and inbred animals. Alcohol Clin Exp Res 14:141–151
31. Hegmann JP, Possidente B (1981) Estimating genetic correlations from inbred strains. Behav Genet 11:103–114
32. Mogil JS (2000) Genetic correlations among common nociceptive assays in the mouse: how many types of pain? In: Devor M, Rowbotham MC, Wiesenfeld-Hallin Z (eds) Proceedings of the 9th World Congress on Pain, IASP Press, Seattle, pp 455–470
33. Lariviere WR, Chesler EJ, Mogil JS (2001) Transgenic studies of pain and analgesia: mutation or background phenotype? J Pharmacol Exp Ther 297:467–473
34. Lander ES, Schork NJ (1994) Genetic dissection of complex traits. Science 265:2037–2048
35. Broman KW, Wu H, Sen S, Churchill GA (2003) R/qtl: QTL mapping in experimental crosses. Bioinformatics 19:889–890
36. Darvasi A, Soller M (1997) A simple method to calculate resolving power and confidence interval of QTL map location. Behav Genet 27:125–132
37. Chesler EJ, Miller DR, Branstetter LR, Galloway LD, Jackson BL, Philip VM, Voy BH, Culiat CT, Threadgill DW, Williams RW, Churchill GA, Johnson DK, Manly KF (2008) The Collaborative Cross at Oak Ridge National Laboratory: developing a powerful resource for systems genetics. Mamm Genome 19:382–389
38. Bennett B (2000) Congenic strains developed for alcohol- and drug-related phenotypes. Pharmacol Biochem Behav 67:671–681
39. Markel P, Shu P, Ebeling C, Carlson GA, Nagle DL, Smutko JS, Moore KJ (1997) Theoretical and empirical issues for marker-assisted breeding of congenic mouse strains. Nat Genet 17:280–284
40. Nadeau JH, Frankel WN (2000) The roads from phenotypic variation to gene discovery: mutagenesis versus QTLs. Nat Genet 25:381–384
41. Darvasi A (1998) Experimental strategies for the genetic dissection of complex traits in animal models. Nat Genet 18:19–24
42. Bailey DW (1971) Recombinant-inbred strains: an aid to finding identity, linkage and function of histocompatibility and other genes. Transplantation 11:325–327
43. Groot PC, Moen CJA, Dietrich W, Stoye JP, Lander ES, Demant P (1992) The recombinant congenic strains for analysis of multigenic traits: genetic composition. FASEB J 6: 2826–2835
44. Nadeau JH, Singer JB, Matin A, Lander ES (2000) Analysing complex genetic traits with chromosome substitution strains. Nat Genet 24:221–225
45. Belknap JK, Mitchell SR, O'Toole LA, Helms ML, Crabbe JC (1996) Type I and Type II error rates for quantitative trait loci (QTL) mapping studies using recombinant inbred mouse strains. Behav Genet 26:149–160
46. Valdar W, Flint J, Mott R (2006) Simulating the collaborative cross: power of QTL detection and mapping resolution in large sets of recombinant inbred strains of mice. Genetics 172:1783–1797
47. Complex Trait Consortium (2004) The Collaborative Cross, a community resource for the genetic analysis of complex traits. Nat Genet 36:1133–1137
48. Waterston RH et al (2002) Initial sequencing and comparative analysis of the mouse genome. Nature 420:520–562

49. Wang J, Peltz G (2005) Haplotype-based computational genetic analysis in mice. In: Peltz G (ed) Computational genetics and genomics: tools for understanding disease. Humana Press, Inc., Totowa, NJ, pp 51–70
50. Wang J, Liao G, Usuka J, Peltz G (2005) Computational genetics: from mouse to human. Trends Genet 21:526–532
51. Mogil JS, Max MB (2005) The genetics of pain. In: Koltzenburg M, McMahon SB (eds) Wall and Melzack's textbook of pain, 5th edn. Elsevier Churchill Livingstone, London, pp 159–174
52. Mogil JS (2004) Complex trait genetics of pain in the laboratory mouse. In: Mogil JS (ed) The genetics of pain, progress in pain research and management. IASP Press, Seattle, pp 123–149
53. LaCroix-Fralish ML, Mogil JS (2009) Progress in genetic studies of pain and analgesia. Annu Rev Pharmacol Toxicol 49:97–121
54. Max MB, Stewart WF (2008) The molecular epidemiology of pain: a new discipline for drug discovery. Nature Rev Drug Discov 7:647–658
55. Furuse T, Miura Y, Yagasaki K, Shiroishi T, Koide T (2003) Identification of QTLs for differential capsaicin sensitivity between mouse strains KJR and C57BL/6. Pain 105: 169–175
56. Wilson SG, Chesler EJ, Hain H, Rankin AJ, Schwarz JZ, Call SB, Murray MR, West EE, Teuscher C, Rodriguez-Zas S, Belknap JK, Mogil JS (2002) Identification of quantitative trait loci for chemical/inflammatory nociception in mice. Pain 96:385–391
57. Mogil JS, Richards SP, O'Toole LA, Helms ML, Mitchell SR, Kest B, Belknap JK (1997) Identification of a sex-specific quantitative trait locus mediating nonopioid stress-induced analgesia in female mice. J Neurosci 17:7995–8002
58. Bergeson SE, Helms ML, O'Toole LA, Jarvis MW, Hain HS, Mogil JS, Belknap JK (2001) Quantitative trait loci influencing morphine antinociception in four mapping populations. Mamm Genome 12:546–553
59. Hain HS, Belknap JK, Mogil JS (1999) Pharmacogenetic evidence for the involvement of 5-hydroxytryptamine (Serotonin)-1B receptors in the mediation of morphine antinociceptive sensitivity. J Pharmacol Exp Ther 291:444–449
60. Belknap JK, Mogil JS, Helms ML, Richards SP, O'Toole LA, Bergeson SE, Buck KJ (1995) Localization to chromosome 10 of a locus influencing morphine analgesia in crosses derived from C57BL/6 and DBA/2 strains. Life Sci 57:L117–L124
61. Liang DY, Liao G, Lighthall GK, Peltz G, Clark DJ (2006) Genetic variants of the P-glycoprotein gene Abcb1b modulate opioid-induced hyperalgesia, tolerance and dependence. Pharmacogenet genomics 16:825–835
62. Liang DY, Liao G, Wang J, Usuka J, Guo Y, Peltz G, Clark JD (2006) A genetic analysis of opioid-induced hyperalgesia in mice. Anesthesiology 104:1054–1062

Chapter 21

RT-PCR Analysis of Pain Genes: Use of Gel-Based RT-PCR for Studying Induced and Tissue-Enriched Gene Expression

Kendall Mitchell and Michael J. Iadarola

Abstract

Frequently, it is important to ascertain whether a molecule that is involved in one model of pain is also involved in other models of pain. Similarly, it may be important to determine whether a molecule involved in nociception in one tissue is also expressed in other tissues and to ascertain the degree of enrichment. Additionally, before initiating a complex set of experiments or purchasing an expensive immunoassay kit, it may be useful to obtain initial supporting evidence to justify the time and money. Is the transcript for the target receptor, protein, or peptide precursor present in, for example, the dorsal root ganglion? And, if present, how abundant is it? Here is where the power of PCR can be applied to obtain a quick but informative answer. In this chapter, we mainly detail the use of gel-based RT-PCR and also provide suggestions on tissue dissection and interpretation of results. The use of gel-based RT-PCR can address many of the questions of abundance or tissue specificity with a minimum of expense and time.

Key words: RT-PCR, Nociception, mRNA, Gene regulation, Pain, Pirt, Dorsal root ganglion

1. Introduction

Although essential for host survival, pain can become unbearable especially when chronic. Accordingly, a great deal of money is expended for current pain relief medications and treatments, as well as invested to find newer, better treatments. A key to discovering better pain therapeutics inevitably involves understanding the molecules that constitute the pain circuits, starting from damaged peripheral tissue and the peripheral nervous system (1) and ending in cerebral cortex (2). The identification of TRPV1, a channel involved in transduction of nociceptive stimuli in peripheral nerve terminals (3), the expression of which is highly enriched in DRG, serves as an example of how new molecular insights can translate into new therapeutic approaches. For example, the intrathecal

Arpad Szallasi (ed.), *Analgesia: Methods and Protocols*, Methods in Molecular Biology, vol. 617, DOI 10.1007/978-1-60327-323-7_21, © Springer Science+Business Media, LLC 2010

administration of the ultrapotent TRPV1 agonist, resiniferatoxin, selectively depletes TRPV1-expressing ganglionic neurons (4) and results in a dramatic reduction of pain from inflammation, cancer and arthritis in animals (5, 6). TRPV1 antagonists are also capable of controlling pain in experimental models although human clinical trials have encountered problems with drug-induced hyperthermia (7).

There are many known and likely many as yet unrecognized molecules that are involved in nociceptive transmission and the neural processing of pain in general. Depending on the cause of pain (e.g. inflammation or nerve injury), a different cascade of pain-inducing molecules appears to be activated, although there is considerable overlap. These molecular changes can occur in circulating and infiltrating leukocytes, resident cells of the affected peripheral tissues, in nerve endings and axons of dorsal root ganglia neurons, in various layers of the spinal cord and a wide variety of brain regions. Molecular alterations due to peripheral inflammation also occur in the choroid plexus, which makes the cerebrospinal fluid, and changes in secreted factors may influence brain function in a very broad fashion (8). The array and diversity of possible changes, therefore, underscore the range of questions that can be asked in attempting to unravel the roles of these molecules and neural circuits in various painful conditions.

For some of these questions, RT-PCR has proven to be a valuable tool in assessing the involvement of a particular gene in a persistent pain state. The focus of this chapter is to describe the advantages and comparative ease of using gel-based RT-PCR to establish the relative expression level of a particular molecule in a target tissue or its regulation during nociception.

2. Materials

2.1. RNA Isolation

1. Trizol (Invitrogen, Carlsbad, CA).
2. RNeasy Mini Kit (Qiagen, Valencia, CA).
3. ZR-Whole Blood Total RNA Kit™ (Zymo Research, Orange, CA).
4. Sonicator (Sonics and Materials, Inc., Newtown, CT) (see Note 1).
5. RNase-Free DNase Set (Qiagen).

2.2. RNA Quantitation

1. Quant-iT™ Ribogreen RNA assay kit (Invitrogen).
2. SpectraMax Gemini XS Fluorescent plate reader.
3. 96-well plate.

2.3. RT-PCR

1. Access RT-PCR System (Promega, Madison, WI).
2. PCR Strip Tubes (Axygen, Union City, CA).
3. Robocycler (Strategene, La Jolla, CA, the thermal cycler we use in our lab).
4. Tomy Capsulefuge Model PMC-860 (Research Products International Corp., Mt. Prospect, IL).
5. Primers (Operon. $12/pair) (see Notes 2 and 3).

2.4. Making Gels

1. UltraPure Agarose (Invitrogen).
2. Microwave.
3. 500 ml Erlenmeyer flask.
4. Microwavable plastic cap (see Note 4)
5. Gel box and Gel Combs (see Note 5).

2.5. Running Gel

1. 60 well HLA Plate (Nunc, Thermo Fisher Scientific, Rochester, NY).
2. 1 kb DNA Ladder Mix (Crystalgen, Plainview, NY) (see Note 6).
3. 50× Tris–Acetate–EDTA Buffer (TAE).
4. Power Supply Model 250.
5. Casting Tray.
6. Ethidium Bromide 10 mg/ml (Invitrogen).
7. Blue/Orange 6× Loading Dye (Promega) (see Note 7).
8. Aerosol tips (see Note 8)

2.6. Obtaining and Quantitating Gel Image

1. FluorChem 8900 System (Alpha Innotech Corp, San Leandro, CA).
2. A connection to a PC.
3. ImageQuant 5.2 (Molecular Dynamics, Piscataway, NJ).

3. Methods

When deciding to use gel-based RT-PCR (also called traditional RT-PCR) it is important to understand the advantages and disadvantages of the technique, which in part can be explained by the mechanism of PCR. PCR amplifications can be broken down into three phases. The exponential phase occurs when the reaction components are in excess thereby theoretically allowing for a doubling of the PCR product per cycle. In the next phase, the amplification of the PCR product occurs linearly rather exponentially as the reagents are partially depleted. Plateau phase represents the point in which the amplifications have further slowed or have completely stopped.

A minor disadvantage of gel-based RT-PCR is that the reaction generally must proceed into the linear phase before the product can be visualized. Thus, when comparing transcript expression in multiple samples, it is likely that samples that contain higher levels of transcript will enter the linear phase well before the other samples, which are still accumulating product exponentially. In this situation, when too many cycles are used, the gel-based approach can result in a reduced difference in expression between samples (i.e., by the time the lower-expressing samples are visualized the higher-expressing sample may reach a plateau). Conversely, an artificially magnified difference may be inferred if too few cycles are used. Moreover, in cases where the actual change in expression is extremely small, it may be possible that this technique may fail to detect those differences (see Fig. 1).

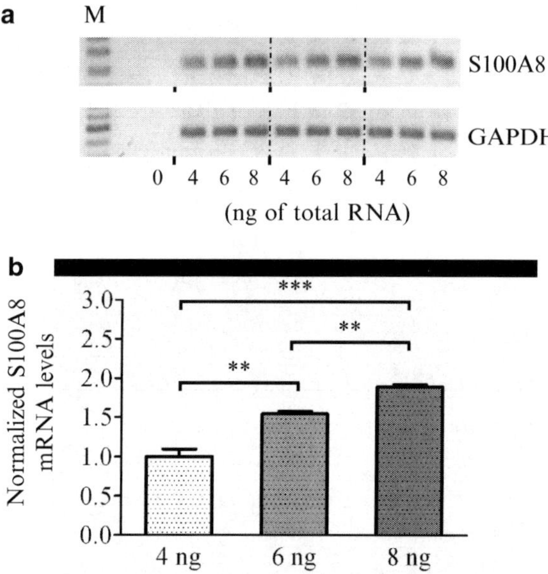

Fig. 1. Ability of gel-based RT-PCR to detect small differences in expression. (**a**) Total RNA from spinal cord was used to amplify S100A8 expression. In triplicate, either 4, 6 or 8 ng of total RNA from one sample was used per RT-PCR reaction. For normalization, GAPDH expression was separately determined by adding 8 ng of the same RNA for all nine reactions. The RT-PCR products for S100A8 and GAPDH were run in three blocks (4, 6, 8 $ng_{first\ set}$, 4, 6, 8 $ng_{second\ set}$, 4, 6, 8 $ng_{third\ set}$) on the gel rather than loading them in a 444, 666 and 888 pattern. The former arrangement is useful in case one side of the gel yields weaker signals than the other side due to non-uniformity of UV transillumination. (**b**) The RT-PCR data in (**a**) were quantified and the fold change is shown. Analysis demonstrated that 6 ng of input RNA resulted in a signal that was 1.54 times higher than that obtained when 4 ng of RNA was used (*1.50 is the expected value*) and 1.23 times lower when 8 ng was used (*1.33 is expected*). Additionally, the 8 ng samples resulted in a signal that was 1.89 times higher than that obtained with 4 ng (*2.00 is expected*). Thus, these data demonstrate that analysis by gel-based RT-PCR can be used to detect small changes in gene expression

Usually, after examination of the expression level in the first RT-PCR amplification by gel electrophoresis, a second amplification starting with a new aliquot of RNA, where the number of cycles is appropriately adjusted up or down, can place the results into the linear range for most studies.

In contrast to gel-based RT-PCR, real time quantitative RT-PCR (qRT-PCR) allows for comparison of samples while each are in the exponential phase, thus, in theory, there is no biasing against samples that start with different expression levels. Despite the advantages of qRT-PCR, it is possible, however, to obtain different quantitative measurements even if performed in the same lab (9). One factor which can contribute to such variation is the failure to appreciate nonspecific amplicons. This is more likely to be seen in the simpler, less expensive SYBR green qRT-PCR assays as compared to Taqman or other qRT-PCR approaches. SYBR green is an intercalating dye and will stain any double-stranded DNA in the RT-PCR tube, thus both specific and nonspecific amplification products will provide signal to the fluorometric detector. Nonspecific amplification, which can vary from sample to sample, also can result in depletion of reaction components and a skewing of data. Although this implies that one should use primers that yield one amplicon (and no primer-dimers), this can sometimes be complicated. When the transcript of interest is expressed at sufficient levels in a sample, it is usually easy to obtain one dominant amplicon. However, when the transcript is expressed at low levels in the samples, it is possible that the primers will latch on to other transcripts giving one or more nonspecific products (see Fig. 2). Visualization of the reaction products on gels can aid in understanding the extent of this artifact. This is very important information to obtain since it can guide choices of qRT-PCR methodology and also be a determinant of one's commitment to the target protein itself:

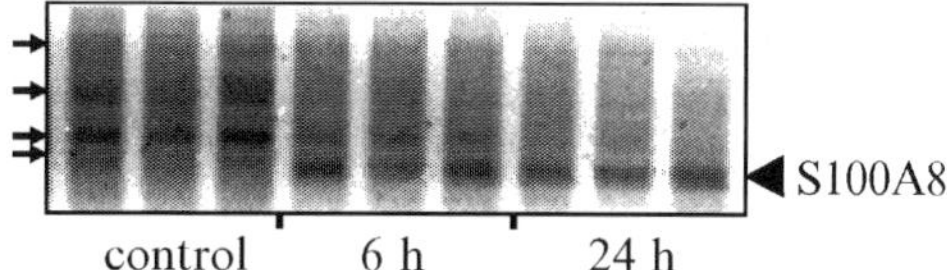

Fig. 2. Potential for amplification of nonspecific PCR-products when target gene is minimally or not expressed in samples. Gel shows PCR products after amplification of S100A8 in spinal cord samples taken from control animals or animals 6 or 24 h after hind paw inflammation. Generally, S100A8 is undetectable in spinal cord samples. However, due to an influx of neutrophils, which highly express S100A8, into the CNS vasculature, the spinal cord samples contain high levels of S100A8 after peripheral inflammation (13). Thus in the 6 and 24 h samples, high levels of S100A8 are detected on the gel. In the control samples, we failed, as expected, to detect an amplicon corresponding to S100A8. Instead, we detected several nonspecific amplicons that were not (or minimally) expressed in the 6 and 24 h samples. Failure to identify these nonspecific amplicons, in for example, the SYBR green qRT-PCR assays can in some cases lead to a misquantification of gene expression changes. Schemes to reduce nonspecific amplicons are described in Notes and Trouble Shooting sections. $^{**}P<0.01$ and $^{**}P<0.001$, as determined by Student's *t*-test

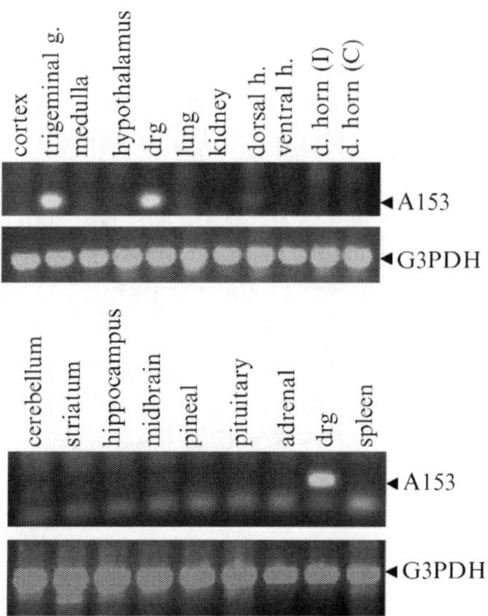

Fig. 3. Gel-based RT-PCR analysis to determine expression profile of a gene in different tissues. After subtraction hybridization analysis (DRG-sciatic nerve genes), we identified numerous clones that were enriched in the DRG as compared to sciatic nerve. Clone A153 (recently identified as the phosphoinositide-binding protein, Pirt, (14) was tested for expression in numerous tissues. Pirt is highly expressed in DRG and trigeminal ganglia. In contrast, its expression is dramatically weaker (or undetectable) in CNS and was not detected at all in nonperipheral nervous tissues. Thirty-three cycles were used to amplify Pirt. GAPDH expression was used to show that the RNA extracted from each tissue sample was intact

if the gene is expressed at very low levels, analysis of the transcript or protein will present challenges when using other methods such as in situ hybridization, western blot, or immunocytochemistry. When little or no prior data are available on the expression level of a particular gene in a specific tissue, a quick evaluation by RT-PCR, as outlined here, can be most informative (see Fig. 3).

Generally, the technique presented provides relative levels of expression. One approach for getting more quantitative data with gel-based RT-PCR is to generate an operationally-defined standard curve. In this case, different amounts (ng) of RNA from a given sample are amplified and run on a gel. The densitometric values are converted back to the amount of sample used. This curve can be used to examine issues of linearity with the amount of input RNA and the number of cycles of amplification and to compare transcript expression in test samples. It is possible to generate single stranded RNA as a template for making a real standard curve, but this will not be covered in this chapter.

The use of gel-based RT-PCR has several advantages. Assuming some of the equipment is already available, this technique is fairly inexpensive and does not require an expensive real-time PCR device to monitor each cycle (as compared to qRT-PCR). It is simple to perform and can be applied without the use of radioactive materials (as compared to Northern Blots). Below, we describe how to perform gel-based RT-PCR with emphasis on using this tool for semi-quantitative purposes.

3.1. Preparation of Samples

1. Dissection of tissue and tissue storage: Dissected tissues are frozen immediately on the bottom of a pre-labeled Eppendorf tube, stored at −80°C and care is taken to prevent thawing (see Note 9).
2. Before sonicating (or homogenizing) samples, push eppendorf tubes containing the entire set of samples deep into dry ice to prevent thawing. Immediately sonicate after the addition of homogenization buffer (done one sample at a time to prevent thawing of subsequent samples).

3.2. Isolation of RNA

Isolation of RNA can be achieved in numerous ways. Below are three common methods to extract RNA from tissue. Note that these are procedures used in our lab, and each kit provides instructions and troubleshooting tips for isolating RNA from tissues and cell cultures.

3.2.1. TRIzol Reagent

1. Sonicate every 50–100 mg of tissue sample in 1 ml of TRIzol Reagent.
2. Incubate at RT for 5 min.
3. Centrifuge at 12,000×*g* for 10 min at 2–8°C.
4. Transfer clear supernatant into a new tube.
5. Add 0.2 ml of chloroform per every 1 ml of TRIzol Reagent.
6. Shake vigorously by hand for 15 s and incubate at RT for 2–3 min.
7. Centrifuge at 12,000×*g* for 15 min at 2–8°C.
8. Gently collect the aqueous phase without disturbing the interphase into a new tube and add 0.5 ml of isopropyl alcohol per 1 ml of TRIzol Reagent.
9. Incubate at RT for 10 min.
10. Centrifuge at 12,000×*g* for 10 min at 2–8°C.
11. Remove supernatant and wash pellet with 1 ml of 75% ethanol per ml of TRIzol Reagent.
12. Vortex and centrifuge at 7,500×*g* for 5 min at 2–8°C.
13. Remove ethanol and let pellet air dry.
14. Add at least 40 μl of RNase-free water and mix thoroughly by pipetting.
15. For RT-PCR, it is especially important that the samples are not contaminated with DNA. Therefore, a DNase digestion step is highly recommended. Our DNA clean up protocol generally uses the RNeasy Mini Kit (see below), where the initial steps are the addition of 300 μl of Buffer RLT containing 1% β-mercapethanol to a tube containing an equal volume of

the RNA sample and ethanol (whose concentration in this tube should be 70%). For example, 210 μl of 100% EtOH and 50 μl of RNase/DNase-free water are added to 40 μl of RNA sample followed by the addition of RLT. The rest of the steps are described in Subheading 3.2.2 (see *).

16. Store at −80°C. We generally freeze samples once before quantifying RNA.

3.2.2. RNeasy Mini Kit

1. Sonicate 20–30 mg of tissue in 600 ml of Buffer RLT containing 1% β-mercapethanol.
2. Centrifuge lysate at maximum speed with table-top centrifuge for 3 min.
3. Transfer supernatant into a new tube.
4. Add 1 volume of 70% ethanol and mix immediately by pipetting.
5. *Apply 700 μl of sample to a pre-labeled RNeasy mini column placed in a 2 ml collection tube.
6. Centrifuge for 15 s at 8,000×*g* at RT.
7. Discard flow-through.
8. Repeat steps 5–7 if the initial volume of sample was greater than 700 μl.
9. Add 350 μl of Buffer RW1.
10. Centrifuge for 15 s at 8,000×*g* at RT.
11. Add 80 μl of freshly prepared DNase I solution (prepared in buffer RDD).
12. Incubate at RT for 15 min.
13. Add 350 μl of Buffer RW1.
14. Centrifuge for 15 s at 8,000×*g*.
15. Discard flow-through.
16. Transfer column into new 2 ml collection tube.
17. Add 500 μl of RPE.
18. Centrifuge for 15 s at 8,000×*g*.
19. Discard flow-through. Add 500 μl of RPE.
20. Centrifuge for 2 min at 8,000×*g*.
21. Place column into new 2 ml collection tube.
22. Centrifuge at maximum speed for 1 min.
23. Transfer column into a pre-labeled RNase/DNase-free 1.5 ml tube (provided).
24. Add 40 μl of RNase/DNase-free water.
25. Centrifuge for 1 min at 8,000×*g*.
26. Store at −80°C.

3.2.3. ZR Whole-Blood Total RNA Kit™

1. Add 700 μl of ZR buffer to 100 μl of blood.
2. Mix and transfer to Zymo-spin IIIC™ column in a collection tube.
3. Centrifuge for 60 s at 12,000×*g* at RT.
4. Discard collection tube containing flow-through.
5. Add 400 μl of RNA prewash buffer to the column in a new collection tube.
6. Centrifuge for 60 s at 12,000×*g*.
7. Discard flow-through.
8. Add 400 μl of RNA wash buffer to column in a new collection tube.
9. Centrifuge for 60 s at 12,000×*g*.
10. Discard flow-through.
11. Transfer column into a 1.5 ml tube.
12. Add 50 μl of RNase/DNase-free water.
13. Centrifuge for 1 min at 8,000×*g*.
14. As describe above, it may be important to perform a DNase digestion step.
15. Store samples at –80°C.

3.3. Quantification of RNA by Fluorescence

1. A standard curve is generated with known concentrations of RNA (generally ranging from 0.0 to 1.0 ng/μl) totaling a volume of 250 μl in RNase free TE buffer (pH 7.4). After mixing, duplicates of each concentration are added to a standard 96 well plate at a volume of 100 μl.
2. RNA samples are diluted (generally 1:100 in RNase-free TE buffer). Per sample, 5 μl of diluted RNA is added to 95 μl of RNase-free TE buffer in the 96 well-plate. Again, this should be done in duplicate.
3. 100 μl of diluted RiboGreen reagent is carefully, but quickly, added to the known standards and to the RNA samples.
4. The 96 well-plate is gently mixed, stored in dark, and read between 5 and 30 min with a fluorometic plate reader. It takes some time for the dye to intercalate thoroughly into the RNA strands.

3.4. Setup of RT-PCR Assay

1. If using the Access RT-PCR System, the reaction is set up as following in an RNase-free environment (see Note 10).
2. Gently mix, quick spin and pipette 21.0 μl into PCR tubes (see Note 11).
3. Add 8 ng of RNA (2 ng/μl) to each tube while on ice (see Note 12).

Table1
RT-PCR Reaction Mixture

Reagents	Per reaction	Master mix 10
DNAse/RNAse Free H2O	8.5 μl	85.0 μl
AMV/Tfl 5× buffer	5.0 μl	50.0 μl
dNTP (10 μM)	0.5 μl	5.0 μl
$MgSO_4$ (25 mM)	1.0 μl	10.0 μl
AMV RT (5 U/μl)	0.5 μl	5.0 μl
Tfl DNA polymerase (5 U/μl)	0.5 μl	5.0 μl
Forward primer (10 μM)	2.5 μl	25.0 μl
Reverse primer (10 μM)	2.5 μl	25.0 μl
Total volume	21.0 μl 21.0 μl/tube	210.0 μl

4. It should also be mentioned that the concentration of reagents (e.g. magnesium or primer concentrations) may need to be adjusted from that recommended in Table 1 (see Notes 13 and 14).
5. Also, it may be good to run a positive control (see Note 15) as well as a negative control (see Note 16) when analyzing the expression of a gene from RNA obtained from newly tested tissues.

3.5. RT-PCR Conditions

1. The RT-PCR reaction is carried out using a Robocycler thermal cycler according to the manufacturer's instructions.
2. One cycle (45 min at 45°C) is used for reverse transcription. This is followed by one cycle (2 min at 94°C) of transcriptase inactivation and 26–32 cycles of denaturation, annealing and extension (94°C for 30 s, 55°C for 1 min, and 68°C for 2 min; respectively). A final extension cycle is done at 68°C for 7 min.
3. Generally, housekeeping genes such as β-actin and GAPDH only require 21–23 cycles, whereas other genes may require 26–32 cycles.

3.6. Loading and Running Gels

1. Using a HLA tray, 5 μl of RT-PCR product is added to 1 μl of fresh 6× loading dye (see Fig. 4).
2. 50× TAE buffer is diluted to 1× using double distilled H_2O. This buffer is used for electrophoresis and to make 2% agarose gels (2 g of agarose/100 ml of buffer). For other options, see also (10).

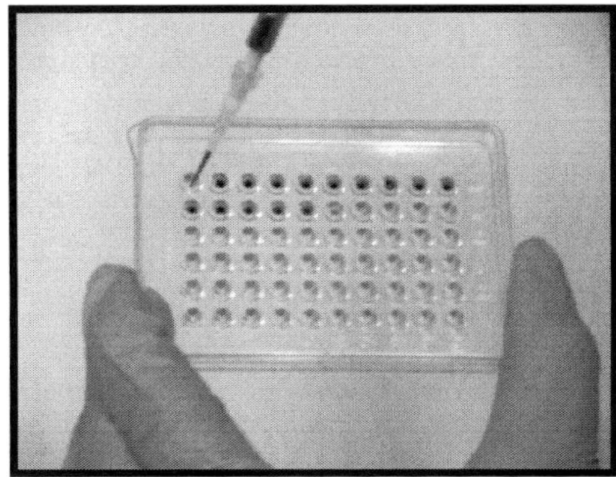

Fig. 4. Mixing RT-PCR products and loading buffer and dye in HLA tray. We have found the HLA tray to be a useful, convenient and inexpensive piece of labware for the preparation of small-volume samples prior to loading on the gel

3. Place gel in electrophoresis chamber and add TAE buffer to cover gel. Load sample to gel and apply 5 V/cm of gel. When the leading dye approaches the end of the gel, discontinue the current.
4. Soak the gel for about 5 min in TAE buffer containing 5 μg/ml ethidium bromide. For simplicity, ethidium bromide can also be added to fresh TAE buffer at a concentration of 0.5 μg/ml to make and run gels without the need of post-incubation. Gloves must be worn when using ethidium bromide as it is a mutagen. If the gel is soaked in ethidium bromide solution, the gel must be soaked in tap water for at least 5 min to remove excess ethidium bromide. The tap water must be discarded in proper chemical waste container, whereas the ethidium bromide solution can be reused as long as it is sealed and stored in the dark.

3.7. Inspecting the Gel and Acquiring Image

1. Ideally, the gel should have one major band at the correct MW. The appearance of primer-dimers is possible. It is acceptable to have some nonspecific bands as long as they are not close in MW to the target band, which could prevent quantification.
2. AlphaEase(FC) software (included with FluorChem 8900) allows for easy capture of a transilluminated gel image (see Note 17). Turn camera and UV transilluminator on and open software. After setting exposure time (auto-exposure or manual exposure), the image can be previewed and acquired. There are many devices of this type for digital capture of the gel image.

3.8. Quantification of the Image

1. The gel image is opened with ImageQuant 5.2 software.
2. A rectangle is drawn just large enough to encompass the largest band (or region of interest – ROI). The ROI is then copied and placed over the corresponding band in other lanes.

3. Select the auto volume report function under the analysis tool to obtain the volume (sum of the individual pixel intensities over the entire ROI) and the background volume.
4. The volume corresponding to the gene of interest is divided by the volume corresponding to the housekeeping gene to obtain a ratio of target gene to housekeeping gene.
5. Trouble-shooting (see Note 18).

4. Notes

1. Sonicating times and settings have to be determined for each tissue type. It is important to consider that incomplete or insufficient sonication can result in a low RNA yield.
2. For designing primers, we typically input mRNA sequences into primer design programs such as the program found on the following website: http://frodo.wi.mit.edu/. We choose 18–20 mers for primer size, optimal Tm of 60°C, and a GC concentration between 55 and 60%. A more detailed background into the design of primers can be found at http://www.premierbiosoft.com/tech_notes/PCR_Primer_Design.html.
3. We order primers from Operon, which sends back lyophilized primers along with a specification sheet indicating the nanomoles of oligonucleotide, Tm, molecular weight, and OD. This information is also labeled on the tubes. RNase/DNase free water is used to bring the primers to a concentration of 100 μM (thus for every 100 nmole, 1,000 μl of H_2O is used). In a separate, autoclaved Eppendorf tube, an aliquot of the stock is diluted to a working concentration of 10 μM. Primers are stored at –20°C.
4. As described above, the RT-PCR amplicons are run on a 2.0% agarose gel and the resulting images can be used to quantitate the expression of genes. It is therefore important to obtain the highest signal-to-noise ratio as possible. This includes using primer pairs that result in one amplicon or in which the amplicon of interest is not in close proximity to nonspecific amplicons. It is also important to make sure the gel is void of impurities, such as from dust particulates or air bubbles, which can result in significant quantifiable signals. To reduce impurities, make sure that the agarose is sufficiently boiled till the point of no bubbles and to use a microwaveable, clean plastic lid to prevent unwanted particulates from falling into the agarose (which could occur if paper towels are used as a sealant). It is also important to pour the gel before bubbles

reappear but not too hot as to cause warping of the casting tray. Also note that the lid should *loosely* cover the Erlenmeyer flask to prevent a buildup of pressure and spilling of agarose during microwaving. It may also be useful to microwave in intervals, with stirring in between, since a long continuous microwaving may also cause spilling. We use a 12 × 14 cm gel tray with slots for two sets of combs. 100 ml is poured for each run.

5. When using gels for quantification, the amount of space between samples is an important practical consideration. Adequate spacing between the teeth is needed for drawing rectangles around amplicons thus making it easier to perform the quantification. Also the shape of the tooth is a factor; if it is too square the product looks like a circle rather than a rectangle. Rectangles are also easier to line up with the molecular weight markers. We prefer using combs whose teeth are distanced at least 1.5 mm from each other. In addition, it may be good to obtain combs that are at least 1.5 mm thick and nearly 4 mm wide which allows for easy pipetting of sample in to wells (5 μl of RT-PCR product plus 1 μl of loading buffer).

6. Although DNA ladders are a valuable guide for product size, sometimes it may be unclear whether the amplicon is running in the correct position. Here, a positive control, or sequencing the product, may be needed for confirmation. Either of these additional verification tests can be *invaluable* if there is a spurious band being amplified that runs near the molecular weight of the expected band.

7. When loading, mix the samples and loading dye thoroughly with the pipettor. This ensures that the samples are as dense as possible. Also make sure that air is not trapped in the pipette tip which could result in air bubbles and an uneven amount of sample loaded which will affect between-lane comparisons. For sample loading, place the tip just inside the well, slowly expel, and then slowly raise the pipette tip. If one needs to step away while loading samples, it is imperative to tightly cover the HLA tray to prevent evaporation of the PCR product. Similarly, if one needs to rerun the PCR product, then store the PCR product at –20°C in tightly capped PCR tubes.

8. Aerosol tips are highly recommended during many of the steps listed in the Methods. These tips trap liquid and aerosol and thus reduce cross-contamination.

9. Freeze thaws will lyse the cell and organelles, liberating RNase which will then degrade the RNA. Thus, freeze thaws must be avoided. If sub-dissecting the brain or spinal cord (11), one might be tempted, after removal of the tissue, to perform the subdissection on a chilled surface such as a glass Petri dish on ice. However, condensation can be a problem.

If the tissue piece is small and condensation occurs on the plate and comes into contact with the tissue sample, this can lyse the cells and the RNA within will rapidly degrade. At present, we perform dissections at room temperature. If we need to collect a large number of brain areas or perform a complicated dissection (i.e. separate removal of lamina I–II, dorsal columns, lamina X and lamina VII–IX from a transverse slice of spinal cord) keeping the tissue chilled is very helpful. Using chilled saline to lubricate the plate surface can help in these circumstances, but each piece of tissue should be frozen quickly. Each small piece of tissue is placed directly into a pre-labeled tube that is on dry ice. Ideally, 1.5 or 2 ml eppendorf tubes should be used due to the volume of reagents needed in subsequent steps for RNA isolation.

10. Although our lab has never encountered RNase contamination, we still consider this a threat. As a result, we periodically clean the work area and pipettors with RNaseZap or RNase Away. Also, to reduce chances of contamination from DNA sources, it may be helpful to use different pipettors for preparing RT-PCR and applying PCR products to gels.
11. If pipetting master mix with a single pipette tip, do not push the plunger of the pipettor beyond the first resistance point. Doing so may result in unequal volumes of master mix being loaded. Only push the plunger beyond the first resistance point while attempting to pipette excess solution back into the Master Mix tube.
12. When setting up RT-PCR reaction, add reagents and RNA to PCR tubes that are placed on ice in order to prevent reverse transcriptase activity.
13. Optimal $MgSO_4$ concentration can increase the efficiency of reverse transcription and amplification. We generally use a final concentration of 1.0 mM $MgSO_4$ in our initial assays. However, a failure to observe the correct amplicon or the identification of too many products with a set of primers (and template) may suggest the need to vary $MgSO_4$ concentrations until the optimal $MgSO_4$ concentration is attained. If no PCR product is observed, then $MgSO_4$ should be increased. If the gel is full of unwanted bands, then $MgSO_4$ concentration should be decreased, for example, to a final concentration of 0.5 mM. *See* also Trouble shooting tips below.
14. We generally use a final concentration of 1 μM for each primer. As with $MgSO_4$ concentration, the concentration of primers can be optimized. However, our preference would be to design primers from other regions of the mRNA rather than change primer concentrations.
15. It is often important to have a positive control to ensure that the primers amplify the correct product. We always try to do this if

possible. For example, if one designs primers for TRPV1 in order to determine whether the encoding gene is expressed in spinal cord, it would be useful for comparative purposes to use RNA extracted from trigeminal or dorsal root ganglia as a control because of the high abundance of this transcript in ganglia.

16. It is also advisable to run a reaction without RNA to ensure that there is no contamination, which could occur if the working area has been exposed to a plasmid containing the gene of interest or if the amplicon has contaminated the work area and/or pipettors.

17. It is important to obtain equivalent signals when running identical samples in different wells of a gel. Given, however, the nonuniformity of many UV transilluminators (12), this may be a challenge, especially if the repeated samples are loaded on opposite ends of the gel. Thus, before using gel-based RT-PCR for semiquantitative purposes, one should run identical samples across the entire gel to determine whether the signals are the same. If nonuniformity exists, then running the PCR product in blocks may be helpful (see Fig. 1). For example, with four different samples, it may be better to run them in an ABCD, ABCD, ABCD pattern instead of an AAA, BBB, CCC, DDD pattern. The former pattern would prevent samples AAA from being artifactually different from DDD if, for example, the left half of the gel yields weaker signals than the right half of the gel (due to nonuniformity of the transillumination).

18. Trouble shooting tips

    Failure to obtain a product

    Check mRNA integrity and RT-PCR procedure by amplifying another gene, e.g. GAPDH, β-actin or another commonly expressed gene

    Check primer integrity by using mRNA from samples known to express the gene of interest

    If mRNA and primers are good, a very low copy number may be in the test sample

        Increase number of cycles for amplification.

    Use nested PCR (i.e. amplify with one primer pair, take product and amplify again with a primer pair that is within the sequence of the first set of primers).

    If mRNA is good and primers do not work

    Increase $MgSO_4$ concentration in RT-PCR reaction (e.g. to 1.5 mM final concentration)

    Lower the annealing temperature

    Pick primers from different region of mRNA

    If unable to amplify any genes with test mRNA

        Re-quantitate diluted and stock RNA concentrations

        Ensure working concentration of 2 ng/μl

Ensure RT-PCR reagents are not contaminated by RNase

If unable to measure RNA, then sample may be degraded or contaminated:

Check how you dissected the tissue. Did it take too long? Was the dissected piece place in contact with condensation? Was there an unintentional freeze thaw?

Ensure water used for diluting RNA is RNase/DNase free

Ensure proper storage of RNA (–80°C)

Ensure working in RNase free environment, do not touch the tubes with your bare hands, the skin has enough RNase on it to degrade your sample.

Background problems on gel

Too many bands

Lower $MgSO_4$ concentration

Raise the annealing temperature

Pick primers from different region of mRNA

Background too high on gel

Soak in tap water

Change exposure time

If needed for quantification

Use lower cycle numbers to prevent saturation

Run standard curve

Acknowledgments

This research was supported by the Intramural Research Program, NIDCR, NIH, DHHS. We thank Dr. H.-Y. T. Yang for helpful comments.

References

1. Yang HY, Mitchell K, Keller JM, Iadarola MJ (2007) Peripheral inflammation increases Scya2 expression in sensory ganglia and cytokine and endothelial related gene expression in inflamed tissue. J Neurochem 103:1628–1643
2. Coghill RC, McHaffie JG, Yen YF (2003) Neural correlates of interindividual differences in the subjective experience of pain. Proc Natl Acad Sci U S A 100:8538–8542
3. Caterina MJ, Schumacher MA, Tominaga M, Rosen TA, Levine JD, Julius D (1997) The capsaicin receptor: a heat-activated ion channel in the pain pathway. Nature 389: 816–824
4. Olah Z, Szabo T, Karai L, Hough C, Fields RD, Caudle RM, Blumberg PM, Iadarola MJ (2001) Ligand-induced dynamic membrane changes and cell deletion conferred by vanilloid receptor 1. J Biol Chem 276:11021–11030
5. Karai L, Brown DC, Mannes AJ, Connelly ST, Brown J, Gandal M, Wellisch OM, Neubert JK, Olah Z, Iadarola MJ (2004) Deletion of

vanilloid receptor 1-expressing primary afferent neurons for pain control. J Clin Invest 113:1344–1352

6. Brown DC, Iadarola MJ, Perkowski SZ, Erin H, Shofer F, Laszlo KJ, Olah Z, Mannes AJ (2005) Physiologic and antinociceptive effects of intrathecal resiniferatoxin in a canine bone cancer model. Anesthesiology 103: 1052–1059
7. Gavva NR (2008) Body-temperature maintenance as the predominant function of the vanilloid receptor TRPV1. Trends Pharmacol Sci 29:550–557
8. Mitchell K, Yang HY, Berk JD, Tran JH, Iadarola MJ (2009) Monocyte chemoattractant protein-1 in the choroid plexus: a potential link between vascular pro-inflammatory mediators and the CNS during peripheral tissue inflammation. Neuroscience 158: 885–895
9. Ali-Seyed M, Laycock N, Karanam S, Xiao W, Blair ET, Moreno CS (2006) Cross-platform expression profiling demonstrates that SV40 small tumor antigen activates Notch, Hedgehog, and Wnt signaling in human cells. BMC Cancer 6:54
10. Brody JR, Calhoun ES, Gallmeier E, Creavalle TD, Kern SE (2004) Ultra-fast high-resolution agarose electrophoresis of DNA and RNA using low-molarity conductive media. Biotechniques 37:598 600, 602
11. Yang HY, Wilkening S, Iadarola MJ (2001) Spinal cord genes enriched in rat dorsal horn and induced by noxious stimulation identified by subtraction cloning and differential hybridization. Neuroscience 103:493–502
12. Chakravarti B, Louie M, Ratanaprayul W, Raval A, Gallagher S, Chakravarti DN (2008) A highly uniform UV transillumination imaging system for quantitative analysis of nucleic acids and proteins. Proteomics 8: 1789–1797
13. Mitchell K, Yang HY, Tessier PA, Muhly WT, Swaim WD, Szalayova I, Keller JM, Mezey E, Iadarola MJ (2008) Localization of S100A8 and S100A9 expressing neutrophils to spinal cord during peripheral tissue inflammation. Pain 134:216–231
14. Kim AY, Tang Z, Liu Q, Patel KN, Maag D, Geng Y, Dong X (2008) Pirt, a phosphoinositide-binding protein, functions as a regulatory subunit of TRPV1. Cell 133:475–485

Chapter 22

Gene-Based Approaches in the Study of Pathological Pain

Elisa Dominguez, Alice Meunier, and Michel Pohl

Abstract

Chronic pathological pain is characterized by extensive plasticity of the systems involved in pain signal transmission and modulation and tissue remodeling in several CNS structures. These long-lasting alterations are mediated by, or associated with, changes in the production of key molecules of nociceptive processing. Gene-based approaches offer the unique possibility of using local or even cell-type specific interventions to correct the abnormal production of some of these proteins, modulate the activity of signal transduction pathways, or overproduce various therapeutic secreted proteins. We showed that certain viral-derived vectors are particularly suitable for mediating gene transfer highly preferential for instance into the primary sensory neurons or into the spinal cord glial cells that represent particularly pertinent targets in the search for new therapeutic strategies of pathological pain.

Key words: Gene therapy, Pathological pain, Glial cells, Spinal cord, Lentiviral vectors

1. Introduction

Management of some forms of chronic pain, especially those of neuropathic origin, is still a real challenge. One of the possible reasons for this unsatisfactory treatment is that most current treatments focus on attenuating neurotransmission, while glial cells activity, though playing a major role in neuropathic pain development, is not yet considered in clinical practice. Another, and in fact, complementary potential explanation is that neuropathic pain is associated with extensive plasticity of the systems involved in pain signal transmission and modulation. Changes in the production of key proteins of nociceptive processing are frequently found to underlie this complex and long-term adaptation. Gene-based techniques allow targeted in situ correction of the abnormal synthesis of these proteins by the delivery of either genes encoding "pain-reducing" proteins or, conversely, nucleic

Arpad Szallasi (ed.), *Analgesia: Methods and Protocols*, Methods in Molecular Biology, vol. 617,
DOI 10.1007/978-1-60327-323-7_22, © Springer Science+Business Media, LLC 2010

acid sequences designed to suppress "pain-inducing" proteins, offering potential new therapeutic strategies.

Huge advances have been made over the past decade in the identification of molecules involved in pathological pain and in the improvement of vector systems (efficacy, specificity, and safety), making these approaches feasible and realistic. It is clear from the constantly increasing number of studies that we are now beyond the phase of demonstration of the feasibility and real therapeutic effect of these approaches. Experimental gene therapy studies suggest that appropriate (distinct) vector systems are needed, depending on the envisaged therapeutic strategy (integration or not of the transgene into the host cell genome, duration of transgene expression, broad or strongly restricted transgene transfer, targeted cell category, etc.) (1, 2).

This chapter should be considered as a guide for the use and application of gene-based approaches in the study of pathological pain rather than a technical protocol for the production of various types of vectors. Our goal is not to provide a "catalogue" of all experimental trials (vectors, targets, transgenes) already carried out in the field of chronic pain, but to show the broad range of possibilities opened up by these techniques. We will provide a detailed description of the procedure for the construction and use of lentiviral vectors that allow highly selective transgene expression in spinal cord glial cells. However, it should be noted that this protocol is also applicable for the construction of other lentiviral vectors.

2. Materials

2.1. Cell Culture (HEK 293T)

1. Dulbecco's Modified Eagle's Medium (DMEM) (Invitrogen, Cergy-Pontoise, France) supplemented with 10% fetal bovine serum (FBS) (Invitrogen), 50 U/mL penicillin G, and 50 μg/mL streptomycin, pH 7.35.
2. Trypsin, 0.05% (1×) with EDTA 4Na (Invitrogen).

2.2. Plasmid Amplification and Transfection

1. Plasmids:

   Expression plasmid pTrip-CMV-WPRE (Dr. Hamid Mammeri, UMR CNRS 7091, Paris, France) containing the super-repressor IκBα coding sequence.

   Plasmid 8.91 (encoding the transregulation proteins).

   Plasmid MD-G (encoding the envelope glycoprotein of vesicular stomatitis virus).
2. LB medium with 50 μg/mL ampicillin (Invitrogen).
3. EndoFree Plasmid Maxi Kit (QIAGEN, Courtaboeuf, France).

4. HBS 2× (pH 7.05): 280 mM NaCl, 50 mM HEPES, and 1.5 mM Na_2HPO_4.
5. 2.5 M $CaCl_2$ solution: dissolve 36.75 g of $CaCl_2$ in 70 mL double distilled (dd) H_2O. Make the solution up to final volume of 100 mL, then filter through a 0.22-μm filter.
6. Chloroquine diphosphate (Merck, Lyon, France).

2.3. Purification of Viral Particles

1. 0.45 μm filters (Millex-HA 0.45 μm MCE 33 mm EtO Ster 50/Pk, Millipore, Guyancourt, France).
2. Dnase I (1 mg/L) (Invitrogen).
3. $MgCl_2$ (2 M).
4. Ultracentrifuge Beckmann with SW48 swinging bucket rotor.
5. Ultracentrifuge tubes and adapter.
6. Phosphate-buffered saline (PBS) (Invitrogen).

2.4. Titration of Lentiviral Vectors

1. p24 ELISA kit (Beckmann Coulter, Roissy, France).
2. HEK 293T cell cultures.
3. 24-Well plates (Nunc, ATGC, Marne la Vallée, France).
4. Microscope cover glasses (Marienfeld GmbH & Co., Dominique Dutcher, Brumath, France) sterilized in an oven at 200°C.
5. Rabbit anti-IκBα antibodies (1/100, Santa Cruz Biotechnology, Santa Cruz, CA).

3. Methods

Before setting up an experimental protocol involving gene-based approaches, several important questions should be answered:

1. Do I seek a broad, restricted (local) or highly targeted gene transfer?
2. Do I need long-term or temporary transgene production?
3. Do I want to assess the potential implication of a target gene in a physiological process or do I want to set up a real (although experimental in its first phase in animals) gene therapy strategy?
4. What is the safety status of a given vector and are there particular security limitations associated with its use?

Wherever possible, the use of "synthetic vectors" (naked or complexed expression plasmid DNA) is beneficial (rapid preparation, minimal technical constraints, safe and easy to handle). One example of a relevant and potentially interesting application of plasmid DNA is the intrathecal administration of a plasmid bearing a secreted therapeutic protein (3). No specific cell type is targeted in this approach and there is no need for focal transgene expression; in fact, this strategy provides a large vector spread, presumably leading to a broad release of "therapeutic" protein into the intrathecal space.

Recent technical advances may also help circumvent the limitations associated with synthetic vectors. In particular, strategies for improved stability of these vectors in physiological fluids (serum, CSF) and offering the possibility of receptor targeting (thus probably targeting various cell types) are currently being developed. However, issues such as limited penetration in some tissues or the relatively short duration of transgene production are still problematic and may rapidly hamper the potential use of synthetic vectors.

Currently, viral-derived vectors seem to be preferred for many applications, despite some associated constraints (construction procedures, handling, possible toxicity). Viral vector-induced immune response is a major potential drawback, leading to cell toxicity and blockade of transgene expression. However, the deletion of several genes from viral genomic DNA (or even the majority of genes from some viruses) greatly improves the safety of viral vectors and reduces their capacity to elicit an immune response. Interestingly, although intrathecal or intracisternal administration of some vectors (e.g. adenoviral-derived vectors) may stimulate a substantial systemic immune response, direct intraparenchymal injection of these vectors is, in most cases, devoid of such an effect.

Viral-derived vectors thus appear to be beneficial for a number of experimental protocols, as they allow good tissue penetration, gene transfer into post-mitotic cells, targeting of several particular cell types, sustained and high-level transgene expression, eventual transgene integration into the host genome.

The anatomical and functional organization of the system of pain signal transmission and modulation allows intervention to be envisaged at several levels.

Peripheral tissues

Peripheral structures may be considered as targets per se or as a means of accessing the central nervous system (departure point of motor or sensory neurons). Various gene transfer techniques have thus been tested in peripheral tissues that are, in principle, easily accessible. These transfer approaches include gene-gun delivery of DNA, direct injection (or electroporation) of plasmid (naked, complexed) DNA and the use of different viral vectors. Thus, for instance, rat skin was transfected with plasmid DNA using gene-gun delivery (4), peripheral nerves (sciatic nerve) were directly injected with adeno-associated viral (AAV) vectors (5), the bladder wall was injected with plasmid DNA or Herpes simplex virus (HSV)-derived vectors (6, 7), joints were injected with HSV- (8), lentivirus- (9) or adenovirus-derived vectors (10), skeletal muscles were electroporated with plasmid DNA (11) or injected with adenoviral vector (12).

Primary sensory neurons (spinal, trigeminal)

Primary sensory neurons are naturally a target of choice. Direct injection of AAV vectors into the sciatic nerve may be envisaged, as mentioned above, and primary sensory neurons may be targeted using HSV-derived vectors. HSV are not only strongly neurotropic but, in addition, primary sensory neurons are their natural targets. Peripheral administration of HSV vectors leads to viral entry into the nerve terminals, followed by rapid retrograde transport to the cell bodies of sensory neurons in sensory ganglia, where HSV remains episomal. HSV vectors may therefore be administered at various sites, depending on the targeted structure. Administration on facial skin (13) allows the efficient transfection of trigeminal sensory ganglia. Dorsal root ganglia may be targeted by HSV vectors administered in skin on the feet (14–18) or back (19), into the bladder wall (6) or pancreas surface (20), or by vectors injected into the sciatic nerve (21) or joint capsule (22). Recently, infection of sensory neurons with AAV serotype 8-derived vector using intrathecal delivery was reported (23), but the actual capacity of these vectors to selectively (or, at least, preferentially) target primary sensory neurons needs to be explored further. The subcutaneous injection of synthetic vectors is also a possible means of targeting primary sensory neurons (24).

Central nervous system (spinal cord, brain)

The spinal cord is another potential site of intervention. Studies over the past decade have clearly demonstrated that neurons are not the only possible targets for novel therapies; indeed, spinal glial cells (and perhaps other cell types, such as pia mater cells), with important roles in pain processing, are of great interest. Several trials have been undertaken, using intrathecal administration of vectors to efficiently transduce spinal cord neurons. Once again, the injection of naked or complexed plasmid DNA (combined with electroporation technique or not) (3, 25, 26) or administration of various types of viral vectors were tested (27–30). Overall, these studies concluded that intrathecal administration of currently available vectors is not an optimal way to transfer a transgene into the spinal cord parenchyma, at least at the present time. Indeed, in most cases, intrathecal administration of vectors resulted in marked transgene expression in pia mater cells, nerve roots or in DRG, but only moderate to weak transgene production in spinal cord parenchyma. The direct intraparenchymal injection of vectors appears necessary for potent transgene transfer into the spinal cord tissue (31–35). For many technical and, possibly, "ethical" reasons, few gene-based studies specifically concerning pain have been performed in the brain. Studies addressing this site of intervention used HSV-derived vectors (36, 37).

As discussed above, spinal cord glial cells are important targets for potential gene-based intervention. Lentiviral vectors could be useful for preferential gene transfer into these cells in the spinal cord. Interestingly, HIV (*human immunodeficiency virus*)- and EIAV (*equine infectious anemia virus*)-derived vectors display differences in tropism in the spinal cord, despite being pseudotyped with identical glycoprotein envelope proteins (VSV) (34). In a comparison of various combinations of envelope proteins and promoters, we showed that HIV-derived vectors pseudotyped with VSV and driving transgene expression under CMV promoter led, both in vitro and in vivo, to strongly preferential transgene expression in rat spinal cord glial cells (38, 39). Here, we provide a detailed protocol for the production of this type of vector.

The sequence of interest (super-repressor IκBα) is subcloned into an expression plasmid (pTrip-CMV-WPRE) containing the CMV promoter and the *cis*-acting woodchuck hepatitis virus post-transcriptional regulatory element (WPRE). Lentiviral vectors are generated by co-transfecting (using calcium phosphate precipitation method) three plasmids into HEK293T cells: pTrip-IκBα and plasmids encoding envelope proteins (vesicular stomatitis virus glycoprotein, pMD-G) and trans-regulation proteins (p8.91). Supernatants containing lentiviral vectors are concentrated by ultracentrifugation and then resuspended in phosphate buffered saline (PBS) and frozen (–80°C) until use. It is important to ensure a good quality of viral suspension during vector preparation. Several steps of purification are performed throughout the preparation to minimize the presence of cellular debris. Because of the capacity of IκBα to interfere with HIV-derived vector production, this protocol differs slightly from the classical protocol for production of lentiviral vectors (40). Twice as many plates (40) of HEK 293 T cells are co-transfected with p8.91 and pTrip-IκBα at a ratio of 2:1 (p8.91: pTrip-IκBα).

3.1. Plasmid Preparation and Plating of HEK 293 T Cells

1. Plasmids pTrip-IκBα, pMD-G and p8.91 should be prepared under endotoxin-free conditions to improve the quality of transfection (see Note 1).
2. Plate HEK 293 T cells (2×10^6) onto forty 10 cm^2 plates to be transfected 48 h later (see Note 2).

3.2. Co-transfection

1. Remove half of the culture medium (5 mL) 1 h (minimum) before co-transfection, and replace with 4 mL of fresh culture medium.
2. To obtain a calcium-phosphate/DNA precipitate:

   All products must be at room temperature before starting.

   For 40 plates of HEK 293 T cells, mix:

- 400 μg of pTrip-IκBα
- 800 μg of p8.91
- 200 μg of pMD-G
- 2 mL of $CaCl_2$ (2.5M)
- Add sterile water to give a final volume of 20 mL

Prepare four Falcon tubes containing 5 mL of HBS 2× and divide the 20 mL of $CaCl_2$/DNA preparation between these four tubes drop by drop (5 mL/tube), while bubbling air through the HBS with a Pasteur pipette, to form 40 mL of precipitate at the end.

The obtained precipitate could be shaken if bubbles are not fine enough (see Note 3).

3. Add 100 μl of chloroquin, drop by drop across each plate of HEK 293 T cells (this enhances the transfection efficiency by inhibiting DNA degradation by lysosomes).
4. Add 1 mL of precipitate, drop by drop, to each plate. Swirl the plates gently before return in cell incubator (5% CO_2; 37°C).
5. Culture medium should be changed 6 h after transfection to avoid toxicity (~9 mL).

3.3. Preparation of Viral Particles

1. Forty-eight hours after transfection, harvest the culture media of 20 plates and centrifuge to remove cellular debris (1,000 g, 8 min) (see Note 4).
2. To further eliminate cellular debris, pass supernatants through 0.45 μm filter.
3. To avoid DNA/protein aggregates in the stocks, add 50 μl of Dnase I (1 mg/l) and 50 μl $MgCl_2$ (2 M) per 50 mL of supernatant. Mix by inverting the tube four times and incubate at 37°C for 20 min.
4. Vectors are concentrated by ultracentrifugation (56,000×*g*, 1.5 h, 4°C).
5. Discard supernatant and invert the tube on paper towels. Carefully dry the tube walls with Kimwipes® or Q-type. Avoid any contact with the viral pellet.
6. Add filtered culture media from resting 20 plates (processed as described above) in ultracentrifuge tubes containing concentrate viral suspension and centrifuge (56,000×*g*, 1.5 h, 4°C) once more.
7. Discard supernatant, invert the tube on paper towels and dry the tubes walls.
8. Apply 75 μl of PBS 1× onto the pellet and place at 4°C for a minimum of 2 h.
9. Gently resuspend the pellets and pool them together in 1.5 mL microcentrifuge Eppendorf® tube.

10. Briefly centrifuge (~6,000×g) the solution containing viral particles and the resting cellular debris and resuspend (using pipette with 200 μl tips) the pellet to separate aggregates; the pellet should be completely solubilized.
11. To eliminate remaining cellular debris, centrifuge briefly at low speed (~6,000×g) and carefully remove the supernatant (=viral suspension). This step must be repeated until the smallest cellular debris disappears (~10 times) (see Note 5).
12. Aliquot the final viral suspension (aliquots of 10 μl are appropriate for most applications) in prechilled 0.5 mL Eppendorf® tubes and store them at −80°C until use.

3.4. Titration of Lentiviral Vectors

Two types of titration procedure can be performed to check the quality of lentiviral vector production.

- p24 protein, a viral capsid protein, may be assayed by enzyme-linked immunosorbent assay (ELISA) in triplicate, according to the manufacturer's instruction (Beckmann Coulter) (see Note 6).
- Alternatively, the viral suspension could be titrated by transducing HEK 293T cells with successive (1/10) dilutions of the stock. Titration can then be evaluated by FACS, detecting Green Fluorescent Protein (GFP) in cells expressing the transgene, or by immunocytochemistry with antibodies targeting the transgene product. The following protocol describes viral vector titration using immunocytochemistry detection of transgene-derived protein (transgene construct not containing a GFP marker).

1. Plate HEK 293T cells onto a 24-well plate (6×10^6 cells/well) on sterilized glass coverslips.
2. After 24 h, prepare successive dilutions of the viral stock, ranging from ~10^{-5} to 10^{-12}/mL in duplicate.

   Ex: add 10 μl of viral stock to 990 μl of culture medium (10^{-5}) and mix well. Take 90 μl of the first dilution and add 810 μl of culture medium (10^{-6}).
3. Remove culture medium and replace it with 500 μl of fresh medium containing appropriate viral dilution.
4. Forty-eight hours after cell transduction, cells are washed in PBS 1× and fixed with 4% paraformaldehyde (5 min); they are then washed three times with PBS 1× and prepared for classical immunocytochemistry with IκBα antibodies (see Note 7).
5. Count the number of plaques of immunoreactive cells per well, starting with the highest dilution. Note that correct lentiviral vector production should have a titer of about 10^{-9} (see Note 8).

3.5. Verification of the Production of Transgene-Derived Protein from the Viral Vector and of its Functional Efficacy

Verification of correct production of transgene-derived protein is fundamental before any experimental procedure with constructed vectors. Immunocytochemistry experiments used to estimate viral titer demonstrate that an immunoreactive material recognized with specific antibodies is indeed produced from vectors. However, western blots are then needed to determine whether the molecular weight of the vector-derived protein corresponds to the expected size. The relationship between the viral titer and the level of transgene-derived protein produced should also be checked. Finally, wherever possible, and depending on the nature of transgene, the functional efficacy of the product should be assessed in in vitro experiments before using the vector in vivo (see Note 9). Upon completion of these preliminary checks the vector can be moved to the animal. In vivo experiments should start with the demonstration of vector spread, identification of the cell type(s) effectively transduced, evaluation of the tissue levels of the transgene-derived molecule and its production over time (short-lasting versus sustained production).

4. Notes

1. The quality of DNA is important for a successful [homogeneous and without excessive cell mortality] co-transfection of cells. Unlike some other plasmid preparation kits, the EndoFree Plasmid Maxi Kit, QIAGEN gives consistent preparations of high quality DNA in several laboratories dealing with these techniques.
2. HEK 293 T cells grow rapidly and cover the plate surface without being firmly attached; be gentle when handling plates and changing the medium.
3. Bubbling with a Pasteur pipette is recommended to reduce the bubble size and improve the quality of the precipitate. You may use a source of compressed air or simply plug your Pasteur pipette on an automatic "pipette boy".
4. The culture media of the remaining 20 plates are processed later, during the first ultracentrifugation step.
5. This step is particularly important because cellular debris can elicit an immune response and, in our case for instance, could lead to glial activation after intraparenchymal injection of vector suspension.
6. The concentration of p24 protein reflects the quantity of total viral particles, including both empty particles and those containing viral ARN (with desired transgene).

7. Cells continue to multiply after transduction with lentiviral vector and will thus form the so-called plaques of transduction.
8. Ex: five plaques of transduction are counted for the dilution 10^{-9}. The viral suspension thus has a titer of 5×10^{9} TU/ml.
9. Thus, for instance, you should demonstrate that a vector producing a secreted protein is able to induce internalization of its specific receptor or modify associated ionic currents, that a vector synthesizing a protein targeting some intracellular pathway is really able to modify the activity of this pathway, or that a vector bearing a shRNA is able to knock-down its target protein.

Acknowledgments

This work was supported by grants from INSERM, Université Pierre et Marie Curie-Paris 6, Institut UPSA de la Douleur and Institut pour la Recherche sur la Moelle épinière et l'Encéphale.

References

1. Lowenstein PR, Castro MG (2004) Recent advances in the pharmacology of neurological gene therapy. Curr Opin Pharmacol 4:91–97
2. Schubert M, Breakefield X, Federoff H, Frederickson M, Lowenstein PR (2008) Gene delivery to the nervous system. Mol Ther 16:640–646
3. Milligan ED, Sloane EM, Langer SJ, Hughes TS, Jekich BM, Frank MG, Mahoney JH, Levkoff LH, Maier SF, Cruz PE, Flotte TR, Johnson KW, Mahoney MM, Chavez RA, Leinwand LA, Watkins LR (2006) Repeated intrathecal injections of plasmid DNA encoding interleukin-10 produce prolonged reversal of neuropathic pain. Pain 126:294–308
4. Lu CY, Chou AK, Wu CL, Yang CH, Chen JT, Wu PC, Lin SH, Muhammad R, Yang LC (2002) Gene-gun particle with pro-opiomelanocortin cDNA produces analgesia against formalin-induced pain in rats. Gene Ther 9:1008–1014
5. Xu Y, Gu Y, Wu P, Li GW, Huang LY (2003) Efficiencies of transgene expression in nociceptive neurons through different routes of delivery of adeno-associated viral vectors. Hum Gene Ther 14:897–9006
6. Yoshimura N, Franks ME, Sasaki K, Goins WF, Goss J, Yokoyama T, Fraser MO, Seki S, Fink J, Glorioso J, de Groat WC, Chancellor MB (2001) Gene therapy of bladder pain with herpes simplex virus (HSV) vectors expressing preproenkephalin (PPE). Urology 57(6 Suppl. 1):116
7. Chuang YC, Chou AK, Wu PC, Chiang PH, Yu TJ, Yang LC, Yoshimura N, Chancellor MB (2003) Gene therapy for bladder pain with gene gun particle encoding pro-opiomelanocortin cDNA. J Urol 170:2044–2048
8. Oligino T, Ghivizzani S, Wolfe D, Lechman E, Krisky D, Mi Z, Evans C, Robbins P, Glorioso J (1999) Intra-articular delivery of a herpes simplex virus IL-1Ra gene vector reduces inflammation in a rabbit model of arthritis. Gene Ther 6:1713–1720
9. Kyrkanides S, Kambylafkas P, Miller JH, Tallents RH (2004) Non-primate lentiviral vector administration in the TMJ. J Dent Res 83:65–70
10. Woods JM, Amin MA, Katschke KJ Jr, Volin MV, Ruth JH, Connors MA, Woodruff DC, Kurata H, Arai K, Haines GK 3rd, Kumar P, Koch AE (2002) Interleukin-13 gene therapy reduces inflammation, vascularization, and bony destruction in rat adjuvant-induced arthritis. Hum Gene Ther 13:381–393
11. Murakami T, Arai M, Sunada Y, Nakamura A (2006) VEGF 164 gene transfer by electroporation improves diabetic sensory neuropathy in mice. J Gene Med 8:773–781

12. Pradat PF, Kennel P, Naimi-Sadaoui S, Finiels F, Orsini C, Revah F, Delaere P, Mallet J (2001) Continuous delivery of neurotrophin 3 by gene therapy has a neuroprotective effect in experimental models of diabetic and acrylamide neuropathies. Hum Gene Ther 12:2237–2249
13. Meunier A, Latrémolière A, Mauborgne A, Bourgoin S, Kayser V, Cesselin F, Hamon M, Pohl M (2005) Attenuation of pain-related behavior in a rat model of trigeminal neuropathic pain by viral-driven enkephalin overproduction in trigeminal ganglion neurons. Mol Ther 11:608–616
14. Antunes Bras JM, Epstein AE, Bourgoin S, Hamon M, Cesselin F, Pohl M (1998) Herpes simplex virus 1-mediated transfer of preproenkephalin A in rat dorsal root ganglia. J Neurochem 70:1299–1303
15. Wilson SP, Yeomans DC, Bender MA, Lu Y, Goins WF, Glorioso JC (1999) Antihyperalgesic effects of infection with a preproenkephalin-encoding herpes virus. Proc Natl Acad Sci U S A 96:3211–3216
16. Braz J, Beaufour C, Coutaux A, Epstein AL, Cesselin F, Hamon M, Pohl M (2001) Therapeutic efficacy in experimental polyarthritis of viral-driven enkephalin overproduction in sensory neurons. J Neurosci 21: 7881–7888
17. Hao S, Mata M, Goins W, Glorioso JC, Fink DJ (2003) Transgene-mediated enkephalin release enhances the effect of morphine and evades tolerance to produce a sustained antiallodynic effect in neuropathic pain. Pain 102:135–142
18. Zhou Z, Peng X, Hao S, Fink DJ, Mata M (2008) HSV-mediated transfer of interleukin-10 reduces inflammatory pain through modulation of membrane tumor necrosis factor alpha in spinal cord microglia. Gene Ther 15:183–190
19. Yeomans DC, Lu Y, Laurito CE, Peters MC, Vota-Vellis G, Wilson SP, Pappas GD (2006) Recombinant herpes vector-mediated analgesia in a primate model of hyperalgesia. Mol Ther 13:589–597
20. Yang H, McNearney TA, Chu R, Lu Y, Ren Y, Yeomans DC, Wilson SP, Westlund KN (2008) Enkephalin-encoding herpes simplex virus-1 decreases inflammation and hotplate sensitivity in a chronic pancreatitis model. Mol Pain 4. doi:10.1186/1744-8069-4-8
21. Palmer JA, Branston RH, Lilley CE, Robinson MJ, Groutsi F, Smith J, Latchman DS, Coffin RS (2000) Development and optimization of herpes simplex virus vectors for multiple long-term gene delivery to the peripheral nervous system. J Virol 74:5604–5618
22. Lu Y, McNearney TA, Wilson SP, Yeomans DC, Westlund KN (2008) Joint capsule treatment with enkephalin-encoding HSV-1 recombinant vector reduces inflammatory damage and behavioural sequelae in rat CFA monoarthritis. Eur J Neurosci 27: 1153–1165
23. Storek B, Reinhardt M, Wang C, Janssen WG, Harder NM, Banck MS, Morrison JH, Beutler AS (2008) Sensory neuron targeting by self-complementary AAV8 via lumbar puncture for chronic pain. Proc Natl Acad Sci U S A 105:1055–1060
24. Thakor D, Spigelman I, Tabata Y, Nishimura I (2007) Subcutaneous peripheral injection of cationized gelatin/DNA polyplexes as a platform for non-viral gene transfer to sensory neurons. Mol Ther 15:2124–2131
25. Lin CR, Yang LC, Lee TH, Lee CT, Huang HT, Sun WZ, Cheng JT (2002) Electroporation-mediated pain-killer gene therapy for mononeuropathic rats. Gene Ther 9:1247–1253
26. Yao MZ, Gu JF, Wang JH, Sun LY, Lang MF, Liu J, Zhao ZQ, Liu XY (2002) Interleukin-2 gene therapy of chronic neuropathic pain. Neuroscience 112:409–416
27. Finegold AA, Mannes AJ, Iadarola MJ (1999) A paracrine paradigm for in vivo gene therapy in the central nervous system: treatment of chronic pain. Hum Gene Ther 10:1251–1257
28. Milligan ED, Sloane EM, Langer SJ, Cruz PE, Chacur M, Spataro L, Wieseler-Frank J, Hammack SE, Maier SF, Flotte TR, Forsayeth JR, Leinwand LA, Chavez R, Watkins LR (2005) Controlling neuropathic pain by adeno-associated virus driven production of the anti-inflammatory cytokine, interleukin-10. Mol Pain 1. doi:10.1186/1744-8069-1-9
29. Yao MZ, Gu JF, Wang JH, Sun LY, Liu H, Liu XY (2003) Adenovirus-mediated interleukin-2 gene therapy of nociception. Gene Ther 10:1392–1399
30. Storek B, Harder NM, Banck MS, Wang C, McCarty DM, Janssen WG, Morrison JH, Walsh CE, Beutler AS (2006) Intrathecal long-term gene expression by self-complementary adeno-associated virus type 1 suitable for chronic pain studies in rats. Mol Pain 2. doi:10.1186/1744-8069-2-4
31. Eaton MJ, Blits B, Ruitenberg MJ, Verhaagen J, Oudega M (2002) Amelioration of chronic neuropathic pain after partial nerve injury by adeno-associated viral (AAV) vector-mediated

over-expression of BDNF in the rat spinal cord. Gene Ther 9:1387–1395

32. Tang XQ, Tanelian DL, Smith GM (2004) Semaphorin3A inhibits nerve growth factor-induced sprouting of nociceptive afferents in adult rat spinal cord. J Neurosci 24:819–827
33. Tappe A, Klugmann M, Luo C, Hirlinger D, Agarwal N, Benrath J, Ehrengruber MU, During MJ, Kuner R (2006) Synaptic scaffolding protein Homer1a protects against chronic inflammatory pain. Nat Med 12:677–681
34. Pezet S, Krzyzanowska A, Wong LF, Grist J, Mazarakis ND, Georgievska B, McMahon SB (2006) Reversal of neurochemical changes and pain-related behavior in a model of neuropathic pain using modified lentiviral vectors expressing GDNF. Mol Ther 13:1101–1109
35. Chen SL, Ma HI, Han JM, Tao PL, Law PY, Loh HH (2007) dsAAV type 2-mediated gene transfer of MORS196A-EGFP into spinal cord as a pain management paradigm. Proc Natl Acad Sci U S A 104:20096–20101
36. Kang W, Wilson MA, Bender MA, Glorioso JC, Wilson SP (1998) Herpes virus-mediated preproenkephalin gene transfer to the amygdala is antinociceptive. Brain Res 792:133–135
37. Jasmin L, Rabkin SD, Granato A, Boudah A, Ohara PT (2003) Analgesia and hyperalgesia from GABA-mediated modulation of the cerebral cortex. Nature 424:316–320
38. Meunier A, Latrémolière A, Dominguez E, Mauborgne A, Mallet J, Phillipe S, Pohl M (2007) Lentiviral-mediated targeted NF-κB blockade in dorsal spinal cord glia attenuates sciatic nerve injury-induced hyperalgesia in rat. Mol Ther 15:687–697
39. Meunier A, Mauborgne A, Masson J, Mallet J, Pohl M (2008) Lentiviral-mediated targeted transgene expression in dorsal spinal cord glia: tool for the study of glial cell implication in mechanisms underlying chronic pain development. J Neurosci Methods 167:148–159
40. Zennou V, Serguera C, Sarkis C, Colin P, Perret E, Mallet J, Charneau P (2001) The HIV-1 DNA flap stimulates HIV vector-mediated cell transduction in the brain. Nat Biotechnol 19:446–450

Chapter 23

Linkage Analysis and Functional Evaluation of Inherited Clinical Pain Conditions

Johannes J. Krupp, Dennis Hellgren, and Anders B. Eriksson

Abstract

Because ion channel function is a fundamental element of any nociceptive signalling, it is not surprising that numerous channelopathies have recently emerged as likely causes of several inherited clinical pain conditions. For example, numerous missense mutations in the $Na_v1.7$ gene *SCN9A* have recently been linked to a congenital inability to sense pain. Establishing the link between a clinical pain phenotype to an inherited molecular dysfunction of a specific protein has its challenges and requires the collaboration between many specialists. However, once established, such a linkage offers the promise of a powerful and elegant way to mechanistically explain the aspects of the disease studied.

Key words: Channelopathies, Insensitivity to pain, Blood sample, Linkage analysis, Sequencing, Patch-clamp, Heterologous expression

1. Introduction

Recently, three rare clinical pain conditions with a congenital background – erythromelalgia (1, 2), paroxysmal extreme pain disorder (3), and congenital inability to experience pain (4–6) – have been linked to mutations in the gene *SCN9A*, encoding the voltage-gated sodium channel $Na_v1.7$. As expected from congenital inherited diseases, the identified mutations are typically unique to the studied pedigree. Yet, despite the fact that numerous mutations have been identified for each clinical phenotype, the effect of these mutations on the functionality of $Na_v1.7$ can be grouped according to the clinical phenotype. Thus, both erythromelalgia (1, 2) and paroxysmal extreme pain disorder (3) link to mutations that cause hyperactivity of the mutated voltage-gated sodium channels, either by shifting the voltage-dependence of activation in

Arpad Szallasi (ed.), *Analgesia: Methods and Protocols*, Methods in Molecular Biology, vol. 617,
DOI 10.1007/978-1-60327-323-7_23, © Springer Science+Business Media, LLC 2010

the hyperpolarizing direction (7, 8) or by attenuating fast inactivation (3). In contrast, mutations that link to congenital inability to experience pain are all nonsense mutations of $Na_v1.7$, producing truncated, non-functional proteins (4–6). These studies clearly indicate that $Na_v1.7$ is a critical element of peripheral nociception in humans and thus a highly interesting target for pharmacological intervention (9). Considering the preclinical data for several other voltage-gated sodium channels (10, 11), it is, however, somewhat surprising that so far no congenital inherited clinical pain conditions could be linked to other voltage-gated sodium channels.

Here, we describe a procedure for linkage analysis of congenital inherited pain phenotypes and subsequent study of the identified mutation(s). The methods described are not only applicable to the identification of channelopathies associated with *SCN9A*, but also to the possible channelopathies associated with other voltage-gated sodium channels. Furthermore, similar protocols should be useful for any other gene and gene product where an electrophysiological read-out can be established.

2. Materials

2.1. Blood Samples

1. 5 or 10 ml EDTA vacutainer tubes. Blood samples can be frozen if necessary and should be stored at –80°C for long durations. Frozen samples can be shipped on CO_2-ice.
2. Qiaamp DNA Blood Midi or Maxi kit (Qiagen, Germantown, MD).

2.2. Whole Genome Scan

1. Linkage Mapping Set version 2.5 (Applied Biosystems, Foster City, CA). There are two versions available, with 5 or 10 cM spacing between markers.

2.3. Bioinformatics and Literature Analysis

1. A standard computer with internet access.
2. Access to the following web sites:

   ENSEMBL: http://www.ensembl.org/index.html,

   NCBI Genome Biology application: http://www.ncbi.nlm.nih.gov/Genomes/,

   UCSC Genome Browser: http://genome.ucsc.edu/,

   Nucleic Acids Research: http://nar.oxfordjournals.org/,

   Allen Brain Bank: http://www.brain-map.org/,

   Human Protein Atlas: http://www.proteinatlas.org/,

   Gene Expression Omnibus: http://www.ncbi.nlm.nih.gov/projects/geo/

3. Access to these additional websites is also helpful:

   http://www.ncbi.nlm.nih.gov/genome/guide/mouse/

   http://www.informatics.jax.org/

   http://phenome.jax.org/pub-cgi/phenome/mpdcgi?rtn=docs/home

   http://www.ncbi.nlm.nih.gov/genome/guide/rat/

   http://rgd.mcw.edu/

2.4. Bidirectional Sequencing

1. 96-well PCR and sequencing reaction plates (ABgene, Epsom, United Kingdom).
2. Big Dye Terminator v3.1 Cycle Sequencing Kit (Applied Biosystems).
3. Thermal Cycler (MJ Research DNA engine, BioRad, Hercules, CA).
4. Microcentrifuge.
5. Centrifuge with variable speed with microtiter plate holders.
6. QIAquick 96 PCR purification kit (Qiagen).
7. QIAvac 96 vacuum manifold (Qiagen).
8. HAD-GT12 DNA/RNA analyser (eGene, Qiagen).
9. Dye Terminator removal Kit, 96-format spin plates (ABgene).

2.5. Site-Directed Mutagenesis

1. Quick Change II Site Directed Mutagenesis Kit (Stratagene/Agilent, La Jolla, CA).
2. Thermal Cycler (MJ Research DNA engine).
3. QIAprep Spin Miniprep Kit (Qiagen).
4. Microcentrifuge.
5. SOC medium: to 950 ml of double deionized H_2O add 20 g Bacto-tryptone, 5 g Bacto-yeast extract, 0.5 g NaCl, and 2.5 ml of a 1 M KCl-solution, adjust with ddH_2O to a 1 L volume. Adjust pH to 7.0 with 10 N NaOH, autoclave to sterilize, add 20 ml of sterile 1 M glucose solution immediately before use.

2.6. Transient Transfection and Cell Culture

1. HEK293 cells and ND7/23 cells (ATCC, Manassas, VA).
2. Access to a sterile fume hood and a cell culture incubator that allows control of humidity, temperature, and environment.
3. Sterile non-pyrogenic plastic pipettes, Costar Stripette (Corning, New York, NY): 1, 2, 10, 25, and 50 ml.
4. Sterile, non-pyrogenic 25 cm^2 and 75 cm^2 cell culture flasks from polystyrene with vented caps and canted necks.
5. All solutions described below should be stored in a fridge (4°C) when not used. Prior to use warm all solutions to a temperature between 30 and 35°C.

6. DMEM F-12 (Gibco/BRL, Bethesda, MD) for culture of HEK293 cells, supplemented with 10% FBS. This solution is best prepared in advance by adding (under sterile conditions) 50 ml of FBS to a fresh 500 ml bottle of DMEM F-12. For the splitting procedure, trypsin is needed.
7. DMEM/Glutamax (Gibco/BRL) for culture of ND7/23 cells with 10% FBS added. This solution is best prepared in advance by adding (under sterile conditions) 50 ml of FBS to a fresh 500 ml bottle of DMEM + Glutamax. For the splitting procedure, Accutase (Gibco) is used.
8. Lipofectamine 2000 (Invitrogen, Carlsbad, CA).
9. Sterile 15-ml plastic polypropylene Falcon tubes.
10. Plasmid DNA of interest (as prepared in Subheading 3.5); a cDNA encoding a suitable transfection marker like pZsGreen1-N1 (Clontech, Mountain View, CA).
11. 35-mm diameter cell culture petri dishes.

2.7. Electrophysiology

1. Vibration-isolated, conventional whole-cell patch-clamp set-up that includes a high-powered microscope with a filter setting that allows detection of green fluorescence, a micromanipulator, a patch-clamp amplifier, and a computer with applicable software (see Note 1).
2. Pipette puller (e.g. DMZ-Universal Puller, Zeitz-Instrumente, München, Germany).
3. Borosilicate glass (GC150, Harvard Apparatus Ltd., Edenbridge, Kent, UK).
4. Intracellular solution: 140 mM Cs-gluconate, 1.2 mM $MgCl_2$, 10 mM HEPES, 10 mM EGTA 10, pH 7.2 (CsOH).
5. To fill the patch pipettes with intracellular solution, first fill a 1-ml syringe with the intracellular solution. Then attach a syringe-driven filter unit for the clarification of aqueous solutions with a 0.45-μm mixed cellulose ester membrane (25 mm diameter; Millipore, Bedford, MA) and a nonmetallic syringe needle for filling micropipettes (MicroFil 34; World Precision Instruments, Sarasota, FL). Patch pipettes are filled from the back.
6. Extracellular solution: 137 mM NaCl 137, 5 mM KCl, 1 mM $CaCl_2$, 1.2 mM $MgCl_2$, 10 mM HEPES, 10 mM glucose, pH 7.4 (NaOH).
7. A superfusion chamber-insert for the Petri dish (Bioscience Tools, San Diego, CA).
8. Tubings for continuous bath superfusion that connect into the superfusion insert, including an inlet from a reservoir containing extracellular solution and an outlet to a waste container (see Note 2).

3. Methods

Mapping and identifying a gene involved in a genetic disorder is a procedure that requires collaboration between many types of specialists: clinicians, geneticists, statistical genetic expertise, and molecular biologists. We have chosen to give only a brief overview of the mapping step and to give introductory links to bioinformatics resources that can be used later in a candidate selection step. It is advised that at least the initial mapping step is done in collaboration with a genetic group with experience in gene mapping.

The most important factor when trying to identify a gene involved in a genetic disorder is the identification of a suitable family or several families with the same disorder. In the majority of cases, the initial information about such a family will come through contact with a clinician who is aware of or actively treating patients within such a family. Multigeneration families are required as data from such pedigree greatly facilitates statistical analysis. It also allows to address the question whether one is dealing with a monogenic disorder or a multifactorial disorder, i.e. a disorder dependent on more than one gene.

A good clinical characterization of the families in question is important and extremely helpful to correlate the mutations identified with their clinical phenotype. This will be helpful to start an understanding of gene function. Furthermore, expert clinical characterization may allow an early identification of a possible issue of phenocopies, i.e. the presence of mutations in different genes in different families that give rise to an apparently identical clinical phenotype.

3.1. Handling of Samples

1. It should be stressed that before any samples can be obtained and worked on, an informed consent (IC) has to be presented, explained, and signed by every participant. IC should contain information on what the purpose of the study is, how data will be stored, and so forth. An IC needs to be written in an easily readable and understandable style. It is imperative that you involve your local ethics committee into this procedure.
2. Once a suitable family has been identified and IC has been obtained, a blood sample is obtained from as many family members as possible. Blood sampling needs to be done by a licensed nurse or clinician, and it is mandatory that you follow the applicable laws and ethical guidelines.
3. Blood sampling should not be restricted to the affected individuals within the family, but should also include healthy family members, as well as cases with an intermediate phenotype, if such a phenotype is apparent within the family.

Data from healthy family members will serve as a control as these individuals should not have a mutated gene. An intermediate phenotype could be due to a gene dosage effect. For example, in case of a recessive disorder, such individuals may have only one mutated copy of a gene.

4. DNA can then be prepared by using any of the commercial kits available on the market, following the instructions provided by the manufacturer. The DNA is quality controlled using a spectrophotometer and plated on a master plate at a concentration suitable for typing with genetic markers. A master plate is then used for the preparation of daughter plates, which in turn are used for the actual genotyping.

3.2. Whole Genome Scan

1. The next step is mapping of the genetic disorder by typing chromosomal markers. There are commercial sets of markers available. We typically use the linkage mapping set from Applied Biosystems, both the 5 and the 10 cM version. The idea behind these markers is the use of genetic recombination to link a gene to a specific chromosomal marker.
2. Recombination is a process whereby homologous chromosomes exchange segments with each other during meiosis. The exchange is in principle a random process and can occur anywhere along a chromosome. As the distance between a marker and a gene increases, the probability that they will be linked genetically decreases, i.e. the likelihood that a recombination occurs and destroys the link between them increases.
3. Therefore, by having sufficient number of chromosomal markers covering the whole genome and by typing these in a multigeneration family, one can link a disorder to a specific region on a chromosome. There are several programs available that do the necessary statistical analysis of genetic typing data. If several families have been genotyped and one suspects a possible phenocopy problem, data from that family can be removed to investigate if a link to a specific region becomes stronger. One can also test different types of inheritance (dominant, recessive, etc.).
4. Assuming a positive result, the linkage region will often be broad, often many millions of base pairs in size. The next step is therefore a bioinformatics analysis of what genes are present in a region to prioritize candidates for the following analysis.

3.3. Bioinformatics and Literature Analysis

1. There are several genome browsers available for investigating what genes are present in a candidate region. We typically use ENSEMBL, NCBI Genome Biology application, and the UCSC Genome Browser. All three resources have the ability

to export data between defined genomic markers and specific chromosomal positions (for example between positions 1,000,000 and 2,000,000 on human chromosome 1). In this way a list of genes in a chromosomal region of interest can rapidly be obtained.

2. The January issue of Nucleic Acids Research (http://nar.oxfordjournals.org/) every year is a database issue describing the recent updates to ENSEMBL, NCBI, and UCSC genome browsers. Nucleic Acids Research also has a web server issue that can be of interest. We highly recommend that you consult the latest year's issue for such studies.
3. The most straightforward approach to identify the gene mutated in a disorder would be to next re-sequence the entire chromosomal region of interest in an affected individual and several unaffected individuals of a family. Such re-sequencing should identify any possible mutation of a gene in the patient and confirm that the mutation is not present in healthy relatives. Furthermore, the mutation should in a follow-up re-sequencing be present in all cases as expected from family information. The association between a gene and a disorder becomes even stronger if another unrelated family also has a mutation in the same gene. Although the sequencing costs of third generation instruments may become lower in the future and thus may make possible such re-sequencing of an entire region in a number of cases and controls, the approach is at present, however, still cost-prohibitive.
4. Alternatively, one presently tries to rank the list of candidate genes present in the chromosomal region of interest as to his/her likelihood of being involved in the diseases studied, i.e. likely to being mutated in the disorder. Competent bioinformatics support is crucially important for this step (see Note 3).
5. One obvious first tool for the task of ranking the candidate genes is literature. A lot of information is available in the literature that may give clues as to the likelihood of being involved in a specific disorder. However, far from all genes have been investigated and are covered by publications. Even less genes have been knocked out in mice. Therefore, other information resources are often required for the selection of re-sequencing candidates.
6. Expression databases are the second important tool to rank the candidate gene. It is important to know if a candidate protein is expressed in an organ affected by the disorder. If this is not the case, this should lower the priority of it being a candidate for re-sequencing. Databases, we typically consult for such questions, are the Allen Brain Bank, the Human Protein Atlas, and the Gene Expression Omnibus.

7. Animal information may also be used as a guide in prioritizing re-sequencing candidates. Mice and rat mutants may have a similar phenotype or a phenotype that partially resembles the human disorder. Several mouse and rat resources can be used as a starting point for this type of investigation (see Subheading 2.3, point 3).

3.4. Bidirectional Sequencing

1. By far, the fastest way to analyse candidate genes is to sequence both DNA strands of PCR amplified exons, including flanking intron/exon splicing junctions. Examples for results from bidirectional sequencing are shown in Fig. 1.
2. We recommend using the Big Dye Terminator v3.1 Cycle Sequencing Kit which is robust, gives even peak heights, and long sequence read lengths of more than 500 bases.
3. The intron–exon border sequences in any candidate gene are defined by aligning the protein sequence with the genomic sequence obtained from e.g. ENSEMBL using the Genewise package software.
4. PCR primers are then designed for amplification of all exons, including approximately 50 bases of flanking intron sequence. We typically use the Oligo 6 software for PCR primer design. In order to obtain more even and stronger raw data signals and make sequencing of different PCR products more convenient, we tag the PCR primers with M13 forward and reverse sequences, respectively.

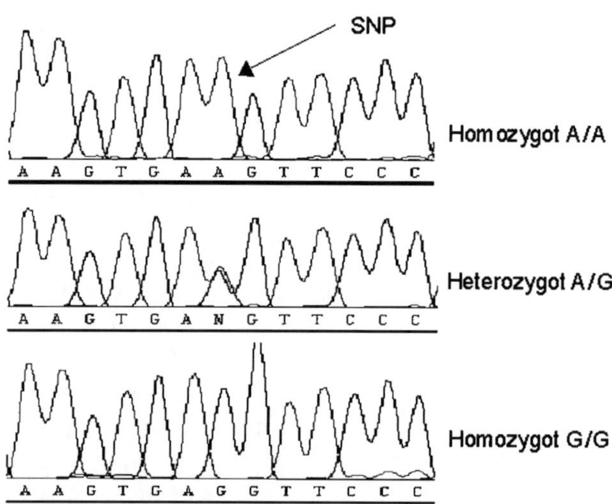

Fig. 1. Example of sequencing results showing the detection of a single-point mutation in a human gene. In the case shown, the sequencing identified a single-nucleotide polymorphism (SNP) in parts of the human population that alters an allelic position from a G to a A in a non-disclosed gene. Homozygotes of both variants can be distinguished, as well as heterozygotic carriers. Figure courtesy of Anna Wallin, AstraZeneca, Södertälje

5. PCR amplification of genomic DNA is set up by pipetting the following into a 96-well plate: 40 ng genomic DNA, 10× buffer, 100 nmol of each oligonucleotide primer, dNTPs, AmpliTaq Gold Polymerase, and H_2O to a final volume of 50 μL.
6. The plate is inserted into a thermal cycler containing a hot top assembly, and the reaction is carried out using the following parameters: 95°C for 30 s then 30–40 cycles of each (95°C for 30 s, 55°C for 30 s and 30 s for 72°C), and finally 4°C until removed.
7. We typically analyse the PCR products by agarose capillary electrophoresis using the HAD-GT12 instrument following the instructions provided by the manufacturer. Analysis can also be done for regular slab gel and gel imaging systems.
8. Purification of PCR products is performed using QIAquick 96 purification kit in combination with QIAvac 96 vacuum manifold following the provided instructions.
9. Before setting up the sequencing reactions, allow the frozen buffers and stocks to thaw carefully at room temperature, mix thoroughly, then centrifuge briefly and keep on ice until further use.
10. In a 96-well plate mix the following: 2 μl Big Dye Sequencing Buffer, 2 μl Ready Reaction Premix (1/2 of the recommended volume of 4 μl could be used w/o decreased sequence quality and length), 3–10 ng of PCR product, 3.2 pmol of M13 sequencing primers and H_2O to a final volume of 20 μl/well.
11. Place the plate in a thermal cycler containing a hot-top assembly and carry out the reaction using the following parameters: 96°C for 60 s, then 25 cycles of each (96°C for 30 s, 50°C for 15 s, and 60°C for 4 min), and finally 4°C until ready to purify.
12. Spin the plate briefly in a centrifuge.
13. Unincorporated dye terminators will now be removed from the reactions prior to electrophoresis. This can be done by ethanol/EDTA precipitation with or without sodium acetate or by spin column purification. We typically use the Dye Terminator Removal kit from Abgene.
14. Take the separation plate out of the bag, and remove the tape sheets from the top and bottom of the plate.
15. Place the separation plate on top of a wash plate and centrifuge for 3 min at 1,000×*g*. Discard the flow through.
16. Place the separation plate on the sample plate.

17. Slowly pipette the 20 μl sequencing reactions onto the center of the gel bed of each well. Avoid touching the surface with the pipette tip.
18. Centrifuge for 3 min at the calculated speed (1,000×*g*).
19. The eluate contains the purified sequencing reactions.
20. Dry the samples in a vacuum centrifuge or uncovered at 70°C in a thermal cycler and dissolve in 20 μl formamide.
21. Analyse the samples by electrophoresis e.g. on the ABI Prism 310 or 3100, 370, 377, 3700 DNA Analyser/Genetic Analyser or ABI 3130 XL Avant Genetic Analyser, which is not described in this chapter.
22. Left over samples can be stored at −20°C for several months.

3.5. Site-Directed Mutagenesis

1. Generation of the identified genomic mutation(s) into the corresponding cDNA sequence can be achieved with high efficiencies using commercially available site directed mutagenesis kits (e.g. Quick Change). Suitable starting material for this is the full length wild type cDNA inserted into mammalian expression vector such as pcDNA3 or pcDNA4. However, we recommend that the mutagenesis is performed on a subcloned fragment that later after complete sequencing is subcloned into the expression vector before functional analysis.
2. Two complementary oligonucleotide primers containing the desired change in nucleotide sequence are first designed. The primers should be 25–45 bp long with 10–15 bp on each side of the site to be mutated, have a GC content of >40%, terminate in at least one C or G, and have a melting temperature (T_M) of ≥78°C. Use the following formula: $T_M = 81.5 + 0.41(\%GC) - 675/N$, where N does not include inserted or deleted bases.
3. The synthesis reaction is set up by pipetting the following into a microcentrifuge tube kept on ice: 5 μl × 10 reaction buffer, 30 ng plasmid DNA, 10 nmol of each oligonucleotide primer, 1 μl dNTP mix, and H_2O to a final volume of 50 μl. Then 1 μl of PfuUltra High-Fidelity DNA polymerase is added, and the mixture is carefully mixed and briefly centrifuged.
4. The tube is inserted into a thermal cycler containing a hot-top assembly and the reaction is carried out using the following parameters: 95°C for 30 s, then 12–18 cycles of each (95°C for 30 s, 55°C for 30 s, and 68°C for 1 min/kb of plasmid length), and finally 4°C until removed.
5. Add 10 units (1 μl) of the *Dpn*I restriction enzyme to the tube, mix gently, centrifuge briefly and incubate at 37°C for 1 h.

6. Before transforming competent bacteria with the digested synthesis reaction, thaw the bacteria carefully on ice.
7. Add 2 μl of the digested synthesis reaction to the supercompetent bacteria, mix carefully by tipping on the tube, and incubate on ice for 30 min.
8. Heat-shock the bacteria by placing the tube in a water bath at 42°C for 30–45 s, and then transfer the tube back on ice for additional 2 min.
9. Add 500 μl of SOC medium at room temperature, and incubate the tube at 37°C for 1 h, shaking at 225 rpm.
10. Place various amounts e.g. 5, 50, and 300 μl of the transformed bacteria on agar plates containing appropriate antibiotic selection.
11. Incubate the plates upside down at 37°C overnight (>16 h)
12. Clones from the plate with well separated colonies should be used for further analysis by DNA sequencing.
13. Pick 8–10 single colonies and inoculate 2 ml LB medium in 14 ml round-bottom tubes containing appropriate antibiotic selection and incubate at 37°C with vigorous shaking for 12–16 h.
14. Harvest bacteria from 1.5 ml of culture to microcentrifuge tubes, centrifuge at 6,800×*g* (>8,000 rpm) for 3 min at room temperature, and remove the supernatants.
15. Prepare plasmid DNA using the QIAprep Spin Miniprep Kit (or corresponding kit from another supplier).
16. Design sequencing oligonucleotide primers covering the complete cDNA insert with 200–300 bp apart on alternating DNA strands.
17. The primers should be 20 bp long, with a Tm of 60°C and GC content around 50%.
18. Proceed with sequencing reactions as described above (see Subheading 3.4) using 200–300 ng plasmid DNA (typically 1 μl of a miniprep). For this, we typically use plasmid preparation kits from Qiagen, following the instructions provided by the manufacturer.

3.6. Transient Transfection and Cell Culture

1. The effects on the function of the generated constructs can be tested by recordings from transfected HEK293 cells, whereas possible effects of the generated constructs on endogenous currents can be tested by transient transfection into a neuroblastoma cell line, like ND7/23 cells. Both cell lines can be cultured in 75 cm^2 cell culture flasks. Cell culture and transfection of HEK293 cells is described below under points 3 and 4, whereas the handling of ND7/23 cells is described below under steps 5 and 6.

2. All cell culture work described should be done in a sterilized fume hood. Wear sterile, one-way gloves throughout all steps.
3. To culture HEK293 cells, add 25 ml of DMEM F-12 containing 10% FBS to a 75 cm^2 flask. Place the capped flasks with their large flat side down into a humidified, sterile incubator set to maintain an atmosphere of 5% CO_2 at 37°C. Control the growth of the cells daily by observing under a low power microscope.
4. Split HEK293 cells between 70 and 80% confluency of cells. For this, first prepare fresh flasks as described above under point 3. Then remove the culture medium from the flask with the cells to be split, and add 1 ml of trypsin with a sterile plastic pipette. Swirl the liquid so that the entire cell sheet is covered. Wait approximately 2 min, then shake the flask gently. Continue to shake the flask until the entire cell sheet has loosened from the plastic. Then add 10 ml of DMEM F-12 containing 10% FBS to the flasks with a sterile 10 ml plastic pipette. This will inactivate the trypsin. Aspirate the cells through the pipette two to three times to produce a suspension of single cells.
5. To culture ND7/23 cells, add 25 ml of DMEM/Glutamax containing 10% FBS to a 75 cm^2 flask. Place the capped flasks with their large flat side down into a humidified, sterile incubator set to maintain an atmosphere of 5% CO_2 at 37°C. Control the growth of the cells daily by observing under a low power microscope.
6. Split ND7/23 cells between 70 and 80% confluency of cells. For this, first prepare fresh flasks as described above under point 5. Then remove the culture medium from the flask with the cells to be split, and add 1 ml of Accutase with a sterile plastic pipette. Swirl the liquid so that the entire cell sheet is covered. Wait approximately 2 min, then shake the flasks gently. Continue to shake the flasks until the entire cell sheet has loosened from the plastic. Then add 10 ml of DMEM/ Glutamax containing 10% FBS to the flasks with a sterile 10 ml plastic pipette. This will inactivate the Accutase. Aspirate the cells through the pipette two to three times to produce a suspension of single cells.
7. For transfection, cells are split approximately 20 h prior to transfection into 25 cm^2 flasks. Both cell lines can be transfected with Lipofectamine 2000. Transfection is done with a cDNA mixture (10:1 relation) of the generated construct and a transfection marker like pZsGreen1-N1. The actual amount of cDNA transfected, as well as the transfection

procedure should follow the manufacturer's description as closely as possible.

8. Approximately 20 h after transfection, both cell lines can be plated for electrophysiology experiments into 35 mm round cell culture dishes filled with 3 ml of DMEM F-12 containing 10% FBS for HEK293 cells, or DMEM/Glutamax containing 10% FBS for ND7/23 cells. For plating, cells are split as described above. One drop of the single cell suspension is then added to each 35 mm culture dish. Gently swirl the fluid in the dishes after adding the cells, put the lids on top, and place the dishes into the humidified incubator. It is recommended to prepare several dishes for electrophysiology experiments. Cells are allowed to recover from plating for an additional 20–48 h prior to electrophysiology experiments.

3.7. Electrophysiology

1. The following is only a short description of the manipulations to obtain a successful whole-cell recording. Before attempting the steps described below, it is highly recommended to read some of the seminal literature on the matter (12–14) and also to try the process of actual patch-clamping under the supervision of an experienced investigator.
2. Prepare the experiment by pulling patch pipettes on a suitable puller such that they have resistances of 2–5 MΩ when filled with the intracellular solution.
3. Patch pipettes are filled with intracellular solution from the back using a 1-ml syringe (see Subheading 2.7, step 5). To remove tiny air bubbles from the very tip of the patch pipette, hold the pipette between two fingers with the back end of the patch pipette upwards and then lightly tap on the side of the patch pipette. Once all air bubbles are removed, mount the patch pipette onto the electrode holder.
4. Remove one of the cell dishes prepared as above (see Subheading 3.6, step 8) from the incubator. At the recording set-up, remove the lid from the dish and push the superfusion insert into the dish. Place the dish onto an appropriate holder mounted onto the stage of the microscope such that the dish can easily be moved in the X and Y direction using the controls of the microscope table.
5. Connect the inlet and outlet of the superfusion system to the superfusion insert in the dish. Adjust flow of inlet and outlet of the extracellular solution to achieve a stable liquid level sufficient to continuously cover the cells in the dish.
6. Place the reference electrode into the bath. Set the recording settings such that the signal is filtered at 10 kHz and digitized at 20 kHz.

7. Apply a continuous short test seal pulse to the patch electrode and monitor the current signal. Using the micromanipulator manoeuvre the tip of the patch electrode into the approximate center of the optical field. Apply positive pressure to the interior of the patch pipette, then using the manipulator manoeuvre the tip of the electrode into the bath. At this point you should see a square wave current deflection that will allow you to calculate the resistance of the patch electrode.
8. Adjust the focus of the microscopic image to have the tip of the patch electrode in sharp focus. Then manipulate the tip of the patch electrode to be in the center of the optical field. After this stepwise lower the focus of the microscopic image closer to the top of the cell layer followed by a lowering of the tip of the patch electrode sharply into the new focus. Repeat this procedure until the focus of the image is just above the cell layer.
9. Focus on the cell layer before switching from normal light settings to fluorescent light setting to identify a cell that expresses the fluorescent transfection marker. Once you have identified such a cell, switch back to normal light setting and, using the microscope stage, manoeuvre the cell exactly below the tip of the patch electrode. Then slowly lower the patch electrode into focus.
10. You will see an indentation of the cell membrane once the tip of the patch electrode touches the cell. Do not further move the patch electrode. Release the positive pressure on the inside of the patch electrode.
11. Follow the current signal on the monitor. Typically you should have already seen a slight increase in the resistance, visible by a smaller deflection of the square wave current signal by now. Apply gentle negative pressure to the inside of the electrode while continuously monitoring the current signal. You will see the formation of a giga seal by a sudden dramatic increase in the resistance, visible by the disappearance of the square wave signal under the previous gain settings.
12. Once a giga seal has been established, adjust the signal for optimal capacitance compensation.
13. Establish whole-cell access by suction or a voltage zap. Once whole-cell access is gained, compensate series resistance.
14. During the recording, continuously monitor cell input resistance and membrane capacitance using a short –10 mV pulse.
15. To study voltage-gated sodium channel, one basic voltage protocol is to start with a holding potential of –100 mV and

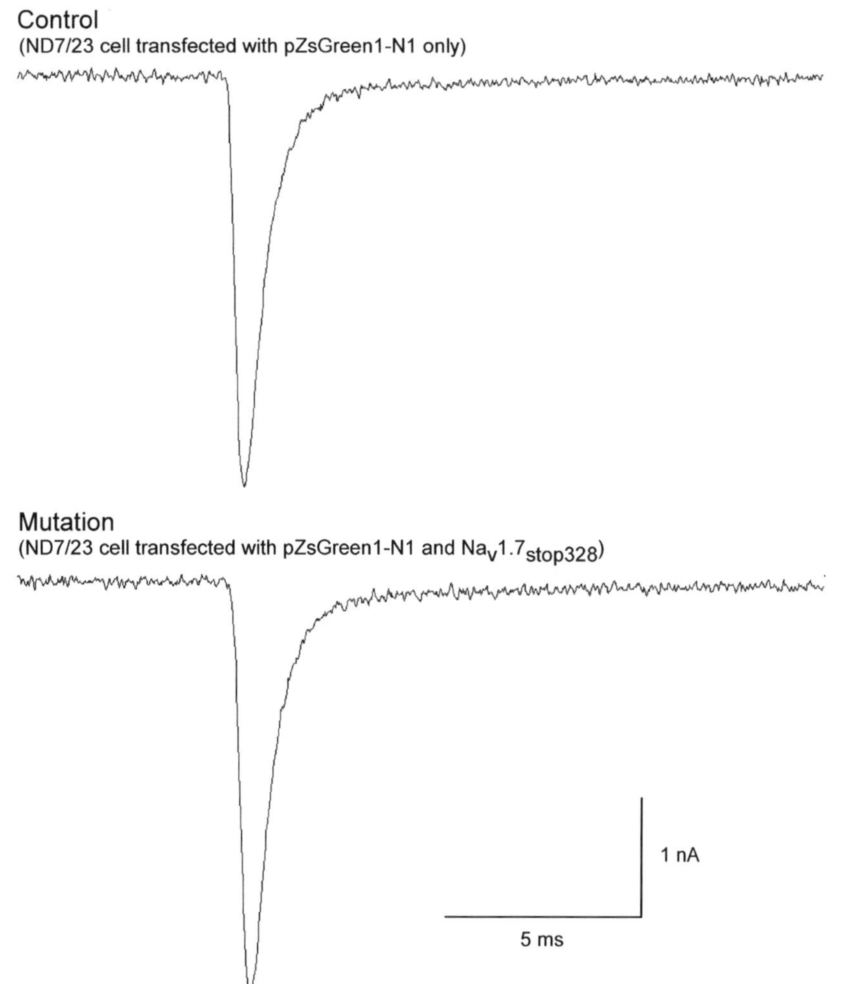

Fig. 2. Examples of endogenous voltage-gated sodium channels obtained from ND7/23 transfected with a truncated $Na_v1.7$ gene and transfection marker (*top*) and with the transfection marker only (*bottom*). The actual voltage protocol was from a holding potential of −100 mV and a 50-ms long step to −15 mV. Transfection of the mutated $Na_v1.7$ gene had no effect on the endogenous voltage-gated sodium currents. Figure courtesy of Per-Eric Lund, AstraZeneca, Södertälje

apply a repeated step protocol consisting of 50 ms long steps to a new holding potential ranging from −90 to +60 mV using 5 mV increments on each repeat. Examples of representative traces obtained with such a protocol are shown in Fig. 2.

16. Dependent on the biophysical properties that one wants to investigate other voltage protocols should be used, as described in the relevant literature (see Note 4).

4. Notes

1. A large variety of options are on the market and most combinations should be fit for purpose. We use the following: an inverted Nikon Eclipse TE2000-S microscope (Nikon) with a 20-fold objective and HEKA Pulse software in combination with a HEKA EPC10/2 amplifier (HEKA Instruments, Bellmore, NY). The electrode holder is attached to a PatchMan NP2 micromanipulator (Eppendorf, Hamburg, Germany).
2. This can be accomplished by several means. We typically use gravity to feed the inlet (reservoir mounted higher than the recording chamber) and flow through the tubing adjusted with a metal clamp pinch (VWR International), while the outlet is driven by a peristaltic pump that continuously removes the liquid above a certain level from the recording chamber.
3. The process of identifying the candidate gene from the genes present in the candidate region is not a mechanistic process, but requires a good deal of disease knowledge and intuition on which proteins could possibly play a role in a pain state. With this in mind, one should not be afraid to challenge decisions made earlier with regard to which gene should be focused on.
4. When it comes to the interpretation of data obtained from overexpressed receptors in cellular expression system, it is prudent to be conservative. For example, the lack of an effect of an overexpressed non-functional $Na_v1.7$ construct on endogenous currents in a neuroblastoma cell line does by no means indicate that the gene product might not have an effect on endogenous currents in DRGs in vivo.

References

1. Yang Y, Wang Y, Li S, Xu H, Li H, Ma L et al (2004) Mutations in *SCN9A*, encoding a sodium channel alpha subunit, in patients with primary erythermalgia. J Med Genet 41:171–174
2. Drenth JPH, te Morsche RHM, Guillet G, Taieb A, Kirby RL, Jansen JBMJ (2005) *SCN9A* mutations define primary erythermalgia as a neuropathic disorder of voltage gated sodium channels. J Invest Dermatol 124:1333–1338
3. Fertleman CR, Baker MD, Parker KA, Moffatt S, Elmslie FV, Abrahamsen B et al (2006) *SCN9A* mutations in paroxysmal extreme pain disorder: allelic variants underlie distinct channel defects and phenotypes. Neuron 52:767–774
4. Cox JJ, Reimann F, Nicholas AK, Thornton G, Roberts E, Springell K et al (2006) An *SCN9A* channelopathy causes congenital inability to experience pain. Nature 444:894–898
5. Goldberg YP, MacFarlane J, MacDonald ML, Thompson J, Dube MP, Mattice M et al (2007) Loss-of-function mutations in the Nav1.7 gene underlie congenital indifference to pain in multiple human populations. Clin Genet 71:311–319
6. Ahmad S, Dahllund L, Eriksson AB, Hellgren D, Karlsson U, Lund P-E et al (2007) A stop codon mutation in *SCN9A* causes lack of pain sensation. Hum Mol Genet 16:2114–2121
7. Cummins TR, Dib-Hajj SD, Waxman SG (2004) Electrophysiological properties of mutant $Na_v1.7$ sodium channels in a painful inherited neuropathy. J Neurosci 24:8232–8236

8. Harty TP, Dib-Hajj SD, Tyrrell L, Blackman R, Hisama FM, Rose JB, Waxman SG (2005) $Na_v1.7$ mutant A863P in erythromelalgia: effects of altered activation and steady-state inactivation on excitability of nociceptive dorsal root ganglion neurons. J Neurosci 26: 12566–12575
9. Chahine M, Chatelier A, Babich O, Krupp JJ (2008) Voltage-gated sodium channels in neurological disorders. CNS Neurol Disord Drug Targets 7:144–158
10. Baker MD, Wood JN (2001) Involvement of Na+ channels in pain pathways. Trends Pharmacol Sci 22:27–31
11. Akopian AN, Souslova V, England S, Okuse K, Ogata N, Ure J et al (1999) The tetrodotoxin-resistant sodium channel SNS has a specialized function in pain pathways. Nat Neurosci 2:541–548
12. Hamill OP, Marty A, Neher E, Sakmann B, Sigworth FJ (1981) Improved patch-clamp techniques for high-resolution current recording from cells and cell-free membrane patches. Pflügers Arch 391:85–100
13. Penner R (1995) A practical guide to patch clamping. In: Neher E, Sakmann B (eds) Single channel recording. Plenum Press, New York and London, pp 3–30
14. Marty A, Neher E (1995) Tight-seal whole-cell recording. In: Neher E, Sakmann B (eds) Single channel recording. Plenum Press, New York and London, pp 31–52

Chapter 24

Rat Bone Marrow Stromal Cells and Oligonucleotides in Pain Research

María Florencia Coronel, Norma Alejandra Chasseing, and Marcelo José Villar

Abstract

In the last years, significant progress has been made in the medical treatment of pain. However, pathological pains, such us neuropathic pain, remain refractory to the currently available analgesics. Therefore, new therapeutic strategies are being evaluated. We have recently shown that both bone marrow stromal cells (MSCs) and the oligonucleotide IMT504 can prevent the development of mechanical and thermal allodynia when they are administered to rats subjected to a sciatic nerve crush. This chapter summarizes the laboratory techniques used to isolate and culture MSCs, administer both MSCs and IMT504, perform the nerve injury and determine mechanical and thermal sensitivities.

Key words: Sciatic nerve injury, Mechanical and thermal allodynia, Oligodeoxynucleotides, Bone marrow stromal cells

1. Introduction

Injuries of the peripheral and central nervous systems often result in neuropathic pain. These injuries may result from major surgeries (amputation, thoracotomy), diabetic neuropathy, viral infection, spinal cord injury and stroke, among other insults (1). Patients with neuropathic pain report spontaneous pain, described as shooting, lancinating or burning pain, as well as pain induced by normally innocuous tactile or thermal stimuli, known as allodynia (2, 3). Neuropathic pain is a chronic, pathological pain that remains refractory to the currently available analgesics (4, 5). Therefore, biomedical researchers continue evaluating new therapeutic strategies. In the last years, exogenously administered bone marrow stromal cells (MSCs) have been shown to participate in the repair

Arpad Szallasi (ed.), *Analgesia: Methods and Protocols*, Methods in Molecular Biology, vol. 617, DOI 10.1007/978-1-60327-323-7_24, © Springer Science+Business Media, LLC 2010

and regeneration of damaged tissues in a variety of animal models (6–9). Moreover, we have recently shown that MSC administration prevents the development of mechanical and thermal allodynia in animals subjected to a sciatic nerve injury (10–12). However, there are some limitations of this therapeutic approach, basically related to the ex vivo cell manipulation procedure (cell isolation, in vitro expansion and cell delivery) (13). IMT504, the prototype of the PyNTTTTGT class of oligodeoxynucleotides (14), is a potent stimulatory signal for MSC expansion both in vitro and in vivo (15). Since systemic treatment with this oligonucleotide can stimulate the animal's own MSCs, inducing their expansion and mobilization (15), we investigated the effect of IMT504 administration on the nociceptive behavior of rats subjected to a sciatic nerve injury. Our results show that IMT504 administration is able to reduce mechanical and thermal allodynia (16), representing a possible therapeutic approach for the treatment of neuropathic pain.

2. Materials

2.1. Animals

1. Adult Sprague–Dawley male rats (200–300 g) kept in a 12 h day/night cycle (light on 6.00 A.M.), with water and food ad libitum and controlled temperature (24°C).
2. Mixture of 4 mL ketamine (50 mg/ml) and 1 mL xylazine (2%). This mixture should be prepared fresh for each experiment.

2.2. Isolation of MSCs

1. Alpha minimal essential medium (α-MEM) (Gibco/BRL, Bethesda, MD) supplemented with 100 IU/ml gentamicine and 2.5 μg/ml amphotericine B.
2. Trypan blue: prepare solution A (trypan blue 0.5% in distilled water), solution B (NaCl 4.25% in distilled water) and trypan blue working solution (4 parts of A and 1 part of B). Store at 4°C.
3. Dulbecco's Modified Eagle's Medium (DMEM) (Gibco/BRL) supplemented with 100 IU/ml gentamicine, 2.5 μg/ml amphotericine, 2 mM L-glutamine, and 20% fetal calf serum.
4. Hoechst 33258 (Sigma, St. Louis, MO) is dissolved at 1 mg/mL (w/v) in sterile distilled water. Protect from light and store at 4°C. Working solutions are stable for at least 6 months. The Hoechst stains are known mutagens and should be handled with care. The dye must be disposed of safely and in accordance with applicable regulations.

5. Trypsin 0.25%.
6. Ethylenediamine tetraacetic acid (EDTA) 1 mM.
7. Phosphate-buffered saline (PBS), 10× stock solution: 1.37 M NaCl, 27 mM KCl, 100 mM Na2HPO4, and 18 mM KH2PO4 (adjust to pH 7.4 with HCl if necessary). Autoclave before storage at room temperature. Prepare working solution by diluting one part of stock solution with nine parts of distilled water.
8. Cell culture plasticware (pipets, flasks, conical tubes, tips, etc.), all sterile.

2.3. Oligonucleotides

1. IMT504 sequence is 5′-TCATCATTTTGTCATTTTGT CATT-3′ (Property of Immunotech SA, Argentina).
2. The HPLC-grade single stranded ODN having phosphorothioate internucleotide linkages (Oligos ETC, Wilsonville, OR).
3. Limulus test (Pyrosate, Associates of Cape Cod, Inc., East Falmouth, MS).

2.4. Nerve Injury Model

1. Sterile surgical instruments.

2.5. IMT and MSC Administration

1. Sterile 1 ml syringes and needles for injection.

2.6. Behavioral Assessment

1. Von Frey hairs (Stoelting, WoodDale, IL).
2. Acetone. Acetone is extremely flammable with a high vapor pressure; use only with good ventilation and avoid all ignition sources.

3. Methods

3.1. Isolation of MSCs

1. All the experiments performed are in accordance to the policy of the Society for Neuroscience and the International Association for the Study of Pain for the use of animals in pain research. Efforts should be made in order to minimize animal discomfort and to use the fewest animals needed for statistical analysis.
2. Anesthetize the animals by an intraperitoneal (i.p.) injection of the mixture of ketamine and xylazine. A 250 g rat should receive 0.3 ml of the mixture (50 mg/kg ketamine and 5 mg/kg xylazine).
3. Dissect out the femoral bones (see Note 1). After removing the epiphyses and gaining access to the marrow cavities, flush out whole bone marrow using a 15-G needle and a 1 ml

syringe with pre-warmed α-MEM supplemented with gentamicine and amphotericine. Collect the bone marrow from at least 8 femoral bones and transfer the suspension to 15 ml conical tubes. Disperse the cells by gentle pipetting up and down (Fig. 1a,b).

4. Centrifuge the cell suspension at 400×*g* for 10 min at room temperature. Discard the supernatant carefully and resuspend the pellet in fresh warm medium. Repeat this procedure twice.
5. Evaluate cell concentration by microscopic cell counting using a Neubauer hemocytometer. It is important to disperse clumps before counting the cells. To check cellular viability, mix 1 volume of the trypan blue working solution with 1 volume of the cell suspension. Wait for 5 min and then load 10 μl of this suspension onto the hemacytometer. View under the microscope (100×). Trypan blue is a vital dye, viable cells remain unstained. Count the number of viable cells in each square grid, calculate the average number of cells per square grid, and finally calculate the number of viable cells per ml (cells/ml = average number of cells per square grid $\times 2 \times 10^4$).
6. Centrifuge again and resuspend the cells at a concentration of 1×10^6 cells/ml in warmed DMEM supplemented with gentamicine, amphotericine, l-glutamine and fetal calf serum, and transfer to 25 cm^2 tissue culture flasks.
7. Place the culture flasks in a humidified 37°C, 5% CO_2 incubator.
8. After 24 h of culture, remove media with a Pasteur pipet in order to discard the non-adherent cells (see Note 2). Add warmed culture medium and incubate the flasks until 90% confluence is reached (approx 12–14 days), renewing the medium every 3–5 days. Check the cells with an inverted microscope once every 2 days (Fig. 1c,d). Cells should not grow further than 90% confluence in order to avoid contact inhibition or transformation.
9. In case you want to localize the cells in the tissues of animals after administration, incubate MSCs with 1 μg/ml bis-benzamide (Hoechst 33258, Sigma) for 24 h prior to harvesting (add 5 μl of Hoechst working solution to 5 ml of culture media) (see Note 3) (Fig. 1e–h).
10. Approximately on day 14, carefully remove media and wash adherent cells with PBS in order to remove residual fetal calf serum which may inhibit trypsin.
11. Add a small volume (0.5–1.0 ml) of trypsin/EDTA solution (enough to cover the monolayer). Place the culture flasks in the incubator at 37°C (to favour the enzymatic activity). Check whether the cells have detached under an inverted microscope every 2–3 min. Cells should not be exposed to trypsin for more

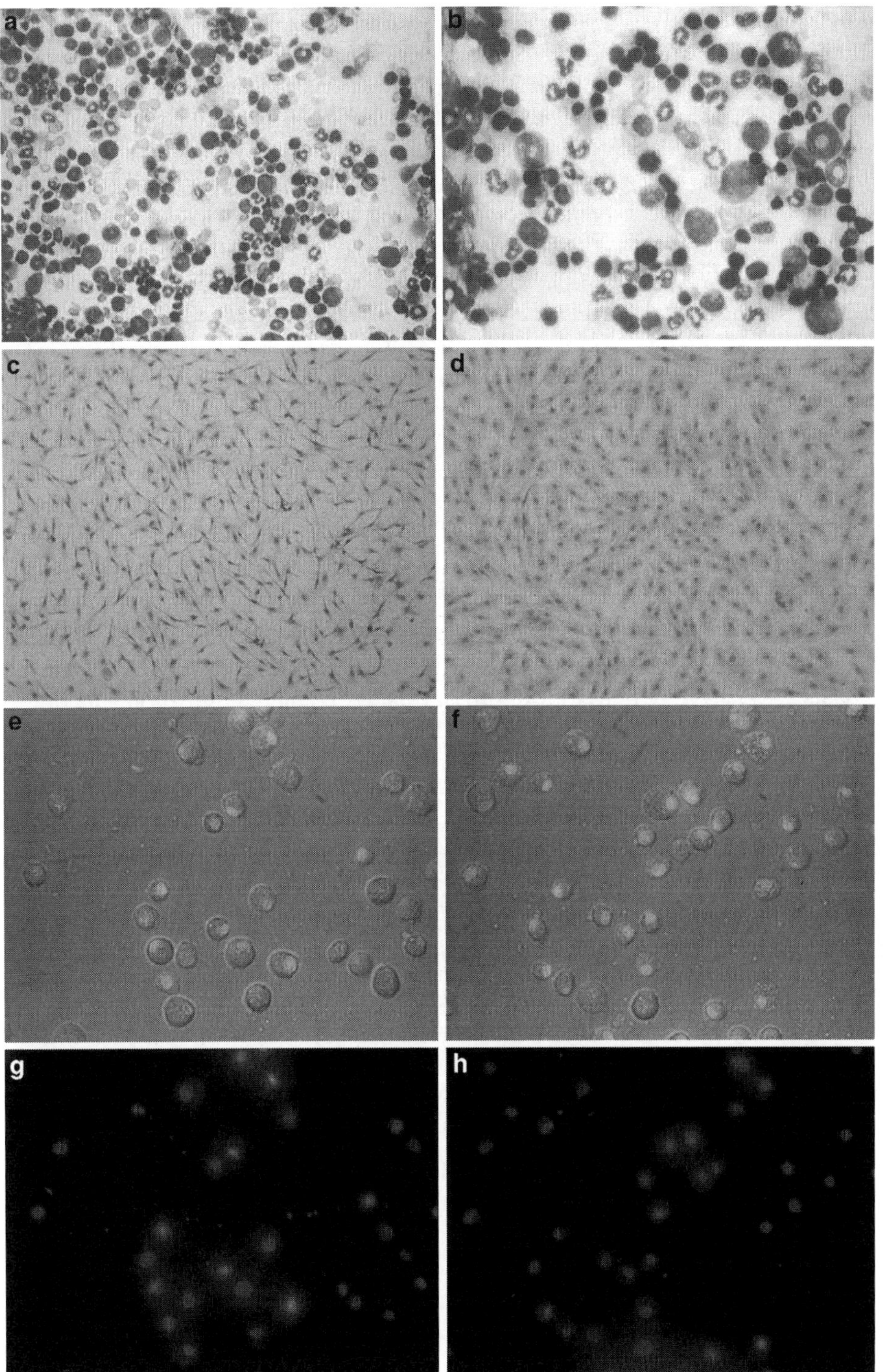

Fig. 1. Microphotographs illustrating different steps in the process of MSC isolation. In (**a**, **b**) whole bone marrow smears obtained from the femoral bones of Sprague–Dawley rats and stained with Giemsa are shown. In culture, MSCs grow in a monolayer as fibroblast-like spindled-shaped cells (**c**, **d**). In (**e**–**h**) a suspension of MSCs stained with Hoechst is shown. Micrographs **e** and **f** were taken under visible and UV illumination, while **g** and **h** were taken under UV illumination only. As it can be observed, Hoechst-positive cells show nuclear fluorescence

than 15 min since prolonged exposure damages them. When cells have detached, add sufficient amount (4–5 ml) of DMEM containing 20% fetal calf serum (to inhibit trypsin), and disperse the cells by gentle pipetting up and down.

12. Check cell number and viability as described previously. Pellet cells for 5 min at 400×*g*, remove supernatant, and resuspend the cells in PBS at a concentration of 3×10^6 cells/ml.

3.2. Preparing Oligonucleotides (ODN)

1. Suspend the ODN in sterile saline (NaCl 0.9%) at a concentration of 10 mg/ml and assay for LPS contamination using the Limulus test. Only ODN preparations with undetectable LPS levels should be used.
2. Keep the ODN at –20°C until used.

3.3. Nerve Injury Model

1. Anesthetize the rats as described previously.
2. Expose the sciatic nerve in the right thigh and dissect it free from the surrounding tissue using sharp microscissors in a 5–8 mm long segment.
3. Crush the nerve for 3 s at the mid thigh level using jeweler's forceps.
4. Mark the site of the lesion using an indelible felt-tip pen.
5. Replace the nerve under the muscle. Suture the skin wound using silk thread and leave the animals to recover under a lamp heating.

3.4. IMT504 and MSC Administration

1. Immediately after performing the nerve injury, inject a group of rats subcutaneously with 500 μl of the ODN IMT504 dissolved in saline (for 250 g rats, dose is 20 mg/kg). This injection should be repeated once daily, for the next four consecutive days.
2. Inject another group of animals with a suspension of MSCs (1.5×10^6/500 μl PBS). These animals should receive one intravascular administration (into the tail vein), immediately after the nerve injury is performed.
3. Include also the following control groups: (1) Animals subjected to the sciatic nerve crush alone. (2) Animals with a sciatic nerve crush receiving five subcutaneous injections of saline, once daily, starting immediately after performing the lesion. (3) Animals with a sciatic nerve crush receiving one intravascular administration of PBS immediately after performing the lesion.

3.5. Behavioral Assessment

1. Perform behavioral testing during daytime (9.00–18.00, preferably always at the same time) in a quiet room. The tests should be performed by blinded investigator. All animals should be tested before surgery (day 0) and at

different time points after the sciatic nerve crush (1, 3, 7, 10, 14 and 21 days, for example). Include in the experiments only rats showing normal responses to mechanical and thermal stimulation before injury.

2. Place the animals in their acrylic testing chambers (8×8×18 cm) on a metal mesh floor (hole size of 3×3 mm), 15 min before starting the test for adaptation (Fig. 2a,b).
3. In order to assess mechanical sensitivity, apply von Frey hairs in ascending order (1, 2, 4, 6, 8, 10, 15, and 26 g) from below the mesh floor to the center of the plantar surface of both ipsilateral and contralateral hindpaws (17) (see Note 4) (Fig. 2b,c).
4. Deliver each hair three times with 5 s intervals and register whether the stimulation induces a brisk foot withdrawal. The lowest force at which application elicits a paw withdrawal is taken as the mechanical response threshold. A paw withdrawal reflex obtained with 6 g or less is considered an allodynic response. See Fig. 3a.
5. In order to determine cold sensitivity, apply 100 μl of acetone to the plantar surface of the paw using a plastic tubule connected to a 1 ml syringe (Choi test) (18). Apply the bubble of acetone five times to each paw with an interval of at least 5 min and record the number of brisk foot withdrawals (from 0 to 5). See Fig. 3b.

4. Notes

1. Sterile conditions must be maintained at all times, and all culture work should be performed under a laminar flow hood. Media, trypsin/EDTA solutions and PBS should be warmed to 37°C in a water bath before use.
2. MSCs grow in a monolayer. Cells with different morphologies are obtained: fibroblast-like spindled-shaped cells, rounded cells and large flat cells (Fig. 1c,d).
3. Hoechst 33258 is a cell permeable nucleic acid stain that emits blue fluorescence when bound to double strand DNA (Fig. 1e–h). This fluorophore is retained for long periods by viable cells.
4. Von Frey hairs are plastic monofilaments that exert an increasing pressure on the skin as they are pressed harder and harder, up to the point where they begin to bend. Pressure on the skin then remains constant over a considerable range of bending. Therefore, filaments should be pressed onto the hindpaws of the animal until they begin to bend (Fig. 3).

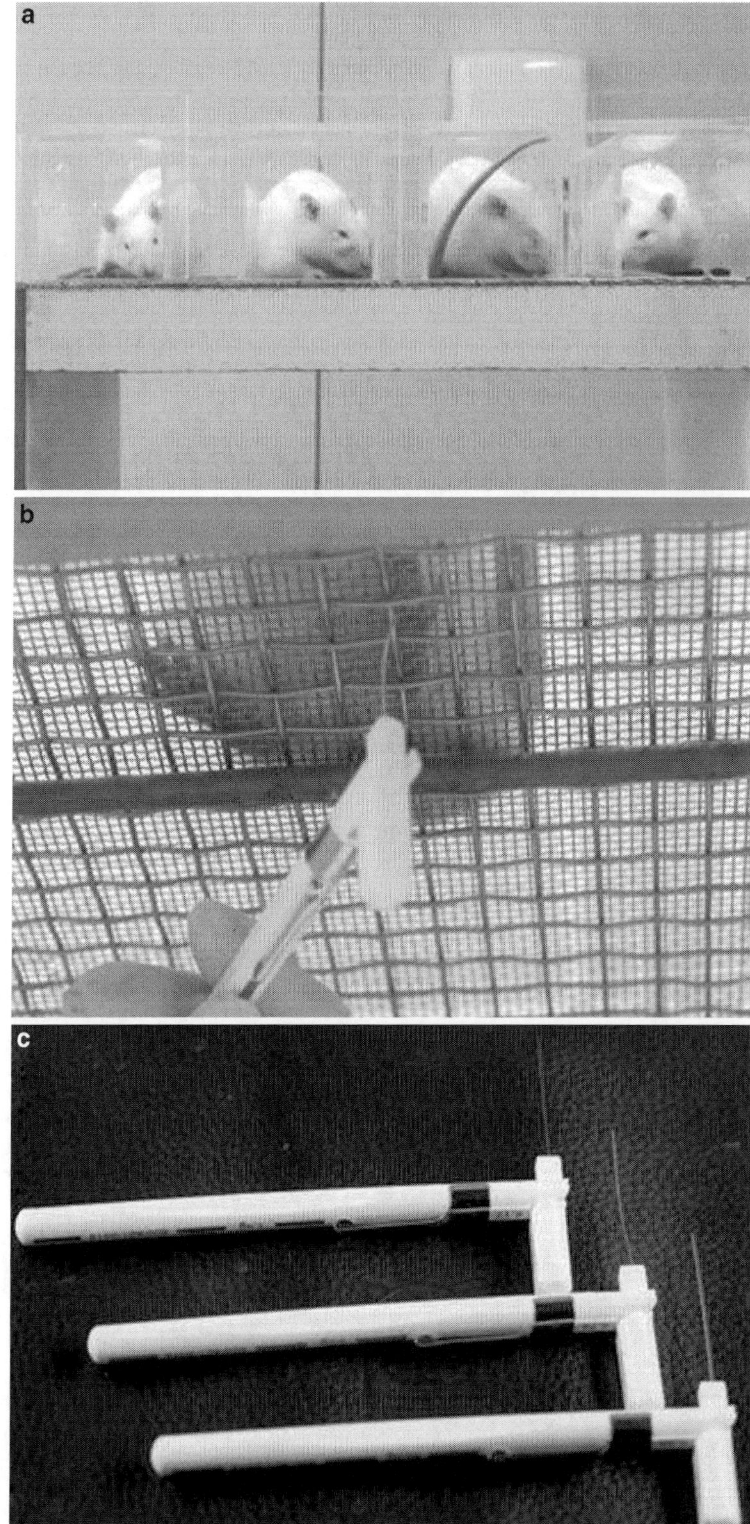

Fig. 2. Photographs showing animals placed in their individual acrylic chambers (**a**) located onto a metal mesh floor (**b**), in order to determine mechanical and thermal sensitivities. In (**c**) three of the von Frey filaments used, corresponding to 1, 6, and 26 g, are shown. Note that the filaments have increasing diameters which result in an increasing applied force. A series of ten filaments is applied in ascending order to both hindpaws. Each hair is applied three times until it begins to bend, as shown in (**b**)

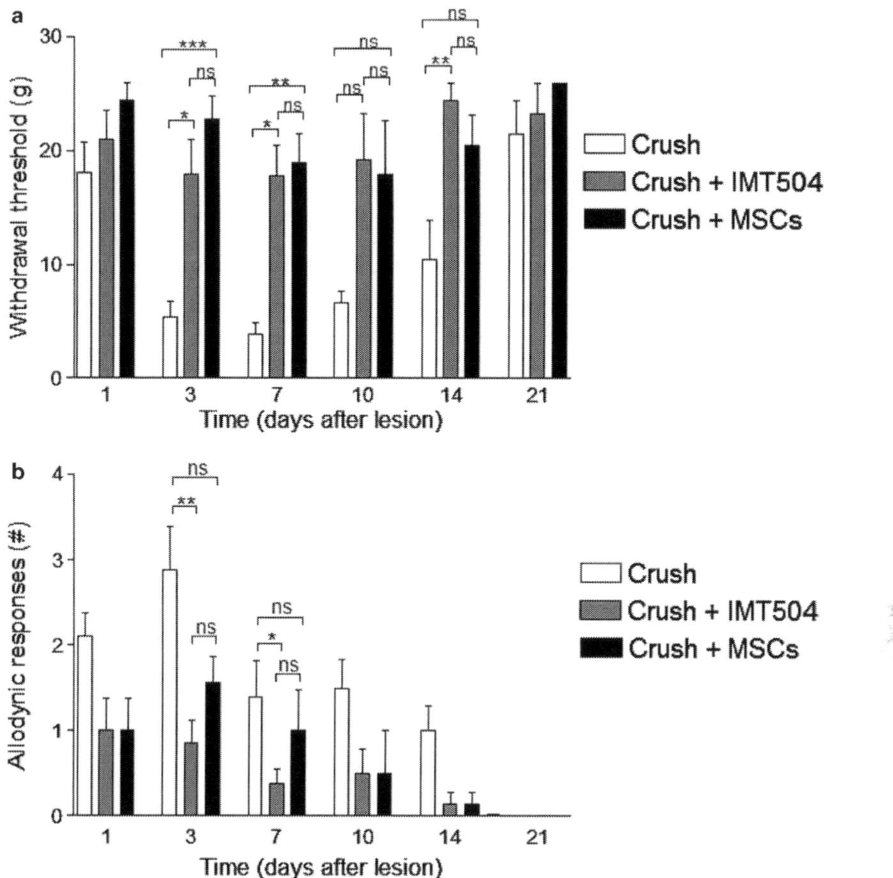

Fig. 3. Effect of either IMT504 or MSC treatment on the development of mechanical (**a**) and thermal (**b**) allodynia in the ipsilateral hindpaw of animals subjected to a sciatic nerve crush. The nociceptive behavior of lesioned animals without any treatment is also shown. These control rats showed a behavioral pattern similar to that of animals receiving either saline or PBS after the sciatic nerve lesion (not shown). (**a**) The sciatic nerve crush induced a significant decrease in paw withdrawal threshold to the von Frey filaments in control animals. Nociceptive responses in the allodynic range were detected 3, 7, and 10 days after the lesion. It is noticeable that the administration of either IMT504 or MSCs prevented the development of mechanical allodynia. Animals receiving either treatment showed similar behavioral responses at all the evaluated time points. (**b**) A significant increase in the number of allodynic responses to cold stimuli was induced in the ipsilateral hindpaw footpad after the sciatic nerve crush. Note that the administration of IMT504 significantly reduces the number of nociceptive responses to cold stimulation, 3 and 7 days after the lesion. MSC administration also results in fewer painful responses when compared to control animals. Values show mean ± S.E.M. Only statistically significant differences between treated and control animals are stated in the graphs, using the following symbols to represent p values: * $0.05 > p > 0.01$; ** $0.01 > p > 0.001$ and *** $p < 0.001$

References

1. Woolf CJ, Mannion RJ (1999) Neuropathic pain: aethiology, mechanisms and management. Lancet 353:1959–1964
2. Jensen TS, Gottrup H, Sindrup SH, Bach FW (2001) The clinical picture of neuropathic pain. Eur J Pharmacol 429:1–11
3. Baron R (2006) Mechanisms of disease: neuropathic pain – a clinical perspective. Nat Clin Pract Neurol 2:95–106
4. Jensen TS, Finnerup NB (2007) Management of neuropathic pain. Curr Opin Support Palliat Care 1:126–131
5. Ossipov MH, Porreca F (2005) Challenges in the development of novel treatment strategies for neuropathic pain. NeuroRx 2:650–661
6. Chen J, Li Y, Wang L, Zhang Z, Lu D, Lu M, Chopp M (2001) Therapeutic benefit of intravenous administration of bone marrow stromal cells after cerebral ischemia in rats. Stroke 32:1005–1011
7. Chopp M, Zhang XH, Li Y, Wang L, Chen J, Lu D, Lu M, Rosenblum M (2000) Spinal cord injury in rat: treatment with bone marrow stromal cell transplantation. Neuroreport 11:3001–3005
8. Piao H, Youn TJ, Kwon JS, Kim YH, Bae JW, Bora-Sohn S, Kim DW, Cho MC, Lee MM, Park YB (2005) Effects of bone marrow derived mesenchymal stem cells transplantation in acutely infarcting myocardium. Eur J Heart Fail 7:730–738
9. Mahmood A, Lu D, Chopp M (2004) Intravenous administration of marrow stromal cells (MSCs) increases the expression of growth factors in rat brain after traumatic brain injury. J Neurotrauma 21:33–39
10. Musolino PL, Coronel MF, Hökfelt T, Villar MJ (2007) Bone marrow stromal cells induce changes in pain behavior after sciatic nerve constriction. Neurosci Lett 418:97–101
11. Coronel MF, Musolino PL, Villar MJ (2006) Selective migration and engraftment of bone marrow mesenchymal stem cells in rat lumbar dorsal root ganglia after sciatic nerve constriction. Neurosci Lett 405:5–9
12. Coronel MF, Musolino PL, Brumovsky PR, Hökfelt T, Villar MJ (2009) Bone marrow stromal cells attenuate injury-induced changes in galanin, NPY and Y1-receptor expression after a sciatic nerve constriction. Neuropeptides 43:125–132
13. Mannello F, Tonti GA (2007) Concise review: no breakthroughs for human mesenchymal and embryonic stem cell culture. Stem Cells 25:1603–1609
14. Elías F, Fló J, López RA, Zorzopulos J, Montaner A, Rodríguez JM (2003) Strong cytosine-guanosine-independent immunostimulation in humans and other primates by synthetic oligodeoxynucleotides with PyNTTTTGT motifs. J Immunol 171:3697–3704
15. Hernando Insúa A, Montaner AD, Rodríguez JM, Elías F, Fló J, López RA, Zorzopulos J, Hofer EL, Chasseing NA (2007) IMT, the prototype of the immunostimulatory oligonucleotides of the PyNTTTTGT class, increases in the number of progenitors of mesenchymal stem cells both in vitro and in vivo: potential use in tissue repair therapy. Stem Cells 25:1047–1054
16. Coronel MF, Hernando-Insúa A, Rodriguez JM, Elías F, Chasseing NA, Montaner AD, Villar MJ (2008) Oligonucleotide IMT504 reduces neuropathic pain after peripheral nerve injury. Neurosci Lett 444:69–73
17. Chaplan S, Bach F, Pogrel J, Chung J, Yaksh T (1994) Quantitative assessment of tactile allodynia in the rat paw. J Neurosci 16: 7711–7724
18. Choi Y, Yoon YW, Na HS, Kim SH, Chung JM (1994) Behavioral signs of ongoing pain and cold allodynia in a rat model of neuropathic pain. Pain 59:369–376

Chapter 25

Transplantation of Human Mesenchymal Stem Cells in the Study of Neuropathic Pain

Dario Siniscalco

Abstract

Neuropathic pain is a complex disease that involves several molecular pathways. Due to its individual character, the treatment of neuropathic pain is extremely difficult. Currently available drugs do not affect the mechanisms underlying the generation and propagation of pain. Therefore, pain research is now focused on molecular approaches such as stem cell therapy. Stem cells mediate neuroprotection in a variety of nervous system injury models. We used spared nerve injury (SNI) model of neuropathic pain to assess the possible use of human mesenchymal stem cells (hMSCs) as neuroprotective tool in the regenerative medicine. We conclude that stem cell transplantation could be a useful therapeutic tool in the future of regenerative medicine.

Key words: Neuropathic pain, Stem cell therapy, Mesenchymal stem cells, Stem cell culture

1. Introduction

Stem cell therapy represents a great promise for the future of molecular medicine (1). The progression of several diseases can be slowed or even blocked by stem cell transplantation. Stem cells could be neuroprotective in a variety of nervous system injury models. Similar to neurodegenerative diseases, neuropathic pain appears to be amenable to stem cell therapy (2). Of stem cell populations, mesenchymal stem cells (MSCs) are believed to have the best potential results in pain–care research. These cells are a population of progenitor cells of mesodermal origin found in the bone marrow of adults, giving rise to skeletal muscle cells, blood, adipose tissue, vascular and urogenital systems, and to connective tissues throughout the body (3, 4). MSCs show a high expansion

Arpad Szallasi (ed.), *Analgesia: Methods and Protocols*, Methods in Molecular Biology, vol. 617, DOI 10.1007/978-1-60327-323-7_25, © Springer Science+Business Media, LLC 2010

potential, genetic stability, stable phenotype, can be easily collected and shipped from the laboratory to the bedside, and are compatible with different delivery methods and formulations (5). In addition, MSCs have two extraordinary characteristics: they are able to migrate to sites of tissue injury and have strong immunosuppressive properties that can be exploited for successful autologous or heterologous transplantation (6). Importantly, MSCs are capable of differentiating into neurons and astrocytes in vitro and in vivo (7). They are able to improve neurological deficits and to promote neuronal networks with functional synaptic transmission when transplanted into animal models of neurological disorders (8).

MSCs have been observed to migrate to the injured tissues and mediate functional recovery following brain, spinal cord, and peripheral nerve lesions, suggesting that MSCs could modulate pain generation after sciatic nerve constriction (9). The molecular mechanisms by which MSCs exert their beneficial actions on pain behaviour are yet to be clarified. MSCs are easily isolated from a small aspirate of bone marrow and expanded with high efficiency. Since MSCs are multipotent cells with a number of potential therapeutic applications, they represent a future powerful tool in regenerative medicine.

We have performed detailed analysis of the effects of human MSC treatment in neuropathic pain by using an experimental mouse mononeuropathy pain model. Reduction in neuropathic pain due to the stem cell transplantation is monitored by pain-like behaviour analysis (thermal hyperalgesia and mechanical allodynia). Motor coordination analysis allows us to exclude the possibility that stem cell transplantation could cause injury to the central nervous system of the neuropathic mice. Fluorescence cell labelling detection allows confirmation that the hMSCs are corrected and transplanted into the key brain areas involved in neuropathic pain.

2. Materials

2.1. Cell Culture

1. Ficoll (see Note 1).
2. Alpha Modified Eagle's Medium (α-MEM) (Lonza, Verviers, Belgium). Store at 4°C (see Note 2).
3. Foetal bovine serum (FBS) (EuroClone-Celbio, Milan, Italy). Store at –20°C (see Note 3).
4. l-glutamine. Store at –20°C.
5. Penicillin and Streptomycin. Store at –20°C.

6. Proliferating medium: α-MEM supplemented with 10% FBS, 2 mM l-glutamine, 100 U/ml penicillin and 100 mg/ml streptomycin. Store at 4°C.
7. Dulbecco's Phosphate Buffered Saline (D-PBS) (Sigma, St. Louis, MO). Store at room temperature; once opened, store at 4°C.
8. Solution of trypsin solution (0.25%) and ethylenediamine tetraacetic acid (EDTA) (1 mM) from Sigma. Store at 4°C.
9. Fibroblast growth factor-basic (b-FGF) (PeproTech, Rocky Hill, NJ) is first dissolved at 1 mg/mL in water and stored in single use aliquots at −20°C, then added to cell culture dishes as required (see Note 4).
10. Vybrant CM-DiI cell labelling solution (Invitrogen, Eugene, OR). Store at −20°C and protect from light.

2.2. Spared Nerve Injury

1. Sodium pentobarbital (Sigma).
2. 5–0 surgical non-absorbable silk.

2.3. Stem Cell Transplantation

1. Sodium pentobarbital.
2. Stereotaxis apparatus.
3. Surgical drill.
4. Hamilton syringe (5 μl).

2.4. Thermal Hyperalgesia

1. Plantar Test Apparatus (Ugo Basile, Varese, Italy).
2. Plastic cage (22 × 17 × 14 cm; length, width, height) with glass door.
3. Infrared bulb (Osram halogen–bellaphot bulb, 8 V, 50 W).

2.5. Mechanical Allodynia

1. Dynamic Plantar Analgesiometer (Ugo Basile).

2.6. Motor Coordination Behaviour

1. Rotarod Apparatus (Ugo Basile).

2.7. Fluorescence Cell Labelling Detection

1. Bouin's fixative is 75 ml picric acid, 25 ml 40% formaldehyde and 5 ml acetic acid glacial for 100 ml volume. Bouin's fixative is stable for two years. The bottles must be kept closed. The advised storage temperature is 18–30°C. Used solutions and solutions that are past their shelf-life must be disposed of, according to local disposal guidelines.
2. Cryostat embedding medium is Killik from Bio-Optica, Milan, Italy. Store at room temperature.
3. Bisbenzimide (Hoechst 33258) from Hoechst, Frankfurt, Germany. Store at −20°C and protect from light.

3. Methods

Human MSCs are isolated from a small aspirate of bone marrow and in vitro expanded in FGF-containing medium (10). Bone marrows are obtained from healthy children after informed consent (biopsy is performed to rule out leukemia) (see Note 5). The experimental procedures were approved by the Ethic Committee of the Second University of Naples.

Human MSCs are transplanted in the following brain areas involved in neuropathic pain controlling: somatosensory cortex, rostral agranular insular cortex, striatum and ventricle. Neuropathic mice are subject to stem cell transplantation after 4 days from sciatic nerve injury (SNI) and are monitored 7, 10, 14, 17 and 21 days after surgery. After each time, the animals are sacrificed and the brain removed for fluorescence microscopy.

3.1. Cell Culture

1. Dilute the aspirate in D-PBS (1:1).
2. Load the solution on 10 ml Ficoll.
3. Spin at 0.4 g for 30 min, room temperature.
4. Collect mononuclear cell fraction in a new tube.
5. Wash with PBS.
6. Spin at 0.4 g for 5 min, room temperature. Discard the supernatant.
7. Seed $1–2.5 \times 10^5$ cells per cm^2 in 100 mm dishes containing proliferating medium. Maintain cell cultures at 37°C with 5% CO_2 (see Note 6).
8. Discard non-adherent cells after 24–48 h to isolate adherent cells representing MSCs along with committed progenitors.
9. Wash twice with PBS.
10. Incubate cells for 7–10 days in proliferating medium to reach confluence.
11. Once to confluence, trypsinize the stem cells with trypsin/EDTA solution for 2 min at 37°C.
12. Stop the reaction with serum. Apply α-MEM with 10% FBS in an equal volume of trypsin/EDTA solution used.
13. Collect cells in a tube.
14. Spin at 0.2 g for 5 min, at room temperature.
15. Discard the supernatant and wash the pellet with PBS (three times).
16. Spin at 0.2 g for 5 min, room temperature. Discard the supernatant.
17. Re-suspend the pellet in 1 ml PBS.

18. Add 5 µl of Vybrant CM-DiI cell labelling solution, incubate for 5 min at 37°C.
19. Spin at 0.2 g for 5 min, room temperature.
20. Discard the supernatant and wash the pellet with PBS (three times).
21. Count cells using a cell counter chamber.
22. Re-suspend cells in PBS with 10% heparin. DiI-labelled hMSCs are now ready to be transplanted.

3.2. Spared Nerve Injury

1. Anaesthetise mice with sodium pentobarbital (60 mg/kg, i.p.) (see Note 7).
2. Expose the sciatic nerve at mid-thigh level distal to the trifurcation and free it of connective tissue (see Note 8).
3. Expose the three peripheral branches (sural, common peroneal, and tibial nerves) of the sciatic nerve without stretching nerve structures.
4. Delicately place a micro-surgical forceps with curved tips below the tibial and common peroneal nerves to slide the thread around the nerves.
5. Loosely tie a chromic gut ligature (5–0 silk) around the tibial and common peroneal branches of the nerve.
6. Axotomise these branches leaving only the sural nerve intact. Remove 1–2 mm section of the two nerves.
7. Close muscle and skin flaps with suture.
8. Apply antibiotic to the exposed tissue to prevent infection.

3.3. Stem Cell Transplantation

1. Anaesthetise mice with sodium pentobarbital (60 mg/kg, i.p.) and place them in a stereotaxic apparatus.
2. The skull is exposed through a longitudinal incision that allows visualisation of the bregma (point of reference for identifying the coordinates of areas of interest anteroposteriority and laterality).
3. The cranial reliquary is then drilled and stem cells are micro-injected into the hole by using a 5 µl Hamilton syringe attached to the stereotaxic apparatus (see Note 9). A volume of 3 µl solution (stem cells + vehicle, or vehicle only) is injected over a period of 5 s (see Note 10). After the administration, antibiotic is applied to the exposed tissue to prevent infection.

3.4. Thermal Hyperalgesia

1. Each animal is placed in a plastic cage with a glass floor.
2. After a 30 min habituation period, the plantar surface of the hind paw is exposed to a beam of radiant heat through the glass floor. The radiant heat source is an infrared bulb.

A photoelectric cell detects light reflected from the paw and turns off the lamp when paw movement interrupts the reflected light. The paw withdrawal latency is automatically displayed to the nearest 0.1 s; the cut-off time is 20 s in order to prevent tissue damage.

3.5. Mechanical Allodynia

1. Mice are allowed to move freely in one of the two compartments of the enclosure positioned on the metal mesh surface.
2. Mice are adapted to the testing environment before any measurements are taken. After that, the mechanical stimulus is delivered to the plantar surface of the hindpaw of the mouse from below the floor of the test chamber by an automated testing device. A steel rod (2 mm) is pushed with electronical ascending force (0–30 g in 10 s). When the animal withdraws its hindpaw, the mechanical stimulus is automatically withdrawn and the force records to the nearest 0.1 g. Nociceptive responses for thermal and mechanical sensitivity are expressed as thermal paw withdrawal latency (PWL) in seconds and mechanical paw withdrawal threshold (PWT) in grams.
3. Each mouse serves as its own control, the responses being measured both before and after surgical procedures.

3.6. Motor Coordination Behaviour

1. Motor coordination is evaluated by the Rotarod test (Ugo Basile, Varese, Italy). The mouse is placed on a rotary cylinder and the time (in second) of its equilibrium before falling is determined. The cylinder is subdivided in five sections, allowing to screen five animals per test (one for section), simultaneously. Below to the cylinder there is a platform in its turn subdivided in five plates (in correspondence of the five sections) each one of which is connected to a magnet that, activated from the fall of the mouse on the plate, allows to record the time of permanence on the cylinder.
2. After a period of adaptation of 30 s ones, the spin speed gradually increases from 5 to 40 rpm for the maximum time of 5 min.
3. In the same day, the animals are analysed by two separate tests from an interval of time of 1 h. The experiment is performed for every group of animals, the day before the behavioural tests in order to avoid useless stress and 1 h after the cell administration. The time of permanence of the mouse on the cylinder is expressed as latency (sec).

3.7. Fluorescence Microscopy

1. Perfuse animals transcardially with 150 ml of saline solution (0.9% NaCl) and 250 ml of Bouin's fixative.
2. Take out the brain and keep it in the fixative for 24 h at 4°C (see Note 11).

3. Wash two times with D-PBS.
4. Keep the tissue in D-PBS + 30% sucrose. Store at 4°C at least overnight.
5. Freeze the tissue, submerging it in cryostat embedding medium. Store at –80°C.
6. Slice serial 15 μm sections of the several brain areas with cryostat.
7. Wash in D-PBS for 5 min, twice.
8. Counterstain sections with bisbenzimide for 5 min at room temperature to stain DNA and identify the nuclei (blue fluorescence).
9. Mount with D-PBS–glycerol (1:1). The slides can be viewed immediately, or be stored in the dark at 4°C for up to a month.
10. The slides are viewed under fluorescence microscopy to locate the cells and identify the brain areas. Software can be used to overlay the fluorescence images. Examples of the labelled stem cells injected are shown in Fig. 1.

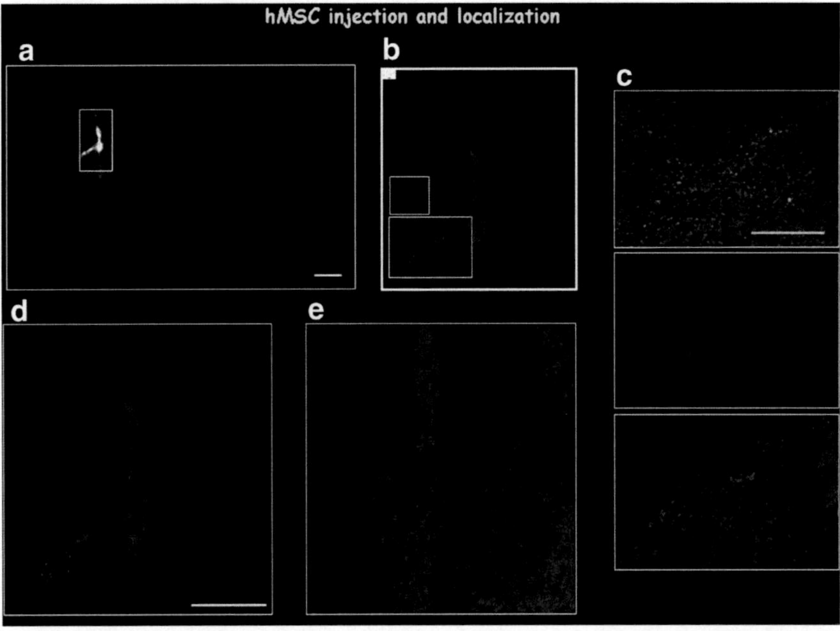

Fig. 1. Representative cross-sections of mouse brain area (*striatum*) from DiI-labelled hMSC-treated mice. (**a**) Human MSCs home at the injection site after transplantation. DiI-labelled hMSCs emit red fluorescence (lighter in the figure). The cell nuclei are counterstained with Hoechst 33258. (**b**) High magnification of (**a**). Subparts (**c**) represent 40× magnification of the area enclosed in the white perimeter in (**b**) (20× magnification). *Top*: The cell nuclei are stained with Hoechst 33258. *Middle*: DiI-labelled hMSCs. *Bottom*: Merge. (**d**) Higher magnification of (**b**). (**e**) Pictures with both DiI (*red*) and Hoechst 33258 (*blue*) fluorescence are merged. Scale bars: 25 μm (**a**), 50 μm (**c**) and 100 μm (**d**)

4. Notes

1. Cell culture: All solutions should be prepared in water that has a resistance of 18.2 MΩ-cm and total organic content of less than five parts per billion.
2. α-MEM and D-PBS: Add penicillin/streptomycin at indicated concentration, once opened. Store at 4°C.
3. FBS: Prepare aliquots and store at –20°C.
4. b-FGF: The lyophilised protein is stable for at least 2 years from date of receipt at –20°C. Reconstituted FGF-basic is stable for several months when stored in working aliquots at –20°C. Avoid repeated freeze/thaw cycles.
5. All children have shown no statistically significant differences in the body mass index and had the same age range (4–6 years old).
6. Stem cells are passaged when approaching confluence with trypsin/EDTA to provide new maintenance cultures on 100 mm; tissue dishes. We use cells till the fourth passage, each time plate 2×10^3 cells per cm^2.
7. Male C57BL/6 N mice (35–40 g) are housed three per cage under controlled illumination (12:12 h light:dark cycle; light on 06:00 h) and environmental conditions (room temperature 20–22° C, humidity 55–60%) for at least 1 week before the commencement of experiments. Mouse chow and tap water are available ad libitum. Behavioural testing is performed before surgery to establish a baseline for comparison with post-surgical values. Mononeuropathy is induced according to the method of Bourquin and Decosterd (11). The experimental procedures must be conformed to the guidelines of the International Association for the Study of Pain (www.iasp-pain.org).
8. Carefully, preserve the sural nerve by avoiding any nerve stretch or nerve contact with surgical tools. Perform sham-operated mice as control. In these animals, the sciatic nerve is exposed, but is not ligated or cut.
9. Transplant 50,000 cells per mouse in a volume of 3 μl using a Hamilton syringe. Cells are suspended in PBS with 10% heparin to avoid cluster formation. Vehicle solution is PBS with 10% heparin. Heparin is added from a stock of 1 KU/ml. Keep gently mixing the final aliquot of stem cells before injection.

10. Microinject hMSCs, controlateral to the sciatic nerve injury, into the following areas of the mouse cortex using coordinates from the Atlas of Paxinos and Watson (12):
    (a) Rostral Agranular Insular Cortex or RAIC: AP=5.6 mm and L=2.5 mm from bregma, V=3.2 mm below the dura;
    (b) Somatosensory 1, Barrel Field or SIBF: AP=4.0 mm and L=3.0 mm from bregma, V=2.0 mm below the dura);
    (c) Striatum (AP=4 mm and L=2 mm from bregma, V=3 mm below the dura);
    (d) Ventricle (AP=3.5 mm and L=1.0 mm from bregma, V=2.5 mm below the dura).
11. Be sure that the brain is completely immerged in the fixative or in the PBS/sucrose solution.

Acknowledgments

The author would like to thank Prof. Franceso Rossi and Sabatino Maione for funding support, Prof. Umberto Galderisi for his advice and encouragement, Dr. Catia Giordano, Nicola Alessio and Livio Luongo for technical assistance.

References

1. Siniscalco D, Rossi F, Maione S (2007) Molecular approaches for neuropathic pain treatment. Curr Med Chem 14:1783–1787
2. Siniscalco D, Rossi F, Maione S (2008) Stem cell therapy for neuropathic pain treatment. Journal of Stem Cells and Regenerative Medicine vol III (1)
3. Beyer Nardi N, da Silva Meirelles L (2006) Mesenchymal stem cells: isolation, in vitro expansion and characterization. Handb Exp Pharmacol 174:249–282
4. Sethe S, Scutt A, Stolzing A (2006) Aging of mesenchymal stem cells. Ageing Res Rev 5:91–116
5. Giordano A, Galderisi U, Marino IR (2007) From the laboratory bench to the patient's bedside: an update on clinical trials with mesenchymal stem cells. J Cell Physiol 211:27–35
6. Le Blanc K, Pittenger M (2005) Mesenchymal stem cells: progress toward promise. Cytotherapy 7:36–45
7. Jori FP, Napolitano MA, Melone MA, Cipollaro M, Cascino A, Altucci L, Peluso G, Giordano A, Galderisi U (2005) Molecular pathways involved in neural in vitro differentiation of marrow stromal stem cells. J Cell Biochem 94:645–655
8. Bae JS, Han HS, Youn DH, Carter JE, Modo M, Schuchman EH, Jin HK (2007) Bone marrow-derived mesenchymal stem cells promote neuronal networks with functional synaptic transmission after transplantation into mice with neurodegeneration. Stem Cells 25:1307–1316
9. Musolino PL, Coronel MF, Hökfelt T, Villar MJ (2007) Bone marrow stromal cells induce changes in pain behavior after sciatic nerve constriction. Neurosci Lett 418: 97–101
10. Squillaro T, Hayek G, Farina E, Cipollaro M, Renieri A, Galderisi U (2008) A case report: bone marrow mesenchymal stem cells from a Rett syndrome patient are prone to senescence and show a lower degree of apoptosis. J Cell Biochem 103:1877–1885
11. Bourquin AF, Süveges M, Pertin M, Gilliard N, Sardy S, Davison AC, Spahn DR, Decosterd I (2006) Assessment and analysis of mechanical allodynia-like behavior induced by spared nerve injury (SNI) in the mouse. Pain 122(14): e1–e14
12. Paxinos G, Watson C (1986) The rat brain in stereotaxic coordinates. Academic, London

Chapter 26

Delivery of RNA Interference to Peripheral Neurons In Vivo Using Herpes Simplex Virus

Anna-Maria Anesti

Abstract

RNA interference (RNAi) has become a powerful tool for modulating gene expression. While delivery of small interfering RNAs (siRNAs) has achieved silencing of pain-related genes in various animal models of nociception, delivery of short-hairpin RNA (shRNA) or artificial miRNA (miRNA) to dorsal root ganglia (DRG) has proven particularly challenging. This chapter describes a highly efficient method for in vivo gene silencing in sensory neurons using replication-defective vectors based on herpes simplex virus (HSV). This method can be utilised to obtain a better understanding of gene function, validate novel gene targets in drug discovery and potentially develop new RNAi-mediated approaches to achieve analgesia.

Key words: RNAi, Herpes simplex virus, Silencing, Sensory neurons, Delivery, shRNA, miRNA

1. Introduction

1.1. RNA Interference

RNA interference (RNAi) is an evolutionary conserved, sequence-specific, post-transcriptional gene silencing mechanism mediated by small dsRNA molecules, including small interfering RNAs (siRNAs) and microRNAs (miRNAs). siRNAs originate from endogenous or exogenous long dsRNA and have been suggested to function in anti-viral defense, silencing of mRNAs that are overproduced or translationally aborted and guarding the genome from disruption by transgenes and transposons. miRNAs are endogenous, regulatory, non-coding RNA molecules involved in almost every developmental and cellular process investigated so far (1, 2). They are transcribed by RNA polymerase (pol) II as part of a long primary miRNA transcript (pri-miRNA) that is processed in the nucleus by the enzyme Drosha into a precursor miRNA (pre-miRNA), which is subsequently exported to the cytoplasm (3–5).

Arpad Szallasi (ed.), *Analgesia: Methods and Protocols*, Methods in Molecular Biology, vol. 617, DOI 10.1007/978-1-60327-323-7_26,

Both siRNAs and miRNAs are generated by Dicer, a cytoplasmic family of RNase III enzymes that cleave long dsRNA or pre-miRNA into 21–23 nt dsRNA molecules with symmetric 2–3 nt 3′ overhangs (6, 7). Following unwinding of the siRNA or miRNA duplex, the strand with the thermodynamically less stable 5′end, termed the guide strand, is incorporated into related RNA-induced silencing complexes (RISCs), while the other strand, termed the passenger strand, is degraded (8). Unlike siRNAs, which generally have perfect complementarity to their mRNA targets and thus mediate silencing by mRNA degradation, animal miRNAs generally have imperfect complementarity to their target mRNAs and thus, direct silencing by repressing translation.

1.2. Induction of RNAi in Mammalian Cells

While effective silencing in *Caenorhabditis elegans* and *Drosophila melanogaster* can be achieved using long dsRNAs, in mammalian systems (9), dsRNA of >30 bp induces the interferon (IFN) response, which leads to non-specific translational inhibition and RNA degradation. RNAi in mammalian cells can be induced by the introduction of synthetic siRNAs and by plasmid or viral vector systems that express short-hairpin RNA (shRNA).

shRNA is most commonly transcribed from a type III RNA pol III promoter, such as U6 or H1, as sense and antisense 19–29 bp long sequences connected by a loop of unpaired nucleotides (Fig. 1a). Following expression in the nucleus, shRNAs are exported to the cytoplasm and are processed by Dicer to generate functional siRNAs. Candidate shRNAs are often designed to target the coding sequence of the target gene that is generally better characterised than the 3′ or 5′ untranslated region (UTR). Moreover, shRNAs may be designed to target orthologs in more than one species or multiple splice variants of the target gene. Different shRNA sequences against a target gene often manifest a spectrum of potency and may non-specifically target unrelated genes to which they anneal with partial complementary, termed off-target effects (10). Computational tools have been developed to increase the likelihood of selecting effective shRNAs and reduce potential off-target effects. Algorithms select candidate shRNA sequences based on the sequence and thermodynamic properties of functional miRNAs and in most cases, a genome-wide BLAST search is automatically performed to identify potential similarities to other mRNAs that may be unintentionally targeted. Nevertheless, experimental validation is necessary to confirm the potency and specificity of the selected shRNAs. Reporter-based assays, which allow the target gene to be fused to a reporter gene and expressed from a plasmid vector, have been developed for rapid validation of shRNA sequences. Although downregulation of reporter activity correlates well with knockdown of target gene expression, it is necessary to test pre-validated shRNAs for their ability to silence endogenous gene expression.

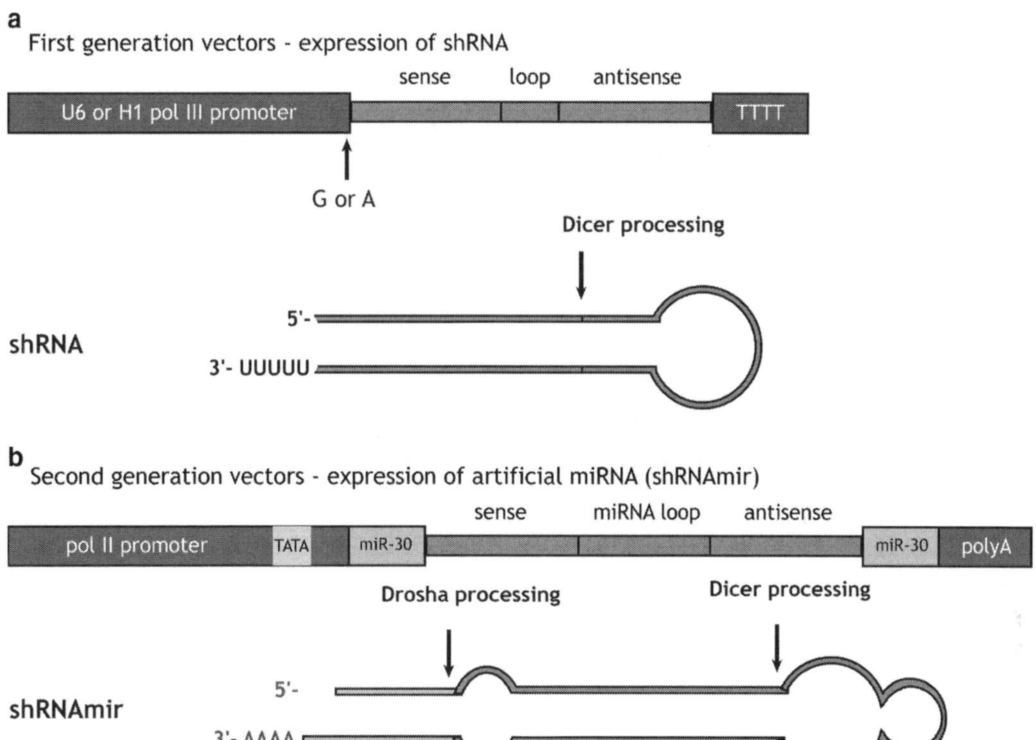

Fig. 1. Expression of shRNA from first- and second-generation vectors. Expression of shRNA under the control of a pol III promoter, such as the U6 or H1 promoter, results in the formation of a stable hairpin with a 3–4 nt 3′ overhang from the RNA pol III transcription termination that resembles an endogenous pre-miRNA. For expression of artificial miRNA, the stem of the pri-miR-30 or pri-miR-155 transcript is replaced with the shRNA sequence, without affecting normal miRNA maturation

In addition to shRNA design, the success of RNAi-mediated gene silencing is also dependent on target gene expression and protein turnover.

As the understanding of miRNA biogenesis advanced, new generation RNAi triggers were developed (Fig. 1b). Artificial miRNAs, also known as shRNAmir, have been most commonly modeled on miR-30 and miR-155 (11–13). The stem of the pri-miRNA, which can be expressed using either pol III or pol II promoters, can be replaced with shRNA sequences against different target genes, without affecting normal miRNA maturation. Drosha excises the engineered stem-loops to generate intermediates that resemble endogenous pre-miRNAs, which are subsequently exported to the cytoplasm and processed by Dicer into functional miRNAs. These artificial miRNAs, which have perfect complementarity to their mRNA targets, have been demonstrated to mediate silencing by mRNA endonucleolytic cleavage rather than translational repression. The use of artificial miRNAs has become a very attractive alternative to the expression of shRNA

(14, 15). Artificial miRNAs are amenable to pol II transcription and polycistronic strategies, which allow delivery of multiple shRNA sequences simultaneously and co-expression of a reporter gene or a biologically active protein together with the shRNA.

Off-target effects have not been reported in systematic studies using shRNA or artificial miRNA. This is most likely due to shRNAs/miRNAs being dependent on endogenous processing by Drosha and Dicer, which are rate-limiting steps in the generation of siRNAs and may therefore limit the concentration-dependent off-target effects observed with synthetic siRNAs. However, expression of shRNA has been shown to cause retraction of synapses and dendritic spines in primary hippocampal neurons by triggering the innate immune response (16), and early embryonic lethality in zygotes that was associated with increased expression of an IFN-induced gene (17). Moreover, specific sequences capable of inducing an IFN response have been identified around the transcription start site in pol III driven shRNA expression systems (18). Induction of an IFN response gene in primary cortical cultures by expression of shRNA was abolished by the introduction of the target sequence into an miR-30 backbone (19). Moreover, neurotoxicity in the mouse striatum caused by expression of shRNAs was significantly attenuated when these sequences were inserted in miR-30-based vectors (20). High levels of shRNA expression, commonly achieved with pol III promoters, can lead to competition with endogenous miRNAs for limiting cellular factors (21–23). This can result in oversaturation of the endogenous miRNA pathway, which has been shown to cause lethality in animals (24). Selection of potent shRNA sequences capable of effective silencing even when expressed at low levels and the use of promoters that mediate moderate levels of shRNA expression are an effective strategy to minimise toxicity. Unlike siRNAs and shRNAs, miRNAs, which are expressed in moderate levels and processed more efficiently than shRNAs, do not compete with the endogenous miRNA pathway and thus, have improved safety profiles (15, 23).

1.3. Induction of RNAi in Peripheral Neurons In Vivo

Most pain-related RNAi approaches published to date involve delivery of synthetic siRNAs by repeated injections or continuous infusion. Silencing of several pain-related genes has been achieved in various animal models of nociception using this experimental design (25–28). However, knockdown is transient lasting only up to several days, requires high doses of siRNAs, and lacks specificity in the sense that uptake of siRNAs cannot be restricted to neurons or a specific subset of neurons. As a more efficient alternative, targeted delivery of RNAi to neurons can be achieved using viral vectors. Although lentiviruses, adenoviruses, and adeno-associated viruses have been engineered to deliver shRNA to the central nervous system (29–33), delivery of shRNA/miRNA to dorsal root ganglia (DRG), which are inaccessible by surgical techniques and thus, not amenable to direct injection with viral vectors, has been particularly challenging.

Herpes simplex virus (HSV-1), which is one of the most common human pathogens causing cold sores, has many unique features that support its development as a vector for the delivery of genes and RNAi to the nervous system. It is a highly infectious, naturally neurotrophic virus and the HSV genome can be easily manipulated, has a high capacity to accept foreign DNA and does not integrate into the host chromosome, thus eliminating the possibility of insertional activation or inactivation of cellular genes. The life cycle of HSV-1 begins in epithelial cells of the skin or mucous membrane. During primary infection, progeny virions enter sensory nerve terminals innervating the infection site, and the nucleocapsid and tegument proteins undergo retrograde axonal transport to the cell bodies in the sensory ganglia, where the viral genomes are retained in a latent state. Periodic reactivation of HSV from latency can occur spontaneously or in response to a variety of stimuli and results in the production of progeny virions that are anterogradely transported back to the nerve terminals. Deletion of essential genes from the HSV-1 genome results in replication-defective viruses that can be directly propagated to high titres in appropriate cell lines, which complement the deleted gene products without the need for a contaminating helper virus. In vivo, the temporal cascade of viral gene expression is incapable of proceeding past the immediate early phase, resulting in recombinants that establish a persistent state very similar to latency, but are unable to reactivate from latency and therefore persist for long periods of time in both neuronal cells and non-neuronal cells in culture.

Replication-defective HSV-1 vectors are safe, non-toxic and allow highly efficient gene delivery to neurons both in vitro and in vivo (34, 35). Moreover, they are particularly efficient at targeting DRG neurons in both mice and rats through retrograde transport following injection into the sciatic nerve. Recently, we have demonstrated that replication-defective HSV-1 vectors can also allow efficient delivery of shRNA and artificial miRNA to peripheral neurons in vivo to induce effective and specific RNAi-mediated silencing of targeted genes (36) (Fig. 2). Several shRNA or miRNA sequences against each target gene are designed using an online algorithm. Up to six candidate sequences per gene are selected, synthesised, annealed, and inserted into plasmid vectors. The shRNA or miRNA sequences are validated in 293 T cells using the pSCREEN-iT/lacZ-DEST Gateway vector kit from Invitrogen, and the most potent sequences are inserted into HSV vectors. Construction of replication-defective HSV-1 vectors involves the introduction of the cassette of interest directly into the HSV-1 genome. This is achieved by insertion of

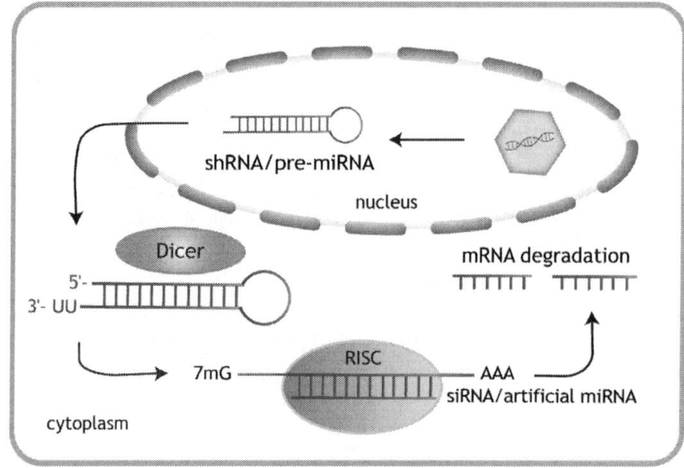

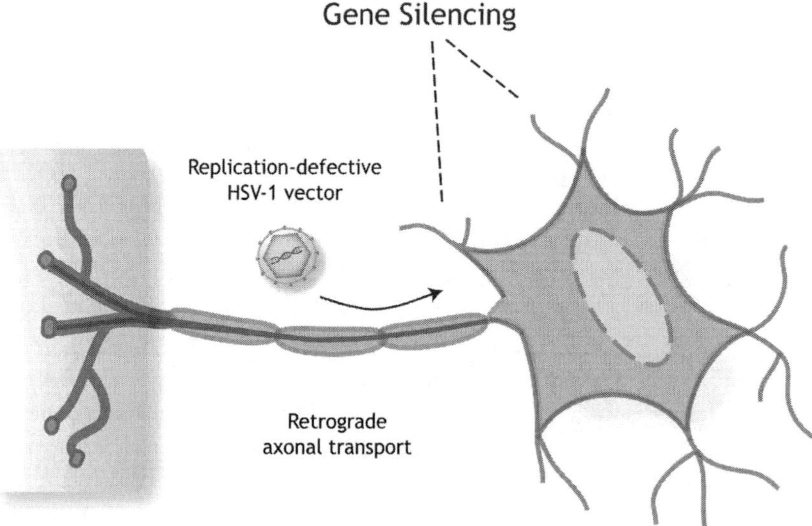

Fig. 2. Silencing in sensory neurons in vivo using replication-defective HSV-1 vectors. Following injection into the sciatic nerve, the virus enters the axons of sensory neurons and gets retrogradely transported to the cell bodies in the DRG, where it expresses shRNA or artificial miRNA, resulting in degradation of target mRNA. Silencing of gene targets can be assessed by western blot analysis on protein extracted from DRG

the shRNA or miRNA sequence into a plasmid that contains the expression cassette flanked by specific HSV sequences. Following co-transfection into complementing cells, the cassette is inserted into the HSV genome by homologous recombination, and the virus is purified and grown to a high titre. Vectors expressing artificial miRNA can be engineered to target multiple genes simultaneously by expressing multiple miRNA sequences. In addition, green fluorescent protein (GFP) is expressed from these vectors to allow labelling of transduced cells.

Replication-defective HSV-1 vectors expressing shRNA or artificial miRNA are available from NeuroVex. Delivery of these vectors to the DRG via injection into the sciatic nerve and assessment target gene silencing using western blot on protein extracted from DRG are described in this chapter.

2. Materials

2.1. Sciatic Nerve Injection

1. Replication-defective HSV-1 (Note 1)
2. Fine forceps (Dumont #55, Dumostar, Williston, VT).
3. Curved tip forceps (Dumont #7, Dumostar).
4. Fine iris straight scissors.
5. Standard scalpel and sterile blades
6. 50 μl microcapillary pipettes
7. 10 μl Hamilton syringe 700 series, cemented needle, blunt end
8. Portex fine bore polythene tubing
9. Silk 5/0 suture
10. Silk 4/0 suture with 16 mm curved needle
11. DMEM (Gibco/BRL, Bethesda, MD)
12. Phosphate buffered saline
13. Carprofen (Rimadyl) (Pfizer Animal Health, New York, NY)
14. Bupivacaine HCl
15. Microcapillary pipettes are polished into fine glass needles and connected to the syringe through fine tubing using super-glue. The needle is washed with PBS and then filled with PBS. Prior to loading the needle with virus, a small air bubble is formed to ensure that PBS and virus do not mix (Note 2).

2.2. Extraction of Protein from DRG

1. Glass homogenizer, 1 ml volume
2. RIPA lysis buffer (Sigma)
3. Protease inhibitors
4. Autoclaved 1.5 ml microcentrifuge tubes
5. Autoclaved cryotubes and liquid nitrogen

2.3. SDS-PAGE

1. Separating gel buffer: 1.5 M Tris–HCl, pH 8.8. Store at room temperature.
2. Stacking gel buffer: 0.5 M Tris–HCl, pH 6.8. Store at room temperature.
3. 30% acrylamide (29.2 g acrylamide and 0.8 g of bis-acrylamide in 100 ml H_2O)
4. 20% SDS (lauryl sodium dodecyl sulfate)

5. 10% Ammonium persulfate (APS)
6. TEMED (N,N,N,N′-Tetramethyl-ethylenediamine)
7. (5×) SDS-PAGE running buffer: 1 g SDS, 3 g Tri-base and 14.4 g Glycine in 1 L H_2O
8. Pre-stained molecular weight markers
9. Laemmli standard loading buffer: 5% β-mercaptoethanol, 50 mM Tris–HCl pH 8.0, 6% (v/v) glycerol, 2% (w/v) SDS, and 0.005% (w/v) bromophenol blue.

2.4. Western Blotting

1. Transfer buffer: 3 g Tris-base and 14.4 Glycine in 800 ml H_2O and add 200 ml methanol
2. Hybond-C nitrocellulose membrane (Amersham, Pittsburgh, PA)
3. 3 mm Whatman paper
4. Tris-buffered saline with Tween (TBS-T), 10× stock: 1.37 M NaCl, 27 mM KCl, 250 mM Tris-HCl, pH 7.4, 1% Tween-20. Dilute 100 ml with 900 ml water for use
5. Blocking buffer: 5% skimmed milk in PBS
6. Antibody dilution buffer: PBST
7. ECL plus reagents (Amersham)

3. Methods

3.1. Sciatic Nerve Injection

1. The animal is injected with Carprofen (10 mg/kg for mouse and 5 mg/kg for rat) at least 1 h prior to the operation. The action of the analgesic lasts for up to 24 h.
2. The animal is removed from the cage and anesthetised in a chamber.
3. A large area of the upper thigh surrounding the operation site is shaved (in a separate room) and sterilised with povidone iodine or chlorhexidine solution and 70% ethanol.
4. The animal is placed on a heated pad to avoid hypothermia and a mask is fitted to maintain anaesthesia. The breathing pattern of the animal should be monitored regularly and the anaesthesia adjusted accordingly. A low amount of anaesthetic is required to maintain anaesthesia, but this may have to be slightly increased when inserting the needle into the sciatic nerve. A drop of local anaesthetic, such as bupivacaine, can be used directly onto the sciatic nerve, but this may interfere with virus transduction.

5. A sterile drape is placed over the whole animal with a small opening over the operation area.
6. Ensure the animal is well anesthetised by testing a reflex such as pinching the web of skin between the toes. If a withdrawal response occurs, the animal is insufficiently anaesthetised and additional anaesthesia should be given, before the test is repeated.
7. A small incision is made in the skin above the upper region of the left femur using a scalpel.
8. Fine scissors are used to pierce the fascia between the biceps femoris and semitendinosus muscles and gently separate the muscles without damaging them in order to expose the sciatic nerve lying beneath.
9. Curved tip forceps are slipped under the sciatic nerve and used to gently lift and position it ready for injection. The forceps hold the nerve during the injection but should not put pressure on the nerve.
10. Fine forceps are used to separate the two main branches of the sciatic nerve (tibial nerve and common peroneal). The tibial nerve is the larger of the two branches and is the nerve injected with virus.
11. A loose ligature is tied around the tibial nerve using 5/0 silk suture.
12. The nerve is carefully pierced with the glass needle, which is inserted a few mm deep and then loosely tied in with the ligature. The virus is slowly injected into the nerve (Note 3).
13. The needle is then carefully withdrawn and the ligature is made slightly taut to prevent any outflow of virus without damaging the nerve (Note 4).
14. The curved tip forceps holding the nerve are removed and the nerve is carefully placed in its original position.
15. Finally, the skin is sutured closed with 4/0 silk suture using a 16-mm curved needle or sealed with tissue glue.
16. The animal is allowed to recover from surgery on the heated pad until the return of major reflexes. It is then placed in a clean cage.
17. The animal should be monitored post-operatively.

An example of delivery to mouse DRG using this method is shown in Fig. 3.

3.2. Extraction of Protein from DRG

1. Injection of the virus into the tibial branch of the sciatic nerve results in delivery mainly to the L4 DRG (Note 5). Dissect the L4 DRG from the injected side of five mice to obtain enough protein for western blotting. If the protein is

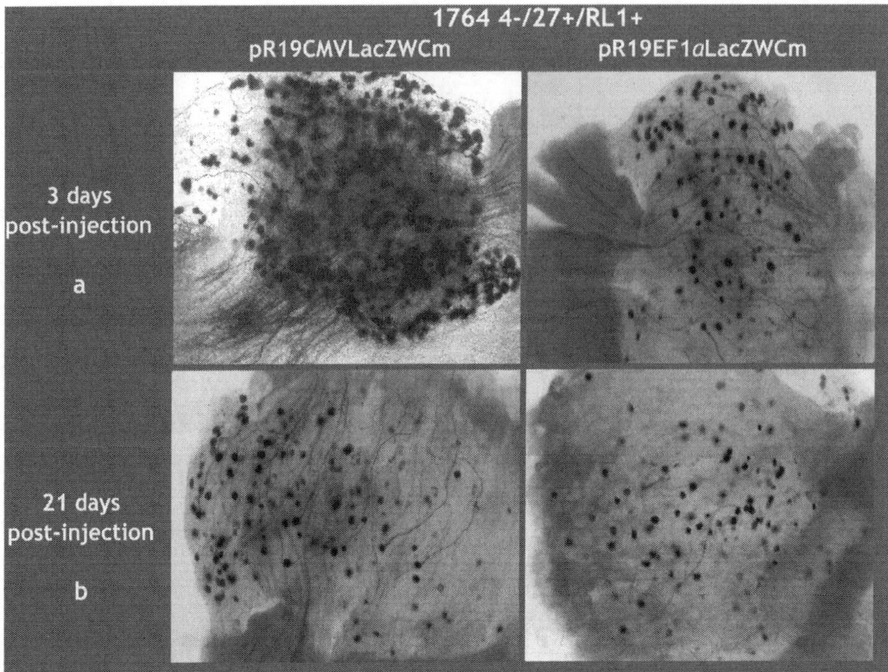

Fig. 3. Evaluation of beta-galactosidase expression in mouse DRG following sciatic nerve injection of a replication-defective HSV-1 virus expressing lacZ either from the CMV or the EF1a promoter. X-gal staining on whole mount L4 DRG preparations at: (**a**) 3 days post-injection demonstrated that the virus allows highly efficient gene delivery to mouse sensory neurons following injection into the sciatic nerve, with the CMV promoter driving considerably higher levels of expression in these neurons than the EF1a promoter. (**b**) 21 days post-injection demonstrated that expression is maintained for long periods of time, but it is reduced compared to that at early times post-injection. (Magnification ×5)

weakly expressed or the antibody results in weak detection of the protein, it may be necessary to extract protein from 10 DRG (Note 6).

2. The DRG are placed into cryotubes and snap-frozen in liquid nitrogen. They can be stored at –80°C or in liquid nitrogen until protein is extracted.
3. Protease inhibitors are added to the lysis buffer. The lysis buffer, glass homogenizer, and all tubes are kept on ice.
4. The frozen DRG are transferred to a single pre-weighted tube. Immediately after they have been weighted, the DRG are transferred to the homogenizer and 300 μl of lysis buffer is added for every 5 mg of tissue. The cell lysate is transferred to a clean tube and the homogenizer is rinsed with 200 μl of lysis buffer.
5. The tube containing 500 μl of cell lysate is placed on an orbital shaker at 4°C for 2 h and then centrifuged at 4°C for 20 min at 12,000 rpm. The supernatant is transferred to a clean tube and kept on ice.

6. The protein extracted from the DRG is concentrated using the MICROCON centrifugal filter device.
7. The concentration of protein is measured using either the BCA or Bradford assay.

3.3. SDS-PAGE

1. The glass plates for the gels are cleaned with ethanol and allowed to dry.
2. 15% separating gel for 4 gels is prepared by mixing 4.7 ml of H_2O, 10 ml 30% acrylamide, 5 ml separating gel buffer, 200 μl 10% APS, 100 μl 20% SDS and 30 μl TEMED. Pour 4 ml gel, leaving space for the stacking gel, and overlay with water. Leave to polymerize for 1 h.
3. Prepare 4% stacking gel for 4 gels by mixing 12.2 ml H_2O, 2.66 ml 30% acrylamide, 5 ml separating gel buffer, 150 μl 10% APS, 100 μl 20% SDS, and 20 μl TEMED. Pour off the water and add the stacking gel. Leave to polymerize for 1 h.
4. Once the gel has set, carefully remove the comb, wash the wells with running buffer using a syringe and place it in the tank.
5. Add running buffer to the upper and lower chambers (Note 7).
6. The cell lysates are denatured in loading buffer at 95°C for 5 min. 10–50 μl of sample and 2–5 μl of marker are loaded to the wells.
7. The gel is run at 20 mA through the stacking gel and then at 40 mA, until the samples have reached the bottom of the gel.

3.4. Western Blotting

1. Whilst the gel is run, the transfer buffer is placed at –20°C.
2. The gel is removed from the tank. The stacking gel is discarded and the separating gel is rinsed in ice-cold transfer buffer.
3. The nitrocellulose membrane and Whatman paper (two sheets per gel) are cut to the size of the gel. The Whatman paper is soaked in ice-cold transfer buffer, whereas the nitrocellulose membrane is placed on the surface of the buffer and is allowed to wet by capillary action.
4. The gel is carefully placed on top of the wet nitrocellulose membrane. The membrane and gel are placed between two sheets of wet Whatman paper, ensuring that no bubbles are trapped between the membrane and gel, and then between two wet foam sheets.
5. The cassette is placed in the tank with the nitrocellulose facing the anode, and the tank is filled with transfer buffer (Note 8).
6. The tank is placed on ice and a magnetic stir bar in the tank is activated to ensure to maintain a temperature of 10–15°C.
7. The samples are transferred at 70 V for 2 h.

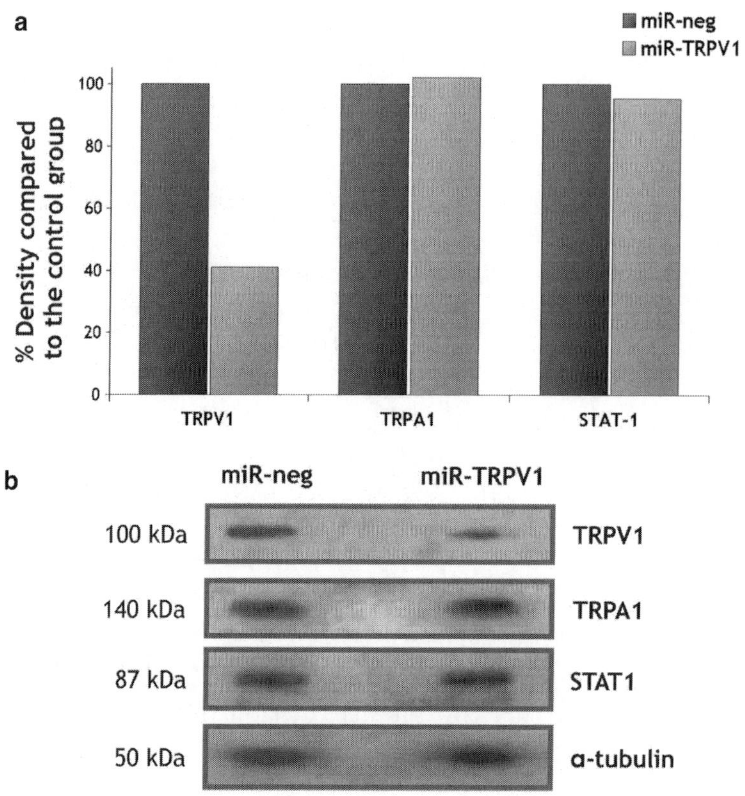

Fig. 4. HSV-mediated silencing of endogenous TrpV1. BALB/c mice were injected once directly into the sciatic nerve with 5×10^6 pfu of either HSV-CMV/EmGFP-miR-TRPV1 ($n=10$) or HSV-CMV/EmGFP-miR-neg ($n=10$), which express miRNA against TrpV1 or an miRNA sequence that is not predicted to target any known vertebrate gene, respectively. At day 8, the L4 DRG isolated from each group were pooled, protein was extracted and western blots were performed for TrpV1, TrpA1, and Stat1. (**a**) The protein levels of α-tubulin were essentially the same between the two groups, indicating that an equal amount of protein was loaded. Whilst the levels of TrpA1 and Stat1 remained the same, the levels of TrpV1 were significantly lower in animals injected with HSV-CMV/EmGFP-miR-TRPV1 compared to animals injected with the negative control. (**b**) The density of the bands was quantified using the Scion Image software. Quantification of band density revealed an average 59% knockdown of TrpV1 protein in animals injected with HSV-CMV/EmGFP-miR-TRPV1 ($n=10$) compared to animals injected with the HSV-CMV/EmGFP-miR-neg control ($n=10$). The levels of TrpA1 and Stat1 were essentially the same between the two groups. Values were normalised against α-tubulin (loading control). Adapted from ref. 36

8. Once the transfer the complete, the nitrocellulose membrane is removed from the cassette and the corner is cut for orientation. The marker should be clearly visible.
9. The membrane is rinsed with PBST and blocked for 1 h at room temperature with gentle agitation (on a shaker).
10. The membranes are rinsed again in PBST and incubated with the primary antibody raised against the target gene (Note 9), STAT1 polyclonal antibody, or α-tubulin polyclonal antibody overnight at 4°C with gentle agitation. STAT-1 is involved in the induction of the IFN response and α-tubulin is a loading control (Note 10).

11. The membranes are washed in PBST 4 times for 5 min at room temperature with constant agitation.
12. The membranes are then incubated for 1 h at room temperature with an HRP-conjugated secondary antibody.
13. The membranes are washed in PBST 4 times for 5 min at room temperature with constant agitation.
14. Immunodetection is performed using the ECL + reagents.
15. The blots are scanned and the pixel count and intensity of each band is quantified using the Scion Image software.
16. Signals are normalised against α-tubulin and the results are expressed as a percentage of the negative control signal. An example of this method is shown in Fig. 4.

4. Notes

1. The HSV vectors are stored in −80°C or liquid nitrogen. The virus to be injected is defrosted and kept on ice. The remaining virus that has been defrosted can be stored at 4°C for up to 1 week. Avoid repeated freeze-thaw cycles as they may considerably affect the titre of the virus and do not store the virus at −20°C.
2. The needle and surgical instruments are autoclaved between injections. Ensure that no bubbles are present in the needle or tubing, as they may affect the pressure at which the virus is injected or completely block the injection.
3. Up to 5 µl of virus can be injected into the mouse and up to 10 µl can be injected into the rat sciatic nerve. If the tubing is blocked and the virus is not being injected despite putting gentle pressure on the plunger of the Hamilton syringe, cut the tubing with scissors, insert an insulin syringe in the tubing and inject very gently.
4. For pain studies, the ligature can be removed 10 min following injection of the virus.
5. HSV vectors expressing miRNA also express GFP co-cistronically with the miRNA. To evaluate the efficiency at which the virus has been delivered to the DRG and estimate the expression levels of miRNA, prior to homogenizing the DRG, assess expression of GFP using a fluorescent microscope. However, it is very important that the time between the DRG being defrosted and lysis buffer being added to them is kept to a minimum.

6. A smaller number of DRG may be isolated from rats to extract a sufficient amount of protein to perform the western blot.
7. The running buffer can be stored at room temperature and used for up to one month.
8. The transfer buffer can be used for up to five transfers in 1 week.
9. We have assessed knockdown of TrpV1 in 30 ng of total protein extracted from mouse DRG using the VR1 polyclonal antibody from Santa Cruz at a 1/200 dilution overnight at 4°C.
10. To assess the specificity of trpV1 silencing, we assessed the levels of trpA1 using the TrpA1 polyclonal antibody from Abcam (ab31486) at a 1/1,000 dilution overnight at 4°C (Fig. 4). If the target gene is a mutant allele, it is recommended that the levels of the wild-type allele are also investigated to determine specificity.

References

1. Lee RC, Feinbaum RL, Ambros V (1993) The *C. elegans* heterochronic gene lin-4 encodes small RNAs with antisense complementarity to lin-14. Cell 75(5):843–854
2. Lewis BP, Burge CB, Bartel DP (2005) Conserved seed pairing, often flanked by adenosines, indicates that thousands of human genes are microrna targets. Cell 120(1):15–20
3. Gregory RI, Yan K-P, Amuthan G, Chendrimada T, Doratotaj B, Cooch N, Shiekhattar R (2004) The microprocessor complex mediates the genesis of micrornas. Nature 432(7014):235–240
4. Lund E, Guttinger S, Calado A, Dahlberg JE, Kutay U (2004) Nuclear export of microrna precursors. Science 303(5654):95–98
5. Han J, Lee Y, Yeom K-H, Kim Y-K, Jin H, Kim VN (2004) The Drosha-DGCR8 complex in primary microrna processing. Genes Dev 18(24):3016–3027
6. Bernstein E, Caudy AA, Hammond SM, Hannon GJ (2001) Role for a bidentate ribonuclease in the initiation step of RNA interference. Nature 409(6818):363–366
7. Hutvagner G, Mclachlan J, Pasquinelli AE, Balint E, Tuschl T, Zamore PD (2001) A cellular function for the RNA-interference enzyme dicer in the maturation of the let-7 small temporal RNA. Science 293(5531):834–838
8. Khvorova A, Reynolds A, Jayasena SD (2003) Functional siRNAs and miRNAs exhibit strand bias. Cell 115(2):209–216
9. Fire A, Xu S, Montgomery MK, Kostas SA, Driver SE, Mello CC (1998) Potent and specific genetic interference by double-stranded RNA in *Caenorhabditis elegans*. Nature 391(6669):806–811
10. Jackson AL, Bartz SR, Schelter J, Kobayashi SV, Burchard J, Mao M, Li B, Cavet G, Linsley PS (2003) Expression profiling reveals off-target gene regulation by RNAi. Nat Biotech 21(6):635–637
11. Zeng Y, Wagner EJ, Cullen BR (2002) Both natural and designed micro RNAs can inhibit the expression of cognate mRNAs when expressed in human cells. Mol Cell 9(6):1327–1333
12. Zeng Y, Cullen BR (2003) Sequence requirements for micro RNA processing and function in human cells. RNA 9(1):112–123
13. Chung KH, Hart CC, Al-Bassam S, Avery A, Taylor J, Patel PD, Vojtek AB, Turner DL (2006) Polycistronic RNA polymerase II expression vectors for RNA interference based on BIC/miR-155. Nucleic Acids Res 34(7):e53
14. Silva JM, Li MZ, Chang K, Ge W, Golding MC, Rickles RJ, Siolas D, Hu G, Paddison PJ, Schlabach MR, Sheth N, Bradshaw J, Burchard J, Kulkarni A, Cavet G, Sachidanandam R, Mccombie WR, Cleary MA, Elledge SJ, Hannon GJ (2005) Second-generation shRNA libraries covering the mouse and human genomes. Nat Genet 37(11):1281–1288
15. Boudreau RL, Martins I, Davidson BL (2008) Artificial microRNAs as siRNA shuttles: improved safety as compared to shRNAs in vitro and in vivo. Mol Ther 17(1):169–175
16. Alvarez VA, Ridenour DA, Sabatini BL (2006) Retraction of synapses and dendritic spines

induced by off-target effects of RNA interference. J Neurosci 26(30):7820–7825

17. Cao W, Hunter R, Strnatka D, Mcqueen CA, Erickson RP (2005) DNA constructs designed to produce short hairpin, interfering RNAs in transgenic mice sometimes show early lethality and an interferon response. J Appl Genet 46(2):217–225
18. Pebernard S, Iggo RD (2004) Determinants of interferon-stimulated gene induction by RNAi vectors. Differentiation 72:103–111
19. Bauer M, Kinkl N, Meixner A, Kremmer E, Riemenschneider M, Forstl H, Gasser T, Ueffing M (2008) Prevention of interferon-stimulated gene expression using microRNA-designed hairpins. Gene Ther 16(1):142–147
20. Mcbride JL, Boudreau RL, Harper SQ, Staber PD, Monteys AM, Martins IS, Gilmore BL, Burstein H, Peluso RW, Polisky B, Carter BJ, Davidson BL (2008) Artificial miRNAs mitigate shRNA-mediated toxicity in the brain: implications for the therapeutic development of RNAi. Proc Natl Acad Sci USA 105(15): 5868–5873
21. Hutvágner G, Mj S, Cc M, Pd Z (2004) Sequence-specific inhibition of small RNA function. PLoS Biol 2(4):e98
22. Yi R, Doehle BP, Qin Y, Macara IG, Cullen BR (2005) Overexpression of exportin 5 enhances RNA interference mediated by short hairpin RNAs and microRNAs. RNA 11(2): 220–226
23. Castanotto D, Sakurai K, Lingeman R, Li H, Shively L, Aagaard L, Soifer H, Gatignol A, Riggs A, Rossi JJ (2007) Combinatorial delivery of small interfering RNAs reduces RNAi efficacy by selective incorporation into RISC. Nucleic Acids Res 35(15):5154–5164
24. Grimm D, Streetz KL, Jopling CL, Storm TA, Pandey K, Davis CR, Marion P, Salazar F, Kay MA (2006) Fatality in mice due to oversaturation of cellular microRNA/short hairpin RNA pathways. Nature 441(7092):537–541
25. Dorn G, Patel S, Wotherspoon G, Hemmings-Mieszczak M, Barclay J, Natt FJC, Martin P, Bevan S, Fox A, Ganju P, Wishart W, Hall J (2004) SiRNA relieves chronic neuropathic pain. Nucleic Acids Res 32(5):e49
26. Luo MC, Zhang DQ, Ma SW, Huang YY, Shuster S, Porreca F, Lai J (2005) An efficient intrathecal delivery of small interfering RNA to the spinal cord and peripheral neurons. Mol Pain 1(1):29
27. Tan PH, Yang LC, Shih HC, Lan KC, Cheng JT (2004) Gene knockdown with intrathecal siRNA of NMDA receptor NR2B subunit reduces formalin-induced nociception in the rat. Gene Ther 12(1):59–66
28. Christoph T, Grünweller A, Mika J, Schäfer MKH, Wade EJ, Weihe E, Erdmann VA, Frank R, Gillen C, Kurreck J (2006) Silencing of vanilloid receptor TRPV1 by RNAi reduces neuropathic and visceral pain in vivo. Biochem Biophys Res Commun 350(1):238–243
29. Ralph GS, Radcliffe PA, Day DM, Carthy JM, Leroux MA, Lee DCP, Wong LF, Bilsland LG, Greensmith L, Kingsman SM, Mitrophanous KA, Mazarakis ND, Azzouz M (2005) Silencing mutant SOD1 using RNAi protects against neurodegeneration and extends survival in an ALS model. Nat Med 11(43):429–433
30. Raoul C, Abbas-Terki T, Bensadoun JC, Guillot S, Haase G, Szulc J, Henderson CE, Aebischer P (2005) Lentiviral-mediated silencing of SOD1 through RNA interference retards disease onset and progression in a mouse model of ALS. Nat Med 11(43):423–428
31. Harper SQ, Staber PD, He X, Eliason SL, Martins ISH, Mao Q, Yang L, Kotin RM, Paulson HL, Davidson BL (2005) RNA interference improves motor and neuropathological abnormalities in a huntington's disease mouse model. Proc Natl Acad Sci USA 102(16):5820–5825
32. Singer O, Marr RA, Rockenstein E, Crews L, Coufal NG, Gage FH, Verma IM, Masliah E (2005) Targeting BACE1 with siRNAs ameliorates Alzheimer disease neuropathology in a transgenic model. Nat Neurosci 8(10): 1343–1349
33. Xia H, Mao Q, Eliason SL, Harper SQ, Martins IH, Orr HT, Paulson HL, Yang L, Kotin RM, Davidson BL (2004) RNAi suppresses polyglutamine-induced neurodegeneration in a model of spinocerebellar ataxia. Nat Med 10(8):816–820
34. Palmer JA, Branston RH, Lilley CE, Robinson MJ, Groutsi F, Smith J, Latchman DS, Coffin RS (2000) Development and optimization of herpes simplex virus vectors for multiple long-term gene delivery to the peripheral nervous system. J Virol 74(12):5604–5618
35. Lilley CE, Groutsi F, Han Z, Palmer JA, Anderson PN, Latchman DS, Coffin RS (2001) Multiple immediate-early gene-deficient herpes simplex virus vectors allowing efficient gene delivery to neurons in culture and widespread gene delivery to the central nervous system in vivo. J Virol 75(9):4343–4356
36. Anesti AM, Peeters PJ, Royaux I, Coffin RS (2008) Efficient delivery of RNA interference to peripheral neurons in vivo using herpes simplex virus. Nucleic Acids Res 36(14):e86

Chapter 27

Combination of Cell Culture Assays and Knockout Mouse Analyses for the Study of Opioid Partial Agonism

Soichiro Ide, Masabumi Minami, Ichiro Sora, and Kazutaka Ikeda

Abstract

Nonselective opioid partial agonists, such as buprenorphine, butorphanol, and pentazocine, have been widely used as analgesics and for anti-addiction therapy. However, the precise molecular mechanisms underlying the therapeutic and rewarding effects of these drugs have not been clearly delineated. Recent success in developing μ-opioid receptor knockout (MOP-KO) mice has elucidated the molecular mechanisms underlying the effects of morphine and other opioids. We have revealed the in vivo roles of MOPs in the effects of opioid partial agonists by using MOP-KO mice for behavioral tests (e.g., several kinds of antinociceptive tests for analgesic effects, conditioned place preference test for dependence). The combination of the cell culture assays using cDNA for μ, δ, and κ opioid receptors and the behavioral tests using MOP-KO mice has provided novel theories on the molecular mechanisms underlying the effects of opioid ligands, especially opioid partial agonists.

Key words: Pain, Knockout mouse, Behavior, Conditioned place preference, Binding assay

1. Introduction

Nonselective opioid partial agonists, such as buprenorphine, butorphanol, and pentazocine, have been widely used as analgesics and for anti-addiction therapy. However, the precise molecular mechanisms underlying the therapeutic and rewarding effects of these drugs have not been clearly delineated, although investigators have estimated their antinociceptive and rewarding effects using selective opioid receptor agonists and antagonists.

Cell culture assays using cDNA for μ (MOP), δ (DOP), and κ (KOP) opioid receptors are useful for investigating the molecular mechanisms underlying the effects of opioid partial agonists. Because the most selective ligands for a specific subtype of opioid

Arpad Szallasi (ed.), *Analgesia: Methods and Protocols*, Methods in Molecular Biology, vol. 617,
DOI 10.1007/978-1-60327-323-7_27,

receptor (e.g., β-funaltrexamine for MOP, naltrindole for DOP, and norbinaltorphimine [nor-BNI] for KOP) possess certain affinities for other subtypes (1), the true affinity, activity, and selectivity of opioid ligands for opioid receptor subtypes should be analyzed using cell lines expressing only one specific opioid receptor subtype.

Recent success in developing MOP knockout (KO) mice has elucidated the molecular mechanisms underlying the effects of opioids (2–5). The analgesic effects of morphine in both the tail-flick and hot-plate tests and the rewarding effects of morphine in self-administration tests are abolished in MOP-KO mice (3–5). By contrast, buprenorphine, a nonselective opioid receptor partial agonist, has no analgesic effect in the tail-flick and hot-plate tests but a significant rewarding effect in the conditioned place preference test in homozygous MOP-KO mice (6). These observations are especially interesting because the distributions of DOP and KOP are not apparently altered in MOP-KO mice (2, 3, 5). Furthermore, using MOP-KO mice in tail-flick and hot-plate tests, the antinociceptive effects of tramadol, an analgesic possessing of both opioid and nonopioid activities, were shown to be mediated mainly by MOPs and adrenergic α_2 receptors (7). Although several compensatory changes might occur in KO animals, they have potential utility in investigating the in vivo roles of specific proteins. Thus, the use of MOP-KO mice has provided novel theories on the molecular mechanisms underlying the effects of opioid ligands, especially opioid partial agonists.

2. Materials

2.1. Cell Culture Assays

1. Cell lines stably expressing MOPs, DOPs, and KOPs.
2. Binding buffer (10×): 500 mM Tris-HCl, pH 7.4, 100 mM $MgCl_2$, 10 mM EDTA. Store at 4°C.
3. Cold and hot [^{3}H]opioid receptor subtype selective ligands (e.g., DAMGO for MOP, DPDPE for DOP, and U69593 for KOP).
4. Whatman GF/C glass fiber filters pretreated with 0.1% polyethyleneimine. Store at 4°C.
5. HEPES-buffered saline (1×): 15 mM HEPES, pH 7.4, 140 mM NaCl, 4.7 mM KCl, 1.2 mM $MgCl_2$, 11 mM glucose. Store at 4°C.
6. 100 μM forskolin. Store at 4°C.
7. 1 mM 3-isobutyl-1-methylxanthine. Store at 4°C.
8. 10% trichloroacetic acid. Store at –20°C.

9. 3′,5′-cyclic adenosine monophosphate (cAMP) assay kit (e.g., Amersham, Buckinghamshire, UK).
10. Homogenizer.
11. Crushed ice.
12. Scintillation cocktail.
13. Liquid scintillation counter.
14. Computer software for nonlinear regression analysis (e.g., GraphPad Prism, GraphPad, San Diego, CA, USA).

2.2. Mice and Genotyping

1. DNA polymerase (e.g., KOD Dash polymerase, Toyobo Co., Ltd., Tokyo, Japan).
2. Buffer for tissue lysis (1×): 70 mM Tris-HCl, pH 8.2, 20 mM EDTA, 100 mM NaCl, 30 mM *N*-lauroylsarcosine sodium salt. Store at 4°C.
3. Proteinase K solution: 20 mg/ml. Store at −20°C.
4. MOP-KO mice (2, 3, 5, 8).
5. Selective primer pairs.
6. Apparatus for polymerase chain reaction (PCR).
7. Apparatus for gel electrophoresis.

2.3. Behavioral Analyses

1. Tail-flick apparatus (MK-330B, Muromachi Kikai Co., Tokyo, Japan).
2. Hot-plate apparatus (MK-350D, Muromachi Kikai Co., Tokyo, Japan).
3. Pressure Analgesy-Meter (Model MK-201D, Muromachi Kikai Co., Tokyo, Japan).
4. Black felt towel.
5. Locomotor activity test apparatus (SUPERMEX, CompACT AMS v. 3, Muromachi Kikai Co., Tokyo, Japan).
6. Conditioned place preference apparatus (SUPERMEX, CompACT CPP, Muromachi Kikai Co., Tokyo, Japan).
7. Morphine hydrochloride (Sankyo Co., Tokyo, Japan).
8. Naloxone hydrochloride (Sigma Chemical Co., St. Louis, MO, USA).
9. Naltrindole hydrochloride (Sigma Chemical Co., St. Louis, MO, USA).
10. norBNI dihydrochloride (Sigma Chemical Co., St. Louis, MO, USA).
11. 0.9% Sterile saline.
12. Acetic acid.

3. Methods

3.1. Cell Culture Assays

In vitro assays using cell lines stably expressing MOPs, DOPs, and KOPs are useful for revealing the characteristics of opioid ligands. Although our previous data in in vitro analyses using cell lines stably expressing human MOPs, DOPs, and KOPs indicated that the most partial opioid ligands show partial agonism for MOP (6, 9), these affinities and efficacies for each subtype would change slightly when the different species of cDNA are used (i.e., mouse, rat). The methods of the representative cell culture assays are specified below and shown in Fig. 1.

3.1.1. Radioligand Binding Assay

1. Harvest cells stably expressing MOPs, DOPs, and KOPs after 65 h in culture.
2. Homogenize harvested cells in ice-cold binding buffer.
3. Pellet by centrifugation for 20 min at 30,000×*g*, and resuspend in binding buffer.
4. For saturation binding assays, incubate the cell membrane suspensions for 60 min at 25°C with various concentrations of [^{3}H]DAMGO for human MOP, [^{3}H]DPDPE for human DOP, or [^{3}H]U69593 for human KOP. Nonspecific binding is determined in the presence of 10 μM unlabeled ligands.
5. For competitive binding assays, incubate the cell membrane suspensions for 60 min at 25°C with 2 nM [^{3}H]DAMGO for human MOP, 2 nM [^{3}H]DADLE for human DOP, or 3 nM [^{3}H]U69593 for human KOP in the presence of various concentrations of ligands (see Note 1).
6. Filtrate membrane suspensions rapidly using glass fiber filters, and wash each filter with binding buffer four times.
7. Add scintillation cocktail for each filter and stay overnight at room temperature.
8. Measure the radioactivity on each filter by liquid scintillation counting.
9. Obtain K_d values of the radiolabeled ligands by Scatchard analysis of the data from the saturation binding assay.
10. Calculate K_i values from the IC_{50} values obtained from the competitive binding assay in accordance with the equation $K_i = IC_{50}/(1 + [\text{radiolabeled ligand}]/K_d)$, where IC_{50} is the concentration of unlabeled ligand producing 50% inhibition of the specific binding of radiolabeled ligand (see Note 2).

3.1.2. cAMP Assay

1. Place 10^5 cells stably expressing MOPs, DOPs, and KOPs into each well of a 24-well plate and grow for 24 h.
2. Wash and incubate with 0.45 ml of HEPES-buffered saline for 10 min at 37°C (see Note 3).

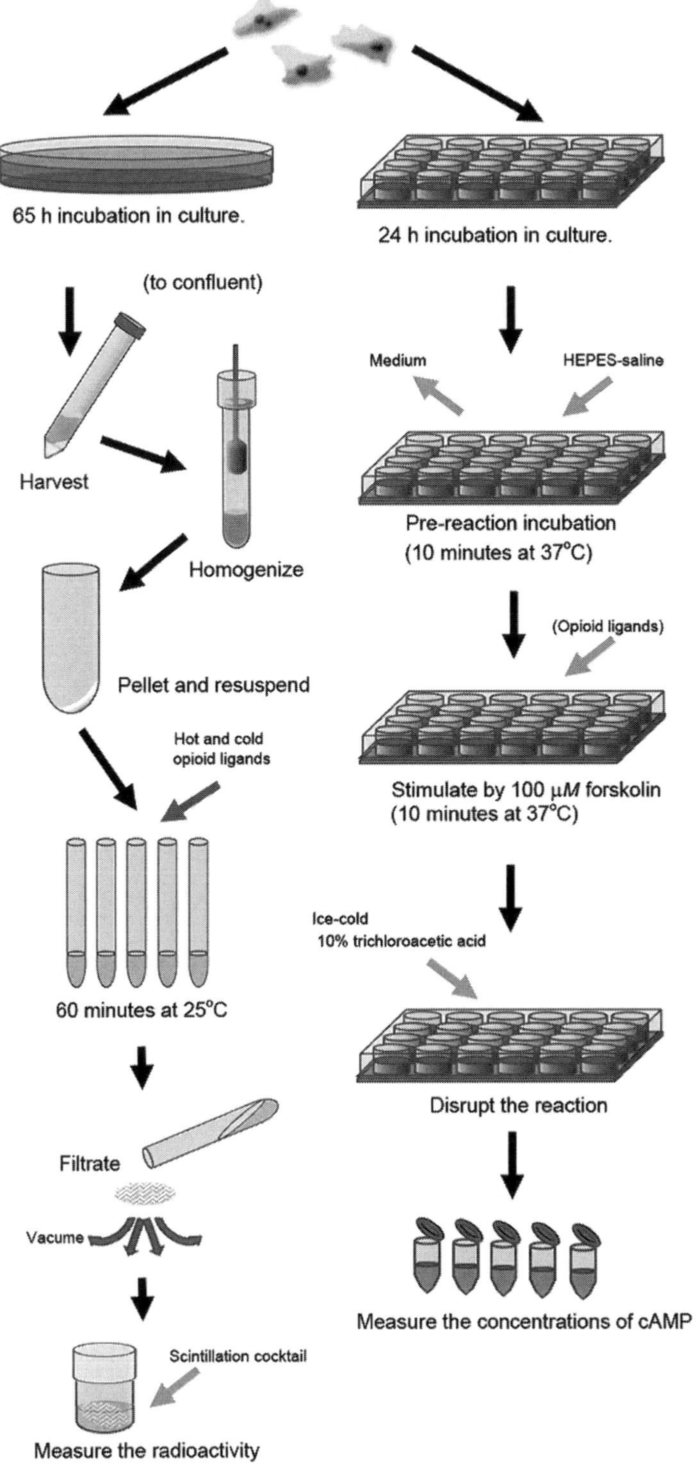

Fig. 1. Experimental procedure for representative in vitro analyses using cell lines stably expressing MOPs, DOPs, and KOPs. *Left flow* is for a binding assay. *Right flow* is for a cAMP accumulation assay

3. Stimulate for 10 min by the addition of 50 μl of HEPES-buffered saline containing 100 μM forskolin and 1 mM 3-isobutyl-1-methylxanthine to each well in the presence or absence of various concentrations of opioid ligands.
4. Disrupt the reaction by adding 0.5 ml of ice-cold 10% trichloroacetic acid to each well.
5. Measure the concentrations of cAMP by immunoassay (Amersham, Buckinghamshire, UK).
6. Calculate IC_{50} values as the concentration of ligand producing 50% of the maximal inhibition of cAMP accumulation.

3.2. Mice and Genotyping

Wildtype, heterozygous, and homozygous MOP-KO mouse littermates are generated from crosses of heterozygous/heterozygous MOP-KO mice. Ideally, mice with a C57BL/6J genetic background are preferable (4) (see Note 4). The method of genotyping is specified below.

1. Cut the tip (approximately 5 mm^2) of the mouse ear (see Note 5).
2. Prepare genomic DNA: Add the 50 μl buffer for tissue lysis (1×) and 0.25 μl proteinase K solution to the mouse ear fragment. Heat at 56°C for 3 h or overnight with continuous shaking or vortexing once per hour. Then heat at 95°C for 15 min and centrifuge at 3,000×*g* for 15 min. The prepared genomic DNA can be stored at –20°C (see Note 6).
3. Amplify the DNA fragment using polymerase chain reaction (PCR) with the pairs of primers.
4. Analyze the DNA fragments by the usual gel electrophoresis method.

3.3. Behavioral Analyses

To evaluate partial agonism of opioid ligands using MOP-KO mice, the analgesic effects should be tested not with just one type of noxious stimulus, but rather with several types (e.g., thermal, mechanical, and chemical) because analgesic efficacy is substantially different among different types of noxious stimuli. Furthermore, examination of locomotor activity and drug preference is also useful. The methods for several representative behavioral tests are described below. Additionally, investigations of opioid partial agonists in MOP-KO mice with selective opioid antagonists (e.g., β-funaltrexamine for MOP, naltrindole for DOP, and nor-BNI for KOP) in these tests are powerful methods (Fig. 2).

3.3.1. Antinociceptive Tests

The hot-plate test is used to evaluate supraspinal thermal antinociception. A commercially available apparatus consisting of an acrylic resin cage and a thermo-controlled aluminum plate (Model MK-350A, Muromachi Kikai Co., Tokyo, Japan) can be used for this test following the methods of Woolfe and MacDonald (10) with slight modifications.

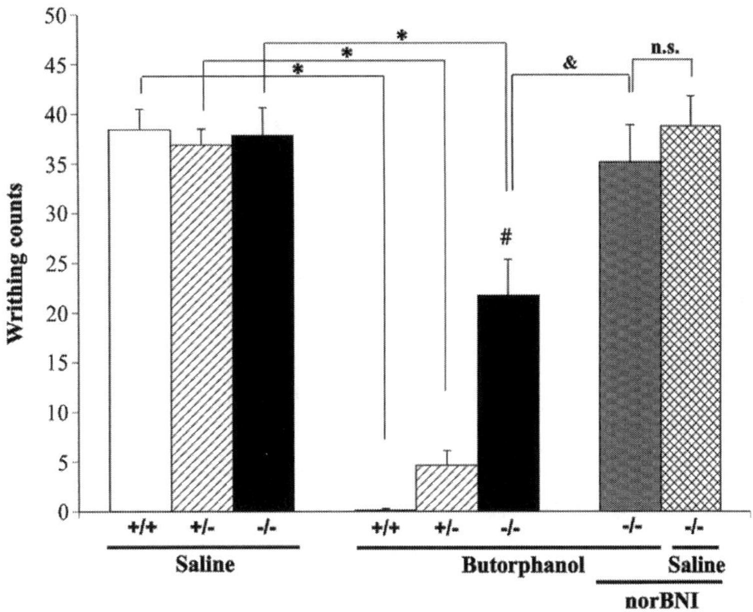

Fig. 2. Visceral chemical antinociceptive effects of butorphanol in wildtype, heterozygous, and homozygous MOP-KO mice. Writhing counts induced by 0.6% acetic acid (i.p.) with saline pretreatment in wildtype [+/+, $n=9$ (male, 5; female, 4)], heterozygous [+/–, $n=10$ (male, 5; female, 5)], and homozygous [–/–, $n=7$ (male, 4; female, 3)] mice, butorphanol pretreatment (3 mg/kg, s.c.) in wildtype [+/+, $n=8$ (male, 5; female, 3)], heterozygous [+/–, $n=8$ (male, 4; female, 4)], and homozygous [–/–, $n=12$ (male, 5; female, 7)] MOP-KO mice, and nor-BNI (5 mg/kg, s.c.), butorphanol (3 mg/kg, s.c.) [–/–, $n=13$ (male, 7; female, 6)], or saline pretreatment [–/–, $n=13$ (male, 4; female, 5)] in homozygous MOP-KO mice. $^{\#}p<0.05$ Significantly different from wildtype mice. $^{*}p<0.05$ Significantly different from saline pretreatment. $^{\&}p<0.05$ Significantly different from nor-BNI pretreatment. *n.s.* Not significant. Data are expressed as mean ± SEM. (Reproduced from ref. 13 with permission from Elsevier Science.)

1. Habituate mouse to the hot-plate apparatus before heating the floor plate (see Notes 7).
2. Place a mouse on a 52 ± 0.2°C hot-plate, and record latency to lick the hind-paw, lift the hind-paw, or jump with a cut-off time of 60 s (see Notes 8).

The tail-flick test is used to evaluate spinal thermal antinociception. A commercially available apparatus consisting of an irradiator for heat stimulation and a photosensor for detecting tail-flick behavior (Model MK-330A, Muromachi Kikai Co., Tokyo, Japan) can be used for this test following the method of D'Amour and Smith (11) with slight modifications.

1. Hold a mouse on the tail-flick apparatus and set the mouse's tail on an irradiator (see Note 9).
2. Heat the mouse's tail, and automatically record tail-flick latencies with a cut-off time of 15 s.

The hind-paw pressure test is used to evaluate mechanical antinociception. A commercially available apparatus (Pressure Analgesy-Meter, Model MK-201D, Muromachi Kikai Co., Tokyo, Japan) can be used following the method of Randall and Selitto (12) with slight modifications.

1. Hold a mouse on the hind-paw pressure apparatus and set the mouse's hind paws on a stage (see Note 9).
2. Gradually press the mouse's hind paws, and automatically record hind-paw withdrawing or struggle latencies with a cut-off pressure at 250 mmHg (see Note 9).

The hot-plate, tail-flick, and hind-paw pressure responses of each mouse in the drug-induced antinociception tests can be evaluated by converting to a percentage of maximal possible effect (%MPE) according to the following formula:

$$\%\,\text{MPE} = (\text{postdrug latency} - \text{predrug latency})/(\text{cut-off time or pressure} - \text{predrug latency}) \times 100\%$$

The writhing test is used to evaluate visceral chemical antinociception.

1. Inject acetic acid (0.6% v/v, 10 ml/kg) intraperitoneally (i.p.).
2. Place the mouse in a large plastic cage.
3. Count the total number of writhes occurring between 0 and 15 min after acetic acid injection. (The writhing response consists of contraction of the abdominal muscles.)
4. Nociception is expressed as writhing scores during the 15 min period.

A large number of KO mice are needed for testing the antinociceptive effects of drugs, and preparation may be troublesome for researchers. Using cumulative dose-response analyses can dramatically reduce the number of mice used in the hot-plate, tail-flick, and hind-paw pressure tests. For example, in the cumulative dose-response analyses, butorphanol is administered subcutaneously (s.c.) at doses of 0.3, 0.7, 2.0, and 7.0 mg/kg, yielding cumulative doses of 0.3, 1.0, 3.0, and 10 mg/kg, respectively. Antinociceptive tests are conducted 20 min after each drug injection. Drug is injected immediately after the previous test (see Note 10). However, although cumulative dose-response analyses have the great advantage of reducing the number of mice required for testing, researchers should pay attention to several points, such as the attenuation of antinociceptive effects by acute tolerance to the test drugs (see Fig. 3). Furthermore, the time-course of drug efficacy should be determined (see Note 11).

3.3.2. Conditioned Place Preference (CPP) Test

The CPP test is used to evaluate the rewarding effect of drugs. Two- or three-compartment Plexiglas chambers are used, in which one compartment is black with a smooth floor, one

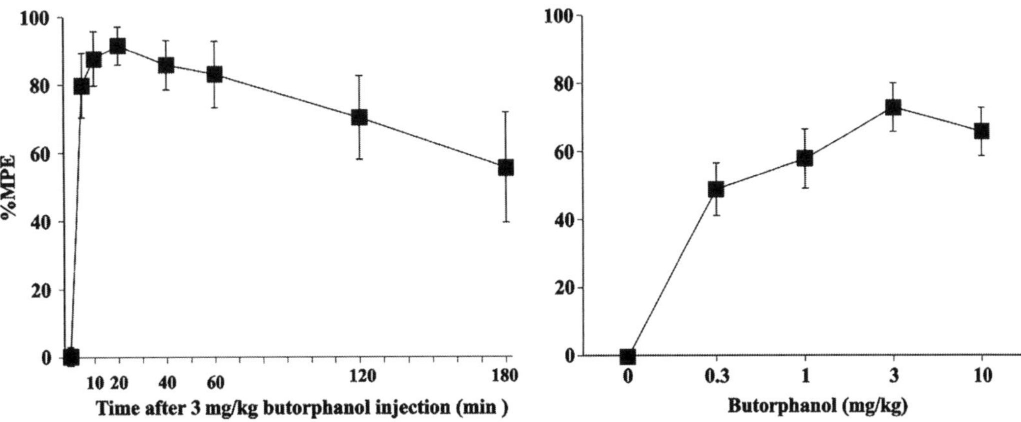

Fig. 3. Thermal antinociceptive effects of butorphanol in wildtype mice in the tail-flick test. (*Left*) Butorphanol (3 mg/kg, s.c.)-induced alterations of %MPE in the tail-flick test in wildtype mice [$n=8$ (male, 4; female, 4)] under the time-course paradigm. (*Right*) Butorphanol-induced alterations of %MPE in the tail-flick test in wildtype mice [$n=11$ (male, 6; female, 5)] under the cumulative dose-response paradigm. (Reproduced from ref. 13 with permission from Elsevier Science.)

compartment is white with a textured floor, and the middle compartment has a gray floor (when a three-compartment model is used). For pre- and post-conditioning test phases, a division with openings allows access to both compartments. During the conditioning phases, the openings are closed to restrict mice to a single compartment. Locomotion and time spent in each compartment are recorded using an animal activity monitoring apparatus (SUPERMEX, CompACT CPP, Muromachi Kikai Co., Tokyo, Japan). The apparatus should be sound- and light-attenuated (see Note 12). Conditioned place preference is assessed by a protocol consisting of three phases, preconditioning, conditioning, and test.

1. Allow mice to freely explore each compartment through the openings for 15 min and acclimatize to the apparatus on days 1 and 2.
2. Perform the same trial on day 3 (preconditioning phase). Measure the time spent in each compartment for 15 min. Determine whether the animal has a preference for a particular compartment before conditioning (see Note 13). When planning a test schedule after the preconditioning phase, a counterbalanced protocol is preferable to nullify each mouse's initial preference, as previously discussed (13).
3. Conditioning is conducted once daily for 4 consecutive days (days 4–7). Perform the assignment of the conditioned compartment randomly, and counterbalance across subjects. Administer drug or saline to the mouse, and immediately confine the mouse to the black or white compartment for 50 min on day 4.

4. Administer the alternate saline or drug to the mouse, and immediately confine the mouse to the opposite compartment for 50 min on day 5.
5. Repeat the same conditioning procedure from days 4 and 5 on days 6 and 7.
6. Measure the time spent in each compartment for 15 min without drug injection during the test phase on day 8.
7. The CPP score is designated as the time spent in the drug-paired compartment on day 8 minus the time spent in the same compartment during the preconditioning phase on day 3.

4. Notes

1. The concentration of radiolabeled ligands used for competitive binding assays is determined from K_d values of the radiolabeled ligands obtained by Scatchard analysis of the data from the saturation binding assay.
2. For the estimation of the inhibitory concentration at 50% (IC_{50}) in the competitive binding assay, a binding model for one-site or two-site competition binding is preferable. Nonlinear regression analysis using computer software (GraphPad Prism, GraphPad, San Diego, CA, USA) can estimate the binding model and the IC_{50} value.
3. All buffers for wash and reaction should be warmed at 37°C before use.
4. To study specific genetic factors for screening behavioral changes and/or drug actions using KO mice, littermate mice are preferable to minimize other genetic effects and nongenetic factors.
5. Although the usual method is cutting the tip of the mouse tail (approximately 5 mm), this should be avoided when mice are tested with noxious stimuli applied to their tails (e.g., tail-immersion test, tail-flick test).
6. After the heat shock at 95°C for 15 min, the genomic DNA solution can be used for PCR without usual phenol extraction. In this procedure, the volume of the genomic DNA solution should be less than 5% of the total volume of the PCR reaction.
7. Mice should be habituated to the hot-plate apparatus before heating the floor plate because mice show exploratory behavior that can cause unstable results when tested without habituation.

8. To evaluate the thermal antinociceptive effects of opioid partial agonists, the temperature of the hot-plate should be set at 52°C or lower (48–52°C) because thermal antinociceptive effects of opioid partial agonists are relatively weak and cannot be clearly analyzed when using a 54°C hot-plate (a temperature usually reserved for rats). If the higher temperature is used to test a full opioid agonist (e.g., morphine, fentanyl), the cut-off time should be 45 s or less.
9. If the mouse struggles and cannot be set on the apparatus, it can be loosely wrapped in a black felt towel.
10. In the cumulative dose-response analyses, the number of drug doses for the test should be less than five. Excessive, repeated testing can have a noxious influence on the mice.
11. The effective duration of tested drugs should be determined before using the cumulative dose-response analyses.
12. Although the compartment usually has dim illumination (about 40 lux), the intensity of light should be adjusted to the condition in which mice show nearly the same time spent in both compartments before the conditioning phase.
13. Biased mice that spend more than 80% of the time (i.e., 12 min) on one side on day 3 or more than 10 min on one side on day 2 and more than 10 min on the other side on day 3 are not recommended to be used for further experiments.

Acknowledgments

We acknowledge Mr. Michael Arends for his assistance with editing the manuscript. This work was supported by grants from the Ministry of Health, Labour and Welfare of Japan (H17-Pharmaco-001, H19-Iyaku-023), the Ministry of Education, Culture, Sports, Science and Technology of Japan (19603021, 20390162, 19659405).

References

1. Newman LC, Sands SS, Wallace DR, Stevens CW (2002) Characterization of μ κ and δ opioid binding in amphibian whole brain tissue homogenates. J Pharmacol Exp Ther 301:364–370
2. Matthes HW, Maldonado R, Simonin F, Valverde O, Slowe S, Kitchen I, Befort K, Dierich A, Le Meur M, Dolle P, Tzavara E, Hanoune J, Roques BP, Kieffer BL (1996) Loss of morphine-induced analgesia, reward effect and withdrawal symptoms in mice lacking the μ-opioid-receptor gene. Nature 383:819–823
3. Sora I, Takahashi N, Funada M, Ujike H, Revay RS, Donovan DM, Miner LL, Uhl GR (1997) Opiate receptor knockout mice define μ receptor roles in endogenous nociceptive responses and morphine-induced analgesia. Proc Natl Acad Sci U S A 94:1544–1549
4. Sora I, Elmer G, Funada M, Pieper J, Li XF, Hall FS, Uhl GR (2001) μ Opiate receptor gene dose effects on different morphine actions: evidence for differential in vivo μ receptor reserve. Neuropsychopharmacology 25:41–54

5. Loh HH, Liu HC, Cavalli A, Yang W, Chen YF, Wei LN (1998) μ Opioid receptor knockout in mice: effects on ligand-induced analgesia and morphine lethality. Brain Res Mol Brain Res 54:321–326
6. Ide S, Minami M, Satoh M, Uhl GR, Sora I, Ikeda K (2004) Buprenorphine antinociception is abolished, but naloxone-sensitive reward is retained, in μ-opioid receptor knockout mice. Neuropsychopharmacology 29:1656–1663
7. Ide S, Minami M, Ishihara K, Uhl GR, Sora I, Ikeda K (2006) Mu opioid receptor-dependent and independent components in effects of tramadol. Neuropharmacology 51:651–658
8. Schuller AG, King MA, Zhang J, Bolan E, Pan YX, Morgan DJ, Chang A, Czick ME, Unterwald EM, Pasternak GW, Pintar JE (1999) Retention of heroin and morphine-6 β-glucuronide analgesia in a new line of mice lacking exon 1 of MOR-1. Nat Neurosci 2:151–156
9. Ide S, Minami M, Ishihara K, Uhl GR, Satoh M, Sora I, Ikeda K (2008) Abolished thermal and mechanical antinociception but retained visceral chemical antinociception induced by butorphanol in μ-opioid receptor knockout mice. Neuropharmacology 54:1182–1188
10. Woolfe G, MacDonald A (1944) The evaluation of the analgesic action of pethidine hydrochloride (demerol). J Pharmacol Exp Ther 80:300–307
11. D'Amour FE, Smith DL (1941) A method for determining loss of pain sensation. J Pharmacol Exp Ther 72:74–79
12. Randall LO, Selitto JJ (1957) A method for measurement of analgesic activity on inflamed tissue. Arch Int Pharmacodyn Ther 111:409–419
13. Tzschentke TM (1998) Measuring reward with the conditioned place preference paradigm: a comprehensive review of drug effects, recent progress and new issues. Prog Neurobiol 56:613–672

Chapter 28

Assessing Potential Functionality of Catechol-*O*-methyltransferase (COMT) Polymorphisms Associated with Pain Sensitivity and Temporomandibular Joint Disorders

Andrea G. Nackley and Luda Diatchenko

Abstract

Catechol-*O*-methyltransferase (COMT) is an enzyme that plays a key role in the modulation of catechol-dependent functions such as cognition, cardiovascular function, and pain processing. Recently, our group demonstrated that three common haplotypes of the human *COMT* gene, divergent in two synonymous and one nonsynonymous position, are associated with experimental pain sensitivity and onset of temporomandibular joint disorder. In order to determine the functional mechanisms whereby these haplotypes contribute to pain processing, a series of *in vitro* experiments were performed. Haplotypes divergent in synonymous changes exhibited the largest difference in COMT enzymatic activity because of reduced amount of translated protein. The major *COMT* haplotypes varied significantly with respect to mRNA local stem-loop structures such that the most stable structure was associated with the lowest protein levels and enzymatic activity. Site-directed mutagenesis that eliminated the stable structure restored the amount of translated protein. These data provide the first demonstration that combinations of commonly observed alleles in the coding region of the human *COMT* gene can significantly affect the secondary structure of corresponding mRNA transcripts, which in turn leads to dramatic alterations in the translation efficiency of enzyme crucial for a variety of essential functions. The protocols applied to the study of these molecular genetic mechanisms are detailed herein.

Key words: COMT, Catecholamine, Pain, mRNA secondary structure, Synonymous polymorphism, Haplotype

1. Introduction

COMT is an enzyme responsible for degrading catecholamines and thus represents a critical component of homeostasis maintenance (1). The human *COMT* gene encodes two distinct proteins: soluble COMT (S-COMT) and membrane-bound COMT

Arpad Szallasi (ed.), *Analgesia: Methods and Protocols*, Methods in Molecular Biology, vol. 617,
DOI 10.1007/978-1-60327-323-7_28, © Springer Science+Business Media, LLC 2010

(MB-COMT) through the use of alternative translation initiation sites and promoters. Recently, COMT has been implicated in the modulation of persistent pain such that low COMT activity is associated with heightened pain states (2–5). Our group demonstrated that three common haplotypes of the human *COMT* gene are associated with pain sensitivity and the likelihood of developing temporomandibular joint disorder (TMD), a common chronic musculoskeletal pain condition (2). Three major haplotypes are formed by three SNPs in the *S*- and *MB-COMT* coding region at codons *his*^{62}*his* (C/T; rs4633), *leu*^{136}*leu* (C/G; rs4818), and *val*^{158}*met* (A/G; rs4680). Based on subjects' pain responsiveness, haplotypes were designated as low (LPS; CGG), average (APS; TCA), or high (HPS; CCG) pain sensitive. Individuals carrying HPS/APS or APS/APS diplotypes were nearly 2.5 times more likely to develop TMD. The ability to predict the downstream effects of APS and HPS haplotypes is critically important for understanding the molecular basis of catechol-dependent diseases and disorders.

The effects of nonsynonymous polymorphisms have been widely characterized; because these variations directly influence protein function, they are relatively easy to study statistically and experimentally (6). However, characterizing polymorphisms located in regulatory regions, which are much more common, has proved to be problematic (7). Therefore, new strategies are required to study regulatory polymorphisms at transcriptional and translational levels. Here, we focus on the mechanism whereby polymorphisms of the *COMT* gene regulate gene expression. *In silico*, mRNA folding was performed to evaluate the effect of LPS, APS, and HPS haplotypes on the stability of the corresponding mRNA secondary structures (8). Subsequent *in vitro* studies were performed to test the molecular modeling results (8). Full-length S- and MB-COMT cDNA clones were constructed in mammalian expression vectors that differed only in three nucleotides corresponding to the LPS, APS, and HPS haplotypes. Rat adrenal (PC-12) cells were transiently transfected with each of these six constructs. COMT enzymatic activity, protein expression, and mRNA abundance were measured using enzyme-linked immunosorbent assay (ELISA), Western blot, and real-time polymerase chain reaction (PCR), respectively. Results from these studies demonstrated that the HPS haplotype exhibited a dramatic decrease in COMT enzymatic activity because of increased stability of its corresponding local mRNA stem-loop structure, which in turn resulted in reduced protein, but not mRNA, levels. Additionally, the APS haplotype exhibited a moderate reduction in COMT enzymatic activity because of *met al*lele-dependent decreases in protein thermostability (8). The vigorous set of molecular and cell biologic experiments permitting these conclusions are provided here.

2. Materials

2.1. Generation of Haplotypic Variants of Human COMT

2.1.1. Purification and Confirmation of COMT cDNA Constructs

1. Full-length pCMV-SPORT6-based cDNA clones (IMAGE clone collection, BG290167, CA489448, BF037202 BI835796) (Open Biosystems, Huntsville, AL).
2. LB plates containing ampicillin: 25 g LB powder and 15 g agar in 1 L H_2O. Autoclave 25 min, cool to 50°C, and add 50 μg/mL ampicillin. Pour 35–40 mL per 10 cm plate, and dry with lids off for 30 min in a laminar flow hood. Store dry wrapped plates at 4°C.
3. LB liquid medium containing ampicillin: 25 g LB powder to 1 L H_2O. Autoclave 25 min and cool. Store at room temperature and add 50 μg/mL ampicillin just prior to use.
4. QIAprep Spin Miniprep Kit (Qiagen, Valencia, CA).
5. SP6 primer: 5′-GATTTAGGTGACACTATAG-3′ (Invitrogen, Carlsbad, CA).
6. COMT-F primer: 5′-TGAACGTGGGCGACAAGAAAGG CAAGAT-3′ (Integrated DNA Technologies, Coralville, IA).
7. EndoFree Plasmid Maxi Kit (Qiagen).
8. 50% glycerol: To prepare, combine 1 part glycerol and 1 part d^2 H_2O.

2.1.2. Construction of S- and MB-COMT Same Length Constructs

1. Confirmed and purified S- and MB-COMT clones from Subheading 2.1.
2. BspMI restriction enzyme (New England Biolabs, Ipswich, MA).
3. TAE electrophoresis buffer (50×): 121 g Tris base, 28.5 mL glacial acetic acid, 18.5 g Na^2 EDTA 2 H_2O, and 500 mL d^2H_2O. To achieve a 1× TAE buffer working solution, dilute 300 mL 50× TAE buffer with 14.7 L d^2H_2O. Store at room temperature.
4. 1.2% agarose gel: 1.2 g agarose, 100 mL 1× TAE buffer, 1 μL ethidium bromide. Store at room temperature. Prior to use, microwave, stir, and cool at 55°C until clear even liquid forms.
5. Prestained 1°Kb molecular weight marker (Invitrogen).
6. 10× gel loading buffer (Invitrogen).
7. QIAquick Gel Extraction Kit (Qiagen, Germantown, MD).
8. Shrimp alkaline phosphatase (Roche Applied Science, Indianapolis, IN).
9. Rapid DNA Ligation Kit (Roche Applied Science).
10. Subcloning efficiency DH5α competent cells (Invitrogen).
11. S.O.C. medium (Invitrogen).

2.1.3. Construction of S- and MB-COMT HPS Constructs with LPS mRNA Secondary Structure

1. S- and MB-COMT same length HPS constructs from Subheading 2.2.
2. QuickChange II XL Site-Directed Mutagenesis Kit (Stratagene, LaJolla, CA).
3. HPS Lsm forward and reverse primers: 5′-CACCATCGA GAT**G**AACCCCGACTGTG-3′ and 5′-CACAGTCGGG GTT**C**ATCTCGATGGTG-3′, respectively (MWG, High Point, NC,).
4. HPS dm forward and reverse primers: 5′-CACCCTTG TGGTT**C**GAGCGTCCCAGG-3′ and 5′-CCTGGGACG CTC**G**AACCACAAGGGTG-3′, respectively (MWG).

2.1.4. Construction of S- and MB-COMT HPS Constructs with APS mRNA Secondary Structure

1. S- and MB-COMT same length HPS constructs from Subheading 2.2.
2. PflF1 restriction enzyme (New England Biolabs).
3. TAE electrophoresis buffer used in Subheading 2.2.
4. 1.2% agarose gel used in Subheading 2.2.
5. Prestained 1 Kb molecular weight marker (Invitrogen).
6. 10× gel loading buffer (Invitrogen).
7. QIAquick Gel Extraction Kit (Qiagen).
8. Shrimp alkaline phosphatase (Roche Applied Science).
9. HPS Asm 78 base pair oligo and reverse complement: 5′-AGGT CACCCTTGTGGTTGGAGCGTCCC AGGACATCATCCC CCAGCTGAAGAAGAAGTATGATGTGGAC ACA**G**TGGACA-3′ and 5′-TGTCCA**C**TGTGTCCACAT CATACTTCTTCTTCAGCTGGGGGATGATGTCCT GGGACGCTCCA ACCACAAGGGTGACCT-3′, respectively (Integrated DNA Technologies).
10. Rapid DNA Ligation Kit (Roche Applied Science).

2.2. Transient Transfection of COMT cDNA Constructs and Isolation of Cell Lysate

1. Rat adrenal PC-12 cells (ATCC, Manassas, VA).
2. PC-12 medium: 250 mL D-MEM media, 250 mL Ham's F-12 media, 56 mL fetal bovine serum (FBS), and 5.6 mL penicillin-streptomycin. Store at 4°C and heat to 37°C in a water bath prior to use.
3. 1× trypsin with EDTA.
4. 1× phosphate-buffered saline (PBS; Invitrogen).
5. DMSO.
6. Serum-free PC-12 media. Prepare as in step 2 above, omitting the fetal bovine serum.
7. Fugene 6 Transfection Reagent (Roche Applied Science).
8. pSV-βGalactosidase vector (Promega, Madison, WI).

9. pSEAP2-control (Clonetech, Mountain View, CA).
10. pCMV SPORT 6 empty vector (Invitrogen).
11. 1× phosphate-buffered saline (Invitrogen).
12. 10 mM trans-1,2-Cyclohexanediaminetetraacetic acid (CDTA; Sigma-Aldrich, St. Louis, MO). Combine 364.35 mg CDTA with 100 mL d² H_2O. Store at 4°C.
13. Trizol (Invitrogen).

2.3. Enzymatic Assay for COMT Activity

1. Cell lysate in 10 mM CDTA isolated from PC-12 cells in Subheading 2.5.
2. BCA Protein Assay kit (Pierce, Milwaukee, WI).
3. βGalactosidase buffer (2×): 542 mg $NaH_2PO_4 \cdot H_2O$, 2,198 mg Na_2HPO4, 40.66 mg $MgCl_2$, 134 mg *O*-nitrophenylgalactopyranoside, 1.56 mL β-mercaptoethanol with d² H_2O up to 100 mL. Make 1.5 mL aliquots and store at –20°C. Thaw to room temperature prior to use.
4. 2 mM $MgCl_2$ in 80 mM PBS: 15.23 mg $MgCL_2$, 40 mL 100 mM PBS, and 10 mL d²H_2O.
5. 7.5 mM L-norepinephrine (NE; Sigma): 26.73 mg NE is dissolved in 2 mL 0.1 M HCl.
6. 6.7 mM *S*-adenosyl-L-methionine (SAMe; ICN Chemicals, Aurora OH). First, prepare 1 M sulfuric acid solution by diluting 1 mL 18 M H_2SO_4 in 17 ml d² H_2O. Second, prepare a 5 mM sulfuric acid solution by diluting 5 ml 1 M solution in 995 ml d² H_2O. Finally, combine 3.5 mg SAMe, 900 μL 5 mM H_2SO_4, and 100 μL 100% ETOH (see Note 1).
7. 0.4 M hydrochloric acid: 40 mL 1 M HCl solution in 60 mL d²H_2O.
8. 330 μM ethylenedinitrilotetraacetic acid (EDTA): 9.64 mg EDTA is dissolved in 100 mL d²H_2O.
9. Normetanephrine ELISA kit (IBL, Hamburg, Germany).

2.4. Western Blotting for COMT Protein Levels

1. Cell lysate in 10 mM CDTA isolated from PC-12 cells in Subheading 2.5.
2. 10% Novex Tris-Glycine gels (Invitrogen).
3. Running buffer (10×): 60.6 g Tris base, 288 g glycine, 20 g SDS, and 2 L d² H_2O. 1× working solution: 1.5 L of 10× running buffer is diluted with 13.5 L d² H_2O.
4. Laemmli buffer (2×): 1.88 g Tris, 2.5 g SDS, 73.75 mg EDTA, 12.5 ml glycerol, and d² H_2O to bring up to 100 ml. Add a few drops of bromphenol blue and pH solution to 6.8. Store at room temperature.

5. β-mercaptoethanol (βME; Sigma).
6. SeeBlue pre-stained standard (Invitrogen).
7. Methanol.
8. Transfer buffer (5×): 30.2 g Tris base, 144 g glycine, and 2 L d^2 H_2O. To achieve a 1× working solution, dilute 3 L of 5× transfer buffer with 2 L d^2 H_2O and add 3 L methanol.
9. TBST buffer: First, prepare a 2 M Tris stock by combining 121.14 g Tris base and 500 mL d^2 H_2O. Second, prepare a 5 M NaCl stock by combining 146 g NaCl in 500 mL d^2 H_2O. Third, prepare a 5× stock solution by combining 50 mL 2 M Tris stock, 300 mL 5 M NaCl stock, 2.5 mL tween, and 2 L d^2 H_2O. To achieve a 1× working solution, dilute 3 L 5× TBST buffer with 12 L d^2 H_2O.
10. Nitrocellulose membranes (Whatman, Florham Park, NJ).
11. Filter paper backing (Bio-Rad, Hercules, CA).
12. 5% nonfat milk: 25 g instant nonfat milk powder in 500 mL TBST buffer.
13. COMT polyclonal 1° antibody (Chemicon, Temecula, CA).
14. Goat Anti-Rabbit IgG HRP polyclonal 2° antibody (1:10, 000; Chemicon).
15. Pierce ECL Western Blotting Substrate (Pierce).
16. Restore western stripping buffer (Pierce).
17. β-actin polyclonal 1° antibody (1:10,000; Santa Cruz Biotechnology, Santa Cruz, CA).
18. Goat Anti-Rabbit IgG HRP polyclonal 2° antibody (1:10,000; Chemicon).

2.5. Real-Time PCR for COMT Transcript Levels

1. Cell lysate in Trizol isolated from PC-12 cells in Subheading 2.5.
2. Chloroform.
3. Isopropyl alcohol.
4. 75% ethanol: 75 ml ethanol is diluted with 25 ml d^2 H_2O.
5. RNase free H_2O (Promega).
6. RNase free-DNase I (Promega).
7. Thermo-X reverse transcriptase (Invitrogen).
8. 50 μM Oligo$(dT)_{20}$ Primer (Invitrogen).
9. 50 mM EDTA (Invitrogen).
10. DyNAmo-SYBRGreen qPCR kit (MJ Research).
11. SEAP (Clonetech).
12. COMT-F and COMT-R primers: 5′-TGAACGTGGGCGA CAAGAAAGGCAAGAT-3′ and 5′-TGACCTTGTCCTT

CACGCCAGCGAAAT-3′, respectively (Integrated DNA Technologies).

13. SEAP-F and SEAP-R primers: 5′-GCCGACCACTCCC ACGTCTT-3′ and 5′-CCCGCTCTCGCTCTCGGTAA-3′, respectively (Integrated DNA Technologies).

3. Methods

3.1. Generation of Haplotypic Variants of Human COMT

A molecular and cell biologic study of human genetic variants requires the generation of corresponding molecular constructs. For variations in the transcribed portion of genes, cDNA expression constructs may often provide comprehensive tools. Although there are a growing number of commercially available sources for cDNA expression constructs, variants of the minor allele are not typically supplied. The common major allele, however, may provide a convenient backbone for necessary constructs.

One such convenient source of full-length cDNA constructs is the NIH initiated I.M.A.G.E. consortium (9). However, even for the *COMT* gene, which is relatively highly expressed, we were not able to find full-length cDNAs in expression vectors for all the common genetic variants. The presence of entire full-length sequences that include complete 5′ and 3′ untranslated regions (UTRs) was crucial for our studies, as its presence affected the mRNA secondary structure as well as enzymatic activity and protein expression under investigation (8). Thus, we obtained the clones that were available at the time of the study and provided the necessary elements for constructing an entire set corresponding to the three major haplotypes in both *S-* and *MB-COMT* constructs. Although several molecular methods could be applied, we found that the approaches described here were the most efficient for *COMT* cDNA, which has a high GC content and strong secondary structure.

3.1.1. Purification and Confirmation of COMT cDNA Constructs

1. Obtain full-length pCMV-SPORT6-based cDNA clones (10) corresponding to the three COMT haplotypes from the IMAGE clone collection. S-COMT clones BG290167, CA489448, and BF037202 represent LPS, APS, and HPS haplotypes, respectively. The MB-COMT clone BI835796 represents the APS haplotype.
2. Grow clone colonies. First, streak clones on ampicillin-resistant LB plates, invert and grow overnight at 37°C. Second, select ~10 colonies, place each in a separate falcon tube containing 5 mL ampicillin-resistant LB liquid media, and grow overnight in a shaker (250 RPM) at 37°C.

3. Purify plasmid DNA corresponding to each selected colony on a small scale as per the QIAprep Spin Miniprep Kit handbook.

4. Confirm purified colony cDNA sequences. First, sequence using SP6 and COMT-F primers as directed by the local sequencing facility. Second, BLAST the result against the GenBank sequence.

5. Purify plasmid DNA corresponding to each of four confirmed constructs on a larger scale. First, expand the confirmed clones by adding 100 μL of each (from the starter culture in step 3) to separate flasks of 100 mL LB liquid media containing ampicillin and allow to grow overnight in a shaker (250 RPM) at 37°C (see Note 2). Second, harvest the bacterial cells by centrifugation at 6,000×*g* for 15 min at 4°C. Finally, proceed with plasmid purification as per the Qiagen Plasmid Purification Handbook.

3.1.2. Construction of S- and MB-COMT Same Length Constructs

1. Digest plasmid DNA corresponding to each of the four clones using the unique restriction enzyme BspMI. BspMI will make one cut 37 base pairs before the first SNP (rs4633) and a second cut 123 base pairs after the last SNP (rs4680) in the haplotype (Fig. 1). Optimal cutting is achieved by incubating 10 μg DNA with 20 μL buffer 3, 2.5 μL BspMI, and d^2 H_2O up to 200 μL at 37°C for 4 h.

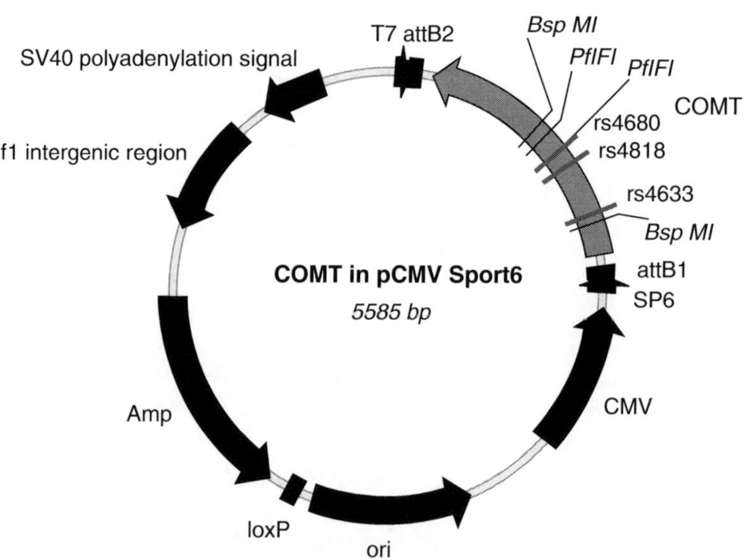

Fig. 1. A schematic illustrates the COMT construct cloned into the pCMV Sport6 vector. pCMV SPORT6-based cDNA clones corresponding to the LPS, APS, and HPS haplotypes were obtained from the IMAGE clone collection. The three SNPs designating LPS, APS, and HPS haplotypes (rs4633, rs4818, and rs4680) are shown in the 1,189 base pair MB-COMT. Additionally, the BspMI and PflFI restriction sites used to generate COMT same-length constructs and HPS APS-like mutants, respectively, are noted

2. Isolate S- and MB-COMT vector and haplotype-specific inserts using gel electrophoresis. Prepare a 1.5 mm thick 1.2% agarose gel, allow to dry (~45 min), and cover with TAE electrophoresis buffer. Load well 1 with the prestained 1 Kb marker and the remaining wells 3, 5, 7, and 9 with digested DNA diluted in the 10× gel loading buffer. Leave wells 2, 4, 6, and 8 empty (see Note 3). Let the gel run at 100 V until the 5.3 Kb vector and 447 base pair insert are clearly separated. Using a razor, excise the vectors (pCMV-SPORT6 vector containing the entire COMT 5′ and 3′ ends) from the S-COMT clone BG290167 and the MB-COMT clone BI835796. Additionally, excise the inserts (coding region of the gene containing all three haplotype-specific SNPs) from the S-COMT clones BG290167, CA489448, and BF037202. Purify the vectors and inserts as per the Qiagen QIAquick Gel Extraction Kit handbook.
3. Dephosphorylate S- and MB-COMT vectors using shrimp alkaline phosphatase according to the Roche protocol.
4. Ligate S- and MB-COMT vectors and inserts. Specifically, ligate the S-COMT BG290167 vector and the MB-COMT BI835796 vector with each of the BG290167, CA489448, and BF037202 inserts. Use the Rapid DNA Ligation Kit according to the Roche protocol.
5. Clone the 3S-COMT and 3MB-COMT constructs by transforming the corresponding plasmid DNA into subcloning efficiency DH5α competent cells according to the Invitrogen protocol.
6. Confirm and purify same length constructs as in Subheading 3.1, steps 2–5.

3.1.3. Construction of S- and MB-COMT Constructs with LPS mRNA Secondary Structure

1. To make the HPS single and double mutants, perform site-directed mutagenesis using the QuickChange II XL Site-Directed Mutagenesis Kit according to the manufacturer's instructions. To generate the HPS LPS-like single mutant, take the S- and MB-COMT same length HPS constructs and introduce the 403C to G mutation in S-COMT and the 625C to G mutation in MB-COMT using HPS Lsm forward and reverse primers.
2. To generate the HPS double mutant, with restored original HPS stem-loop structure, take the HPS LPS-like single mutant and introduce a second 479G to C mutation in S-COMT and the 701G to C mutation in MB-COMT using HPS dm forward and reverse primers.
3. Clone the HPS LPS-like mutants and double mutants as in Subheading 3.2, step 5.
4. Confirm and purify HPS mutants as in Subheading 3.1, steps 2–5.

3.1.4. Construction of S- and MB-COMT Constructs with APS mRNA Secondary Structure

1. Digest the S- and MB-COMT same length HPS constructs with the unique restriction enzyme PflFI. PflFI will make one cut 71 base pairs before and a second cut 6 base pairs after the 533C nucleotide in S-COMT and the 755C nucleotide in the MB-COMT. Optimal cutting is achieved by incubating 2 μg DNA with 5 μL buffer 4, 0.5 μL BSA, 2 μL PflFI, and d^2 H_2O up to 50 μL at 37°C for 1 h.
2. Isolate the S- and MB-COMT vectors (~5 Kb) using gel electrophoresis as in Subheading 3.2, step 2. Purify the vectors as per the Qiagen QIAquick Gel Extraction Kit handbook.
3. Dephosphorylate S- and MB-COMT vectors using shrimp alkaline phosphatase according to the Roche protocol.
4. Ligate S- and MB-COMT vectors with the HPS Asm 78 base pair oligo and reverse complement that contains the 533C to G substitution in S-COMT and the 755C to G substitution in MB-COMT. Use the Rapid DNA Ligation Kit according to the Roche protocol.
5. Clone the HPS APS-like mutants as in Subheading 3.2, step 5.
6. Confirm and purify HPS mutants as in Subheading 3.1, steps 2–5.

3.2. Transient Transfection of COMT cDNA Constructs and Isolation of Cell Lysate

A transient transfection is a quick way to deliver expressed gene variants to cells in order to study their potential functional effects. Stable transfection with the variants of interest may be a more robust choice when only the activity of the corresponding protein is altered; however, when expression of the genes is studied, stable transfection results are difficult to interpret as each transfected clone displays different expression levels, largely driven by genetic content at the site of construct insertion. Transient transfection, however, requires tight control for the efficiency of transfection that may drive the observed differences in expression of the variants. We cotransfected the variants of interest with the expression vector for βGalactosidase, the activity of which in the cell lysates can be quickly and robustly measured, for activity and protein assays. We also co-transfected the variants of interest with the SEAP vector as a control for transfection efficiency in real-time PCR experiments, as we found SEAP cDNA has a robust quantitative pattern of amplification.

The choice of the cell line for construct transfection can be a very crucial step, as activation of the majority of transduction pathways displays cell-specific characteristics. Thus, the genetic variants under investigation should be tested in the cell system that has an active corresponding pathway. However, endogenous expression of the gene should not be too high, allowing for differences in the transfected endogenous variants' activities to be observed. We generally recommend that several cell lines initially be tested.

For COMT expression, we found that the PC-12 cell line, a widely used model of neuronal cells, provided the best test system.

1. Plate frozen rat adrenal PC-12 cells. Place a 1 mL aliquot of frozen cells in FBS and DMSO (see Note 4) in a 37°C water bath until thawed (~1 min) and then add to 9 mL PC-12 media in a 100 mm dish. Change media after cells adhere (~1–2 h).
2. Passage cells. When cells become confluent, aspirate media, wash cells with 1× PBS, add 1 mL trypsin, and gently rock so trypsin covers the plate. Place the dish in a 37°C incubator for 3–5 min or until cells move freely when dish is gently tapped. Add 10 mL fresh media to the cells and gently pipette up and down (~10 times) to break up clumps of cells. Plate cells at a 1:10 dilution by adding 1 mL cells to 9 mL media in a 100 mm dish. Passage cells ~2–3 times to establish normal growth prior to experiment. It is important to note that cell passage number significantly affects experimental results (Fig. 2). Thus, we do not recommend using cells with passage number exceeding 40.
3. Prepare cells for transfection. When passaging cells immediately prior to transfection, plate them in 35 mm 6-well dishes with 2 mL media per well. Prepare enough dishes to account for duplicates for enzymatic activity, and protein expression assays (in which cells are collected in 10 mM CDTA) and RNA

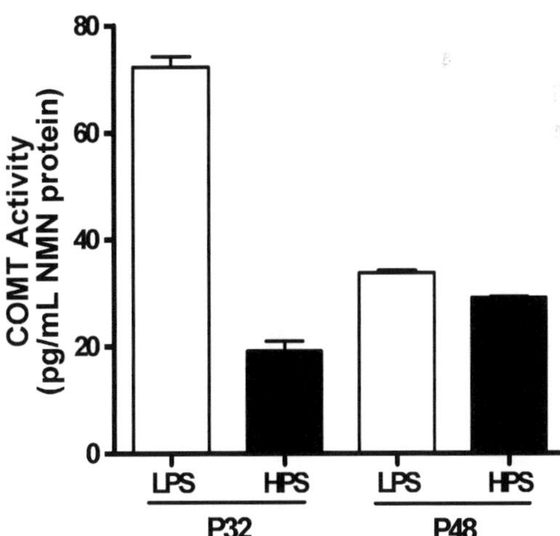

Fig. 2. The PC-12 cell passage number at the time of transfection affects COMT enzymatic activity. PC-12 cells from ATCC were acquired through the UNC tissue culture facility at passage 30 (P30). Younger cells used closer to this passage time demonstrated significant haplotype-dependent differences in S-COMT enzymatic activity relative to older cells that were passaged numerous times. As illustrated above, the LPS haplotype exhibited a fourfold increase in activity compared with the HPS haplotype when constructs were transfected in P32 cells. However, no differences between LPS and HPS haplotypes were found when the constructs were transfected in P48 cells. Data represent Mean ± SEM

abundance assays (in which cells are collected in Trizol). One hour prior to transfection, remove 1 mL media per well so that only 1 mL media remains.

4. Transfect cells. A 1:10 split of PC-12 cells will provide experimental cultures that are approaching optimal 60–70% confluence after 12 h. Combine COMT plasmid (2 μg/well) and control bGalactosidase and SEAP cDNA plasmids for transfection efficiency (0.1 μg each/well). Transiently transfect cells using SuperFect Reagent in accordance with manufacture's recommendations. Transfection with the pCMV SPORT 6 vector lacking the insert should be done for each experiment. Change media ~12 h following transfection.
5. Collect cell lysates ~40 h posttransfection. To collect cells for measurement of enzymatic activity and protein expression, remove media, wash cells 2 times with PBS (~2 mL per well), then add 300 μL 10 mM CDTA per well, and store dishes at −80°C. To collect cells for measurement of RNA abundance, remove media, add 500 μL Trizol per well, pipette several times to remove all adherent cells, transfer cells in Trizol to 1.7 mL conical tubes, and store at 4°C (see Note 5).

3.3. Enzymatic Assay for COMT Activity

The assay for biologic activity of the gene product is the most relevant for assessing the potential functionality of genetic variants. It is also most difficult for generalization, as the majority of gene products require their own specific assay depending on the nature of their biological activity. As COMT methylates catecholamines, we developed an enzymatic assay that applies the ELISA for measuring the amount of normetanephrine (NMN) in cell lysates. Although there are other approaches to measure methylated catecholamines with even higher sensitivity, such as HPLC, commercial availability of the ELISA for NMN provides significant convenience. The ELISA measuring metanephrine and metadopamine can also be used for the assessment of COMT enzymatic activity.

1. Lyse cells collected in 10 mM CDTA by repeatedly freezing/thawing five times at −80°C and room temperature, respectively. Collect the cells in 1.7 mL tubes, centrifuge at 2,000×*g* for 10 min, and remove filtrate.
2. Normalize for protein concentration using the Pierce BCA kit according to the Pierce protocol.
3. Evaluate transfection efficiency. Combine 50 μL normalized cell lysate from step 2 with 50 μL 2× βGalactosidase buffer in a clear 96-well plate and incubate at 37°C for 20–30 min or until lysate begins to turn yellow. Quantify absorbance using a luminometer with a 405 nM filter (see Note 6).

4. The COMT enzymatic assay is based on the method described by Masuda's group (11). Purified lysates (8 μl) are incubated with 11 μl 2 mM $MgCl_2$ in 80 mM PBS, 0.5 μl 7.5 mM NE, 0.5 μl 6.7 nM SAMe, and 1 μl d^2H_2O for 60 min. The reaction is terminated using 20 μl of 0.4 M HCl and 1 μl of 330 mM EDTA. The same reaction in the presence of 15 mM EDTA should be carried out in parallel for each lysate to bind Mg^{+2} ions required for COMT activity – this provides a negative control.
5. COMT activity is assessed as measurement of NMN by Normetanephrine ELISA kit in accordance with manufacture's recommendations using 10 μl of reaction mixture from step 3 above. COMT activity is determined after subtracting the amount of NMN produced by endogenous enzymatic activity (transfection with empty vector). COMT activity is then normalized for transfection efficiency based on β-galactosidase activity quantified for each lysate.

3.4. Western Blotting for COMT Protein Levels

As one finds that genetic variants alter activity of the corresponding protein, the next critical question is the level of the regulation. To determine if genetic variants differentially control gene expression at the level of translation, relative protein amounts should be measured. Probably the most common approach is the Western blot analysis described here.

1. Prepare a 10% Novex Tris-Glycine gel by washing individual wells with running buffer. Assemble the gel in Western electrophoresis chamber. Fill chamber with running buffer and then wash individual wells with running buffer a second time by gently pipetting up and down several times. Importantly, remove any bubbles remaining in wells with a pipette tip.
2. Prepare purified lysates normalized for protein concentration obtained in Section 3.3, step 2. Dilute samples (10–50 μg per well) in 2× Laemmli buffer and 5% βME (e.g., 95 μL Laemmli buffer and 5 μL βME) for a final volume of 30 μL (see Note 7). Vortex samples and boil for 5 min at 95°C to denature proteins.
3. Run protein samples. Load ~7 μL SeeBlue marker in well 1 and 30 μL of samples in Laemmli buffer in the remaining wells. Add Laemmli buffer to any remaining empty wells. Run the gel at 90 V for 2 h or 80 V for 3 h (see Note 8).
4. Transfer protein samples from the gel to a nitrocellulose membrane. In advance, soak the membrane in methanol and the transfer sponges and filter paper in transfer buffer for 5–10 min. Prepare a "transfer sandwich" in a shallow plastic container filled with transfer buffer by placing the transfer cassette bottom-side down then layering (1) 1 sponge, (2) several sheets of filter paper, (3) gel removed from plastic

case, (4) membrane, (5) several sheets of filter paper, and (6) 1 sponge. Importantly, make sure there are no bubbles between the gel and membrane (see Note 9). Close the cassette and place it in the transfer chamber so the gel side is toward the cathode and the membrane side is toward the anode. Place a magnetic stir bar at the bottom in the middle of the chamber, add the ice bucket, and fill chamber with transfer buffer. Run on magnetic mixer at 85 V for 2 h or 25 V overnight at 4°C.

5. Stain the membrane for COMT protein. Rinse the membrane with TBST buffer and then, block it in 5% nonfat milk for 1 h at room temperature. Wash the membrane three times for 5 min each in TBST at room temperature. Incubate the membrane with COMT polyclonal 1° antibody overnight at 4°C and then with Goat Anti-rabbit IgG HRP polyclonal 2° antibody for 1 h at room temperature.
6. Measure COMT protein. Wash the membrane with TBST for 10 min at room temperature and then expose it to western blotting substrate as per Pierce's guidelines. Cover the membrane in plastic and then measure electrochemiluminescence using the GE ImageQuant or similar imager.
7. Verify equal loading of samples by measuring β-actin. Strip the membrane using Restore western stripping buffer, wash two times for 15 each in TBST, and block in 5% nonfat milk for 30 min at room temperature. Incubate the membrane with β-actin polyclonal 1° antibody for 1 h at room temperature followed by Goat Anti-Rabbit IgG HRP polyclonal 2° antibody for 1 h at room temperature. Measure β-actin protein as in step 7 above.

3.5. Real-Time PCR for COMT Transcript Levels

If expression levels of the variants are altered at the protein level, it is highly likely that these differences are driven by differences in mRNA transcription. Expression constructs are not suitable for studying differences in transcription efficiency because they contain an artificial strong viral promoter instead of a natural promoter of the gene under investigation. To study genetic variants that alter transcription, corresponding variant promoter regions should be cloned in one of the reporter vectors that allow the study of transcription efficiency. However, expression constructs may display different mRNA levels due to difference in mRNA degradation rates. An application of real-time PCR for measuring mRNA levels that is much more efficient than alternative approaches such as Northern blot analysis or 5′ extension assay is described here. However, as we show here, the experimenter should be aware that relative abundance of the amplified regions reflects relative abundance of corresponding mRNA only if genetic variants do not differentially affect cDNA synthesis or PCR efficiency.

In the case of COMT, we show that genetic variants possess alternative secondary structures that affect the efficiency of transcription in the condition routinely used for cDNA synthesis and require specific reverse transcriptases and enzymatic reaction conditions that are insensitive to mRNA secondary structures.

1. Isolate RNA. Take 1.7 mL tube of cells collected in Trizol from Subheading 3.5, step 5. Add 200 μL chloroform, vortex ~1 min, and centrifuge at 13,000×*g* for 15 min at 4°C. The RNA is present in the top colorless aqueous phase. Transfer the aqueous phase to a new 1.7 mL tube, add 500 μL isopropyl alcohol, vortex, incubate 10 min at room temperature, and centrifuge at 13,000×*g* for 10 min at 4°C. RNA appears as a gel-like pellet on the side of the tube towards the bottom. Remove supernatant, add 1 mL 75% ethanol, vortex, and centrifuge at 7,500×*g* for 5 min at 4°C. Remove supernatant and allow RNA pellet to dry (~20 min). Reconstitute dry pellet in ~30 μL RNase-free H_2O to achieve a concentration of ~800–1,600 ng/μL. Use a spectrometer to determine final RNA concentration and store RNA at −80°C until ready to use. Note that the length of time the samples remain in Trizol prior to purification will affect the total amount of RNA (Fig. 3).
2. Purify RNA with RNase-free-DNase I according to the Promega protocol.
3. Perform first strand cDNA synthesis using Thermo-X reverse transcriptase according to a modified version of the Invitrogen protocol. For the annealing step, combine the RNA sample

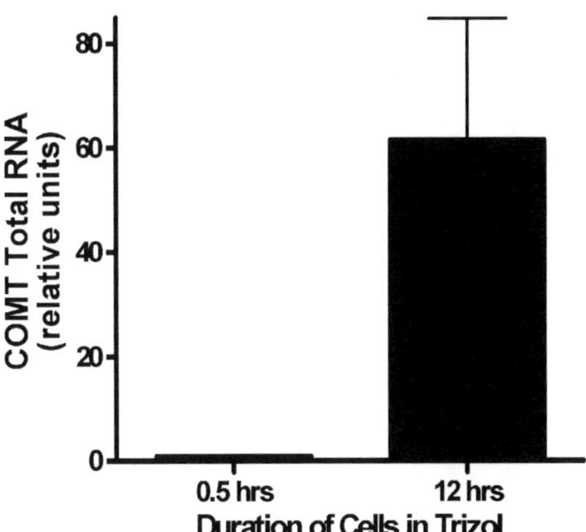

Fig. 3. The duration of PC-12 cells in Trizol prior to purification affects RNA abundance. Cells transfected with S-COMT constructs were incubated in Trizol for either 0.5 or 12 h prior to isolation of total RNA. Cells incubated in Trizol for 12 h at 4°C exhibited an approximately 60-fold increase in RNA yield relative to cells incubated in Trizol for only 0.5 h. Data represent Mean ± SEM

(1 ng to 5 μg), 1 μL 50 μM Oligo(dT)$_{20}$, 1 μL 10 mM dNTP mix, and nuclease-free H_2O for a final volume of 10 μL. Mix, incubate for 5 min at 65°C, and then cool on ice for 1 min or longer. For the extension step, add the following to each tube of annealed RNA: 4 μL Thermo-X buffer, 5 μL nuclease free H_2O, and 1 μL Thermo-X reverse transcriptase. Mix, incubate for 30 min at 64°C, add 2 μL 50 mM EDTA, incubate for 5 min at 90°C. Store samples at –20°C until ready to use. Prior to real-time PCR, dilute samples 1:10 in nuclease-free H_2O. Note that the type of reverse transcriptase used may affect real-time PCR results (Fig. 4).

4. Prepare COMT and SEAP standards for real-time PCR. To prepare the COMT standards, first prepare a 100 pg/mL stock solution from one of the purified COMT constructs. Then, make 5 fivefold serial dilutions (20 μL 100 pg/mL plasmid diluted in 80 μL TE buffer = 20 pg/mL, 20 μL 20 pg/mL plasmid diluted in 80 μL TE buffer = 4 pg/mL, etc.) to yield a total of 7 standards: 100, 20, 4, 0.8, 0.16, 0.04, and 0 pg/mL. To prepare the SEAP standards, first make a 50 pg/mL stock solution from the Clonetech SEAP plasmid. Then, make 5 fivefold serial dilutions (20 μL 50 pg/mL plasmid diluted in 80 μL TE buffer = 10 pg/mL, 20 μL 10 pg/mL plasmid diluted in 80 μL TE buffer = 2 pg/mL, etc.) to yield a total of 7 standards: 50, 10, 2, 0.4, 0.08, 0.016, and 0 pg/mL.

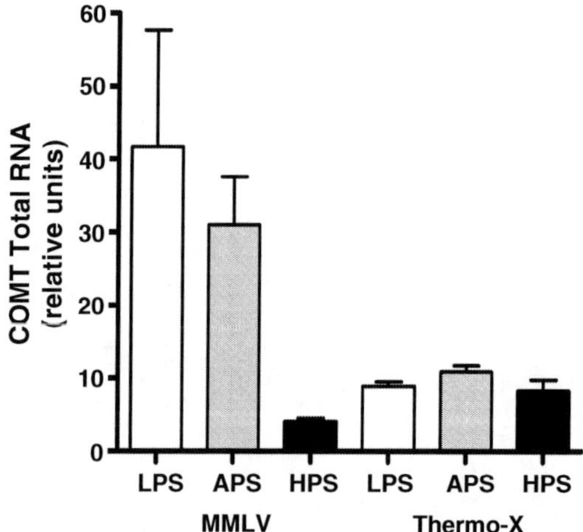

Fig. 4. RNA secondary structure influences the ability of reverse transcriptase to synthesize cDNA. First strand synthesis performed using MMLV reverse transcriptase yields an artificial tenfold difference observed in relative RNA abundance between the S-COMT LPS and HPS haplotypes. This artificial difference driven by the more stable secondary structure associated with the HPS haplotype (8, 12) was eliminated when first strand synthesis was performed using Thermo-X, which is a reverse transcriptase designed to synthesize cDNA from more challenging templates with high GC content or extensive secondary structure. Data represent normalized Mean values ± SEM

5. Prepare real-time PCR pates. Each RNA sample is tested for both COMT (experimental sample) and SEAP (experimental control) mRNA amount. For each COMT sample, standard, or negative control well, combine 12 µL SYBR Green dye, 0.5 µL 20 µM COMT-F primer, 0.5 µL 20 µM COMT-R primer, 5 µL nuclease-free H_2O, and 2 µL template from step 3 or 2 µL standard from step 4. For each SEAP sample or standard well, combine the same ingredients but substitute SEAP-F and SEAP-R for COMT-F and COMT-R primers (see Note 10). After filling the wells, spin the plate so that no bubbles remain, and then carefully cap the wells.
6. Perform real-time PCR. Enter the following routine in the PCR machine: Step 1: Initial denaturation 95°C for 12 min, Step 2: Denaturation 95°C for 30 s, Step 3: Annealing 55°C for 30 s, Step 4: Extension 71°C for 30 s, Step 5: Read, Step 6: Repeat cycles two to four 40 times, Step 7: Incubate 10°C forever, and Step 8: End. Calculate COMT mRNA abundance for each sample and then normalize for transfection efficiency based on SEAP mRNA abundance (see Note 11).

4. Notes

1. SAMe is very unstable, even stored as powder at –80°C. The half life is 30 min at room temperature and activity diminishes rapidly with repeated freeze thawing. Over time, the white powder turns to a brown "glue" that is no longer usable.
2. After growing plasmids and prior to purification, it is important to save an aliquot of each plasmid for long-term storage. Place 1 ml of plasmid in a cryo-safe tube and add 150 µL of 50% glycerol to achieve a final dilution of 7% glycerol. Gently mix by inverting the tube several times, then store in liquid nitrogen.
3. When purifying DNA from agarose gel, it is important to leave wells between samples empty in order to prevent cross-contamination that may occur when cutting bands close together.
4. After passaging cells 2–3 times, it is important to save aliquots for long-term storage. Once cells are confluent, trypsinize them, collect in 1 mL PC-12 media, and place in a 15 mL tube. Add 8 mL FBS and 1 mL DMSO. Mix well by gently pipetting several times and aliquot 1 mL cells per cryotube. Store in liquid nitrogen.
5. Cells can remain in Trizol at 4°C for up to 2 weeks. If a longer storage time is needed prior to purification of RNA, place cells in Trizol solution at –80°C, where they can remain indefinitely.

6. Obtaining a relative measure of transfection efficiency for each sample is important as it allows for normalization of enzymatic assay results. If transfection efficiency is low, the incubation time may need to be extended for several hours or even overnight.
7. For best results, do not store Laemmli buffer with β-mercapto-ethanol.
8. If protein bands do not run evenly on the gel, it could be due to an expired gel, low level of buffer, or too high a voltage.
9. Air bubbles between the gel and membrane will disrupt the transfer of protein. To eliminate bubbles, gently force them to the closest edge of the gel. Test tubes, pipettes, or gel rollers may also be used for this purpose.
10. To achieve the most uniform results, calculate the total number of COMT standard, SEAP standard, COMT sample, and SEAP sample wells required for the experiment and prepare COMT and SEAP master mixes that contain enough dye, appropriate primer, and water for that total number of wells. Pipette 18 μL master mix in each well, then add 2 μL sample to the master mix in each well. For a standard experiment, estimate running duplicate wells for 7 COMT standards, 7 SEAP standards, and single wells for DNase-treated RNA samples that did not undergo first strand cDNA synthesis (negative control). The remaining wells can be used to amplify COMT or SEAP for each experimental sample in duplicate.
11. The experiments studying differences in mRNA levels can be modified for more exact identification of mRNA degradation rates. Actinomycin D, a nonspecific inhibitor of mRNA transcription, should be added to cells transfected with the variants under investigation, several time points collected, and RNA isolated and measured by real-time PCR as described above.

Acknowledgments

The authors would like to thank Dr. Inna Tchivileva and Katherine Satterfield for their help in developing the HPS LPS-like and HPS APS-like mutants and Drs. Svetlana Shabalina and William Maixner for their support in the development of these studies. Additionally, the authors would like to thank IBL Hamburg for their generous gift of normetanephrine ELISA kit components. This work was supported by the NIH/NCRR KL2-RR025746 and NIH/OBSSR R24-DK067674 awards to Andrea Nackley and the NIH/NIDCR R01-DE016558, PO1-NS065685, and U01-DE017018 awards Luda Diatchenko.

References

1. Mannisto PT, Kaakkola S (1999) Catechol-O-methyltransferase (COMT): biochemistry, molecular biology, pharmacology, and clinical efficacy of the new selective COMT inhibitors. Pharmacol Rev 51:593–628
2. Diatchenko L, Slade GD, Nackley AG, Bhalang K, Sigurdsson A, Belfer I, Goldman D, Xu K, Shabalina SA, Shagin D et al (2005) Genetic basis for individual variations in pain perception and the development of a chronic pain condition. Hum Mol Genet 14:135–143
3. Marbach JJ, Levitt M (1976) Erythrocyte catechol-O-methyltransferase activity in facial pain patients. J Dent Res 55:711
4. Rakvag TT, Klepstad P, Baar C, Kvam TM, Dale O, Kaasa S, Krokan HE, Skorpen F (2005) The Val158Met polymorphism of the human catechol-O-methyltransferase (COMT) gene may influence morphine requirements in cancer pain patients. Pain 116:73–78
5. Zubieta JK, Heitzeg MM, Smith YR, Bueller JA, Xu K, Xu Y, Koeppe RA, Stohler CS, Goldman D (2003) COMT val158met genotype affects mu-opioid neurotransmitter responses to a pain stressor. Science 299: 1240–1243
6. Yampolsky LY, Kondrashov FA, Kondrashov AS (2005) Distribution of the strength of selection against amino acid replacements in human proteins. Hum Mol Genet 14:3191–3201
7. Knight JC (2005) Regulatory polymorphisms underlying complex disease traits. J Mol Med 83:97–109
8. Nackley AG, Shabalina SA, Tchivileva IE, Satterfield K, Korchynskyi O, Makarov SS, Maixner W, Diatchenko L (2006) Human catechol-O-methyltransferase haplotypes modulate protein expression by altering mRNA secondary structure. Science 314:1930–1933
9. Lennon G, Auffray C, Polymeropoulos M, Soares MB (1996) The I.M.A.G.E. Consortium: an integrated molecular analysis of genomes and their expression. Genomics 33:151–152
10. Strausberg RL, Feingold EA, Grouse LH, Derge JG, Klausner RD, Collins FS, Wagner L, Shenmen CM, Schuler GD, Altschul SF et al (2002) Generation and initial analysis of more than 15,000 full-length human and mouse cDNA sequences. Proc Natl Acad Sci U S A 99:16899–16903
11. Masuda M, Tsunoda M, Yusa Y, Yamada S, Imai K (2002) Assay of catechol-O-methyltransferase activity in human erythrocytes using norepinephrine as a natural substrate. Ann Clin Biochem 39:589–594
12. Harrison GP, Mayo MS, Hunter E, Lever AM (1998) Pausing of reverse transcriptase on retroviral RNA templates is influenced by secondary structures both 5′ and 3′ of the catalytic site. Nucleic Acids Res 26:3433–3442

Chapter 29

Genetic Polymorphisms and Human Sensitivity to Opioid Analgesics

Daisuke Nishizawa, Masakazu Hayashida, Makoto Nagashima, Hisashi Koga, and Kazutaka Ikeda

Abstract

Opioid analgesics are commonly used for the treatment of acute as well as chronic, moderate to severe pain. Well-known, however, is the wide interindividual variability in sensitivity to opioids that exists, which has often been a critical problem in pain treatment. To date, only a limited number of studies have addressed the relationship between human genetic variations and sensitivity to opioids, and such studies are still in their early stages. Therefore, revealing the relationship between genetic variations in many candidate genes and individual differences in sensitivity to opioids will provide valuable information for appropriate individualization of opioid doses required for adequate pain control. Although the methodologies for such association studies can be diverse, here we summarize protocols for investigating the association between genetic polymorphisms and sensitivity to opioids in human volunteers and patients undergoing painful surgery.

Key words: Analgesics, Genetic polymorphisms, Single nucleotide polymorphism (SNP), Genotype–phenotype association, Haplotype, Opioids, Opiates, Pain relief, Personalized medicine, Pharmacogenomics

1. Introduction

Opioid analgesics are commonly used for the treatment of acute or chronic, moderate to severe pain. However, wide interindividual variability exists in sensitivity to opioid analgesics (1). Because of this variability, a dose of an opioid that can produce satisfactory pain relief without significant adverse effects in some patients might cause underdosing or overdosing in others. Individual differences can be attributed to both genetic and environmental factors,

Arpad Szallasi (ed.), *Analgesia: Methods and Protocols*, Methods in Molecular Biology, vol. 617,
DOI 10.1007/978-1-60327-323-7_29, © Springer Science+Business Media, LLC 2010

although the relative influence of each of these factors is diverse (2). Genetic variations in many genes involved in opioid pharmacokinetics and pharmacodynamics might be responsible, at least partially, for the individual differences in phenotypes related to analgesic efficacy of opioids.

Numerous molecules are known to be involved in the pharmacological effects of opioids. The genes encoding these molecules are candidates for exploring the relationships between genetic variations and individual differences in phenotype traits related to opioid actions. Recently, several studies in humans have investigated the relationships between the individual genetic variations in the μ-opioid receptor gene (*OPRM1*) and sensitivity to opioids (2–8). However, such studies are still in their early stages and await future meta-analyses for clarification of the precise phenotype-to-genotype relationships.

Therefore, revealing the relationships between genetic variations in many candidate genes and interindividual differences in sensitivity to opioids will facilitate a better understanding of how human genetic polymorphisms can cause differences in sensitivity to opioids. Data from such studies will provide valuable information for appropriate individualization of opioid doses to achieve adequate pain control and open new avenues for personalized pain treatment.

2. Materials

2.1. Collecting Clinical Data

1. A form describing the design of the study approved by each Institutional Review Board (IRB) at the respective institutions.
2. Letters to the candidate subjects explaining the outline or details of the study and reply cards on which the candidates indicate whether they are interested in participating in the study.
3. Packages to be sent to participating subjects that include explanatory leaflets describing the detailed study protocol, written informed consent forms, instructions for collecting oral mucosa samples (see section 3.2.1.), cotton swabs to collect oral mucosa samples, test tubes to enclose the samples, and stamped return-mail envelopes.
4. In the case of retrospective studies, lists of ex-patient or patient candidates who had previously undergone surgery (e.g., major open abdominal surgery) and received opioids (e.g., fentanyl or morphine) postoperatively during a specific period (e.g., the first 24 h postoperative period) at the hospitals where clinical data are collected.

5. Several references of papers or books describing the method of properly converting the dose of an opioid analgesic to the equivalent dose of another opioid analgesic. For example, to allow for intersubject comparisons of opioid doses required during the specific period, doses of opioid analgesics used during this period were converted to an equivalent dose of systemic fentanyl in our study.

2.2. Preparation of Genomic DNA

1. Four cotton swabs for each subject (see Note 1).
2. Screw-cap centrifuge tube for each subject in which to enclose swabs (e.g., Corning® 15 mL PP Centrifuge Tubes; Corning Inc., Corning, NY).
3. Cup of water to rinse out subject's mouth.
4. DNA extraction kit (e.g., QIAamp DNA Mini Kit; QIAGEN, Hilden, Germany).
5. Phosphate buffered saline (PBS): 1 tablet of Phosphate Buffered Salts Tablets (Takara Bio, Otsu, Japan) is dissolved in 100 mL of distilled water.
6. Whole genomic DNA amplification kit (e.g., illustra GenomiPhi V2 Kit, 100rxns; GE Healthcare UK, Buckinghamshire, United Kingdom).
7. TE buffer: 300 μL of 1 M tris base, 60 μL of 0.5 M EDTA (pH 8.0), and distilled water to a total volume of 30 mL.
8. Spectrophotometer for measurement of the concentration of genomic DNA (e.g., NanoDrop ND-1000 Spectrophotometer; NanoDrop Technologies, Wilmington, DE).

2.3. Genotyping

2.3.1. Polymerase Chain Reaction–Restriction Fragment Length Polymorphism (PCR–RFLP)

1. Purified 5–50 ng genomic DNA.
2. Forward and reverse oligonucleotide primer set encompassing the specific region, including the polymorphic site for PCR amplification.
3. Reaction buffer for PCR including DNA polymerase, dioxyribonucleoside triphosphate (dNTP), and $MgCl_2$ (e.g., GoTaq® Master Mix; Promega, Madison, WI).
4. Thermal cycler (e.g., PROGRAM TEMP CONTROL SYSTEM PC-818-02; Astec, Fukuoka, Japan).
5. Agarose (e.g., Agarose ME, Classic Type; Nacalai Tesque, Kyoto, Japan), stored at room temperature.
6. TAE buffer (50×): 242 g of tris base, 57.1 mL of glacial acetic acid, 100 mL of 0.5 M EDTA (pH 8.0), and water to a total volume of 1,000 mL, stored at room temperature.
7. DNA size marker (e.g., Loading Quick® 100 bp DNA Ladder; Toyobo, Osaka, Japan), stored at –20°C.

8. Ethidium bromide solution (Sigma-Aldrich, St. Louis, MO), stored at 4°C.
9. Appropriate restriction enzymes for digestion of PCR products.

2.3.2. Allele–Specific PCR (AS–PCR)

1. Purified 5–50 ng genomic DNA.
2. Two forward oligonucleotide primers, whose 3′ ends are specific for detecting each of the two alleles at the polymorphic site, and a reverse oligonucleotide primer.
3. DNA polymerase attached with reaction buffer, dNTP, and $MgCl_2$ (e.g., GoTaq® Master Mix; Promega) (see Note 2).
4. Thermal cycler (e.g., PROGRAM TEMP CONTROL SYSTEM PC-818-02; Astec, Fukuoka, Japan).
5. Agarose (e.g., Agarose ME, Classic Type; nacalai tesque), stored at room temperature.
6. TAE buffer (50×): 242 g of tris base, 57.1 mL of glacial acetic acid, 100 mL of 0.5 M EDTA (pH 8.0), and water to a total volume of 1,000 mL, stored at room temperature.
7. DNA size marker (e.g., Loading Quick® 100 bp DNA Ladder; Toyobo), stored at –20°C.
8. Ethidium bromide solution (Sigma-Aldrich), stored at 4°C.

2.3.3. TaqMan® SNP Genotyping Assays

1. Purified 5–50 ng genomic DNA.
2. 40× (or 20× or 80×) SNP Genotyping Assay containing sequence-specific forward and reverse primers to amplify the polymorphic sequence of interest and two TaqMan® MGB probes labeled with VIC® dye to detect the sequence of one allele and with FAM™ dye to detect the sequence of another allele.
3. TaqMan® Universal PCR Master Mix (Applied Biosystems, Foster City, CA).
4. Real-time PCR system (e.g., 7300 Real-Time PCR System; Applied Biosystems).

2.3.4. Multiple Primer Extension (MPEX)

2.3.4.1. Oligonucleotide Module Fabrication

1. S-Bio® PrimeSurface® (BS-11608) consisting of COC grafted with an original biocompatible phospholipid polymer, poly [2-methacryloyloxyethyl phosphorylcholine (MPC)-co-n-butyl methacrylate (BMA)-co-p-nitrophenyloxycarbonyl polyethyleneglycol methacrylate (MEONP)] (PMBN) hydrophilic polymer (Sumitomo Bakelite, Tokyo, Japan).
2. Oligonucleotide probes (see Note 3) designed to hybridize allele-specific PCR products of the arbitrary gene (e.g., *OPRM1*).

3. Spotting solution (250 mM sodium carbonate buffer, pH 9.0), stored at room temperature.
4. BioChip Arrayer® spotting robot (Filgen, Nagoya, Japan).
5. Oligonucleotide modules (gasket-type hybridization cassettes; one module consisting of 16 [8 × 2 lanes] hybridization wells; Sumitomo Bakelite).
6. Blocking buffer solution (0.5 N NaOH), stored at room temperature.

2.3.4.2. Preparation of Template Multiplex PCR Products and Their Confirmation

1. Multiplex PCR Mix® (TaKaRa Bio), stored at –30°C.
2. Primer pairs designed to amplify allele-specific PCR products of the arbitrary gene (e.g., *OPRM1*).
3. Thermal cycler (e.g., TaKaRa PCR Thermal Cycler Dice® Model TP600; TaKaRa Bio).
4. Wizard® SV 96 PCR Clean-Up System (Promega), stored at room temperature (22–25°C).
5. 80% ethanol, stored at room temperature.
6. Agarose (e.g., Agarose S; Nippon Gene, Tokyo, Japan), stored at room temperature.
7. TAE buffer (50×): 242 g of tris base, 57.1 mL of glacial acetic acid, 100 mL of 0.5 M EDTA (pH 8.0), and water to a total volume of 1,000 mL, stored at room temperature.
8. DNA size marker (e.g., 100 bp DNA Ladder; New England Biolabs, Ipswich, MA), stored at –20°C.
9. Ethidium bromide (Nippon Gene), stored at 4°C.

2.3.4.3. Modified MPEX Reaction

1. dNTP Set: 100 mM Solutions (GE Healthcare UK; working solution 1 mM for each dNTP), stored at –30°C.
2. HotStar Taq™ DNA polymerase (QIAGEN), stored at –30°C.
3. Biotin-11-dUTP (PerkinElmer, Wellesley, MA; working solution 1 mM), stored at –30°C and protected from prolonged exposure to light, with minimal freeze-thaw cycles.
4. 10× MPEX Buffer A: 1% TritonX100, stored at room temperature.
5. 2× MPEX Buffer B: 0.1 M phosphate buffer, pH 7.0, stored at room temperature.
6. Hybridization oven (e.g., Hybaid Midi Dual-14; Hybaid, Middlesex, United Kingdom).

2.3.4.4. Visualization by Colorimetric Reaction

1. Washing Buffer A: 10 mM Tris–HCl, pH 7.6, 150 mM NaCl, 0.1% Tween 20, stored at room temperature.
2. Washing Buffer B: 0.1% Tween 20, stored at room temperature.

3. Streptavidin-AP (PerkinElmer), stored at –20°C, and then stored at 4°C after thawing, without refreezing.
4. BCIP/NBT substrate solution (PerkinElmer), stored at 2–8°C.
5. Scanner (e.g., GT-9700F personal image scanner; Epson, Tokyo, Japan).

2.4. Statistical Analyses

1. Suitable commonly used statistical software such as SPSS (SPSS Inc., Chicago, IL), SAS (SAS Institute, Cary, NC), JMP (SAS Institute, Cary, NC), R (freely available; http://www.r-project.org/), and/or software programs for genetic analyses (Table 1) to perform tests of Hardy–Weinberg equilibrium and linkage disequilibrium (LD) and association analyses.
2. Computer environment capable of accessing any websites of the databases of interest.

3. Methods

There are many ways of designing studies to explore the relationship between polymorphisms in some candidate genes and human sensitivity to opiates. In study designs, research subjects can be human volunteers undergoing standardized pain tests before and after administration of a given opioid, or patients undergoing standardized surgery and receiving opioids for postoperative pain control. Endpoint data that may represent the phenotypic traits related to analgesic efficacy of opioids can include the analgesic effect of the opioid evaluated by a standardized pain test or opioid requirements during and/or after standardized surgery as well as postoperative pain scores. Below are examples of an experimental study enrolling human volunteers, a prospective clinical study enrolling patients who are scheduled to have elective surgery of a given type, and a retrospective clinical study enrolling patients or ex-patients who previously underwent surgery of a given type. Research subjects are human volunteers or patients with American Society of Anesthesiologists Physical Status I or II ((9); Table 2) who do not have serious coexisting disease or a history of using opioids or other psychoneurotic agents.

3.1. Clinical Data Collection

The quality of clinical data is critical for accurately detecting polymorphisms associated with human sensitivity to opiates. Researchers may design many ways of collecting clinical data. We describe examples of our procedures and some points or issues that should be noted.

Table 1
Useful software programs for genetic analyses

Name	Application (main characteristics)	Platform	URL	Reference
Haplotype/Linkage disequilibrium analysis				
GENEPOP	A population genetics software package	–	http://genepop.curtin.edu.au	(33)
PHASE	Reconstructing haplotypes from population genotype data	–	http://www.stat.washington.edu/stephens/software.html	(34)
HAPLOVIEW	Haplotype analysis; single SNP haplotype association tests	Win/Mac/Unix	http://www.broad.mit.edu/mpg/haploview/index.php	(35)
LDSELECT	Analyses on patterns of linkage LD between polymorphic sites in a locus	–	http://droog.gs.washington.edu/ldSelect.html	(25)
GOLD	A software package that provides a graphical summary of LD in human genetic data	–	http://www.sph.umich.edu/csg/abecasis/GOLD	(36)
HAPLOTYPER	Estimation of haplotypes by MCMC	–	http://www.people.fas.harvard.edu/~junliu/Haplo/docMain.htm	(37)
Tagger	A tool for the selection and evaluation of tag SNPs from genotype data	web-based	http://www.broad.mit.edu/mpg/tagger	(38)
HAPLOBLOCKFINDER	A package for haplotype block identification, visualization and htSNP selection	UNIX/Win	http://cgi.uc.edu/cgi-bin/kzbang/haploBlockFinder.cgi	(39)
GENECOUNTING	Haplotype analysis with permutation tests for global association and specific haplotypes	Win/UNIX (Solaris)/Linux	http://www.mrc-epid.cam.ac.uk/Personal/jinghua.zhao/software.htm http://www.mrc-epid.cam.ac.uk/Personal/jinghua.zhao/software/	(40)

(continued)

Table 1 (continued)

Name	Application (main characteristics)	Platform	URL	Reference
HAPBLOCK	Dynamic programming algorithms for haplotype block partitioning and tag SNPs selection	Win/Linux/UNIX(Solaris)	http://www-hto.usc.edu/msms/HapBlock/	(41)
HAPLOBLOCK	Haplotype block identification, haplotype resolution and linkage disequilibrium mapping	UNIX(Solaris)/Linux/MacOS X	http://bioinfo.cs.technion.ac.il/haploblock/	(42)
SNPAlyze	A SNP and disease association analysis software	Win(98Me/NT4.0/2000/XP)	http://www.dynacom.co.jp/e/products/package/snpalyze/index.html	(43)
EH (EHPLUS, EH+)	Estimation of haplotypes and case–control study based on estimated haplotypes	MS-DOS/UNIX	http://www.genemapping.cn/eh.htm http://linkage.rockefeller.edu/software/eh	(44)
SNPHAP	A program for estimating frequencies of haplotypes of large numbers of diallelic markers	–	http://www-gene.cimr.cam.ac.uk/clayton/software	–
Arlequin	An exploratory population genetics software environment able to handle large samples of molecular data	Win	http://cmpg.unibe.ch/software/arlequin3/ http://lgb.unige.ch/arlequin/	(45)
HelixTree	Comprehensive toolset for population-based association studies	Win/Linux/MacOS X	http://www.goldenhelix.com/SNP_Variation/HelixTree/index.html	(46)
Association study				
HARDY	MCMC program for association in two-dimensional contingency tables	UNIX (DEC-UNIX/..)	http://www.stat.washington.edu/thompson/Genepi/Hardy.shtml	(47)

haplo.stats (formerly haplo.score)	A suite of routines for the analysis of indirectly measured haplotypes	UNIX	http://mayoresearch.mayo.edu/mayo/research/biostat/schaid.cfm	(48)
UNPHASED	A suite of programs for association analysis of multilocus haplotypes from unphased genotype data	UNIX(Solaris)/Linux/Win	http://www.mrc-bsu.cam.ac.uk/personal/frank/software/unphased/	(49)
HTR	Haplotype association mapping using unrelated individuals; "fixed" and "sliding" window analysis	Win/UNIX(Solaris)	http://statgen.ncsu.edu/zaykin/htr.html http://statgen.ncsu.edu/pub/zaykin/htr/	(46)
GENETIC POWER CALCULATOR	Automated power analysis for VC QTL linkage and other common tests	–	http://pngu.mgh.harvard.edu/~purcell/gpc/	(50)
CHAPLIN	Identifying specific haplotypes or haplotype features that are associated with disease	Win(2000/XP)	http://www.genetics.emory.edu/labs/epstein/software/chaplin/index.html	(51)
PAWE	Power and sample size calculations for genetic case–control association studies allowing for errors	–	http://linkage.rockefeller.edu/pawe/	(52)
Quanto	A program that computes sample size or power for association studies	Win (98/NT 2000/..)	http://hydra.usc.edu/GxE/	(53)
Hplus	Performing haplotype estimation on genetic markers and handling datasets that include case–control status	MS-Windows/Linux	http://cougar.fhcrc.org/hplus/	(54)
PLINK	A whole-genome association analysis toolset focusing purely on analysis of genotype/phenotype data	–	http://pngu.mgh.harvard.edu/purcell/plink/	(55)

SNP single nucleotide polymorphism, *LD* linkage disequilibrium, *MCMC* Markov chain Monte Carlo, *htSNP* haplotype tagging SNP, *VC* variance components, *QTL* quantitative trait locus

Table 2
American Society of Anesthesiologists Physical Status Classification System

P1:	A normal healthy patient
P2:	A patient with mild systemic disease
P3:	A patient with severe systemic disease
P4:	A patient with severe systemic disease that is a constant threat to life
P5:	A moribund patient who is not expected to survive without the operation
P6:	A declared brain-dead patient whose organs are being removed for donor purposes

3.1.1. Ethical Issues and Study Designs

1. Plan study protocol such that it meets all requirements imposed by the laws and guidelines regarding studies that handle human genomes (see Note 4).
2. Obtain approval from each respective institutional IRB for the study protocol.
3. Obtain written informed consent from each human subject after appropriately explaining, in written form, the clinical data sampling and DNA analysis.
4. A personal information manager responsible for managing personal information of the research subjects and making such information unidentifiable based on instructions from the head of the respective research institution should anonymize the collected samples before and after researchers handle the data to ensure the protection of personal information. Fig. 1 shows an example of the procedure in which personal information is protected.

3.1.2. Collecting Data in an Experimental Study Enrolling Human Volunteers

1. A given dose of a given opioid analgesic (e.g., intravenous [i.v.] injection of fentanyl, 2 μg/kg; i.v. injection of morphine, 0.2 mg/kg; i.v. infusion of remifentanil, 0.2 μg/kg/min over hours) is administered to human volunteers.
2. A standardized pain test, such as for thermal, mechanical, or electrical pain, is performed before, during, and after opioid administration (10).
3. An appropriate cutoff point is set to avoid tissue damage.
4. The pain test can be performed repeatedly, at a given interval, during and/or after opioid administration (e.g., every hour during and after i.v. infusion of remifentanil) over 4 h (10).
5. End-points can be latency to pain perception and/or pain tolerance, or pain perception and/or pain tolerance thresholds.

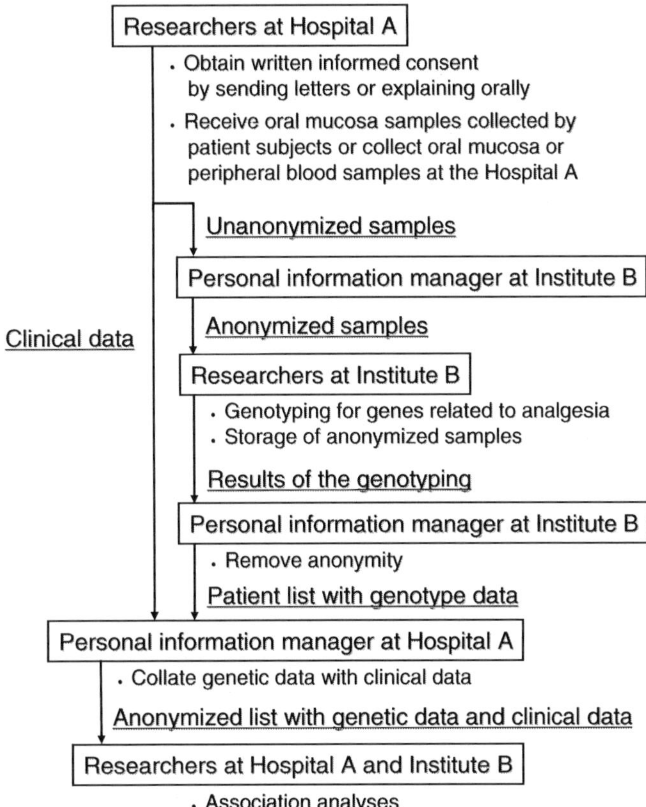

Fig. 1. Example of the procedure in which the personal information of research subjects is properly preserved. In this case, clinical data are collected at Hospital A, and genetic data are collected at Institute B.

6. The percent maximum possible effect (%MPE) can be calculated as an easy-to-interpret indicator of analgesic efficacy of the opioid: *%MPE = (cutoff value – maximum value during or after opioid administration)/(cutoff value – value before opioid administration) × 100.*
7. Whole blood (10 ml) or oral mucosa is sampled for genomic DNA analysis.

3.1.3. Collecting Clinical Data in a Prospective Study

1. Subjects are patients who are scheduled to have surgery of a given type that involves well-standardized procedures (e.g., distal gastrectomy for gastric cancer) under standardized anesthesia (e.g., sevoflurane–remifentanil anesthesia with or without epidural anesthesia).
2. Postoperative pain is managed with a single opioid analgesic according to a standardized protocol using a patient-controlled analgesia (PCA) pump (e.g., fentanyl, 20 μg per

demand dose with a lockout interval of 5 min; morphine, 2 mg per demand dose with a lockout interval of 10 min) (11).

3. Rescue analgesics (e.g., nonsteroidal antiinflammatory drugs) should be prescribed whenever the analgesic effect of the opioid is inadequate or the use of the opioid is discontinued because of significant adverse effects.
4. Postoperative pain scores are recorded at given postoperative time-points (e.g., 3, 6, 12, and 24 h after surgery) using an appropriate pain scale (e.g., visual analog scale, verbal pain rating scale, numerical pain rating scale) (11).
5. Presence/absence and severity (if present) of adverse effects of the opioid (e.g., nausea/vomiting and respiratory depression) are recorded.
6. Clinical data that may relate to analgesic efficacy of the opioid are recorded, including age, gender, type of surgery, duration of surgery, type of anesthesia, intraoperative opioid requirements, postoperative opioid requirements, rescue analgesic requirements during a given postoperative period (e.g., during the first 24 h after surgery), and postoperative pain scores.
7. Whole blood (10 ml) or oral mucosa is sampled for genomic DNA analysis.

3.1.4. Collecting Clinical Data in a Retrospective Study

1. A researcher in charge of clinical data collection (Researcher C) lists ex-patient or patient candidates who previously underwent surgery of a given type and received opioids for postoperative pain control at a particular hospital.
2. Researcher C mails letters to these candidates explaining the outline of the study protocol and reply cards on which the candidates can indicate their interest in participating in the study.
3. A researcher in charge of genomic DNA analysis (Researcher D) receives the reply cards from the candidates who are willing to participate in the study.
4. Researcher D sends packages to these candidates that include explanatory leaflets describing the detailed study protocol, written informed consent forms, instructions to collect oral mucosa samples, cotton swabs to collect oral mucosa samples, test tubes to enclose the samples, and stamped return-mail envelopes.
5. Researcher D receives signed informed consent forms and oral mucosa samples from the candidates who have been determined to be research subjects.
6. Researcher C collects clinical data from the hospital records of the research subjects that may relate to analgesic efficacy of opioids (see Subheading 3.1.3).

7. Ideally, for further analyses, postoperative pain should be managed with a standardized protocol employing a single opioid analgesic (e.g., i.v. PCA fentanyl). However, if multiple opioids were used postoperatively, intersubject comparisons of postoperative opioid requirements are possible by converting the dose of one opioid to an equivalent dose of another, based on published data showing equipotent doses of various opioid analgesics. For example, epidural fentanyl 100 μg, systemic morphine 10 mg, epidural morphine 2 mg, systemic pentazocine 30–60 mg, and systemic buprenorphine 333 μg can be converted to an equivalent systemic fentanyl dose of 100 μg (7). The total opioid requirements in the first 24 h postoperative period are determined as the sum of equivalent systemic fentanyl doses of all opioids used during this period.
8. If postoperative pain scores are not documented in hospital records, the researchers can ask the research subjects, by mail, to rate the pain intensity they had at rest during the particular period (e.g., during the first 24 h postoperative period) using a 5-point verbal pain rating scale (0 = no pain, 1 = mild pain, 2 = moderate pain, 3 = severe pain, 4 = the most severe pain imaginable).

3.2. Preparation of Genomic DNA

Before genotyping specific polymorphisms, genomic DNA of the subjects should be collected and purified. Although genomic DNA can be extracted from various cells or tissues in humans, we describe here the methods of extracting it from cells of oral mucosa. Only a small amount of DNA is usually extracted from the oral mucosa of each subject; therefore, the oral mucosa might not be durable for repeated use intended to genotype many candidate polymorphisms. However, recent whole genome amplification technology has enabled us to investigate genotypes of many genetic polymorphisms in the candidate loci without repeatedly collecting DNA samples from subjects.

3.2.1. Collection of Oral Mucosa

1. Rinse mouth with clean water.
2. Press the first swab onto the upper right buccal mucosa and roll it on the mucosa 25 times, slightly changing its position (see Fig. 2).
3. Put the swab into a centrifuge tube. Hold the tube and swab upright and let the swab fall down directly onto the bottom of the tube, avoiding contact between the swab and the inner wall of the tube (see Fig. 2).
4. Similarly, press the second, third, and forth swabs onto the lower left, lower right, and upper left buccal mucosa, respectively, and roll each of them 25 times on the mucosa of each site. Put the swab sticks, one at a time, into the same test tube as the first swab (see Fig. 2). Rinse mouth with clean water each time.

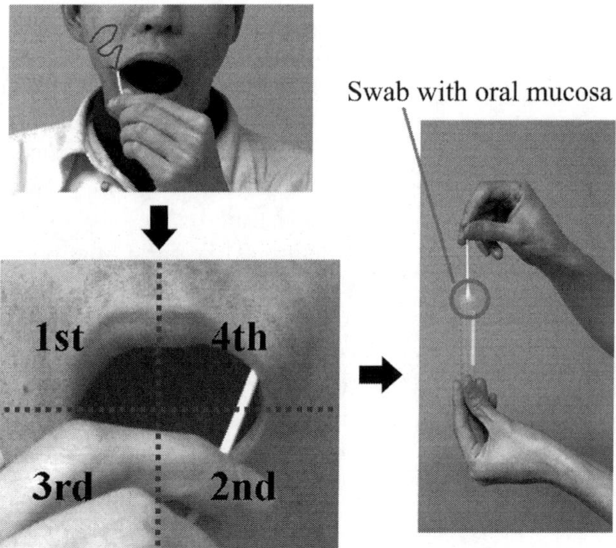

Fig. 2. Procedure for collecting oral mucosa (see Subheading 3.2.1).

5. Finally, rinse mouth with clean water or drink something.
6. Cap the centrifuge tube firmly and send it back to the researchers as soon as possible so that the researchers can store it at 4°C until DNA extraction.

3.2.2. Purification of Genomic DNA

1. After separating four swabs with oral mucosa from the sticks using scissors, if needed, and placing them in a 2 mL microcentrifuge tube, dry them up for 2 h at room temperature, and add 500 μL PBS to the sample (see Note 5).
2. Extract total genomic DNA using the DNA purification kit according to the manufacturer's instructions. Each buffer used in each purification step is 500 μL.
3. Store eluted genomic DNA at 4°C until used. If not used for an extended length of time, storage at −20°C is recommended.

3.2.3. Whole Genome Amplification (WGA)

1. Amplify the total genomic DNA using a whole genomic DNA amplification kit. 10 ng of purified template genomic DNA is sufficient.
2. Purify the amplified genomic DNA by conventional ethanol precipitation and dissolve in 300–400 μL TE buffer.
3. Measure the concentration of the purified DNA (see Note 6) and store it at 4°C until use. If not used for an extended length of time, storage at −20°C is recommended.

3.3. Genotyping

To date, many technologies of genotyping polymorphisms, most often single nucleotide polymorphisms (SNPs), have been developed and advanced. We do not describe all of these details here because the respective features of each of these methods have been discussed extensively elsewhere (12–16). Generally, most genotyping methods consist of forming allele-specific products v a detection procedure to identify them (15). The biochemical techniques involved or reagents and instruments required in each step differ among various genotyping methods, impacting accuracy, cost, throughput, and laboratory availability. Researchers must choose the most suitable method that meets their requirements. In the following subsections, we briefly describe the protocol for several genotyping methods.

3.3.1. PCR–RFLP

PCR–RFLP is one of the methods utilizing endonuclease (restriction enzyme) in the allelic discrimination steps. It does not require costly equipment and thus is feasible in most molecular biology laboratories. Additionally, throughput is not diminished if the numbers of samples per SNP are not extensive. The commonly recognized drawbacks of this technique are that it is labor-intensive, not suitable for large-scale clinical applications, and applicable only when the SNPs alter a restriction enzyme cutting site (12, 16).

1. Perform PCR in a total of 10 μL solution containing 5–50 ng purified genomic DNA as the template, DNase-free water, forward and reverse primers to amplify the region encompassing the polymorphic site, DNA polymerase, and reaction buffer including dNTP and $MgCl_2$. During the PCR reactions, control the temperature, such as with PROGRAM TEMP CONTROL SYSTEM PC-818-02. For example, the PCR program for amplifying the region of the A1032G SNP in the G-protein-activated inwardly rectifying potassium (GIRK) channel gene, *GIRK2*, is the following: 95°C for 2 min, followed by 35–40 cycles of 95°C for 30 s, 50°C for 30 s, and 72°C for 1 min, with a final extension at 72°C for 8 min (17).
2. Digest the amplified DNA fragments with the restriction enzyme in a reaction solution containing buffer, the restriction enzyme to discriminate the genotypes, and the PCR product as the substrate.
3. Separate the digestion products by electrophoresis using 1–2% agarose gel in 1× TAE buffer and stain with ethidium bromide for visualization under ultraviolet illumination. Detect the DNA fragment size pattern specific to the genotype of the loaded sample.

3.3.2. AS–PCR

AS-PCR utilizes the difference in the extension efficacy of DNA polymerases depending on whether the 3′ ends of the primers are matched or mismatched for hybridization at the polymorphic site.

Although the allele-specific primers used in this method often bear labeling tags, such as fluorescence (18, 19), we describe here a method in which such tags are not involved, and detection of allele-specific products are carried out by gel electrophoresis, which is more labor-intensive for large-scale genotyping but has lower initial set-up costs.

1. Perform PCR in a total of 10 μl solution containing 5–50 ng purified genomic DNA as the template, DNase-free water, forward and reverse primers to amplify the region including the polymorphic site, DNA polymerase, and reaction buffer including dNTP and $MgCl_2$. During the PCR reactions, control the temperature, such as with PROGRAM TEMP CONTROL SYSTEM PC-818-02. For example, the allele-specific PCR program for the A118G SNP in the *OPRM1* is the following: 95°C for 2 min, followed by 35 cycles of 95°C for 30 s, 62°C and 64°C for 30 s for the forward primer specific for A and G, respectively, and 72°C for 1 min, with a final extension at 72°C for 8 min (20).
2. Separate the presence of allele-specific PCR products by electrophoresis using 1–2% agarose gel in 1× TAE buffer and stain with ethidium bromide for visualization under UV illumination. For example, Fig. 3 shows the detection of the allele-specific PCR products for the A118G SNP.

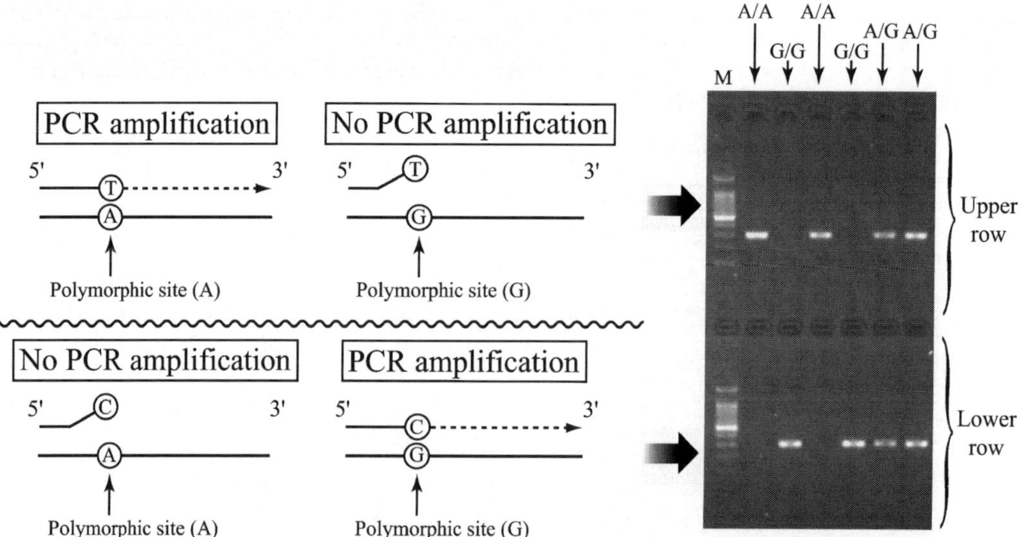

Fig. 3. Detection of allele-specific PCR products for the A118G SNP in the μ-opioid receptor gene (*OPRM1*). The principle as well as the results of AS-PCR is illustrated. Upper and lower rows in each lane indicate the A allele- and G allele-specific PCR products for each sample, respectively. The presence of only A-specific and G-specific products indicates the A/A genotype and G/G genotype, respectively, whereas the presence of both products indicates the A/G genotype. M, 100 bp DNA size marker.

3.3.3. TaqMan® SNP Genotyping Assays

TaqMan Assays are representative genotyping methods that utilize hybridization with allele-specific oligonucleotide probes at the region including the polymorphic site. It also utilizes 5′ exonucleotide activity of DNA polymerase in PCR reactions and techniques of fluorescence resonance energy transfer (FRET) in the detection step. This technique was developed by Applied Biosystems and supports ready-to-use, validated assays providing both the reagents and instrumentation for genotyping common SNPs (16, 21). Although the initial cost of this method is high, the running cost of this method is relatively low. Therefore, this method is useful for analyses of small numbers of SNPs using large-size samples, such as analyses in clinical and diagnostic settings (15).

1. Perform PCR in a total of 5 μl solution containing 5–50 ng purified genomic DNA as the template, with 40× (or 20× or 80×) SNP Genotyping Assay TaqMan® Universal PCR Master Mix. The PCR program is the following: 95°C for 10 min, followed by 40 cycles of 92°C for 15 s and 60°C for 1 min.
2. Perform the post-PCR plate read using a real-time PCR system. Genotyping is determined after generating standard curves to quantify the amount of DNA in each sample and identifying allele types.

3.3.4. MPEX

The modified MPEX is a recently developed, allele-specific extension (ASE) method (22). In the modified MPEX, hybridization and extension reactions are only performed on the substrate, a plastic S-BIO® PrimeSurface® with a biocompatible polymer whose surface chemistry offers extraordinarily stable thermal properties and chemical properties advantageous for enzymatic reactions on the surface (22). At least 50 oligonucleotides for different SNPs can be spotted onto the same surface area (22), and this method appears to be suitable for restricted SNP analysis focused on a moderate number of candidate genes that might affect human sensitivity to opiates. We demonstrate here the significance of this method combined with multiplex PCR by analyzing representative SNPs on different LD blocks of *OPRM1* (23).

3.3.4.1. Oligonucleotide Module Fabrication

1. The oligonucleotide probes are designed to hybridize allele-specific PCR products of *OPRM1* and are dissolved in spotting solution to a final concentration of 0.2 μM.
2. The oligonucleotides are spotted (approximately 600 μm in diameter, approximately 12.5 nl/spot) on the surface of S-Bio® PrimeSurface® (BS-11608) using a BioChip Arrayer® spotting robot.
3. The modules (gasket-type hybridization cassettes) are incubated overnight in a humid chamber with 250 mM sodium phosphate buffer at room temperature.

4. The excess amine-reactive group (MEONP) is inactivated for 5 min at room temperature in blocking buffer solution.
5. After the modules are washed in boiling water for 2 min, they are washed in water at room temperature for 2 min and then dried by centrifugation.
6. The oligonucleotide modules are stored in a desiccated state at 4°C until use.

3.3.4.2. Preparation of Template Multiplex PCR Products and Their Confirmation

1. PCR reactions are carried out using Multiplex PCR Mix® in a 20 μL total reaction volume containing 10 μL Multiplex PCR Mix 1, 0.1 μL Multiplex PCR Mix 2, 1 μL template genomic DNA (0.5–19.75 ng), and an appropriate concentration of each primer (G5953A, A2109G: 5.0 μM; C691G, A118G: 1.0 μM). PCR is performed for 40 cycles consisting of denaturation at 94°C for 30 s, annealing at 54°C for 90 s, and extension at 72°C for 90 s.
2. After the PCR reaction, the multiplex PCR products are purified with the Wizard® SV 96 PCR Clean-Up System according to the manufacturer's instructions (http://www.promega.com/tbs/tb311/tb311.pdf). To reduce residual primers, an optional wash protocol using 80% ethanol is also performed.
3. The amplified products are electrophoresed on 2.0% agarose gels and then visualized by ethidium bromide staining.
4. An 8/10 volume of purified PCR product is used for the further modified MPEX reaction.

3.3.4.3. Modified MPEX Reaction

1. After the template PCR products have been denatured at 95°C for 20 min on a thermal cycler, the PCR products are subjected to an annealing reaction with immobilized oligonucleotides on the modules in a 100 μL reaction volume containing 1× PCR buffer supplied by QIAGEN (information regarding the components is not available), 0.1% TritonX100, 0.04 mM dNTP, and 2.5 U HotStar TaqTM DNA polymerase (QIAGEN).
2. The modules are rinsed three times with MPEX Buffer A.
3. The samples are further incubated at 66°C for 3 h, and biotin-dUTP is incorporated during the extension of the complementary strand. This reaction is performed in a hybridization oven that should be prewarmed at least 1 h before the reaction. To avoid a decrease in temperature, the modules are covered with aluminum foil.
4. The residual reaction mixture is removed by decantation, and the modules are then agitated with 100 μL of MPEX Buffer

A for 1 min on a Double Shaker NR-3 (65 r/min; Taitec, Saitama, Japan).

5. After the removal of MPEX Buffer A, the modules are further agitated with 100 μL of MPEX Buffer B for 1 min.
6. The MPEX Buffer B is completely removed by decantation and centrifugation.

3.3.4.4. Visualization by Colorimetric Reaction

1. A working solution of Streptavidin-AP should be prepared immediately before the reaction (0.15 μL of Streptavidin-AP, 15 μL of 10× MPEX Buffer A, 75 μL of 2× MPEX Buffer B, to a volume of 150 μL with distilled water).
2. The working solution is added to the modules, and the samples are incubated at 37°C for 10 min. During this reaction, the modules are covered with aluminum foil.
3. The residual reaction mixture is removed by decantation, and the modules then are agitated with 100 μL of MPEX Buffer A for 1 min on a Double Shaker NR-3 (65 r/min; Taitec, Saitama, Japan).
4. After the removal of MPEX Buffer A, the modules are further agitated with 100 μL of MPEX Buffer B for 1 min.
5. The MPEX Buffer B is completely removed by decantation and centrifugation.
6. The colorimetric detection of the AP-labeled complementary strand is performed in BCIP/NBT substrate solution at 37°C for 30 min.
7. The BCIP/NBT substrate solution is removed, and the modules then are agitated with 100 μL of distilled water for 1 min on a Double Shaker NR-3 (65 r/min; Taitec, Saitama, Japan).
8. For the purpose of taking photographs, the modules are immediately dried by centrifugation.
9. The dark purple stains are scanned on a GT-9700F personal image scanner.
10. The scanned data are stored using the free software Epson TWAIN 5 (http://www.epson.jp/dl_soft/list/1379.htm) and then graphically manipulated using Adobe® Photoshop Elements v. 4.0. The recommended resolution of the graphics is more than 600 dpi.
11. The SNPs are assessed principally by visual inspection of the signal intensities.

3.4. Statistical Analyses

The statistical methodologies for detecting genetic polymorphisms affecting human sensitivity to opiates can be diverse, depending on how the study is designed by researchers and what variables and covariables are incorporated into the analyses from the clinical data of the subjects. In the following subsections, we concisely describe our protocol for investigating the association between genetic polymorphisms and human sensitivity to opiates. Here we cover only population association studies for quantitative traits in which unrelated individuals without population stratification who were treated with analgesics are genotyped at a number of polymorphisms. We do not address family-based association studies and case–control studies, which have an important role in efforts to understand the effects of genes on disease but require different types of statistical analyses. For more information, recent review articles have discussed association studies using various statistical approaches (24). All of the statistical analyses we describe can be performed using one or more of the software programs listed in Table 1, all of which can be found at the Genetic Analysis Software website (http://www.nslij-genetics.org/soft/).

3.4.1. Data Validation

Before beginning an association analysis, the genotype data should be appropriately formatted to be inputted into the software.

1. Check the genotyped polymorphism data. To perform precise and unbiased haplotype estimation, remove individual data in which genotypes for most of the polymorphisms of interest were not successfully determined due to inherent problems of such DNA samples. (Some software may automatically remove such genotype data or predict such data based on the observed genotypes at neighboring SNPs.)
2. Perform a statistical test to check the genotype data for deviation from Hardy-Weinberg Equilibrium (HWE). In most cases, deviation from HWE in healthy subjects indicates a genotyping error, inbreeding, stratification, or natural selection of the population, and thus further analysis using the genotype data for that SNP may be abandoned.
3. Format the genotype data to be inputted into the statistical analysis software or genetic analysis software (Table 1). Many software programs for analyzing haplotype-based associations might require the genotype data to be in a specific format (e.g., linkage format).
4. For a haplotype-based association study, perform haplotype phasing of the samples using genotype data and one of the suitable genetic analysis software programs (Table 1).

3.4.2. Linkage Disequilibrium (LD) Analysis

Information of LD between the SNPs at the region of interest is important in several ways. Even if the causal SNP is not directly genotyped, one could capture the association between other SNPs that show a strong LD with the causal SNP and a specific phenotype.

Additionally, if two SNPs are in strong LD, and almost no recombination is assumed between them, genotyping only one of the SNPs is sufficient. The strength of LD between two SNPs is often measured by the values *D'* and r^2, both of which are commonly used together but calculated by different formulas. Furthermore, a subset of the SNPs that is selected based on the information of LD relationships and tags the representative haplotypes at the region appropriately (25) are termed "haplotype tagging SNPs" or "tag SNPs" and might promote the efficiency of genotyping and further analyses without reducing the power to detect the expected association.

1. Estimate the strength of LD between the SNPs by calculating the values *D'* and r^2 based on the genotype data of the subjects using the suitable genetic analysis software programs (Table 1).
2. Select the tag SNPs that best represent the haplotypes at the region by using the suitable genetic analysis software programs, such as "Tagger" ((36); Table 1).

3.4.3. Association Study for Distinct SNPs

To explore the association between SNPs and some quantitative traits with normal distribution, several types of statistical analysis are possible, such as analysis of variance (ANOVA) and linear regression, which assumes a linear relationship between the mean value of the trait and the genotype.

1. Perform the statistical tests by running a software program to investigate the association between each distinct SNP and the phenotypic traits of interest. In the case of ANOVA, phenotypic traits and genotypes of a SNP should be treated as dependent and independent variables, respectively. Most software programs can also accept covariable data as well as genotype and phenotype data such as age, sex, and other characteristics of the subjects.
2. Check whether the output *P*-value achieves the level of significance for detecting a positive association.
3. In many cases, corrections of multiple testing might be required for the number of SNPs tested to avoid a type I error. However, corrections such as Bonferroni might not be required in some cases to avoid a type II error (26, 27).

3.4.4. Association Study for Haplotypes

Relatively few software programs are available for analyzing association between haplotypes and quantitative traits such as analgesic requirements compared with software programs that are available for case–control studies. Furthermore, estimated haplotypes of individuals or haplotype frequencies of the population tend to differ among the software used, depending on the algorithms employed by the programs. Minor differences in haplotype frequency estimates can produce very large differences in statistical tests (28). Therefore, comparing the outcomes of similar analyses carried out by different software programs is advisable to confirm the results.

1. Perform the statistical tests by running a software program to investigate the association between one or more haplotypes and the phenotypic traits of interest. In many cases, haplotype-based association studies might be completed concurrently with haplotype estimations of the populations involved.
2. Check whether the output *P*-value achieves the level of significance for detecting a positive association.
3. In some cases, corrections of multiple testing might be required for the number of haplotypes tested to avoid a type I error. However, corrections such as Bonferroni might not be required in some cases to avoid a type II error (26, 27).

3.4.5. Utilization of Databases

Numerous databases have become openly available that are helpful for designing a study and for analyzing the results. Below are a few databases that are useful for surveying genes and genetic polymorphisms and downloading data that could expedite study analyses. A recent review article discusses bioinformatics approaches for SNP analyses (29).

1. To obtain overall information of any SNP, consult the dbSNP database ((30); http://www.ncbi.nlm.nih.gov/SNP/), which contains the largest amount of data on genetic variations, including SNPs.
2. To obtain Genotype-to-Phenotype information, consult HGVbase (Human Genome Variation database; http://hgvbase.cgb.ki.se; formerly known as HGBASE), which provides a high-quality, nonredundant database of available genomic variation data of all types (31).
3. To obtain information of SNPs related to drug response, consult the PharmGED database (http://bidd.cz3.nus.edu.sg/phg/), which provides information about the effects of a particular protein polymorphism, noncoding region mutation, splicing alteration, or expression variation on the response of a particular drug.
4. To obtain overall information about the haplotype map of the human genome or to download genotype data for linkage disequilibrium analysis or other purposes, consult the HapMap database ((32); http://www.hapmap.org/index.html.en), which helps researchers find genes associated with human disease and pharmaceutical response.

4. Notes

1. Any form of clean cotton swab can be used, such as the commercially available Sterile Omni Swab (Whatman plc, Kent, United Kingdom) or a commonly used small wad of cotton wrapped around the end of a small rod made of wood, rolled paper, or plastic. To maintain cleanliness, each swab should be packaged before use.
2. The DNA polymerase used in the AS-PCR should be the one that lacks proofreading activity because the polymerase with proofreading activity could substitute a mismatched base for the correct base at the polymorphic site, owing to its exonuclease activity from 3′ to 5′.
3. The oligonucleotides used here were single-stranded 19–27 mer 5′-C6-amino-oligonucleotides. The oligonucleotides were designed and synthesized by NovusGene (Tokyo, Japan).
4. All researchers handling human genomes must observe the laws and guidelines set forth in their respective countries. Such laws and guidelines may be enacted based on the Declaration of Helsinki, World Medical Association (WMA), and Universal Declaration on the Human Genome and Human Rights adopted by the UNESCO Bioethics Programme General Conference in 1997. For example, researchers in Japan must observe the "Ethical Guidelines for Analytical Research on the Human Genome/Genes" issued by the Japanese Ministry of Education, Culture, Sports, Science and Technology, the Ministry of Health, Labour and Welfare, and the Ministry of Economy, Trade and Industry.
5. Clean the scissors used to separate the swab from the sticks with ethanol each time to avoid genomic DNA contamination from the previous sample.
6. The concentration of the purified DNA should be similar among samples because heterogeneity in the concentration of genomic DNA could increase the generation of false products in the AS-PCR, leading to misjudging the genotype of the sample.

Acknowledgments

We acknowledge Mr. Michael Arends for his assistance with editing the manuscript. This work was supported by grants from the Ministry of Health, Labour and Welfare of Japan (H17-Pharmaco-001, H19-Iyaku-023), the Ministry of Education,

Culture, Sports, Science and Technology of Japan (20602020, 19659405, 20390162), The Naito Foundation, and The Mitsubishi Foundation.

References

1. Ikeda K, Ide S, Han W, Hayashida M, Uhl GR, Sora I (2005) How individual sensitivity to opiates can be predicted by gene analyses. Trends Pharmacol Sci 26:311–317
2. Coulbault L, Beaussier M, Verstuyft C, Weickmans H, Dubert L, Trégouet D, Descot C, Parc Y, Lienhart A, Jaillon P, Becquemont L (2006) Environmental and genetic factors associated with morphine response in the postoperative period. Clin Pharmacol Ther 79:316–324
3. Bruehl S, Chung OY, Donahue BS, Burns JW (2006) Anger regulation style, postoperative pain, and relationship to the A118G mu opioid receptor gene polymorphism: a preliminary study. J Behav Med 29:161–169
4. Chou WY, Wang CH, Liu PH, Liu CC, Tseng CC, Jawan B (2006) Human opioid receptor A118G polymorphism affects intravenous patient-controlled analgesia morphine consumption after total abdominal hysterectomy. Anesthesiology 105:334–337
5. Chou WY, Yang LC, Lu HF, Ko JY, Wang CH, Lin SH, Lee TH, Concejero A, Hsu CJ (2006) Association of μ-opioid receptor gene polymorphism (A118G) with variations in morphine consumption for analgesia after total knee arthroplasty. Acta Anaesthesiol Scand 50:787–792
6. Klepstad P, Rakvåg TT, Kaasa S, Holthe M, Dale O, Borchgrevink PC, Baar C, Vikan T, Krokan HE, Skorpen F (2004) The 118 A > G polymorphism in the human μ-opioid receptor gene may increase morphine requirements in patients with pain caused by malignant disease. Acta Anaesthesiol Scand 48: 1232–1239
7. Hayashida M, Nagashima M, Satoh Y, Katoh R, Tagami M, Ide S, Kasai S, Nishizawa D, Ogai Y, Hasegawa J, Komatsu H, Sora I, Fukuda K, Koga H, Hanaoka K, Ikeda K (2008) Analgesic requirements after major abdominal surgery are associated with *OPRM1* gene polymorphism genotype and haplotype. Pharmacogenomics 9:1605–1616
8. Fukuda K, Hayashida M, Ide S, Saita N, Kokita Y, Kasai S, Nishizawa D, Ogai Y, Hasegawa J, Nagashima M, Tagami M, Komatsu H, Sora I, Koga H, Kaneko Y, Ikeda K (2009) Association between *OPRM1* gene polymorphisms and fentanyl sensitivity in patients undergoing painful cosmetic surgery. Pain 147:194–201
9. Dripps RD (1963) New classification of physical status. Anesthesiology 24:111
10. Vinik HR, Kissin I (1998) Rapid development of tolerance to analgesia during remifentanil infusion in humans. Anesth Analg 86: 1307–1311
11. Wu CL (2005) Acute postoperative pain. In: Miller RD (ed) Miller's anesthesia, 6th edn. Elsevier/Churchill-Livingstone, Philadelphia, pp 2729–2762
12. Shi MM, Bleavins MR, de la Iglesia FA (1999) Technologies for detecting genetic polymorphisms in pharmacogenomics. Mol Diagn 4:343–351
13. Syvänen AC (2001) Accessing genetic variation: genotyping single nucleotide polymorphisms. Nat Rev Genet 2:930–942
14. Shi MM (2001) Enabling large-scale pharmacogenetic studies by high-throughput mutation detection and genotyping technologies. Clin Chem 47:164–172
15. Chen X, Sullivan PF (2003) Single nucleotide polymorphism genotyping: biochemistry, protocol, cost and throughput. Pharmacogenomics J 3:77–96
16. Jannetto PJ, Laleli-Sahin E, Wong SH (2004) Pharmacogenomic genotyping methodologies. Clin Chem Lab Med 42:1256–1264
17. Nishizawa D, Nagashima M, Katoh R, Satoh Y, Tagami M, Kasai S, Ogai Y, Han W, Hasegawa J, Shimoyama N, Sora I, Hayashida M, Ikeda K (2009) Association between *KCNJ6* (*GIRK2*) gene polymorphisms and postoperative analgesic requirements after major abdominal surgery. PLoS ONE 4:e7060
18. Germer S, Higuchi R (1999) Single-tube genotyping without oligonucleotide probes. Genome Res 9:72–78
19. Myakishev MV, Khripin Y, Hu S, Hamer DH (2001) High-throughput SNP genotyping by allele-specific PCR with universal energy-transfer-labeled primers. Genome Res 11:163–169
20. Nishizawa D, Han W, Hasegawa J, Ishida T, Numata Y, Sato T, Kawai A, Ikeda K (2006) Association of μ-opioid receptor gene polymorphism A118G with alcohol dependence in a Japanese population. Neuropsychobiology 53:137–141
21. Livak KJ, Flood SJ, Marmaro J, Giusti W, Deetz K (1995) Oligonucleotides with fluores-

cent dyes at opposite ends provide a quenched probe system useful for detecting PCR product and nucleic acid hybridization. PCR Methods Appl 4:357–362

22. Imai K, Ogai Y, Nishizawa D, Kasai S, Ikeda K, Koga H (2007) A novel SNP detection technique utilizing a multiple primer extension (MPEX) on a phospholipid polymer-coated surface. Mol Biosyst 3:547–553
23. Ide S, Kobayashi H, Ujike H, Ozaki N, Sekine Y, Inada T, Harano M, Komiyama T, Yamada M, Iyo M, Iwata N, Tanaka K, Shen H, Iwahashi K, Itokawa M, Minami M, Satoh M, Ikeda K, Sora I (2006) Linkage disequilibrium and association with methamphetamine dependence/psychosis of μ-opioid receptor gene polymorphisms. Pharmacogenomics J 6:179–188
24. Balding DJ (2006) A tutorial on statistical methods for population association studies. Nat Rev Genet 7:781–791
25. Carlson CS, Eberle MA, Rieder MJ, Yi Q, Kruglyak L, Nickerson DA (2004) Selecting a maximally informative set of single-nucleotide polymorphisms for association analyses using linkage disequilibrium. Am J Hum Genet 74:106–120
26. Nyholt DR (2001) Genetic case–control association studies: correcting for multiple testing. Hum Genet 109:564–567
27. Perneger TV (1998) What's wrong with Bonferroni adjustments. BMJ 316:1236–1238
28. Curtis D, Xu K (2007) Minor differences in haplotype frequency estimates can produce very large differences in heterogeneity test statistics. BMC Genet 8:38
29. Mooney S (2005) Bioinformatics approaches and resources for single nucleotide polymorphism functional analysis. Brief Bioinform 6:44–56
30. Smigielski EM, Sirotkin K, Ward M, Sherry ST (2000) dbSNP: a database of single nucleotide polymorphisms. Nucleic Acids Res 28: 352–355
31. Fredman D, Siegfried M, Yuan YP, Bork P, Lehväslaiho H, Brookes AJ (2002) HGVbase: a human sequence variation database emphasizing data quality and a broad spectrum of data sources. Nucleic Acids Res 30:387–391
32. International HapMap Consortium (2005) A haplotype map of the human genome. Nature 437:1299–1320
33. Raymond M, Rousset F (1995) GENEPOP (version 1.2): population genetics software for exact tests and ecumenicism. *J.* Heredity 86:248–249
34. Stephens M, Smith NJ, Donnelly P (2001) A new statistical method for haplotype reconstruction from population data. Am J Hum Genet 68:978–989
35. Barrett JC, Fry B, Maller J, Daly MJ (2005) Haploview: analysis and visualization of LD and haplotype maps. Bioinformatics 21: 263–265
36. Abecasis GR, Cookson WO (2000) GOLD: graphical overview of linkage disequilibrium. Bioinformatics 16:182–183
37. Niu T, Qin ZS, Xu X, Liu JS (2002) Bayesian haplotype inference for multiple linked single-nucleotide polymorphisms. Am J Hum Genet 70:157–169
38. de Bakker PI, Yelensky R, Pe'er I, Gabriel SB, Daly MJ, Altshuler D (2005) Efficiency and power in genetic association studies. Nat Genet 37:1217–1223
39. Zhang K, Jin L (2003) HaploBlockFinder: haplotype block analyses. Bioinformatics 19: 1300–1301
40. Zhao JH, Lissarrague S, Essioux L, Sham PC (2002) GENECOUNTING: haplotype analysis with missing genotypes. Bioinformatics 18: 1694–1695
41. Zhang K, Qin Z, Chen T, Liu JS, Waterman MS, Sun F (2005) HapBlock: haplotype block partitioning and tag SNP selection software using a set of dynamic programming algorithms. Bioinformatics 21:131–134
42. Greenspan G, Geiger D (2004) High density linkage disequilibrium mapping using models of haplotype block variation. Bioinformatics 20(Suppl 1):i137–i144
43. Shimo-onoda K, Tanaka T, Furushima K, Nakajima T, Toh S, Harata S, Yone K, Komiya S, Adachi H, Nakamura E, Fujimiya H, Inoue I (2002) Akaike's information criterion for a measure of linkage disequilibrium. J Hum Genet 47:649–655
44. Zhao JH, Curtis D, Sham PC (2000) Model-free analysis and permutation tests for allelic associations. Hum Hered 50:133–139
45. Excoffier L, Laval G, Schneider S (2005) Arlequin ver. 3.0: an integrated software package for population genetics data analysis. Evol Bioinform Online 1:47–50
46. Zaykin DV, Westfall PH, Young SS, Karnoub MA, Wagner MJ, Ehm MG (2002) Testing association of statistically inferred haplotypes with discrete and continuous traits in samples of unrelated individuals. Hum Hered 53:79–91
47. Guo SW, Thompson EA (1992) Performing the exact test of Hardy–Weinberg proportion for multiple alleles. Biometrics 48:361–372
48. Schaid DJ, Rowland CM, Tines DE, Jacobson RM, Poland GA (2002) Score tests

for association between traits and haplotypes when linkage phase is ambiguous. Am J Hum Genet 70:425–434

49. Dudbridge F (2003) Pedigree disequilibrium tests for multilocus haplotypes. Genet Epidemiol 25:115–121

50. Purcell S, Cherny SS, Sham PC (2003) Genetic Power Calculator: design of linkage and association genetic mapping studies of complex traits. Bioinformatics 19:149–150

51. Epstein MP, Satten GA (2003) Inference on haplotype effects in case–control studies using unphased genotype data. Am J Hum Genet 73:1316–1329

52. Gordon D, Finch SJ, Nothnagel M, Ott J (2002) Power and sample size calculations for case–control genetic association tests when errors are present: application to single nucleotide polymorphisms. Hum Hered 54:22–33

53. Gauderman WJ (2002) Sample size requirements for matched case–control studies of gene-environment interaction. Stat Med 21:35–50

54. Zhao LP, Li SS, Khalid N (2003) A method for the assessment of disease associations with single-nucleotide polymorphism haplotypes and environmental variables in case–control studies. Am J Hum Genet 72:1231–1250

55. Purcell S, Neale B, Todd-Brown K, Thomas L, Ferreira MA, Bender D, Maller J, Sklar P, de Bakker PI, Daly MJ, Sham PC (2007) PLINK: a tool set for whole-genome association and population-based linkage analyses. Am J Hum Genet 81:559–575

Chapter 30

Molecular Assays for Characterization of Alternatively Spliced Isoforms of the Mu Opioid Receptor (MOR)

Pavel Gris, Philip Cheng, John Pierson, William Maixner, and Luda Diatchenko

Abstract

Mu-opioid receptor (MOR) belongs to a family of heptahelical G-protein-coupled receptors (GPCRs). Studies in humans and rodents demonstrated that the *OPRM1* gene coding for MOR undergoes extensive alternative splicing afforded by the genetic complexity of *OPRM1*. Evidence from rodent studies also demonstrates an important role of these alternatively spliced forms in mediating opiate analgesia via their differential signaling properties. MOR signaling is predominantly $G_{i\alpha}$ coupled. Release of the α subunit from G-protein complex results in the inhibition of adenylyl cyclase/cAMP pathway, whereas release of the βγ subunits activates G-protein-activated inwardly rectifying potassium channels and inhibits voltage-dependent calcium channels. These molecular events result in the suppression of cellular activities that diminish pain sensations. Recently, a new isoform of *OPRM1*, MOR3, has been identified that shows an increase in the production of nitric oxide (NO) upon stimulation with morphine. Hence, there is a need to describe molecular techniques that enable the functional characterization of MOR isoforms. In this review, we describe the methodologies used to assay key mediators of MOR activation including cellular assays for cAMP, free Ca^{2+}, and NO, all of which have been implicated in the pharmacological effects of MOR agonists.

Key words: Alternative splicing, OPRM1, Opioid, Calcium, cAMP, Nitric oxide, Fluo-4, Fluo-3, GPCR, FSK, Capsaicin

1. Introduction

The major form of *OPRM1*, called MOR-1, is coded by exons 1, 2, 3, and 4 (1). Exon 1 codes for first transmembrane domain (TMH1) and exons 2 and 3 code for the TMH2 through TMH7. However, many 5′- end and 3′-end alternatively spliced forms of *OPRM1* have also been cloned (2). A common splicing pattern among the 3′-end alternatively spliced forms involves the alternative

Arpad Szallasi (ed.), *Analgesia: Methods and Protocols*, Methods in Molecular Biology, vol. 617, DOI 10.1007/978-1-60327-323-7_30, © Springer Science+Business Media, LLC 2010

C-terminus, coded by various exons, while all seven transmembrane domains that form the binding pocket are coded by exons 1, 2, and 3, stay intact. The structural difference at the C-terminus has been proposed to drive differential cellular signaling in response to receptor activation (1–5). Alternative splicing at the 5′-end results either in an alternative TMH1 domain (via alternative exon 11) or in isoforms that start from exon 2 (6, 7), which lack an amino acid sequence of approximately 90 amino acids (N-terminus, TMH1 and part of the first intracellular loop) (8) but retain the ligand binding pocket distributed across the conserved TMH2, TMH3, and TMH7 domains.

The binding of an agonist to MORs usually results in the inhibition of cellular activity; however, there is a growing body of research demonstrating excitatory events downstream to MOR receptor stimulation (9, 10). Both cell culture and animal experiments suggest that opioid-induced analgesia is a consequence of inhibitory cellular effects resulting from the binding of μ-opioid agonists to MOR (11). Since MOR is predominately coupled to G_i, the resulting molecular cascade leads to decreased levels of cAMP (12) and intracellular calcium (13–15) with a resulting inhibition of neuronal activity. The analgesic effect of MOR activation has also been attributed to the release of the $G_{\beta\gamma}$ dimer from $G_{i/o}$, which activates inwardly rectifying potassium (GIRK) channels (16) and inhibits voltage-dependent calcium channels (VDCCs) (17). The resulting hyperpolarization suppresses neuronal activity. Adenylyl cyclase inhibition may also contribute to opioid analgesia, since its activation has been suggested to elicit analgesic tolerance or tolerance-associated hyperalgesia (18, 19).

Conversely, the pronociceptive effects of μ-opioid agonists are associated with excitatory cellular events: increase in levels of cAMP (20) and intracellular Ca^{2+} (21). Excitatory cellular events have been implicated in molecular mechanism of opioid receptor-mediated hyperalgesia, tolerance, and dependence (22). Both extremely low and extremely high doses of morphine, as well as chronic administration of opioids, can elicit a hyperalgesia in both human clinical and animal models of pain (22–24). A dual effect of opioids on cAMP and Ca^{2+} levels in vitro has been corroborated by Rubovitvh and coworkers (9). It has been proposed that a switch in the G-protein coupling profile of the OPRM1 from G_i to both G_s and G_q as well as adenylyl cyclase (AC) activation by $G_{\beta\gamma}$ explains the phenomenon of opioid induced excitation (9, 25, 26). It has also been established that the activation of cAMP and cGMP cascades through Ca^{2+}-dependent activation of nitric oxide synthase leads to activation of protein kinases A (PKA) and G (PKG) and establishment of a pronociceptive phenotype (27). The increased influx of Ca^{2+} leads to activation of nitric oxide synthase through Ca-calmodulin dependent mechanism resulting in increased production of NO (28). In turn, increased levels of

NO stimulate guanylyl cyclase, leading to the production of cGMP, activation of PKG, and establishment of a pro-nociceptive phenotype (28). In agreement with this, the newly cloned human 5′-end alternatively spliced isoform of MOR-3 that codes for six transmembrane variant rather than the classic seven transmembrane variant, exhibited a dose-dependent release of NO following treatment with morphine (8). The effect was abrogated by administration of naloxone (8).

The present report reviews techniques used to assay the levels of cAMP, Ca^{2+}, and released NO produced by μ-opioid receptor agonists in in vitro cellular assays designed to characterize the functional properties of alternatively-spliced isoforms of MOR.

2. Materials

2.1. Measurement of cAMP Levels in Forskolin (FSK) Stimulated Cells

1. Geneticin and hygromycin (Invitrogen, Carlsbad, CA).
2. Lipofectamine 2000 (Invitrogen).
3. 2-(2-(Bis(carboxymethyl)amino)ethyl-(carboxymethyl) amino)acetic acid (EDTA).
4. Trypsin (Gibco/BRL, Bethesda, MD).
5. Capsaicin (Sigma St. Louis, MO) is dissolved in 100% ethanol to make 10,000× (3 mM) stock solution. Toxic if inhaled, irritant. Store at 4°C. If stock solution is made, store at 4°C as well. Stock solution is stable indefinitely.
6. IBMX3-Isobutyl-1-methyl-xanthine (Sigma).
7. 7β-Acetoxy-8,13-epoxy-1α,6β,9α-trihydroxylabd-14-en-11-one (Forskolin) (Sigma).
8. Cyclic AMP EIA Kit (Cayman Chemicals Ann Arbor, MI).

2.2. Measurement of cAMP Levels in PGE2 Stimulated Cells

1. Hanks' balanced salt solution (HBSS, pH 7.3 at 4°C): 17 mM NaCl, 6 mM KCl, 1.6 mM NaHPO, 0.5 mM KHPO, 6 mM D-glucose, and 0.01% phenol red.
2. Collagenase (Sigma).
3. Tripsin (Gibco).
4. Dulbecco's Modified Eagle's Medium (DMEM) (Gibco/BRL).
5. Nerve growth factor (NGF) (Harlan, Indianapolis, IN).
6. Fetal bovine serum (FBS) (Gibco/BRL).
7. Penicillin–Streptomycin (PenStrep) 50–100 U of penicillin, 50–100 μg of streptomycin (Gibco/BRL).
8. Ellman's reagent (5,5′-dithiobis-(2-nitrobenzoic acid), DTNB) (Thermo Scientific, Rockford, IL).

9. Uridine 5′-diphosphate disodium salt hydrate.
10. 5-fluoro-2′-deoxyuridine.
11. 4-(3-cyclopentyloxy-4-methoxy-phenyl)pyrrolidin-2-one Rolipram (Peninsula Laboratories, Torrance, CA).
12. (d-Ala^2,*N*-MePhe^4,Gly-ol^5) enkephalin (DAMGO) (Peninsula Laboratories).
13. Morphine sulfate is dissolved in ddH2O to make 1,000× (1 mM) stock solution. Store at 4°C.
14. Naloxone hydrochloride dehydrate.
15. Prostaglandin E2 (PGE_2) (Cayman Chemicals).

2.3. Microplate Reader Measurement of Intracellular Ca^{2+} (Flou-3)

1. Capsaicin (Sigma).
2. IBMX3-Isobutyl-1-methyl-xanthine (Sigma).
3. NOVOstar fluorescence microplate reader (BMG Offenburg, Germany).
4. Morphine sulfate.
5. Fluo-3 AM (Sigma).
6. PSS buffer (pH 7.4): 5.9 mM KCl, 1.5 mM $MgCl_2$, 1.2 mM NaH_2PO_4, 5 mM $NaHCO_3$, 140 mM NaCl, 11.5 mM glucose, 1.8 mM $CaCl_2$, and 10 mM HEPES.

2.4. Microplate Reader Measurement of Intracellular Ca^{2+} (Fluo-4)

1. Fluo-4 NW Calcium Assay Starter Kit (Invitrogen). Store and desiccate contents (assay buffer, probenecid, Fluo-4 NW dye mix) at −20°C. Protect contents from light.
2. Microplate reader Wallac1420 Victor3 (PerkinElmer Waltham, MA) with 500 nm excitation and 515 nm emission filters.

2.5. Measurement of Nitric Oxide Release from Transfected Cells

1. Clonfectin Transfection Kit (Clontech Palo Alto, CA).
2. Multilineage progenitor cells (MLPC) (St. Paul, MN).
3. Puromycin (Sigma).
4. Fetal Bovine Serum.
5. 96 well plates (Falcon San Jose, CA).
6. DMEM (Invitrogen).
7. Micromanipulator (World Precision Instruments Sarasota, FL).
8. *S*-nitroso-*N*-acetyl-D,L-penicillamine (World Precision Instruments).
9. NO-specific amperometric probe (30 μm, 0.5 mm; World Precision Instruments).
10. Inverted microscope (Diaphot Nikon, Tokyo, Japan).
11. 4-channel ESA BioStat with an NO-selective amperometric 600 μm nanoprobe (Innovative Instruments).

3. Methods

Signaling through GPCRs can lead to a variety of cellular responses via changing intracellular levels of second messengers and gene transcription (reviewed by (29)). Activation of MOR that is coupled to G_i inhibits adenylate cyclase (30), decreasing the production of cAMP (31). Due to variable levels of cAMP in cultured cells, the activity of GPCRs coupled to G_i is assayed in cells with artificially elevated cAMP levels. The levels of cAMP are usually stimulated by either PGE2 of FSK. A mu-opioid receptor agonist is then administered at varying concentrations. The extent of decrease in cAMP levels indicates the efficacy of receptor–ligand interaction.

To determine the optimal concentration of the mu-opioid agonist (see Note 1), it is often necessary to asses its effect across a range of the doses. This is especially true when characterizing a newly identified receptor isoform or working with variable tissues and cell types. An in-depth discussion of the construction of concentration curves is beyond the scope of the present paper as excellent reviews on this topic already exist (32). A simple way to prepare a dose response curve for morphine to assay cAMP levels in vitro is provided (see Note 2).

As activation of the opioid receptors decreases Ca^{2+} uptake (36, 37) and inhibits voltage-dependent calcium channels (13), measuring intracellular Ca^{2+} levels is an important assay for characterizing MOR signaling. Fluorescent Ca^{2+} detection was developed in the late eighties (33). This approach allows for optical detection and quantification analysis of intracellular calcium levels. Due to the inhibitory nature of GPCRs coupled to G_i, Ca^{2+} levels are assayed in cells with artificially (capsaicin) elevated Ca^{2+} levels (13, 34, 35). Since not all cell types express capsaicin receptor TRPV1, the cells are transfected with TRPV1 expressing construct. In the experiment described below, the HEK293 cells that do not express either MOR or TRPV1 are transfected with these receptors prior to the experiments.

Mu-opioids signaling also involves production and release of NO via Ca^{2+}-stimulated activation of constitutive nitric oxide synthase that has been specifically linked to MOR-3 isoform of *OPRM1*. (8) The following technique developed to rapidly evaluate MOR agonist NO stimulating activity in vitro.

3.1. Stimulation of cAMP by FSK

1. Human embryonic kidney cells (*HEK293*) are transfected with full-length MOR expression construct in pcDNA3 tagged with FLAG using Lipofectamine 2000 (Invitrogen) according to the manufacturer's protocol, and stable FLAG-MOR expressants are selected with 0.5 mg/ml geneticin (see Note 3).

2. Colonies originating from a single cell are selected and FLAG-MOR expression is verified by Western Blotting.
3. Stable FLAG-MOR expressants are split every 4–6 days using trypsin/EDTA and maintained at 37°C in a 5% humidified CO_2 incubator in DMEM medium containing 10% heat-inactivated fetal bovine serum (FBS), 2 mM l-glutamine, and 110 mg pyridoxine.
4. For the cAMP accumulation assay, FLAG-MOR expressants are plated on 12 well plates and grown to 90% confluency.
5. Twenty-four hours prior to sample preparation, media are changed to DMEM supplemented with 0.5% heat-inactivated FBS.
6. On the day of sample preparation, cells are washed with DMEM to remove serum and incubated with serum-free DMEM containing the phosphodiesterase inhibitor IBMX (100 μM) for 30 min, mu-opioid agonist (see Note 1) is then added and cells incubated for a further 15 min.
7. Following this, FSK (50 μM) is added to the wells and the cells are incubated for 15 min to stimulate cAMP production. DMSO alone is used as a vehicle control.
8. After incubation, reactions are terminated by aspiration of the medium and addition of 0.1 M HCl followed by 20 min incubation at room temperature. After centrifugation of the cell samples at 10,000×*g* for 10 min, the protein content of the supernatant is assessed and the samples are diluted to protein concentrations of 20 μg/ml using *e*nzyme *i*mmuno*a*ssay (EIA) buffer supplied with the cAMP EIA kit.
9. 100 μl of EIA Buffer is added to Nonspecific Binding wells, and 50 μl to Maximum Binding wells.
10. 50 μl from the tubes containing cAMP standard is added into the wells allocated for the 8 point standard curve. Two aliquots of 50 μl each should be taken from each tube, as the standard is being run in duplicate.
11. 50 μl of sample is added per well. Each sample is assayed in at a minimum of two dilutions. Each dilution is assayed in duplicate or triplicate.
12. 50 μl of cAMP Tracer is placed into to each well except the Total Activity and Blank wells.
13. 50 μl of rabbit anti-AMP antibody is added to each well except the Total Activity, Non-specific Binding, and Blank wells.
14. The plate is incubated for 18 h at 4°C after covering each plate with a plastic film.
15. The wells are rinsed five times with Wash Buffer.
16. 200 μl of Ellman's Reagent is added to each well.

17. 5 μl of tracer is added to the Total Activity wells.
18. The plate is covered with plastic film and placed on orbital shaker in the dark. Allow the plate to develop for 90–120 min.
19. Intracellular cAMP levels are measured with a competitive cAMP EIA kit in triplicate. An example result is shown in Fig. 1 (13).

3.2. Stimulation of cAMP Levels by PGE2

1. Fresh trigeminal ganglion neurons (TG) are washed with HBSS (Ca^{2+}, Mg^{2+} free), digested with 3 mg/ml collagenase for 30 min at 37°C and centrifuged to pellet cells/tissue as described by Vasko and coworkers (36).
2. The pellet is resuspended following further digestion with 0.1% trypsin (15 min) and 167 μg/ml DNase (10 min) at 37°C in the same solution.
3. Cells are pelleted by centrifugation (5 min at 5000×*g*) and resuspended in DMEM (high glucose) containing 250 ng/ml NGF, 10% FBS, 1× Pen/Strep, 1× l-glutamine and the mitotic inhibitors: 7.5 μg/ml uridine and 17.5 μg/ml 5-fluoro-2′-deoxyuridine.

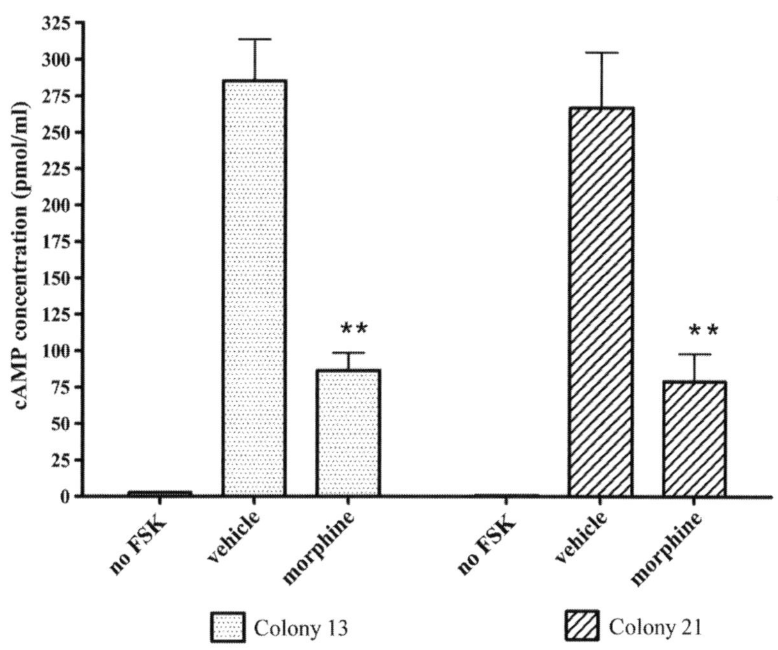

Fig. 1. Inhibition of FSK-stimulated cAMP accumulation by morphine (1 μM). cAMP levels in FLAG-MOP stable colonies were measured using an enzyme-immunoassay kit either in unstimulated cells (no FSK), or in cells treated with FSK (50 μM) and IBMX (100 μM). Morphine (1 μM) significantly reduced cAMP levels in FSK-stimulated cells (morphine) compared to stimulated cells treated with water (vehicle). Morphine inhibited cAMP production by 67.0 ± 4.6% for FLAG-MOP/TRPV1 colony 13 (dotted bars) and 79.2 ± 7.4% for colony 21 (cross-hatched bars). Data are presented as mean ± SEM from $n = 3$ samples read in triplicate. **$p < 0.01$ compared to vehicle. (Vetter et al. Molecular Pain 2006 2:22)

4. After triturating to disrupt tissue, the cell suspension is seeded on poly-d-lysine-coated 0.17 mm glass inserts in 24-well plates or polylysine-coated 48-well plates (3 TG per plate).
5. Media are changed at 24 h and then every 48 h after plating. Cells are used after 5 or 6 days in culture and serum and NGF are removed from the media 24 h before experimentation.
6. TG cultures are washed twice with HBSS containing 10 mM Hepes and 4 mM sodium bicarbonate, pH 7.4 wash buffer.
7. Cells are preequilibrated in 250–500 μl wash buffer per well of 48 well plate for 30 min at 37°C in 5% CO_2. Where indicated, inhibitors are added during the preequilibration period.
8. To determine MOR-mediated effects, cells are incubated with the phosphodiesterase inhibitor, rolipram (10 μM), along with mu-opioid agonist (see Note 1) for15 min at 37°C.
9. PGE_2 (1 μM) is added, followed by incubation for a further 15 min.
10. Incubations are terminated by aspiration of the wash buffer and addition of 500 μl ice cold absolute ethanol.
11. The ethanol extracts from individual wells are dried under a gentle air stream and reconstituted in 100 μl of 50 mM sodium acetate, pH 6.2.
12. The cAMP content of each 100 μl sample is determined by radioactive immune assay RIA or EIA. (37, 38)

3.3. Measuring of Intracellular Ca^{2+} Levels with Fluo-3

1. FLAG-MOR/TRPV1 expressants are plated on poly-D-lysine -coated 96-well plates at a cell density of approximately $3–4 \times 10^5$ cells/ml 3–5 days prior to experiments and used at 70–90% confluency (see Note 4).
2. Cells are loaded with Fluo-3 AM (6 μM) in loading buffer (pH 7.4, composition as PSS plus 3 mg/ml bovine serum albumin (BSA)) for 20–30 min at 37°C.
3. Wells containing FLAG-MOR/TRPV1 double expressants are then washed three times with PSS buffer and incubated for 15 min with PSS or mu-opioid agonist followed by 15 min of incubation with PSS or kinas activators with mu-opioid agonist as appropriate.
4. Preincubation steps and Ca^{2+} imaging are carried out at 29°C in order to avoid subcellular dye compartmentalization while maintaining constant experimental conditions.
5. Fluo-3 loaded cells are excited at 420 nm and emission is recorded at 510 nm using a NOVOstar fluorescence microplate reader.
6. Fluorescent emission readings are recorded every 0.5 s. Raw fluorescence data are normalized by subtracting the average

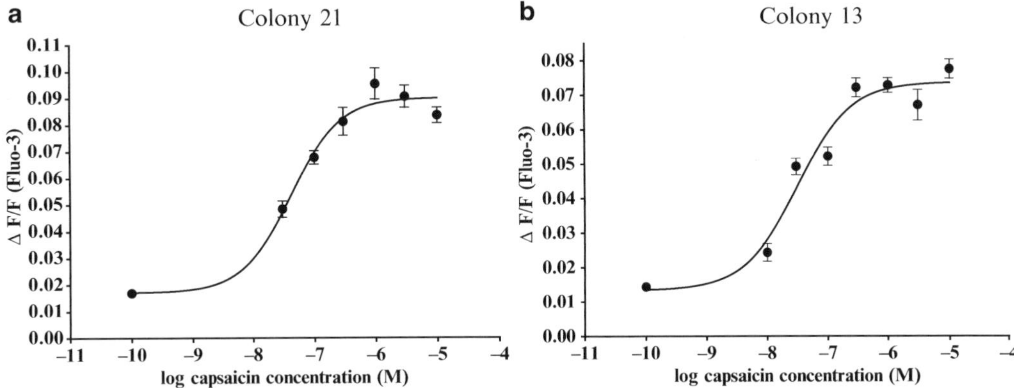

Fig. 2. Capsaicin dose-response curves from two independent FLAG-MOP/TRPV1 expressants. Ca2+ responses of Fluo-3-loaded cells to injection of capsaicin were measured using a fluorescent Microplate reader and maximum change in fluorescence, expressed as ΔF/F, was plotted as a function of capsaicin concentration. A 4-parameter Hill function was fitted to the data using GraphPad Prism. (**a**) Capsaicin dose-response from FLAG-MOP/TRPV1 double expressant colony 13. (**b**) Capsaicin dose–response from FLAG-MOP/TRPV1 double expressant colony 21. (Data are expressed as mean ± SEM with *n* = 8.) Vetter et al. Molecular Pain 2006 2:22

fluorescence from 4 recordings just prior to addition of agonist from all subsequent time points. The data are analyzed using a 4-parameter logistic Hill equation (see Note 8) and plotted using GraphPad Prism. An example result is shown in Fig. 2 (13).

3.4. Microplate Reader Measurement of Intracellular Ca^{2+} with Fluo-4 Reagent

1. BE2C human neuroblastoma cells are grown to near confluence in black 96-well poly-d-lysine coated plates. The cell cultures are grown in DMEM/F12 media (see Note 3).
2. The indicator Fluo-4 NW dye is prepared as outlined in manufacturer instructions (see Notes 4 and 5).
3. Cell culture medium is removed from all wells except three, which will serve as controls, 100 μL of capsaicin then is added to the wells (see Note 5)
4. After 20 s the treatments are removed from all wells as well as the DMEM/F12 medium from the control wells (see Note 6).
5. Quickly, but carefully, 100 μL of Fluo-4 NW dye is added to each well.
6. The plate is then incubated with the lid on at 37°C for 30 min, then at room temperature for an additional 30 min (see Note 6).
7. The fluorescence is measured using a microplate reader with settings for emission at 515 nm and excitation at 500 nm (see Notes 7 and 9). An example result is shown in Fig. 3.

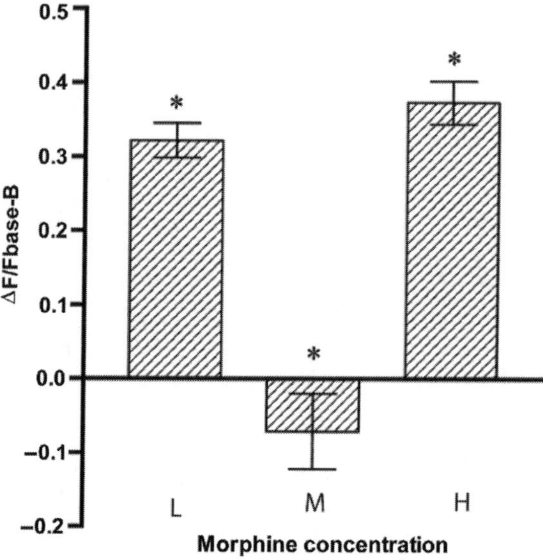

Fig. 3. Effect of the different doses of morphine on the Ca^{2+} levels in BE(2)C cells. The low doses (L) of morphine (10^{-3} μM) and high (H) doses (10^{2} μM) result in increase in Ca^{2+} levels in BE2C cells. The 1 μM dose (M) of morphine caused a small decrease in Ca^{2+} levels. Data are presented as mean ± SEM from $n=8$ $*p<0.01$ compared to vehicle

3.5. Measuring of NO Production

1. COS-1 cells are stably transfected (see Note 2) with an expression vector (see Note 10) with cloned MOR-3 cDNA using the Clonfectin Transfection Kit.
2. Stable cell lines are selected with puromycin at a concentration of 7.5 μg/ml. The stable transfectants are grown in DMEM supplemented with 10% FBS at 37°C and then screened by RT-PCR for the MOR-3 opiate receptor variant transcript. The cells are subsequently used for functional analysis. For NO determination, 2.5×10^5 of COS1 cells are placed in each well of a 96-well plate and allowed to adhere overnight in 200 μl of DMEM supplemented with 2% FBS.
3. Before NO determination, the medium is removed and replaced with 200 μl of PBS solution. Transfected COS-1 cells as well as nontransfected cells are plated and tested (see Fig. 4).
4. NO release from the transfected and untransfected cell lines is directly measured using an NO-specific amperometric probe.
5. A micromanipulator, which is attached to the stage of an inverted microscope, is used to position the amperometric probe 15 μm above the cells (see Note 11).

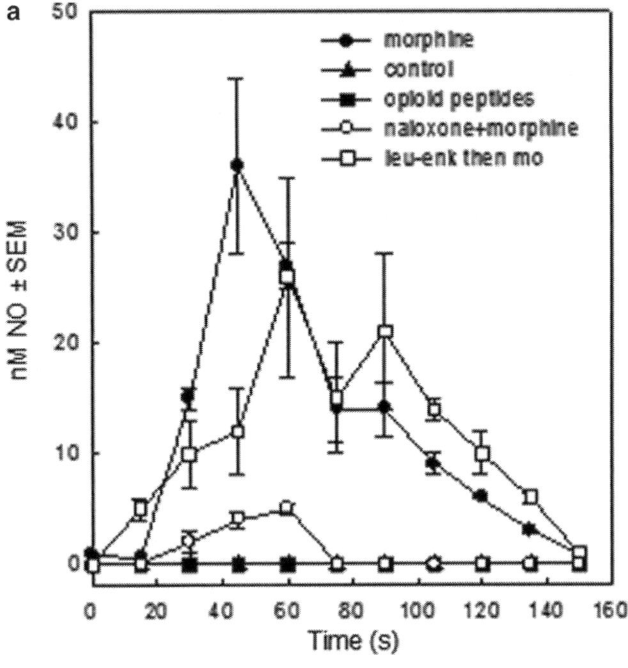

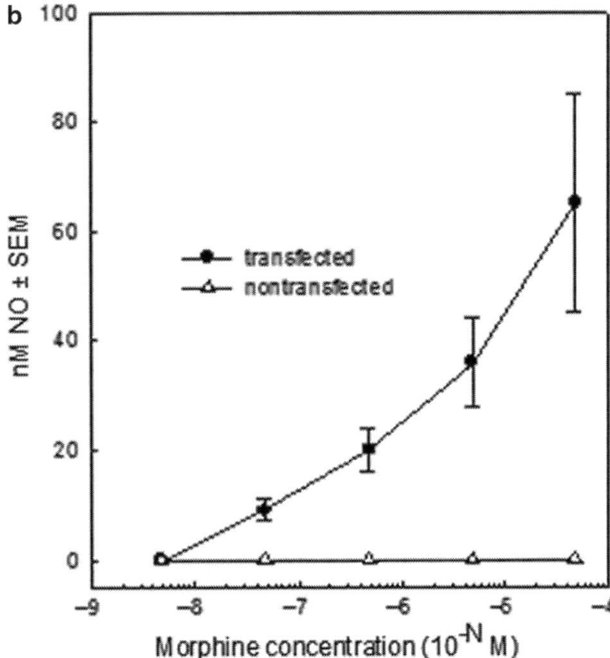

Fig. 4. (**a**) Real-time NO production measurements in μ3-transfected COS-1 cells after addition of the opiate alkaloid, morphine, or the opioid peptides, Met- and Leu-enkephalin. The control represents the addition of PBS to the cells. Each experiment was replicated four times ± SEM. (**b**), Peak concentration-dependent morphine-stimulated NO release from COS-1 cells and μ3-transfected COS-1 cells. Each experiment was replicated four times; results shown are the mean ± SEM. (Copyright 2003 The American Association of Immunologists, Inc.)

6. The amperometric probe is allowed to equilibrate for at least 10 min before being transferred to the well containing the cells.
7. Morphine-stimulated NO release is evaluated in response to increasing morphine concentrations, such as in the range of 10^{-5}–10^{-9} M (see Note 1). Each experiment is repeated four times along with a control (cells transfected with vector alone).
8. Real-time release of NO from multilineage progenitor cells (MLPC) is quantified using a 4-channel ESA BioStat with an NO-selective amperometric 600 μm nanoprobe (see Note 14). MLPCs are used in this assay because they demonstrate high endogenous level of MOR-3 activity (39).
9. The amperometric probe is allowed to equilibrate for at least 10 min before being transferred to the well containing the cells.
10. Baseline levels of NO release are determined by evaluation of real-time NO concentration in PBS. Evoked release of NO from MLPC is evaluated at final concentrations of 10^{-5} M to 10^{-7} M morphine (see Note 13). Using μ opioid receptor antagonist to confirm specificity of agonist binding is recommended (see Note 12) (39).

4. Notes

1. Mu-opioid agonists, such as morphine or DAMGO (d-Ala[2], *N*-MePhe[4],Gly-ol[5]) enkephalin should be used to test for dose-dependent responses. Importantly, MOR isoforms demonstrate a range of both specificity and selectivity towards different mu-opioid agonists. For instance, MOR-3 was shown to be insensitive to opioid peptides (8, 39).
2. A simple way to prepare a dose response curve for morphine to assay cAMP levels in vitro is presented here as an example. Initially, 100 μL of a 1,000× stock solution of agonist (1 mM morphine) is added to a test tube containing 900 μL of cell culture media. The resulting 100 μM preparation is vortexed for 15 s to ensure complete mixing. 100 μL of the 100 μM solution is pipetted into another test tube containing 900 μL of media. Repetition of this step yields a serial dilution of the ligand.

   To demonstrate the receptor specificity of agonist-stimulation, one arm of the experimental protocol should include pretreatment of the cell culture with a selective mu-receptor antagonist such as naloxone.

3. Transient transfection can also be used.
4. Black 96-well plates are used because the fluorescence measurements made by the microplate reader are taken from the top of the wells, and if the plates are not black, they will reflect light and ruin the measurements.
5. It is best to add the capsaicin as quickly, but carefully, as possible as the exposure time of the cells to capsaicin should only be 20–45 s. Be ready to remove the capsaicin from the wells as soon as the 20 s has passed.
6. It is important to remove as much of the medium as possible to eliminate sources of background fluorescence.
7. It is assumed that fluorescence measurements will be done at room temperature. If you plan on doing fluorescence measurements at 37°C, you only need to incubate the plate for 30–45 min at 37°C before taking fluorescence measurements.
8. A 488 nm argon laser line works as well as the microplate reader if you want to use that instead.
9. $\frac{\Delta F}{F} = \frac{(F - F_{\text{base}})}{(F_{\text{base}} - B)}$ Where F is the measured fluorescence of the samples exposed to capsaicin F_{base} is the measured fluorescence of the controls, and B is the background signal. The ratio
   $\frac{\Delta F}{F}$ is thought to approximately reflect calcium concentration levels if there is no change in dye concentration, intracellular environment, or path length (40).
10. The optimal concentration of capsaicin to use will fall within the linear range of the drug–response curve. We found that range to be approximately 100–500 nM, and settled on 300 nM as an optimal concentration (7).
11. The authors used vector pExP1 (Clontech, Palo Alto, CA).
12. The well-established NO donor *S*-nitroso-*N*-acetyl-dl-penicillamine is used to calibrate the system daily.
13. The authors used naloxone or d-Phe-Cys-Tyr-Trp-Orn-Thr-Pen-Thr-NH_2) at 10^{-7} M. Other antagonists (naltrexone) can also be used.
14. Although different opioid agonists can be used in these types of experiments, it is important to bear in mind that not all MOR isoforms are equally responsive to opioid peptides. For instance, MOR-3 (μ-3 as it is named by the group that reported it) was shown to be insensitive to opioid peptides (8, 39).

References

1. Pasternak GW (2004) Multiple opiate receptors: deja vu all over again. Neuropharmacology 47(Suppl. 1):312–323
2. Pan YX et al (2003) Identification and characterization of two new human mu opioid receptor splice variants, hMOR-1O and hMOR-1X. Biochem Biophys Res Commun 301(4):1057–1061
3. Pasternak DA et al (2004) Identification of three new alternatively spliced variants of the rat mu opioid receptor gene: dissociation of affinity and efficacy. J Neurochem 91(4):881–890
4. Pan YX et al (2005) Identification of four novel exon 5 splice variants of the mouse mu-opioid receptor gene: functional consequences of C-terminal splicing. Mol Pharmacol 68(3):866–875
5. Pan L et al (2005) Identification and characterization of six new alternatively spliced variants of the human mu opioid receptor gene, *Oprm*. Neuroscience 133(1):209–220
6. Shabalina SA et al (2008) Expansion of the human {micro}-opioid receptor gene architecture: novel functional variants. Hum Mol Genet. 2009 Mar 15;18(6):1037–51
7. Gris P, Cheng P, Pierson J, Gauthier J, Shabalina S, Spiridonov N, Maixner W, Diatchenko L (2008) Functional characterization of the novel alternatively spliced form of mu-opioid receptor *OPRM1*. In: 12th World congress on pain. Glasgow, UK
8. Cadet P, Mantione KJ, Stefano GB (2003) Molecular identification and functional expression of mu 3, a novel alternatively spliced variant of the human mu opiate receptor gene. J Immunol 170(10):5118–5123
9. Rubovitch V, Gafni M, Sarne Y (2003) The mu opioid agonist DAMGO stimulates cAMP production in SK-N-SH cells through a PLC-PKC-Ca^{++} pathway. Brain Res Mol Brain Res 110(2):261–266
10. Galeotti N et al (2006) Signaling pathway of morphine induced acute thermal hyperalgesia in mice. Pain 123(3):294–305
11. Costigan M, Woolf CJ (2000) Pain: molecular mechanisms. J Pain 1(3 Suppl):35–44
12. Dolan S, Nolan AM (2001) Biphasic modulation of nociceptive processing by the cyclic AMP-protein kinase A signalling pathway in sheep spinal cord. Neurosci Lett 309(3): 157–160
13. Vetter I et al (2006) The mu opioid agonist morphine modulates potentiation of capsaicin-evoked TRPV1 responses through a cyclic AMP-dependent protein kinase A pathway. Mol Pain 2:22
14. North RA et al (1987) Mu and delta receptors belong to a family of receptors that are coupled to potassium channels. Proc Natl Acad Sci U S A 84(15):5487–5491
15. Chieng BC et al (2008) Functional coupling of mu-receptor-Galphai-tethered proteins in AtT20 cells. Neuroreport 19(18):1793–1796
16. Ikeda K et al (2000) Involvement of G-protein-activated inwardly rectifying K (GIRK) channels in opioid-induced analgesia. Neurosci Res 38(1):113–116
17. Saegusa H et al (2000) Altered pain responses in mice lacking alpha 1E subunit of the voltage-dependent Ca2+ channel. Proc Natl Acad Sci U S A 97(11):6132–6137
18. Wang L, Gintzler AR (1997) Altered mu-opiate receptor-G protein signal transduction following chronic morphine exposure. J Neurochem 68(1):248–254
19. Ito A et al (2000) Mechanisms for ovariectomy-induced hyperalgesia and its relief by calcitonin: participation of 5-HT1A-like receptor on C-afferent terminals in substantia gelatinosa of the rat spinal cord. J Neurosci 20(16): 6302–6308
20. Fields A, Sarne Y (1997) The stimulatory effect of opioids on cyclic AMP production in SK-N-SH cells is mediated by calcium ions. Life Sci 61(6):595–602
21. Sarne Y et al (1998) Dissociation between the inhibitory and stimulatory effects of opioid peptides on cAMP formation in SK-N-SH neuroblastoma cells. Biochem Biophys Res Commun 246(1):128–131
22. Crain SM, Shen KF (2000) Antagonists of excitatory opioid receptor functions enhance morphine's analgesic potency and attenuate opioid tolerance/dependence liability. Pain 84(2–3):121–131
23. Olmstead MC, Burns LH (2005) Ultra-low-dose naltrexone suppresses rewarding effects of opiates and aversive effects of opiate withdrawal in rats. Psychopharmacology (Berl) 181(3): 576–581
24. Crain SM, Shen KF (2001) Acute thermal hyperalgesia elicited by low-dose morphine in normal mice is blocked by ultra-low-dose naltrexone, unmasking potent opioid analgesia. Brain Res 888(1):75–82
25. Martin NP et al (2004) PKA-mediated phosphorylation of the beta1-adrenergic receptor promotes Gs/Gi switching. Cell Signal 16(12):1397–1403
26. Hill SJ, Baker JG (2003) The ups and downs of Gs- to Gi-protein switching. Br J Pharmacol 138(7):1188–1189

27. Malmberg AB et al (1997) Diminished inflammation and nociceptive pain with preservation of neuropathic pain in mice with a targeted mutation of the type I regulatory subunit of cAMP-dependent protein kinase. J Neurosci 17(19):7462–7470
28. Chen GD et al (2008) Calcium/calmodulin-dependent kinase II mediates NO-elicited PKG activation to participate in spinal reflex potentiation in anesthetized rats. Am J Physiol Regul Integr Comp Physiol 294(2): R487–R493
29. Selbie LA, Hill SJ (1998) G protein-coupled-receptor cross-talk: the fine-tuning of multiple receptor-signalling pathways. Trends Pharmacol Sci 19(3):87–93
30. Tell GP, Pasternak GW, Cuatrecasas P (1975) Brain and caudate nucleus adenylate cyclase: effects of dopamine, GTP, E prostaglandins and morphine. FEBS Lett 51(1):242–245
31. Connor M, Christie MD (1999) Opioid receptor signalling mechanisms. Clin Exp Pharmacol Physiol 26(7):493–499
32. Aronson JK (2007) Concentration-effect and dose–response relations in clinical pharmacology. Br J Clin Pharmacol 63(3): 255–257
33. Minta A, Kao JP, Tsien RY (1989) Fluorescent indicators for cytosolic calcium based on rhodamine and fluorescein chromophores. J Biol Chem 264(14):8171–8178
34. Vetter I et al (2008) Mechanisms involved in potentiation of transient receptor potential vanilloid 1 responses by ethanol. Eur J Pain 12(4):441–454
35. Vetter I et al (2008) Rapid, opioid-sensitive mechanisms involved in transient receptor potential vanilloid 1 sensitization. J Biol Chem 283(28):19540–19550
36. Vasko MR, Campbell WB, Waite KJ (1994) Prostaglandin E2 enhances bradykinin-stimulated release of neuropeptides from rat sensory neurons in culture. J Neurosci 14(8): 4987–4997
37. Berg KA et al (2007) Integrins regulate opioid receptor signaling in trigeminal ganglion neurons. Neuroscience 144(3):889–897
38. Berg KA et al (1994) Signal transduction differences between 5-hydroxytryptamine type 2A and type 2C receptor systems. Mol Pharmacol 46(3):477–484
39. Cadet P et al (2007) A functionally coupled mu3-like opiate receptor/nitric oxide regulatory pathway in human multi-lineage progenitor cells. J Immunol 179(9):5839–5844
40. Takahashi A et al (1999) Measurement of intracellular calcium. Physiol Rev 79(4): 1089–1125

Chapter 31

Inhalational Anesthetic Photolabeling

Roderic G. Eckenhoff, Jin Xi, and William P. Dailey

Abstract

Photolabeling has allowed considerable progress in the understanding of anesthetic binding to proteins, of target identity, and of site localization. There are, however, few groups doing this work, so this article is an attempt to demystify the method. We will discuss the theory, method, and limitations of this useful experimental approach.

Key words: Inhaled anesthetics, Photolabeling, Halothane

1. Introduction

The inhaled anesthetics are a particularly troublesome group of drugs for investigators. Their small size, volatility, and few interactive features result in weak binding constants making it difficult to discover targets and binding sites for further drug refinement (1). Photolabeling allows conversion of these rapid binding constants into stable covalent bonds for subsequent identification with conventional biochemistry. Initially applied with the drug halothane, the toolbox of probes now contains several novel, small volatile diazirine compounds.

1.1. Theory

Halothane (1-Bromo-1-Chloro-2,2,2-trifluoroethane). This halogenated ethane has a weakened C-Br bond because of the adjacent trifluoromethyl group. Cleaved by 254 nm illumination, a carbon-centered-free radical is generated, which then reacts with adjacent electrophilic groups to form a stable adduct. By virtue of a radiolabeled carbon, the adduct can be detected and monitored through any subsequent chemistry (2, 3). The carbon-centered radical is not reactive enough to label nonselectively; aromatics are preferred (3).

Arpad Szallasi (ed.), *Analgesia: Methods and Protocols*, Methods in Molecular Biology, vol. 617, DOI 10.1007/978-1-60327-323-7_31, © Springer Science+Business Media, LLC 2010

Halothane photolysis is complex, however, in that the predicted reaction produces two reactive moieties (chlorotrifluoroethyl radical and free Br); the potential for subsequent reactions is high. In addition, 254 nm illumination causes direct photolytic damage to the target, and combined with the chain reaction initiators from halothane photolysis, considerable cross-linking occurs. This limits the subsequent identification approach to fairly crude techniques such as gel and column chromatography, limited proteolysis, and if lucky, the laborious Edman degradation (3, 4). Edman chemistry can be blocked by backbone atom adduction by this small molecule. The principal advantage of halothane photolabeling, is, of course, that it is an unmodified general inhalational anesthetic with an extensive literature and clinical history.

Anesthetic/diazirine compounds. Because of the above technical problems with halothane photolabeling, compounds that retain anesthetic character, yet include the diazirine group, have been designed, synthesized, and tested. Both halogenated alkanes (5) and ethers (6) have now been validated. These compounds have the large advantage of requiring longer UV photolysis (320–350 nm), inducing less target damage and the release of only a single and very reactive intermediate, a halogenated carbene. The carbene is predicted to react with target sites more quickly than the carbon-centered radical and demonstrates considerably less photoselectivity toward amino acids, both important features in interpreting the adduction site. Because of the somewhat cleaner chemistry, more sophisticated detection and analysis approaches like mass spectroscopy can be employed. This considerably reduces the cost and increases the safety of the below approaches. Nevertheless, appropriate design of the compound can include an exchangeable hydrogen atom, so that tritiation can occur through base-catalyzed exchange.

2. Materials

2.1. Photolabels

It is important to note at the outset that *not a single photoaffinity anesthetic label* is commercially available, limiting the current implementation of this approach to custom synthesis or collaboration with one of only two or three academic groups. Detailed description of the synthetic routes to these compounds is considered beyond the scope of this paper; the methods for synthesis of these novel compounds are contained in the original references for those courageous investigators with organic synthesis capability.

1. *Halothane* – (1-bromo-1-chloro-2,2,2-trifluoroethane). This can be custom synthesized with a ^{14}C on the trifluoromethyl, but

is extremely expensive. Further, there is a risk of β-degradation; the β-particle liberated by decay of the ^{14}C atom has enough energy to occasionally cleave the C-Br bond, and initiate chain reactions.

2. *Halothane mimic.* (3-(2-bromo-2-chloro-1,1-difluoroethyl)-3H-diazirine)(Fig. 1a)(5).
3. *H-diaziflurane.* (3-(difluoro(2,2,2-trifluoroethoxy)methyl)-3H-diazirine)(Fig. 1b) (6).
4. *Azi-isoflurane.* (3-((1-chloro-2,2,2-trifluoroethoxy)difluoromethyl)-3H-diazirine)(Fig 1c)(7).

2.2. Other Components

1. *Buffers.* All buffers have not been tested, but the inorganic buffers are generally preferred (e.g., phosphate) to avoid scavenging reactions (see below). The labels are tolerant of pH values in the biologic range.
2. Target (tissues, proteins, membranes, etc.). To achieve high labeling efficiency, reasonable UV penetrance is required. Thus, protein concentration of tissue homogenates is generally kept below 1 mg/ml, and samples are continuously mixed during photolysis.
3. Nitrogen/Argon source with air stone or equivalent means of deoxygenating buffers.
4. UV source. 254 nm – Oriel 6035 Low Pressure Hg(Ar) Calibration lamp driven at 18 mA.

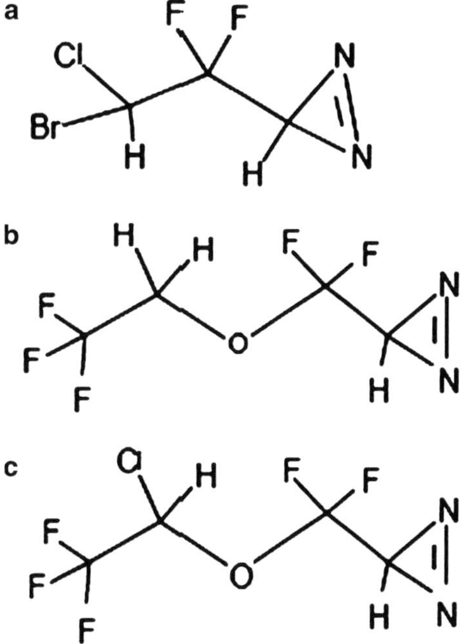

Fig. 1. Volatile anesthetic photolabels. Shown are the stick structures for the halothane mimic (**a**), the H-diazrithane (**b**) and azi-isoflurane (**c**)

300–350 nm – Rayonet reactor with appropriate bulbs (300 or 350 nm).

5. Hamilton Gas Tight syringes of various sizes, with removable blunt needles and Teflon seals. Extra Teflon washers. These are wonderful vessels for handling hydrophobic, volatile chemicals like the anesthetics. Plasticware should be avoided.
6. *Quartz cuvettes.* The Teflon-stoppered varieties are preferred, and path length should be limited to 5 mm or less owing to poor penetrance of UV. The 1 × 0.5 × 4 cm cuvettes hold 2 ml, and accommodate microstir bars for mixing during photolysis.
7. *Filters and centrifuges.* This will depend on the desired separations, proteolysis and biochemistry to be employed postphotolysis.

3. Methods

1. Buffers for suspension of the protein or tissue should be deoxygenated with either argon or nitrogen bubbling. This reduces reactions between molecular oxygen and the radical or carbene, and effectively increases efficiency of the desired adduction. The deoxygenated buffer is drawn up into Hamilton gas-tight syringes that contain Teflon microstir bars.
2. The anesthetic photolabel is drawn up into Hamilton microsyringes and injected into the larger gas-tight syringe containing buffer through the removable needle port. The extra Teflon washer under the well- tightened knurled nut is necessary to get a good seal around the injecting needle. The syringe is then placed on a magnetic stirrer and allowed to stir for several hours in the dark. Solubilization of the label can be facilitated by connecting two syringes via the removable needle (as above) and passing the buffer back and forth through the narrow needle lumen. In such cases, adequate anesthetic dissolution can be achieved in less than 15 min. At this point, the anesthetic solution can be aliquoted into Teflon (or better yet, foil) -sealed glass vials and stored at –80°C for later use, or used immediately.
3. If using radioactivity, a small aliquot (1–2 μl) of the solubilized label is injected into scintillation vials filled with cocktail for counting to determine anesthetic concentration from the known specific activity. If not using radioactivity, this step can be ignored.

4. We use 2 ml 10 × 5 × 40 mm Teflon-stoppered quartz cuvettes for most experiments. These easily accommodate a microstir bar for mixing during photolysis if the apparatus is held at about a 15° angle from horizontal. A shuttered housing provides exact illumination times, and close proximity between lamp and cuvette. In our system, the lamp is about 1 cm from the cuvette surface. For very small volume samples due to scarcity of either ligand or target, cuvettes as small as 300 μl are commercially available, and smaller can be designed. We have also photolabeled slide-mounted brain sections by fabricating a thin aluminum and quartz cuvette into which is inserted the entire slide (8). Of greatest concern here, however, is the homogeneity of illumination, which has proven difficult for some light sources (notably the Oriel calibration lamp).
5. If labeling tissue homogenate or protein solutions, a predetermined amount is added to quartz cuvettes, with or without added buffer, to bring the protein to 1 mg/ml or less (to facilitate UV penetrance) or to introduce other components (like agonists, antagonists, etc.) leaving just enough headspace for the final addition of volatile photolabel. Cuvettes are tightly sealed with Teflon stoppers, and then mixed by inversion several times and immediately exposed to the appropriate wavelength (300–350 nm for diazirines, 254 nm for halothane). Distances are kept small to maximize illumination amplitude. Illumination times for 254 nm light are kept to less than 60 s because of target damage, while we often expose to 350 nm illumination for 5–10 min with little evidence of target damage.
6. In some cases, it is useful to determine specificity of labeling by adding potential competitor ligands to the cuvette. Further, estimates of the IC_{50} can be achieved by varying the concentration of competitor in the cuvette, as long as it is understood by the investigator that the system is nonequilibrium and the results, therefore, are only a rough (generally low) estimate of the IC_{50}.
7. We generally do not include scavenging molecules, such as reduced glutathione, in the photolysis mixture because this unexpectedly reduces specific binding with little effect on nonspecific binding. In the case of halothane, photolysis of the molecule in the bulk, unbound aqueous phase creates two species that are thought to recombine to reform halothane. On the other hand, if bound in a site with a photochemical partner, then the desired adduction (labeling) occurs. Thus, providing a photochemical partner in solution, such as glutathione, reduces the mass of halothane capable of entering and labeling sites of interest during the photolysis period

(which is very long relative to binding and unbinding rates for these molecules). In the case of the carbene, since it can react with water (albeit at lower rates), the inclusion of glutathione makes little difference.

8. After photolysis, the labeled material is separated from unbound aqueous phase by any of several approaches: dialysis, centrifugation, filtration, column chromatography, SDS-PAGE, 2D-electrophoresis (9), etc., depending on the subsequent approach used for identification of labeling magnitude, labeled target, or labeled site. For example, if simply measuring incorporated radioactive label in a protein sample, we precipitate the protein with 10–20% trichloroacetic acid (TCA), filter through glass fiber filters (Whatman GFB), and wash with dilute (1%) TCA. The filter is then equilibrated with scintillant and counted. Although the free ligand was initially volatile, one cannot rely on vacuum extraction to rid the labeled mixture of free label. The photolysis often creates a variety of small water soluble by products.
9. To determine radiolabel incorporation into gel bands (intact proteins or proteolytic fragments), the band of interest is excised with a scalpel blade, placed in scintillation vials with 30% H_2O_2, capped tightly and heated to 60°C for several hours (or until the gel slice liquefies). Scintillation fluid is then added and the sample counted. The β radiation from either ^{14}C or ^{3}H lacks sufficient energy to escape the gel – even if cut or ground into small pieces.
10. For samples that are expected to be analyzed for label incorporation by mass spectroscopy, it is critical to purify to near homogeneity to avoid contaminating sequences. Recent progress with LC/MS approaches reduces this need somewhat. Further, it is important to compare proteins and peptides to samples that have been exposed to UV alone.
11. We have found that anesthetic photolabeling is of reasonably high efficiency – demonstrated by the unprecedented ability to observe electron density of the adduct within an anesthetic binding site by X-ray diffraction (6).

4. Notes

1. *Warning note*: The diazirines are relatively unstable molecules and need to be handled with some caution. Phase changes, impact, and pressure spikes can cause an explosion. For example,

Hamilton microsyringes can generate large hydraulic forces, and if containing a diazirine, can trigger an explosion. Handle only limited quantities and wear appropriate protection when dealing with the neat compound. Further, all such novel and/or radiolabeled volatile compounds should be handled in a well-functioning fume hood.

2. For determining concentrations, the diazirine compounds have a characteristic double peak of absorbance at 300–340 nm, with extinction coefficients between 100 and 150 $M^{-1}.cm^{-1}$.
3. Photolysis is occasionally divided into two or more sessions in order to switch cuvette sides for greater penetrance or invert cuvettes for greater mixing. This results in somewhat greater efficiency of label incorporation.
4. With the diazirines, successful photolysis can be verified by the generation of small, readily observed bubbles (released nitrogen) in the cuvette.
5. Glass fiber filters equilibrate (become saturated) with scintillant very slowly. Equilibration can be accelerated by vigorous shaking to break the filter apart, but still requires more than 12–24 h.
6. After proteolysis, some fragments in the UV plus ligand sample "disappear" from the mass spectrum, rather than just shift in mass, as compared to the UV alone sample. This is probably due to increased adherence (MALDI) or hydrophobicity (LC/MS) as a result of an adduction event. The matrix used for MALDI may have to be altered, or in the case of LC/MS, the elution gradient changed for the labeled samples.

References

1. Eckenhoff RG, Johansson JS (1997) Molecular interactions between inhaled anesthetics and proteins. Pharmacol Rev 49:343–367
2. Eckenhoff RG, Shuman H (1993) Halothane binding to soluble proteins determined by photoaffinity labeling. Anesthesiology 79:96–106
3. Eckenhoff RG (1996) An inhalational anesthetic binding domain in the nicotinic acetylcholine receptor. Proc Natl Acad Sci U S A 93: 2807–2810
4. Ishizawa Y, Pidikiti R, Liebman PA, Eckenhoff RG (2002) G protein coupled receptors as direct targets of general volatile anesthetics. Mol Pharmacol 61:945–952
5. Eckenhoff RG, Knoll FL, Greenblatt EP, Dailey WP (2002) Halogenated diazirines as photolabel mimics of the inhaled haloalkane anesthetics. J Med Chem 45:1879–1886
6. Xi J, Liu R, Rossi M, Yang J, Loll PJ, Dailey WP, Eckenhoff RG (2006) Photoactive analogues of the haloether anesthetics provide high resolution features from low affinity.interactions. ACS Chem Biol 1:377–384
7. Eckenhoff RG, Xi J, Shimaoka M, Bhattacharji A, Covarrubias M, Dailey WP(2009) Azi-isoflurane, a photolabel analog of the commonly used inhaled general anesthetic, isoflurane. ACS: Chemical Neuroscience doi:10.1021
8. Eckenhoff MF, Eckenhoff RG (1998) Quantitative autoradiography of halothane binding in rat brain. J Pharmacol Exp Ther 285:371–376
9. Pan JZ, Xi J, Tobias JW, Eckenhoff MF, Eckenhoff RG (2007) Halothane binding proteome in human brain cortex. J Proteome Res 6:582–592

Chapter 32

Measuring Membrane Protein Interactions Using Optical Biosensors

Joseph Rucker, Candice Davidoff, and Benjamin J. Doranz

Abstract

Membrane proteins, such as G protein-coupled receptors (GPCRs) and ion channels, represent important but technically challenging targets for the management of pain and other diseases. Studying their interactions has enabled the development of new therapeutics, diagnostics, and research reagents, but biophysical manipulation of membrane proteins is often difficult because of the requirement of most membrane proteins for an intact lipid bilayer. Here, we describe the use of virus-like particles as presentation vehicles for cellular membrane proteins ("Lipoparticles"). The methods for using Lipoparticles on optical biosensors, such as the BioRad ProteOn XPR36, are discussed as a means to characterize the kinetics, affinity, and specificity of antibody interactions using surface plasmon resonance detection.

Key words: Biosensor, Virus-like particle, Membrane protein, GPCR

1. Introduction

G protein-coupled receptors (GPCRs) and ion channels represent the largest and most diverse family of cell surface receptors. Both are widely distributed in the peripheral and central nervous systems and these protein families represent some of the most important therapeutic targets in pain medicine. For example, both GPCRs and ion channels are present on the plasma membrane of neurons and their terminals along the nociceptive pathways and many can modulate pain transmission (1). All GPCRs share a similar structure, which consists of seven transmembrane domains linked by alternating intracellular and extracellular loops, and most ion channels contain between six and twenty-four membrane spanning domains. Because of their structural dependence on a lipid bilayer, integral membrane proteins are usually studied

Arpad Szallasi (ed.), *Analgesia: Methods and Protocols*, Methods in Molecular Biology, vol. 617,
DOI 10.1007/978-1-60327-323-7_32, © Springer Science+Business Media, LLC 2010

within whole cells or crude membrane preparations that make the proteins difficult to purify to homogeneity while retaining their native structure (2–5).

Membrane proteins interact with a variety of ligands that initiate a signal. GPCRs, for example, can induce intracellular G protein signaling after contact with ligands as diverse as single atoms (e.g. Ca^{2+} activates the Calcium-sensing receptor (CaSR), small molecules (5HT activates serotonin receptors), or peptides and proteins (e.g. cyclosporine activates the formylpeptide receptor). In addition to native ligands, man-made agonists and antagonists, including monoclonal antibodies (MAbs), are of interest for therapeutic purposes. Such molecules often interact with membrane proteins with very high affinity to modulate the function of the membrane proteins for therapeutic purposes. For example, functional MAbs against the human β2-adrenergic receptor have been used to modulate these GPCRs both in vitro and in vivo (6–8). MAbs that react with disease-associated proteins or specific epitopes on these proteins can also be of value for diagnostics.

Characterizing the interactions of ligands with their target membrane proteins is of interest in both basic and applied research. For example, optimizing such interactions is an important part of the drug optimization process within the pharmaceutical industry, and is routinely applied to both small molecule (medicinal chemistry) and antibody (protein engineering) therapeutics. The most potent and desirable therapeutic candidates typically have very strong affinities for their target. Moreover, the kinetics of interaction that describe the rates of binding and dissociation of the best candidates typically favor very slow off-rates that prevent the therapeutic molecule from dissociating once bound (9). Typical optimization programs can result in hundreds or thousands of variants, and characterizing all of them quickly and efficiently to assess their interaction potential with target proteins can be difficult. For membrane proteins, which require a lipid bilayer to maintain their structure, characterization of the affinity and kinetics of interactions is substantially more difficult because of the limited number of methods to study structurally intact membrane proteins.

A novel approach to studying membrane proteins in their native lipid bilayer is by incorporating them onto virus-like particles that bud from the cell plasma membrane, a technology referred to as Lipoparticles. Lipoparticles retain the native structure of integral membrane proteins and routinely incorporate 10 to 100-fold more concentrated membrane proteins than can be found in whole cells or membrane preparations. Because of this increase in purity, Lipoparticles can be used for applications in which other sources of membrane proteins have proven difficult, such as characterizing affinity and kinetic interactions using optical biosensors.

Optical biosensors have been in use for over 15 years and are now routinely used in basic, diagnostic, and applied research laboratories for measuring affinity, specificity, and kinetics of interactions. Optical biosensors typically provide real-time information about interactions using label-free detection techniques such as surface plasmon resonance (SPR), which measures changes in refractive index at surfaces (10). By attaching the protein of interest (the "ligand") to the surface of an optical biosensor (typically a derivatized gold film on glass) and flowing over the interacting molecule of interest (an "analyte"), binding to the target protein can be detected as an increase in refractive index proportional to the change in mass. By monitoring such changes in real-time and by using defined quantities of analyte, association, and dissociation rate constants (k_{on} and k_{off}) as well as binding equilibrium constants (K_D) can be accurately calculated.

For soluble proteins, the methodology for measuring interactions on biosensors has been well developed. For membrane proteins, however, measuring such interactions has proven exceptionally challenging because of the difficulty of attaching membrane proteins to surfaces or of using them as soluble reagents without damaging their structural integrity. Lipoparticle technology provides a novel approach to studying membrane protein interactions using optical biosensors. Here, the methodology of using Lipoparticles as ligands attached to the chip surface is discussed. The use of Lipoparticles as analytes in solution provides an alternative, highly sensitive means to rapidly detect membrane protein interactions, but does not provide detailed kinetic information as discussed elsewhere (11). While a number of optical biosensors are now commercially available, the BioRad ProteOn XPR36, an array-based biosensor based on surface plasmon resonance, is used in our methodology because of its advantages in speed, ease of use, and unique analysis capabilities offered by its array-based format (e.g. "One-Shot kinetics") (12). Other optical biosensors, including the popular Biacore biosensors, have also been readily used with Lipoparticles using similar methodology discussed here for the ProteOn (11, 13, 14).

2. Materials

2.1. Preparation of Biosensor Surfaces for Attachment

1. ProteOn optical biosensor (BioRad, Hercules, CA) (see Note 1).
2. ProteOn GLC or GLM chip (see Note 2).
3. PBS (0.2 μm filtered, extensively degassed, and *without* Tween-20) (see Note 3 and 4).
4. 0.5% SDS.

5. 50 mM NaOH.
6. 100 mM HCl.

2.2. Attachment of Lipoparticles to a Biosensor Surface by Capture Antibody

1. PBS (0.2 μm filtered, degassed, and *without* Tween-20).
2. 16 mM 1-ethyl-3-(3-dimethylaminopropyl)carbodiimide hydrochloride (EDC).
3. 4 mM N-hydroxysulfosuccinimide (Sulfo-NHS) (see Note 5).
4. JS-81 (anti-CD81 antibody) (see Note 6).
5. 10 mM sodium acetate, pH 5.0.
6. 1 M ethanolamine.
7. 100 Units Lipoparticles per channel (Integral Molecular, Philadelphia, PA).

2.3. Biosensor Binding Experiments

1. PBS (0.2 μm filtered) supplemented with 0.2 mg/ml BSA (Fraction V ~99%; Sigma).
2. Receptor-specific and control antibodies.
3. Regeneration solution 1:1% Empigen (VWR).
4. Regeneration solution 2: 100 mM H_3PO_4.

3. Methods

Detection of specific binding is achieved within biosensor experiments by using control surfaces, ligands, and analytes within the experiment. For the ProteOn, each of the 36 interactions spots can be internally referenced against an adjacent region. In addition, at least one horizontal channel (one ligand) and one vertical channel (one analyte) are used as negative controls to provide double-referencing data in which multiple negative controls are subtracted from the test interaction of interest. For example, Null Lipoparticles (without any specific receptor) are typically used as one negative control, and a nonspecific MAb is used as another negative control. To further reduce nonspecific binding, all experiments here are conducted in the presence of 0.2 mg/ml BSA, which significantly lowers background binding to lipid membrane structures (see Note 3). Figure 1 shows an example of Lipoparticle capture and analyte binding on the ProteOn using the GPCR CXCR4.

Quantification of the on-rate, off-rate, and affinity of interactions on optical biosensors requires the measurement of ligand–analyte interactions at a variety of analyte concentrations. Most biosensor experiments achieve these measurements by multiple attachment-regeneration cycles in which progressively increasing

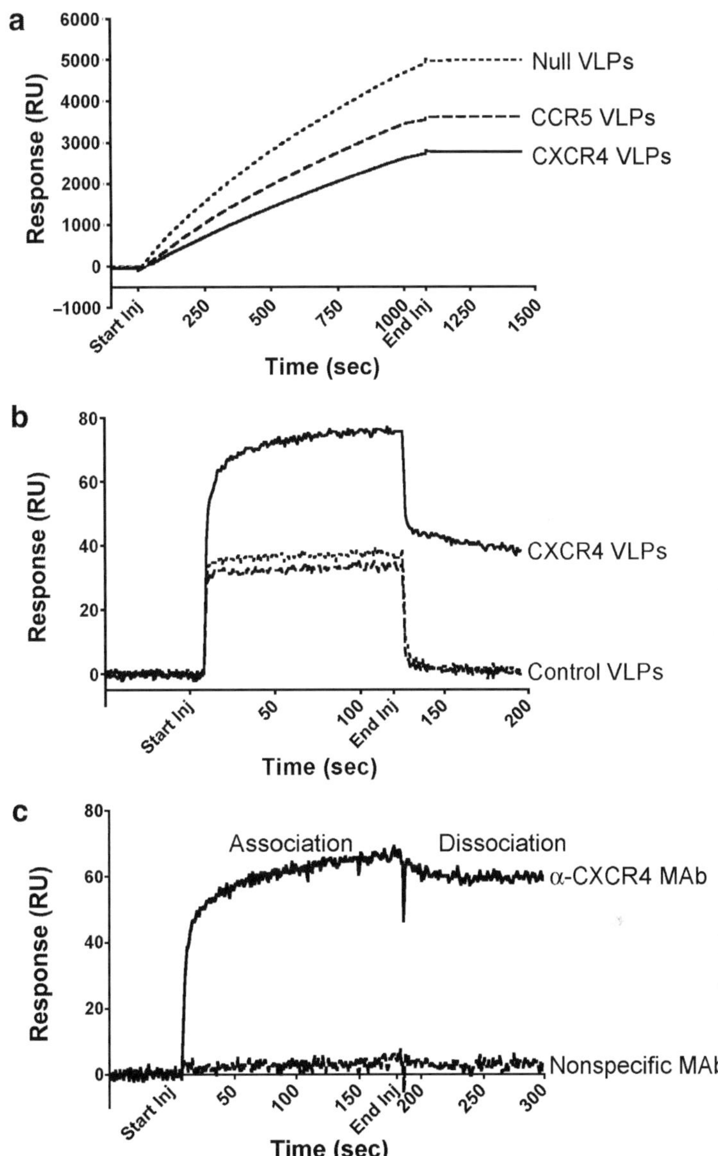

Fig. 1. *Use of Lipoparticles on the ProteOn XPR36 Biosensor.* (**a**) Capture of Lipoparticles onto three different ProteOn ligand channels. (**b**) Injection of a specific monoclonal antibody against CXCR4 (12G5) in the analyte direction across multiple ligand channels. Specific binding is only seen with the CXCR4 Lipoparticle channel. Reactivity against Lipoparticles containing no or other receptors show only a bulk refractive index change. (**c**) A nonspecific antibody (9E10) shows no binding to Lipoparticles or the alginate matrix

amounts of analyte are flowed over a fixed concentration of ligand. The BioRad ProteOn, however, enables six concentrations of analyte to be assessed simultaneously (and against multiple ligands), precluding the need for multiple regeneration cycles

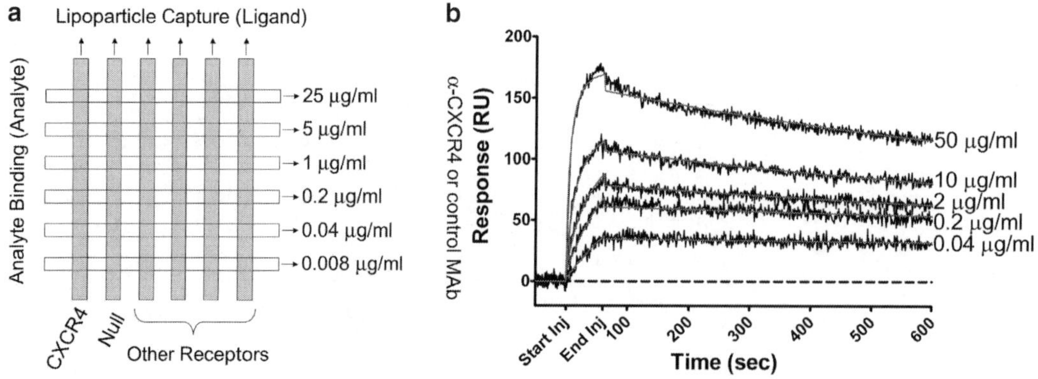

Fig. 2. *One-Shot Kinetic Assay*. (**a**) Schematic of One-Shot Kinetic assay. Vertical (ligand) channels are derivatized with the capture antibody. Different Lipoparticles are then captured on each channel. In the example shown, CXCR4 Lipoparticles and Null lipoparticles (containing no CXCR4) are captured on two of six channels. Lipoparticles containing other receptors can be captured on the remaining channels. A concentration series of antibody (receptor-specific or control) is then flowed in the horizontal (analyte direction). (**b**) Specific binding of a concentration series of an anti-CXCR4 antibody (12G5) against CXCR4 Lipoparticles. The specific response is calculated by subtracting the response to Null Lipoparticles. Curve fits are shown in red

(an analysis strategy called "One-Shot Kinetics"). An example of this type of experiment is shown in Fig. 2. As an alternative, others have also used kinetic titrations in which increasing concentrations of analyte are flowed across the ligand *without* regeneration between concentrations (15).

3.1. Preparation of Biosensor Surfaces for Attachment

1. Chip preparation is performed using degassed PBS (0.2 μm filtered). A GLM or GLC chip is docked to a ProteOn biosensor and is initialized with air.
2. The channels are cleaned using BioRad's recommended preconditioning protocol in the vertical direction (using a Ligand injection, with default injection quality). All injections are 60 s at a flow rate of 30 μl/min. Sequentially inject: 0.5% SDS, 50 mM NaOH, and 100 mM HCl (see Note 7).

3.2. Attachment of Lipoparticles to a Biosensor Surface by Capture Antibody

1. Attachments are performed using degassed PBS (0.2 μm filtered).
2. After the chip has been docked and cleaned as described above, surface carboxyl groups are activated by a 1:1 mixture of EDC and Sulfo-NHS injected in the vertical direction (using a Ligand injection, with default injection quality) for 5 min at a flow rate of 30 μl/min.
3. Lipoparticle capture antibody, JS-81 (anti-CD81), is diluted to 50 μg/ml in 10 mM sodium acetate, pH 5.0 and is injected in the vertical direction over the desired channels for 5 min at a flow rate of 30 μl/min. This should yield approximately 2,000 RU of immobilized antibody (see Note 8).

4. The remaining activated carboxyl groups are blocked by a 5 min injection in the vertical direction of 1 M ethanolamine at 30 μl/min.
5. After all surfaces are derivatized, the machine is washed with running buffer until the baseline has stabilized.
6. The system is switched to a new running buffer, PBS with 0.2 mg/ml BSA (0.2 μm filtered), using a Flush command to exchange the buffer in the microfluidics system.
7. Several 2-min Blank injections in the vertical direction at 100 μl/min will serve to equilibrate the chip surface in the new buffer. Use a Pause command to flow running buffer over the surface until the baseline signal stabilizes.
8. Lipoparticles are diluted to 1:20 in running buffer and are injected *twice* in the vertical direction over the desired channels for 1,078 s (18 min, maximum length injection) each time, at a flow rate of 25 μl/min. Injection quality should be set to minimum to allow for maximum injection length. This should yield approximately 5,000 RU of Lipoparticle binding. Multiple Lipoparticle injections can be used to increase the amount of captured Lipoparticles.
9. It is critical that a negative-control surface containing Lipoparticles not containing the receptor(s) of interest ("Null" Lipoparticles) be included. Care should be taken to attach approximately equivalent amounts (RUs) of Lipoparticles to each channel.
10. After Lipoparticle capture, the instrument is washed with running buffer until the baseline stabilizes.

3.3. Biosensor Binding Experiments

1. As described above, Lipoparticles containing receptor(s) of interest are captured onto the vertical channels of the ProteOn biosensor chips. Up to five different receptor-containing Lipoparticles, plus a control channel, can be analyzed simultaneously using all of the vertical channels. For any channel not used during the experiment, all injections should be replaced by running buffer. The recommended running buffer is PBS with 0.2 mg/ml BSA (0.2 μm filtered).
2. Switch the chip to the horizontal direction. Use several default Blank injections of running buffer in the horizontal direction to stabilize the baseline signal.
3. Each of the six horizontal channels of the ProteOn surface can be used to present a different analyte. It is recommended that one channel be reserved for a negative-control analyte to measure background signal. This negative-control analyte should be closely matched to the analytes of interest (e.g. if testing murine-derived antibodies, the control should be a

murine-derived antibody with an epitope not present on the receptors or Lipoparticles).

4. Introduce the analytes using an Analyte injection in the horizontal direction at a flow rate of 30 μl/min. A typical injection duration is 2–3 min, although longer association phases may be required in those cases where the association rate is very slow or where equilibrium binding is being measured. Set the dissociation time to 5–10 min, although longer periods can be used in cases of analytes with extremely slow dissociation rates.
5. Use a 2-min Blank injection at 100 μl/min in the horizontal direction to rinse any excess analyte from the system using running buffer.
6. Steps 4 and 5 can be repeated with a new analyte set. Channels can be regenerated back to capture antibody at least five times (see Note 9).
7. After all analytes have been tested, channel(s) are regenerated back to the JS-81 baseline values using several short, high flow rate injections of regeneration buffer in the vertical direction. Lipoparticles are effectively removed by two cycles of the following regeneration: duplicate 30 s pulses of 1% Empigen at 100 μl/min followed by two additional pulses of 100 mM H_3PO_4.
8. The binding data can be collected and processed (subtraction of background signal and removal of injection artifacts) using the ProteOn's built-in software (ProteOn Manager 2.1).

3.4. One-Shot Kinetics

Rather than sequential injections of increasing analyte concentration, BioRad's ProteOn enables simultaneous injection of an entire range of analyte to perform all required kinetic curves simultaneously ("One-Shot Kinetics"). In One-Shot Kinetics, each of the six horizontal channels of the ProteOn surface is used to present a different concentration of the same analyte, diluted in running buffer. Optimally, analyte concentrations should cover a wide range bracketing the K_d of the analyte. Background signal and injection artifacts can be measured either by reserving one analyte channel for running buffer alone or by injecting a separate concentration series using a non-specific antibody.

1. Inject the antibody concentration series using an Analyte injection in the horizontal direction at a flow rate of 30 μl/min. A typical injection duration is 2–3 min, although longer association phases may be required in those cases where the association rate is very slow or where equilibrium binding is being measured. Set the dissociation time to 5–10 min, although longer periods can be used in cases of analytes with extremely slow dissociation rates.

2. Use a 2-min Blank injection at 100 µl/min in the horizontal direction to rinse any excess analyte from the system with running buffer.
3. Steps 1 and 2 should be repeated with an analyte that is not expected to bind to the surface to provide a reference of nonspecific binding. This negative-control analyte should be closely matched to the analyte of interest (e.g. if testing a murine-derived antibody, the control should be a murine-derived antibody with an epitope not present on the receptors or Lipoparticles). The negative-control analyte should be used at the same concentration set as the experimental analyte.
4. After all analytes have been tested, channel(s) are regenerated back to the JS-81 baseline values using several short, high flow rate injections of regeneration buffer in the vertical direction. Lipoparticles are effectively removed by two cycles of the following regeneration: duplicate 30 s pulses of 1% Empigen at 100 µl/min followed by two additional pulses of 100 mM H_3PO_4.
5. Once data are collected and processed (subtraction of background signal and removal of injection artifacts), equilibrium and rate constants can be extracted using the ProteOn's built-in fitting software. Equilibrium and kinetic analysis of biosensor data is often performed globally (all data sets simultaneously); however, the use of multiple independent flow channels requires the R_{max} values to be fitted. Data analysis requires a choice of a particular binding model. A common default is the assumption of 1:1 binding, meaning that one analyte molecule binds to one receptor molecule, although MAbs can often bind bivalently. More complicated but sometimes more accurate models can be used, taking into account mass-transport (See Note 10), bivalent binding (See Note 11), or conformational changes.

4. Notes

1. BioRad ProteOn, Biacore BiaX, and Biacore Bia2000 optical biosensors have been used for Lipoparticle experiments. Other commercial biosensors should also be adaptable using the methods here.
2. The ProteOn GLC and GLM chips are both gold surfaces derivatized with a modified alginate; they differ in the thickness of the matrix. Other chips with diverse chemistries, such as the C1 chip from Biacore, also work very well with Lipoparticles.

The Biacore carboxydextran chip (CM5) can work but demonstrates reduced Lipoparticle attachment in comparison, likely due to the poor penetration of Lipoparticles into the dextran matrix or to charge effects.

3. PBS containing 0.005% Tween-20 is commonly used in biosensor experiments to reduce nonspecific binding. However, Tween-20 can potentially disrupt Lipoparticle membranes so this and other detergents should be avoided. In addition to BSA, DMEM supplemented with 0.1% w/v Pluronics F-127 can also reduce nonspecific binding in certain applications (13). This is a reference number. Pluronics have been extensively studied for their ability to reduce nonspecific binding of proteins to surfaces (16). However, because SPR (and other optical biosensor technologies) detects all interactions at the biosensor surface, binding of blocking agents will increase the baseline signal and can sometimes lead to baseline artifacts, e.g., caused by pump pulsing. This can be avoided by using the minimal concentrations of blocking agents.
4. We have found extensive degassing, 15–30 min, of sample buffer to be critical for obtaining high-quality injections on the ProteOn.
5. Amine-coupling to carboxylated surfaces commonly uses N-hydroxysuccinimide (NHS) rather than N-hydroxysulfosuccinimide (Sulfo-NHS). The ProteOn alginate surface shows increased coupling activity with sulfo-NHS in comparison with NHS. However, NHS can easily substitute for sulfo-NHS in these assays.
6. CD81 is a endogenous cell surface molecule found at high densities on Lipoparticles produced from HEK-293 cells (17). We have found the binding of Lipoparticles via the antibody JS-81 to be a robust method for Lipoparticle capture. It should be noted that not all antibodies against CD81 are suitable for capture.
7. Sample volume for the ProteOn is increased roughly sixfold over the reagent usage for a single-injection system, such as the Biacore 2000.
8. Greater levels of antibody immobilization do not necessarily yield greater Lipoparticle capture levels.
9. Due to the presence of the lipid membrane, Lipoparticle structure and integrity is sensitive to many reagents that are commonly used for regeneration. For this reason, assays that do not require regeneration (such as kinetic titrations and One-shot kinetics) are preferred. If needed, however, bound analytes can be regenerated from the Lipoparticle surface without Lipoparticle disruption (13).

10. Mass transport effects can, in cases of extremely high or low rates, affect binding measurements. For example, rapid association and dissociation rates can be limited by the diffusion of analytes to the biosensor surface and rapid rebinding of analyte (18). Mass transport effects can be reduced mathematically during data analysis or by using high flow rates and reducing the number of binding sites on the biosensor surface (e.g. fewer attached Lipoparticles).
11. In general, antibody binding to Lipoparticle-expressed receptors is best fit to a bivalent model, consistent with antibody structure and with the presence of multiple copies of the receptor per Lipoparticle.

Acknowledgments

We thank Sharon Willis for her help with Lipoparticle production and biosensor optimization and Laura Moriarty (BioRad) and Mohammed Yousef (BioRad) for their helpful discussions.

References

1. Woolf CJ, Ma Q (2007) Nociceptors–noxious stimulus detectors. Neuron 55(3):353–364
2. Navratilova I, Dioszegi M, Myszka DG (2006) Analyzing ligand and small molecule binding activity of solubilized GPCRs using biosensor technology. Anal Biochem 355(1):132–139
3. Navratilova I, Sodroski J, Myszka DG (2005) Solubilization, stabilization, and purification of chemokine receptors using biosensor technology. Anal Biochem 339(2):271–281
4. Rice PJ et al (2002) Human monocyte scavenger receptors are pattern recognition receptors for (1–>3)-beta-D-glucans. J Leukoc Biol 72(1):140–146
5. Stenlund P, Babcock GJ, Sodroski J, Myszka DG (2003) Capture and reconstitution of G protein-coupled receptors on a biosensor surface. Anal Biochem 316(2):243–250
6. Mobini R et al (2000) A monoclonal antibody directed against an autoimmune epitope on the human beta1-adrenergic receptor recognized in idiopathic dilated cardiomyopathy. . Hybridoma 19(2):135–142 (in eng)
7. Peter JC, Eftekhari P, Billiald P, Wallukat G, Hoebeke J (2003) scFv single chain antibody variable fragment as inverse agonist of the beta2-adrenergic receptor. (Translated from eng). J Biol Chem 278(38):36740–36747 (in eng)
8. Day PW et al (2007) A monoclonal antibody for G protein-coupled receptor crystallography. Nat Methods 4(11):927–929
9. Tummino PJ, Copeland RA (2008) Residence time of receptor-ligand complexes and its effect on biological function. (Translated from eng). Biochemistry 47(20):5481–5492 (in eng)
10. Canziani G et al (1999) Exploring biomolecular recognition using optical biosensors. (Translated from eng). Methods 19(2):253–269 (in eng)
11. Willis S et al (2008) Virus-like particles as quantitative probes of membrane protein interactions. Biochemistry 47(27):6988–6990
12. Bravman T et al (2006) Exploring "one-shot" kinetics and small molecule analysis using the ProteOn XPR36 array biosensor. (Translated from eng). Anal Biochem 358(2):281–288 (in eng)
13. Hoffman TL, Canziani G, Jia L, Rucker J, Doms RW (2000) A biosensor assay for studying ligand-membrane receptor interactions: binding of antibodies and HIV-1 Env to chemokine receptors. (Translated from eng). Proc Natl Acad Sci USA 97(21):11215–11220 (in eng)
14. Rucker J (2003) Optical biosensor assay using retroviral receptor pseudotypes. Methods Mol Biol 228:317–328

15. Karlsson R, Katsamba PS, Nordin H, Pol E, Myszka DG (2006) Analyzing a kinetic titration series using affinity biosensors. (Translated from eng). Anal Biochem 349(1):136–147 (in eng)
16. Green RJ, Davies MC, Roberts CJ, Tendler SJ (1998) A surface plasmon resonance study of albumin adsorption to PEO-PPO-PEO triblock copolymers. (Translated from eng). J Biomed Mater Res 42(2):165–171 (in eng)
17. Segura MM et al (2008) Identification of host proteins associated with retroviral vector particles by proteomic analysis of highly purified vector preparations. J Virol 82(3):1107–1117
18. Myszka DG, He X, Dembo M, Morton TA, Goldstein B (1998) Extending the range of rate constants available from BIACORE: interpreting mass transport-influenced binding data. (Translated from eng). Biophys J 75(2):583–594 (in eng)

Chapter 33

Proteomics and Metabolomics and Their Application to Analgesia Research

Nichole A. Reisdorph and Richard Reisdorph

Abstract

Technological innovations have increased our potential to evaluate global changes in protein and small molecule levels in a rapid and comprehensive manner. This is especially true in mass spectrometry-based research where improvements, including ease-of-use, in high performance liquid chromatography (HPLC), column chemistries, instruments, software, and molecular databases have advanced the fields of proteomics and metabolomics considerably. Applications of these technologies in clinical research include biomarker discovery, drug targeting, and elucidating molecular networks, and a systems-based approach, utilizing multiple "omics," can also be taken. While the exact choice of workflow can dramatically impact the results of a study, the basic steps are similar, both within and between metabolomics and proteomics experiments. Although gel-based methods of quantitation are still widely used, our laboratory focuses on mass spectrometry-based methods, specifically protein and small molecule profiling.

Key words: Proteomics, Metabolomics, Mass Spectrometry, Protein Digest, Metabolite Profiling, Label-free Quantitation

1. Introduction

Liquid chromatography mass spectrometry (LCMS)-based methods have become powerful and popular means of profiling clinical samples for the purpose of biomarker discovery. Biomarkers can be used in several areas of clinical research and patient care, including disease detection and diagnosis, drug monitoring, and assessing drug efficacy. A wide range of biomolecules can be profiled using LCMS, including proteins, peptides, and various classes of endogenous or exogenous small molecules and metabolites. Appropriately, there are a vast number of methods and workflows that can be used to compare relative quantities of molecules within a system. For example, in several recent analgesic

Arpad Szallasi (ed.), *Analgesia: Methods and Protocols*, Methods in Molecular Biology, vol. 617,
DOI 10.1007/978-1-60327-323-7_33, © Springer Science+Business Media, LLC 2010

proteomics studies, proteins extracted from mouse brain tissue were analyzed using two-dimensional gel electrophoresis (2DGE) followed by LCMS to identify proteins of interest (1). Other recent studies utilized a gel-free approach, namely LCMS (2). In fact, a variety of proteomic methods are being applied to analgesic research (3–5). Furthermore, many proteomics studies now focus on a subproteome. In the case of brain samples, microproteomics (6), which focus on a particular cell type, is highly appropriate given the heterogeneity of the tissue, whereas examination of the glycoproteome of plasma may lessen the challenges associated with high abundant proteins in that particular biofluid. Importantly, for global proteomic studies, fractionation or simplification of the sample is generally required. Similarly, for metabolomics studies, sample preparation must be geared to enrich molecules of interest. Although metabolomics is arguably the most nascent of the three major "omics," it is already being applied to clinical research (7, 8). The current work will focus on general LCMS-based profiling methods which for both metabolomics and proteomics a general workflow consists of sample preparation → data acquisition → data analysis. Because there are many options at each step of these workflows, alternatives are included throughout.

Metabolomics is the global analysis of all metabolites in a system and can be influenced by several environmental, dietary, and genetic factors. While numerous nuclear magnetic resonance metabolomics studies have been performed (9), LC/MS has more recently begun to be applied to metabolomics due to major advances in chromatography, instrumentation, and software. The basic LCMS metabolomics workflow consists of the following basic components:

1. *Sample preparation* – extraction of small molecules and protein removal.
2. *Mass spectrometry* – to detect "features" (i.e. small molecules) in a sample which are defined by mass and retention time on a column.
3. *Data analysis* – comparison of "features" to determine differences. The result is a list of masses that are used to query a database.
4. *Database search* – a mass list is searched against a database of known and often well-characterized small molecules. A list of potential matches, i.e., candidate biomarkers, is the result.
5. *Purification/enrichment and Identification* – small molecule candidate biomarkers are purified from the starting material and structural studies are performed. If available, standards are purchased and their chemistry is compared to that of the purified compound.
6. *Validation* – following identification of a candidate biomarker, large-scale clinical validation studies must be performed.

Challenges include the large differences between classes of small molecules, the lack of complete small molecule databases, and large, inherent variability in human and animal samples. Conversely, a great body of work exists for targeted analysis of specific small molecules, including lipids, amino acids, organic acids, steroids, etc. Experiments involved in the first four steps of a typical metabolomics workflow are included herein.

Proteomics profiling studies generally focus on one of the two basic workflows: (1) Two-dimensional gel electrophoresis (2DGE) to resolve and relatively quantitate proteins followed by mass spectrometryor (2) quantitative mass spectrometry approaches including metabolic and post-metabolic labeling and nonlabeling strategies (10, 11). In addition, proteomics workflows can be further divided based on the sample type. For example, analysis of plasma generally requires removal of high abundant proteins using affinity chromatography as a first step. Conversely, cells can be fractionated based on organelle, for example, nuclear or mitochondria, and proteins are further fractionated based on chemistry, for example, using ion exchange chromatography. A nonlabeling strategy, including fractionation, suitable for profiling of tissues or cells is included herein with the following steps:

1. *Cell lysis and protein solubilization* – A variety of methods can be used to extract and solubilize proteins, depending on the sample type. Options include subcellular fractionation, precipitation, addition of various detergents, and centrifugation. In some cases, samples can be immediately denatured and digested (See Note 1).
2. *Fractionation* – Chromatography is often used to fractionate samples via chemistries, such as strong cation exchange, in part because the step can be automated, although size exclusion or other methods can be used. Affinity chromatography, such as antibody-based immunoprecipitation, or glycoprotein enrichment, or removal of high abundant proteins is also used.
3. *Protein digest* – Although quantitative LC/MS methods exist for intact proteins, such as molecular imaging and profiling (12), most often proteins are further solubilized and digested with the protease trypsin prior to analysis by mass spectrometry. Alternatives in this step include choice of proteolytic enzyme and buffer components (See Note 2).
4. *Mass spectrometry* – There are several classes of mass spectrometers and a variety that are used in proteomics such as quadrupole time-of-flight (QTOF), ion trap, ion cyclotron resonance, and matrix assisted laser desorption ionization time-of-flight (MALDI-TOF). The choice of instrument is based on the application and the features of the instrument itself.

5. *Data analysis* – Two general workflows exist for data analysis: protein identification followed by quantitation by comparing either the peptide intensities or number of mass spectra; quantitation and comparison of the peptide intensities followed by a targeted mass spectrometry analysis resulting in identification. In both cases protein sequence databases are queried using a protein database search program.

Following biomarker discovery, whether for proteins or small molecules, a targeted analysis can be developed using similar sample preparation and data acquisition parameters. A technique commonly used in small molecule analysis, for example in newborn screening (13), is now being applied to targeted protein analysis (9). Termed multiple reaction monitoring (MRM), this directed approach uses mass spectrometry and stable isotope-labeled internal standards. MRM is performed on both the labeled and the endogenous molecules and their amounts compared, providing quantitative information. This method is more precise than antibody-based assays, which are often complicated by non-specific reactions. MRM assays can be cost- and time-effective means of conducting large-scale validation studies for both proteomics and metabolomics.

2. Materials

2.1. Label-Free Quantitative Proteomics: Cell lysis, protein solubilization, and protein concentration determination

1. Extraction buffer: To 900 μl HPLC-grade water, add 0.087 g NaCl (1500 mM) and 100 μl of Tris–HCl, pH 8.0.
2. PPS Silent Surfactant (Protein Discovery, Knoxville, TN). Once reconstituted, the PPS must be used within 12 h. Because PPS is not stable, it is recommended to read the PPS package insert for more information (see Note 3).
3. Protease Inhibitor HALT (Pierce, Rockford, IL). This can be divided into 100 μl aliquots and stored at –20°C.
4. Non-interfering protein assay (Calbiochem, San Diego, CA).
5. PBS (Sigma, St. Louis, MO) dissolved in 1 L MilliQ water or 100 mM Tris–HCl, pH 7.5 to wash cells.

2.2. Fractionation

1. High performance liquid chromatography system (Agilent 1200 with binary pump), autosampler with thermostat, diode array detector, and fraction collector with thermostat.
2. Sample dilution buffer: 6M Urea in 1% acetic acid. Dissolve 36 g urea (Sigma) in 80 ml HPLC-grade water. Add 1.0 ml acetic acid and bring up to a total volume of 100 ml in HPLC-grade water (see Note 4). Make fresh just prior to using. Do not heat urea above 30°C. Do not freeze or re-use after 1 day.

3. Macroporous reverse-phase C18 column (Agilent Technologies).
4. Buffer A: 0.1% trifluoracetic acid (TFA). Add 1 ml of TFA to 999 ml HPLC-grade water.
5. Buffer B: 0.08% TFA in acetonitrile (ACN). Add 800 μl TFA to 999.2 ml ACN (See Note 5).

2.3. In Solution Protein Digestion

1. Urea is dissolved at 8 M in 100 mM Tris–HCl, pH 8.5. Dissolve 480 mg urea (Sigma) in 700 μl of 100 mM Tris–HCl (pH 8.5). A 500 ml solution of 100 mM Tris–HCl can be made in advance by dissolving 6.05 g of Tris base in 300 ml HPLC-grade water and pH-ing to 8.5 using HCl. Add water for a final volume of 500 ml.
2. 1M Tris (2-carboxyethyl) phosphine (TCEP, reducing agent). Dissolve 287 mg TCEP (Pierce) in 1 ml HPLC-grade water. Aliquot in 10 μl and store at –20°C.
3. 500 mM Iodoacetamide (IAA, alkylating agent). Dissolve 92 mg IAA (BioRad) in 1 ml HPLC-grade water. Make fresh just prior to use.
4. 1 μg/ul Trypsin solution. Add 100 μl ice-cold, HPLC-grade water to 1 @ 100 μg vial of Trypsin Gold (Promega). Store immediately in 5 μl aliquots at –80°C. (See Note 6).

2.4. Sample Clean up

1. C18 clean up tips (Agilent) or columns (Pierce).
2. Equilibration, Wash, and Elution Solutions require the following: trifluoroacetic acid (TFA), acetonitrile (ACN), and HPLC-grade water. Solutions can be made in advance according to the manufacturer's instructions and placed in wide-mouth glass bottles. Solutions can be aliquoted into 1.5 ml microfuge tubes just prior to use for easy access and limiting cross contamination between experiments.

2.5. Mass Spectrometry

1. LC/MS/MS instrument such as quadrupole time-of-flight (QTOF) (Agilent) or ion trap (Agilent) equipped with nanoflow electrospray (ESI) source. The source could be a nano-ESI with separate enrichment column module and switching valve, or an HPLC-Chip Cube system (Agilent). An attached HPLC (Agilent) should include nanopump with degasser, capillary pump with degasser, and microautosampler with thermostat.
2. Buffer A: 0.1% formic acid. Add 4 ml of formic acid to 4 L bottle of HPLC-grade water.
3. Buffer B: 90% acetonitrile (ACN) and 0.1% formic acid. Combine 900 ml ACN, 100 ml HPLC-grade water, and 1 ml formic acid.

4. C18 enrichment column and analytical column, which are integrated in the HPLC Chip. Separation column is 75 mm × 150 mm, packed with Zorbax 300SB-C18 5 mm material, 300 A pore size.

2.6. Data Analysis

1. Feature extraction software such as Mass Hunter (Agilent Technologies). Generally, this software will be included with the instrument. In some cases, the software can be used for proteins and small molecules.
2. Data analysis software such as Genespring MS (Agilent Technologies). Generally this software is similar to that used for gene expression studies, another technique where high-dimensional data analysis is required. Major vendors carry similar software and freeware can be found on-line.
3. Database searching program such as MASCOT (Matrix Sciences) or SpectrumMill (Agilent Technologies). Programs often are packaged with instruments and free versions can be found on-line. Resources can be found at www.expasy.org.

2.7. Liquid-Chromatography Mass Spectrometry-Based Metabolomics Profiling: Sample Preparation

1. Sample resuspension buffer: 0.1% formic acid in HPLC-grade water. Add 100 µl formic acid to 100 ml water. Store in wide-mouth glass container.
2. Fresh or frozen urine.
3. 5,000 Dalton molecular weight cut-off filters.
4. For plasma preparation, HPLC-grade methanol and water are used.

2.8. Mass Spectrometry

1. Liquid chromatography time-of-flight mass spectrometer (LC-TOF, Agilent 6210) with electrospray source. Alternative high mass accuracy instruments include Waters, Orbitrap or LTQ-FT (Thermo), and QTrap (ABI).
2. High performance liquid chromatography system: Agilent 1200 with binary pump with degasser, autosampler with thermostat, and column compartment. For reference mass infusion, a separate isocratic pump with splitter is recommended but not required.
3. Column: Agilent SB-AQ 2.1 × 50 mm, 1.8 µm column. Alternatives include: ZORBAX XDB C18.
4. Buffer A: 0.1% formic acid in HPLC grade water. Combine 1 ml formic acid with 1 l HPLC-grade water.
5. Buffer B: 90% acetonitrile (ACN), 0.1% formic acid in HPLC grade water. Combine 1 ml formic acid with 900 ml ACN and 99 ml HPLC-grade water.

2.9. Data Analysis

1. Feature extraction and data analysis software.
2. Small molecule databases are available on-line and many are free: Metlin (http://metlin.scripps.edu/) and Human metabolome database (http://www.hmdb.ca/) are two examples. A partial listing of additional resources is available at the Metlin site. A commercial version of Metlin (Personalized Metlin, Agilent Technologies) is also available.

3. Methods

3.1. Label-Free Quantitative Proteomics: Cell lysis and protein extraction

1. Prepare 1 ml extraction buffer. Just prior to pelleting cells, add 100 μl extraction buffer to one 10 mg PPS vial for a final concentration of 10% PPS (See Note 1).
2. Methods for removing cells from plates vary according to cell type. Therefore, it is recommended to use, for example, a scraper, media, or trypsin to remove cells from the plate according to your previous methods. This protocol is generally appropriate for approximately one 35 mm plate of confluent cells. Enough starting material to yield approximately 500 μg of protein is required and may have to be determined empirically after a trial experiment (See Note 3).
3. Remove media and wash plates 2–3 times with PBS or 100 mM Tris pH 7.5 to remove any remaining media. Alternatively, cells that detach easily can be pelleted and washed in a microfuge tube. Pellet cells by spinning at 3,000×*g* at 4°C for 5 min. Try to remove as much PBS as possible without disturbing cells in a final spin.
4. Resuspend pelleted cells in 90 μl extraction buffer. Volumes may have to be adjusted depending on cell type.
5. Add 10 μl PPS in extraction buffer plus 1 μl protease inhibitor (HALT) to resuspended cells for a final concentration of 1% PPS. Volumes may have to be adjusted depending on cell type.
6. Vortex sample on high speed for 30 s, then place on ice for 30 min. Vortex sample again on high speed for 30 s prior to centrifugation.
7. Centrifuge 13,000×*g* at 4°C for 10 min. Place supernatant in new tube, discarding pellet. Store at –80°C or proceed to fractionation.

3.2. Fractionation

1. Prepare lysates for fractionation:
   (a) Determine protein concentration using non-interfering protein assay according to the manufacturer's instructions.

(b) Dilute up to 340 mg protein in 6M Urea, 1% acetic acid (final concentration) to a total volume between 100 ml and 900 ml.

2. Fractionate by macroporous reverse-phase C18 chromatography:

   (a) Set up a HPLC method using the parameters shown in the table below.

Time	Solvent B%	Solvent C%	Solvent D%	Flow	Pressure
0.00	20.0	0.0	0.0	0.750 ml/min	250
40.00	50.0	0.0	0.0	0.750 ml/min	250
50.00	100.0	0.0	0.0	0.750 ml/min	250
55.00	100.0	0.0	0.0	0.750 ml/min	250
65.00	0.0	100.0	0.0	0.750 ml/min	250
70.00	0.0	0.0	100.0	0.750 ml/min	250
75.00	0.0	0.0	100.0	0.750 ml/min	250
80.00	20.0	0.0	0.0	0.750 ml/min	250

3. Set the column temperature to 80°C. Collect data at 210 and 280 nm. Collect equivalent fractions (≥20 for complex mixtures). Freeze fractions at –80°C for a minimum of 4 h, or flash freeze in liquid nitrogen, and lyophilize in a freeze dryer overnight. An example of the resulting UV chromatogram is shown in Fig. 1.

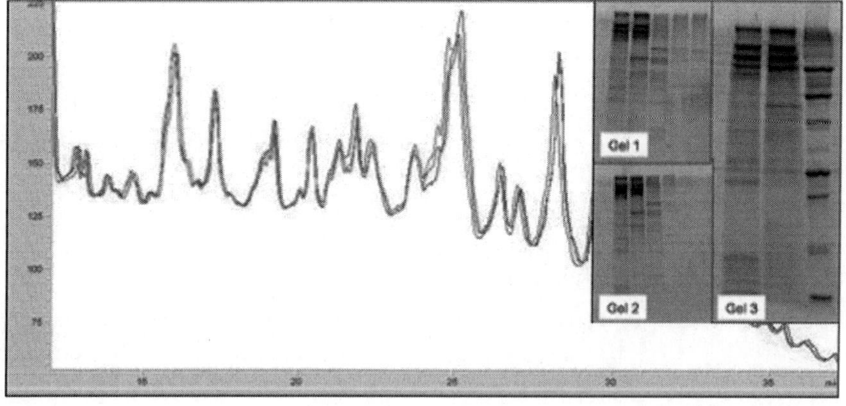

Fig. 1. Fractionation of mitochondrial proteins on C18 macroporous column (rMP) is reproducible. UV chromatogram and SDS-PAGE of mitochondrial proteins from rat skeletal muscle ($n = 3$). Intact proteins were separated using C18 designed for intact proteins and the fractionations collected. In one experiment, fractions were resolved using SDS-PAGE to assess carryover and reproducibility

3.3. In-Solution Protein Digestion

1. Reconstitute dried protein sample in 40 μl of 8.0 M urea in 100 mM Tris–HCl (pH 8.5) (See Note 2).
2. Dilute the 1M TCEP 1:10 in HPLC water and add 1.2 μl of 100 mM TCEP (5 mM final concentration) and shake for 20 min at room temperature.
3. Add 0.88 μl of 500 mM IAA (10 mM final concentration) and shake in the dark for 15 min. A piece of aluminum foil placed over a vortexer is adequate for this step. An accessory can be purchased in order to vortex multiple microfuge tubes automatically.
4. Add 120 μl of 100 mM Tris-HCl (pH 8.5) solution to dilute the urea to 2M.
5. Add Trypsin in appropriate ratio (1:30) to approximate amount of protein by weight. (Generally speaking, for a complex sample, such as a whole cell or whole organelle lysate, a good starting point is 0.5 μg.) (See Note 4).
6. Digest overnight at 37°C.

3.4. Sample Clean up using C18 Spin Columns or Zip Tips

1. Prepare samples, bind to C18 resin, wash, and elute according to the manufacturer's protocol. This step is necessary to remove urea or other potential contaminants from the sample.

3.5. Mass Spectrometry

Mass spectrometry parameters and method specifics will vary somewhat depending on the instrument used. The method below is appropriate for an Agilent 6510 QTOF equipped with a HPLC chip nanoflow source.

1. Set up the mass spectrometry method for MS level analysis. The HPLC gradient is shown in the table below.

Time	B%	Flow
0	3	0.45 μl/min
1	3	0.45 μl/min
50	45	0.45 μl/min
54	45	0.45 μl/min
58	80	0.45 μl/min
62	80	0.45 μl/min
62.01	3	0.45 μl/min
65.00	3	0.45 μl/min

2. Set instrument parameters as follows: capillary voltage = 1,750–1,900 (this is empirically determined and is dependent on individual chips and number of hours in use); drying gas

temperature = 300 degrees; flow rate = 4 L/min; acquisition mode = MS; TOF spectra range = 300–3,000; acquisition rate = 1 spectra/s, 1,000 ms/spectra; ion polarity = positive. The acquisition rate can be increased to sample more spectra per cycle but with a trade-off of reduced response.

3. Empirically determine appropriate injection volume for analysis by running 0.5–1.0 μl sample and inspecting the chromatogram. The most abundant peaks should not exceed an intensity of 10^7; note that intensity is an arbitrary unit and set by the manufacturer, the value of 10^7 is appropriate for an Agilent QTOF. Inspect representative extracted ion chromatograms to determine if peaks are saturated. Overloading can result in chromatography artifacts such as retention time shifts and reduced mass accuracy. If necessary, reduce the amount of analyte by lowering the injection volume or diluting samples.
4. Analyze replicate injections of appropriate volumes (e.g. 0.5–1.0 μl). Analyze three replicates as a minimum, 4–5 is recommended.

3.6. Data Analysis

1. Raw data quality control. Prior to performing detailed analyses, inspect total ion chromatograms (TIC) for abundance and retention time (RT) reproducibility. Abundance variance should be within 10–15%. Retention time variance should be less than 0.5 min. Exclude runs with poor reproducibility from further analysis and repeat injections if necessary. An example of the data analysis workflow is shown in Fig. 2.
2. Molecular feature alignment, filtering, and statistical analysis. Prior to performing subsequent analysis, molecular features must be aligned for RT and mass. GeneSpring MS performs this function during data import. A detailed description of data import and analysis in GeneSpring is beyond the scope of this chapter. Basic parameters and considerations are included here.
   (a) Molecular feature alignment: Retention Time Tolerance. If your chromatographic reproducibility is good, i.e., variation <0.5 min, the default RT alignment values can be used: Before RT Correction– Intercept = 0.5 min, Slope = 0.5 min; After RT Correction – Intercept = 0.3 min, Slope = 0.0 min; RT Correction Method = without standards. Mass Tolerance. Intercept = 2.0 mDa; Slope = 10 ppm. Mass tolerance is dependent on the performance of the instrument used to collect the data.
   (b) Pre-alignment Filters: Mass Defect = peptide-like; Number of ions >2, Charge State = multiple charge required, Minimum Abundance = 1,000.

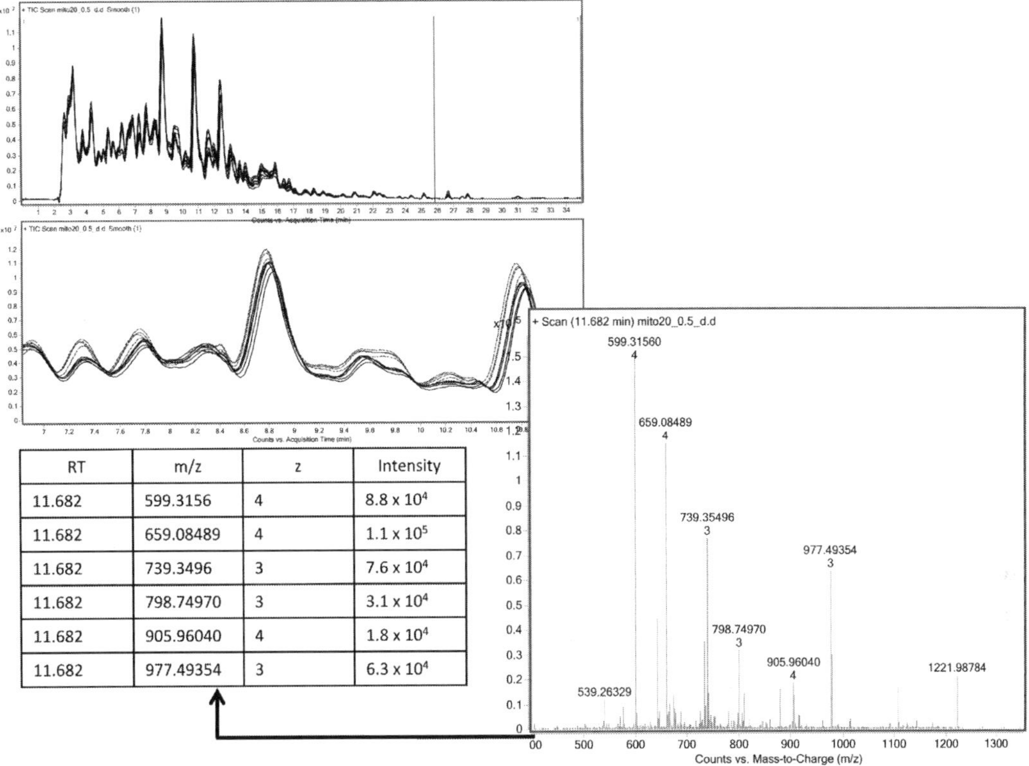

RT	m/z	z	Intensity
11.682	599.3156	4	8.8×10^4
11.682	659.08489	4	1.1×10^5
11.682	739.3496	3	7.6×10^4
11.682	798.74970	3	3.1×10^4
11.682	905.96040	4	1.8×10^4
11.682	977.49354	3	6.3×10^4

Fig. 2. The LC/MS portion of analysis is reproducible as shown with overlaid total ion chromatograms (TIC) for five replicate analyses. The TIC represents the intensity for all peptides and noise (collectively called ions) present for any given QTOF scan. For example, for the scan that represents what is eluting from the column at 5.302 min, shown in the bottom panel, several peptides/features are present. These are extracted and exported based on the criteria detailed below. Samples were obtained from obese prone (OP-*Dark Grey*) and obese resistant (OR-*Light Grey*) rats

(c) Normalization: Use the Standard MS scenario, select Use Recommended Order.

3. Data Quality control: To assess the quality of the aligned data, co-variance analysis and/or unsupervised clustering should be performed. Both can be accomplished in GeneSpring MS with principal components analysis (PCA) and Condition Tree clustering, respectively. It is useful to perform these analyses before and after the filtering steps described below. An example of resulting data is shown in Fig. 3.

4. Filtering: The following filter steps work well for a variety of data sets. Use discretion and tailor filters appropriately if required. Perform these steps sequentially, with each successive step being performed on the mass list resulting from the previous filter step.

   (a) Relative Frequency: Force the feature to be present in 70% of in least one condition.

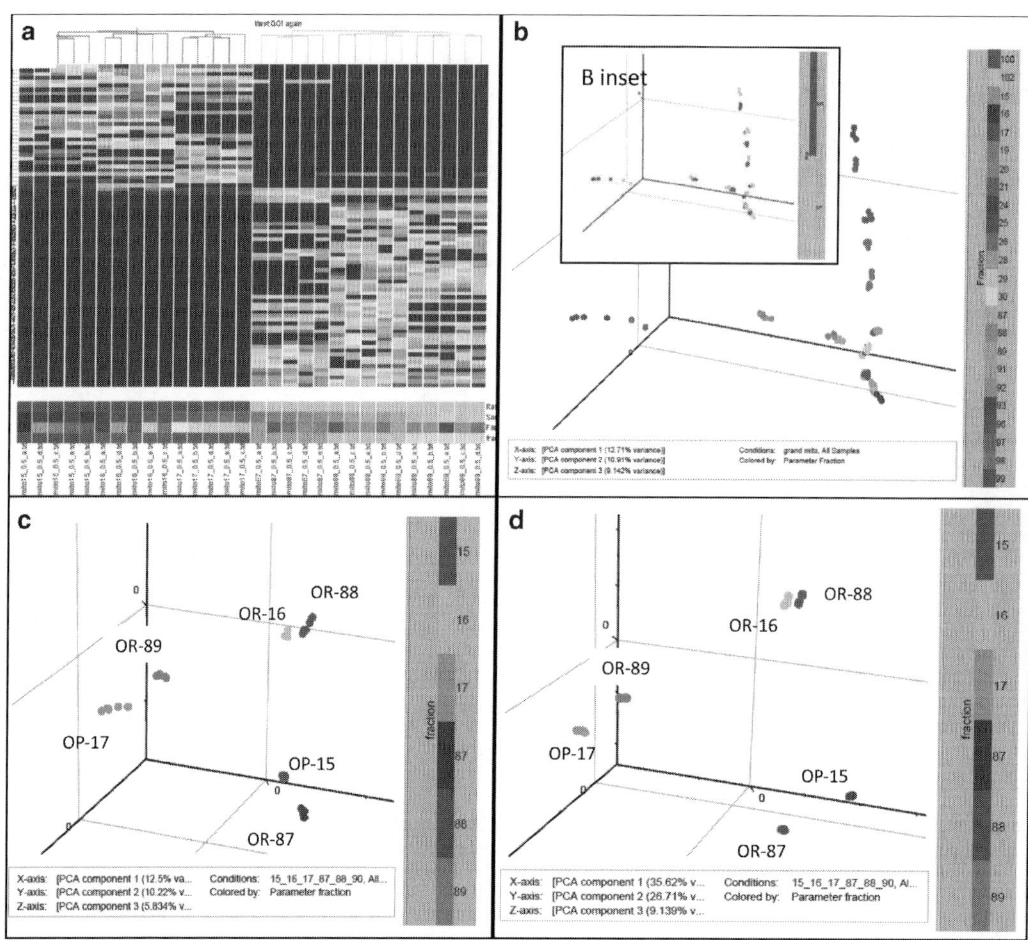

Fig. 3. Clustering and principle component analysis (PCA) of a total of 12 fractions (panels **a** and **b**) and fractions 15–17 and corresponding fractions 87–89 (**c** and **d**) from OP and OR rats, respectively. Mitochondria were isolated, lysed, and fractionated according to the text. Fractions were run in quintuplicate on a QTOF, resulting data extracted, and the data analyzed in GenespringMS software. Panel **a** shows clustering of MS data from analysis of all 12 fractions. *Dark Grey*= OP and *Light Grey*= OR. PCA on 12 fractions shows reproducibility of the analysis, with like colors clustering together (panel **b**). Panel **b** inset shows the same PCA color coded for phenotype with *Dark Grey*= OP and *Light Grey*= OR. Clustering is more clear when only three fractions are analyzed (**c** and **d**) where PCA was performed both before (**c**) and after (**d**) ANOVA to demonstrate the reproducibility of the method. The colored bars on the right corresponds to fraction numbers. *OP* Obese prone, *OR* Obese resistant

(b) Error: Set the Error Type to coefficient of variation. For biological replicates, particularly clinical samples, the CV value may need to be set between 30 and 40%. For technical replicates, the CV should be set between 15 and 20%.

(c) ANOVA/*T*-test. Depending on the number of experimental parameters, perform either an ANOVA or *t*-test. The *p*-value can be left at the default value of 0.05. However, remember that a *p*-value of 0.05 means that 5%

of the molecular features analyzed will appear to be different by chance. For example, if 1,000 features were analyzed using a *p*-value of 0.05, 50 would be expected to appear to be significantly different and would actually be due to chance. The appropriate *p*-value should be set according to your experimental questions, the sample source and your comfort level.

(d) Fold Change. Filter the ANOVA mass list using a fold change filter suitable for your analysis. Each saved fold change mass list can be exported for targeted MSMS analysis.

5. Export inclusion lists for targeted MSMS analyses: Select a Fold Change mass list. From the Tools menu, select Export Inclusion List. Set the RT tolerance appropriately for your data set. This value should be determined by inspection of raw chromatograms. A tolerance value of 0.3 min will result in MSMS acquisition 0.15 min on either side of the RT value assigned to the molecular feature. Ion selection criteria: start with All Z states and alter if necessary. For example if, on average, the number of features co-eluting within a give RT window exceeds the acquisition rate in the instrument MSMS parameters, you will need to simplify the list. Choosing Most Abundant will reduce the number of features. Alternatively, you may need to edit the inclusion list manually to create multiple lists.

3.7. Targeted MSMS Analysis

1. Set up a method for targeted analysis of molecular features in the exported inclusion list. Except for acquisition parameters, this method should be identical to that used to collect MS level data. It is important that the same LC buffer preparations and LC chip (columns) are used for both MS and targeted MSMS analyses. Successful targeted analysis is dependent on consistent feature elution.
2. Data acquisition parameters for the instrument are as follows: Spectral Parameters: MS = 300–3,000; MSMS = 100–1,800; MS Acquisition rate = 8 spectra/s, 125 ms/spectra; MSMS Acquisition rate = 3 spectra/s, 333 spectra/s; Collision Energy = 3.0; Offset = 2.2. Import the inclusion list. In the Targeted table, leave the collision energy field blank.
3. For the targeted analysis, inject 5–10 times more sample than was analyzed during MS acquisition. Adjust the amount as needed based on initial results.
4. Verify successful acquisition of targeted features by examining spectra. If targeted features were not properly selected within designated RT windows, inspect extracted ion chromatograms to determine if RT drift occurred.

3.8. Protein Identification

1. Spectrum Mill: Data extraction and database searching.
   (a) Extract spectra from the targeted MSMS raw data files using the following parameters: signal-to-noise = 25:1, maximum charge state allowed = 4, precursor charge assignment = Find.
   (b) Search parameters: SwissProt species-specific database (e.g. Human), carbamidomethylation as a fixed modification (if IAA used during digest), Digest = trypsin, maximum of one missed cleavage, instrument = Agilent ESI Q-TOF, precursor mass tolerance = 20 ppm, product mass tolerance = 50 ppm, maximum ambiguous precursor charge = 3.
   (c) Validate protein identifications using a minimum of two peptides per protein, protein score > 20, individual peptide scores of at least 10, and Scored Percent Intensity (SPI) of at least 70%. The SPI provides an indication of the percent of the total ion intensity that matches the peptide's MS/MS spectrum.
   (d) Perform manual inspection of spectra to validate spectrum match to predicted peptide fragmentation pattern as necessary to increase confidence in protein identifications.
2. Further validation should be performed by checking identified peptides against molecular features and retention times in the inclusion list. (See Note 6).

3.9. Liquid-Chromatography Mass Spectrometry-Based Metabolomics Profiling: Sample preparation

1. Immediately after sample collection, urine is placed in a 15–45 ml falcon tube and centrifuged at 3,000×*g*, for 10 min at 4°C.
   (a) If necessary, the sample can remain at 4°C (or on ice) for up to 1 h prior to processing.
   (b) Make certain the centrifuge is at 4°C before spinning samples.
   (c) The supernatant is aliquoted and placed in new 15 ml tubes or into microfuge tubes and immediately frozen at –80°C. The sample can also be analyzed fresh.
2. Add 1 μl of 1% formic acid to 10 μl urine. Mix gently with vortex and place in autosampler vial for MS analysis.
3. (Optional) Rinse 5 kDa molecular weight cut-off (MWCO) filter with HPLC grade or MilliQ water.
   (a) Add 100 μl water to the filter. Spin for 14,000×*g* for 10 min at 4°C. Discard any remaining fluid but do not let filter dry out
   (b) This step is necessary to remove contaminants from the filter that will be detected by your mass spectrometer.

(c) Add 100 μl urine to rinsed filter. Spin for 14,000×*g* for 10 min at 4°C. Discard the retentate and place filtered sample in new tube. The sample can be aliquoted and frozen at −80°C until further use.

(d) If internal standards are used, they are added before processing.

4. (Alternative) For plasma samples, add 300 μl ice-cold methanol to 100 μl plasma and vortex for 30 s. Incubate at −20°C for 30 min with vortexing every 10 min. Centrifuge at 14,000×*g* for 10 min at 4°C. Place supernatant in new tube and discard the pellet. The sample can be aliquoted and frozen at −80°C until further use.

3.10. Mass Spectrometry

1. Set instrument parameters as follows: drying gas temperature = 250 degrees; flow rate = 10 L/min; nebulizer = 35 psig; TOF spectra range = 50–1,000; ion polarity = positive.
2. Analyze 2 μl of prepared sample in triplicate ($n = 3$, or up to $n = 5$, which is recommended)

(a) HPLC gradient is as follows with 10 min re-equilibration time.

(b) An example of the resulting total ion chromatogram (TIC) is shown in Fig. 4.

Time	B%	Flow
0	2	0.3 ml/min
3	2	0.3 ml/min
13	60	0.3 ml/min
13.01	100	0.3 ml/min
23	100	0.3 ml/min

3.11. Data Extraction and Analysis

1. Data are extracted and analyzed as described in Proteomics subheading 3.6. The final feature list is queried against a metabolomics database such as Metlin.

4. Notes

1. Sample collection and storage: Proteins and small molecules can degrade and/or become modified starting immediately upon collection. Freeze/thaw cycles can also have an effect on certain molecules. Samples should therefore be processed, aliquoted in small volumes, and frozen at −80°C as quickly and as reproducibly as possible.

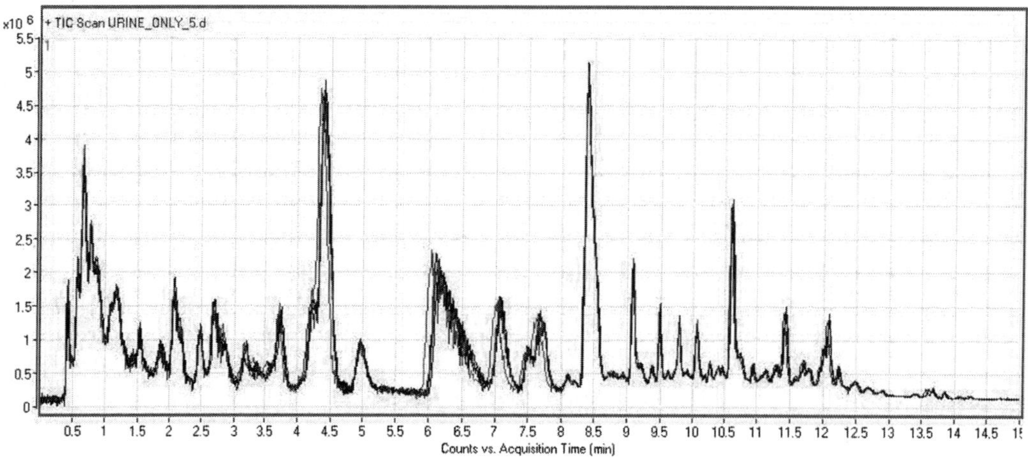

Fig. 4. Overlay of total ion chromatograms of urine following metabolomics sample preparation and analysis by mass spectrometry. The *x*-axis is time and the *y*-axis is arbitrary intensity. The peaks are indicative of small molecules eluting from the column

2. Protein sample processing: Keratin is a major contaminant of proteomics experiments and can not only affect your results, but can prevent identification of low abundant proteins in a mixture. Several resources exist for tips on preventing keratin contamination, including www.Reisdorphlab.org.
3. The protocol describes sample preparation for cells and can be used for tissues, organelles, and biofluids; however, modification of the type and amount of detergent used may be required. The PPS detergent is compatible with subsequent LC/MS steps and modifications to the protocol may require optimization of subsequent chromatography and/or fractionation steps, if used. Low retention microfuge tubes are recommended and some laboratories wash the tubes in 50:50 MeOH:H_2O or ACN prior to use.
4. In all cases, use bottles or consumables that have been designated for mass spec or HPLC use only.
5. Protein Digest: Trypsin will undergo rapid autolysis, especially at room temperature. When aliquoting, keep pre-labeled tubes on ice, work quickly, and freeze immediately at –80°C. When ready to digest, thaw on ice and use immediately. Also, dithiothreitol (DTT) can be used in place of TCEP.
6. Database searching for protein identification: Repeat searches using different parameters; for example, include variable modifications such as phosphorylations. Make note of the database version used and all search parameters. These are required for manuscript submissions (14).

References

1. Kalenka A, Hinkelbein J, Feldmann RE Jr, Kuschinsky W, Waschke KF, Maurer MH (2007) The effects of sevoflurane anesthesia on rat brain proteins: a proteomic time-course analysis. Anesth Analg 104:1129–1135
2. Chiang N, Schwab JM, Fredman G, Kasuga K, Gelman S, Serhan CN (2008) Anesthetics impact the resolution of inflammation. PLoS ONE 3:e1879
3. Atkins JH, Johansson JS (2006) Technologies to shape the future: proteomics applications in anesthesiology and critical care medicine. Anesth Analg 102:1207–1216
4. Niederberger E, Geisslinger G (2008) Proteomics in neuropathic pain research. Anesthesiology 108:314–323
5. LoPachin RM, Jones RC, Patterson TA, Slikker W Jr, Barber DS (2003) Application of proteomics to the study of molecular mechanisms in neurotoxicology. Neurotoxicology 24:761–775
6. Gutstein HB, Morris JS, Annangudi SP, Sweedler JV (2008) Mass Spectrom Rev 27:316–330
7. Oldiges M, Lütz S, Pflug S, Schroer K, Stein N, Wiendahl C (2007) Metabolomics: current state and evolving methodologies and tools. Appl Microbiol Biotechnol 76:495–511
8. Gomase VS, Changbhale SS, Patil SA, Kale KV (2008) Metabolomics. Curr Drug Metab 9:89–98
9. Serkova N, Reisdorph N, Tissot van Patot M (2007) Metabolic markers of hypoxia: systems biology application in biomedicine. Toxicol Mech Methods 18(1):81–95
10. Bowler R, Ellison M, Reisdorph N (2006) Proteomics in pulmonary medicine. Chest 130:567–574
11. Aebersold R, Mann M (2003) Mass spectrometry-based proteomics. Nature 422:198–207
12. Cornett DS, Reyzer ML, Chaurand P, Caprioli RM (2007) MALDI imaging mass spectrometry: molecular snapshots of biochemical systems. Nat Methods 4:828–833
13. Silcken B, Wiley V (2008) Newborn screening. Pathology 40:104–115
14. Carr S, Aebersold R, Baldwin M, Burlingame A, Clauser K, Nesvizhskii A (2004) Mol Cell Proteomics 3:531–533

Chapter 34

Preemptive Analgesia: Problems with Assessment of Clinical Significance

Igor Kissin

Abstract

The results of clinical studies on the value of preemptive analgesia are far from being unanimous. There are a number of potential problems related to preemptive analgesia that could lead to controversy regarding its clinical significance. The following potential problems are analyzed: (1) terminology, (2) approach to reveal the effect of preemptive analgesia, (3) verification of the direct pharmacological effect of a treatment, (4) partial preemptive effect in control, (5) intensity of noxious stimuli, (6) difference in a drug concentration between study groups during postoperative period, and (7) outcome measures.

Key words: Central sensitization, Pain relief, Pathological pain, Postoperative pain, Preemptive analgesia, Preventive analgesia

1. Introduction

Preemptive analgesia is an antinociceptive treatment that prevents the establishment of altered processing of afferent input that amplifies postoperative pain. Preemptive analgesia prevents (or reduces) pathologic pain that is different from physiologic pain in several aspects: it is excessive (in intensity and spread), can be activated by low-intensity stimuli (allodynia, hyperalgesia), and includes hyperpathia. The concept of preemptive analgesia was formulated by Crile (1) at the beginning of previous century on the basis of clinical observations. Crile advocated the use of regional blocks in addition to general anesthesia to prevent pain and the formation of painful scars caused by changes in the central nervous system during surgery owing to unsuppressed access of noxious stimuli to the brain. The revival of this idea was associated with a series of experimental studies started by Woolf (2)

Arpad Szallasi (ed.), *Analgesia: Methods and Protocols*, Methods in Molecular Biology, vol. 617,
DOI 10.1007/978-1-60327-323-7_34, © Springer Science+Business Media, LLC 2010

in 1983 and highlighted by Wall (3) in a 1988 editorial on the prevention of postoperative pain. Views on the concept of preemptive analgesia were summarized by a statement that evidence for the concept derived from experimental studies is overwhelmingly convincing; however, results of clinical studies regarding the value of preemptive analgesia are controversial (4).

Studies on preemptive analgesia are numerous. The PubMed database for the term "preemptive analgesia" has more than 160 clinical trials, of which 67 have been published in the last 5 years. In addition, the PubMed lists 69 reviews on this topic. The results of clinical studies on the value of preemptive analgesia are far from being unanimous. There are a number of potential problems related to preemptive analgesia that could lead to controversy regarding its clinical significance. Here, we will discuss the most important of them.

2. Terminology

Probably, the most important problem with clinical studies on preemptive analgesia is related to terminology. Preemptive analgesia is a misleading term because it creates an impression that the secondary feature associated with the phenomenon represents its basis. The term preemptive analgesia suggests that an antinociceptive intervention provided preoperatively prevents or reduces pain after surgery. With this definition, the main feature of preemptive analgesia is perceived as *preempting the incision*. However, the emphasis should not be on the timing of treatment initiation but on the pathophysiologic phenomenon it should prevent: altered sensory processing. The timing of the treatment should cover the entire duration of high-intensity noxious stimulation that can initiate the altered sensory processing. High-intensity noxious stimulation is generated not only by incisions (primary phase of injury) but also by the release of chemicals and enzymes from damaged tissues (secondary phase of injury extended well into the postoperative period). Noxious stimuli can initiate altered central processing after the surgery during the inflammation caused by incisions. The treatment should *preempt initiation of altered central processing* not only during surgery but also after it (if the inflammatory phase of injury is strong). It has even been suggested to replace "preemptive analgesia" by the term "preventive analgesia" and to use the term "preemptive analgesia" only for the limited effect on sensitization by the part of preventive treatment that begins before surgery and does not include the postoperative periods (5, 6). The other definition for the treatment that prevents central sensitization during both operative and immediate postoperative phases is "protective analgesia" (7). It is clear that in principle, the outcome of the "preventive analgesia" should be more significant than that of "limited preemptive analgesia."

3. Two Approaches to Reveal Effect of Preemptive Analgesia

One approach is to demonstrate a reduction in pain intensity and/or analgesic use beyond the drug presence in the biophase. This approach is based on a study design comparing preoperative treatment and non-treatment groups (PRE versus NO). The other approach is to prove that a treatment applied before surgery is more effective than the same treatment provided at the end of surgery (PRE versus POST). The PRE versus NO approach was commonly used in the initial clinical studies on preemptive analgesia (8); the PRE versus POST approach was introduced later (9).

These two approaches may reflect two different definitions of preemptive analgesia that were discussed previously. The PRE versus POST design has led to a situation in which establishment of sensitization during inflammatory injuries in the initial postoperative period is excluded from consideration; the PRE versus NO design may include the impact of inflammation (if the PRE treatment also covers the postoperative phase). Katz recently compared the outcomes of studies with both approaches designed to reveal the prevention of pain hypersensitivity (6). He reported that the PRE versus NO design resulted in a positive effect more frequently than the PRE versus POST design and that, in general, the effects with the PRE versus NO design were of greater magnitude. These findings illustrate that more complete prevention of sensitization (caused not only by incisional but also inflammatory injuries) has greater clinical value.

The PRE versus POST approach was the most common study design for preemptive analgesia and almost all systematic reviews are based on the studies with this approach. Moiniche et al. published a systematic review of 80 studies based on this design (7). The authors drew a negative conclusion regarding the potential clinical value of preemptive analgesia in the treatment of postoperative pain. At the same time, they noted that the trials of single-dose epidural analgesia resulted in an improvement in pain control in 7 of 11 studies (the best outcome of all types of analgesic interventions in their review). They stated that validity and clinical relevance of the effect of epidural analgesia were questionable and difficult to interpret; therefore, they concluded that the results reveal lack of evidence for any important effect (rather than evidence for lack of effect). The conclusions of Moiniche et al. are largely at odds with those of Ong et al. (10), who presented a meta-analysis using the methodology proposed by the Cochrane Collaboration. The authors analyzed 66 studies related to five groups of interventions: epidural analgesia, peripheral local anesthetic infiltrations, systemic NMDA (N-methyl-D-aspartate) receptor antagonists, systemic nonsteroidal antiinflammatory drugs (NSAID), and systemic opioids. Only studies with the PRE versus POST design were included. The analyzed outcome measures were pain intensity, supplemental analgesic consumption, and time to first analgesic. They found a pronounced preemptive effect with epidural analgesia, local infiltration, and systemic NSAID administration. Most impressive were reductions (from 44 to 58% at very high levels of statistical significance) in supplemental analgesic consumption. With opioids and NMDA receptor antagonists, the results were equivocal. Ong et al. suggested that ten additional new trials (2001–2003, not included in the review by Moiniche et al.), stricter criteria for inclusion into the analysis, and a different approach for calculation of the pain score differences gave them an opportunity to better demonstrate a real value of preemptive analgesia for several types of analgesic interventions. Thus, with the PRE versus POST approach, results regarding clinical value of preemptive analgesia are often controversial.

4. Verification of Direct Pharmacologic Effect of Treatment

Control of the degree of completeness of direct pharmacologic intervention is the other factor contributing to the preemptive analgesia controversy. Such control is very important and can be done in various ways, for example, by verification of the sufficiency of a neural blockade in the assessment of the effect of epidurally administered local anesthetics. The interesting results in this regard are presented by Shir et al. (11). They compared three groups of patients undergoing radical prostatectomy with general, epidural, or combined epidural and general anesthesia. Preemptive analgesia was observed only with epidural anesthesia because this type of anesthesia allows for even minor discomfort to be noticed and treated during surgery. The authors concluded that "complete intraoperative blockade of afferent signals to the CNS is fundamental in decreasing postoperative pain." Another study with well-controlled sufficiency of epidural anesthesia in patients undergoing radical prostatectomy also reported positive results. Gottschalk et al. (12) administered epidural bupivacaine or epidural fentanyl before induction of general anesthesia and throughout the surgery, and compared the pain outcomes with those of similar treatment initiated at the fascial closure. Sufficiency of epidural blockade was verified by measurement of the sensory level (at least the fourth thoracic dermatome) before induction of general anesthesia and also in the postanesthesia care unit. Patients who did not have a T4 sensory level were excluded from the study. The authors reported that the patients who received epidural bupivacaine or epidural fentanyl before surgical incision (preemptive analgesia group) experienced less pain while they were hospitalized (visual analog scale was one-third less, $P=0.007$). At 9.5 weeks, 86% of the patients who received preemptive analgesia were pain-free compared with only 47% of the control patients ($P=0.004$). The authors concluded that, even in the presence of aggressive postoperative pain management, preemptive epidural analgesia decreases postoperative pain during hospitalization and long after discharge (12). In many studies that failed to find any preemptive effect, the effectiveness of the blockade was not controlled. Studies by Kehlet's group (13) have clearly demonstrated difficulties in providing complete blockade of noxious stimuli during surgery, indicated by an increase in plasma cortisol concentration and other metabolic responses. Kehlet's results show that only an extensive epidural blockade from T4 to S5 prevents the cortisol response to lower abdominal surgery (14). Kehlet suggested that conflicting results reported in the literature about the effect of neural blockade on the cortisol response are probably attributable to the insufficient afferent block in most studies. The same argument is related to conflicting results regarding preemptive analgesia.

5. Partial Preemptive Effect in Control

The effect of preemptive analgesia is assessed by measuring the difference between outcomes in control and preemptive groups. However, the use of a routine anesthetic technique used in the control group exploits, to some extent, the advantages of preemptive analgesia. For example, in most of the studies on preemptive analgesia, opioids were used in control groups in the induction of anesthesia and during surgery. Nitrous oxide can also induce preemptive analgesia (15, 16). However, this anesthetic was used for anesthesia maintenance in both control and preemptive groups. Finally, with recovery from anesthesia, the effective antinociceptive treatment in the control group during the initial postoperative period is governed by ethical considerations. As a consequence, the difference between groups in terms of degree of "noxious bombardment" of the spinal cord during general anesthesia and initial postoperative period could become too small to be of clinical significance.

6. Intensity of Noxious Stimuli

Surgery with low-intensity noxious stimuli during surgery and the initial postoperative period may not generate enough difference between preemptive and control groups. In addition, low-intensity stimuli may not trigger the altered central processing of afferent inputs. As a result, postoperative pain will represent only "physiologic," not "pathologic," pain (when pain response is profoundly amplified). If pathologic pain is absent, preemptive analgesia has nothing to prevent. One might argue that preemptive analgesia can be observed only when a control group demonstrates that the surgery was painful enough to have a preemptive effect (17).

7. Difference in Drug Concentrations During Postoperative Period

Because of the drugs' pharmacokinetics, the time difference in drug administration between preemptive (PRE) and control (POST) groups results in significantly larger concentrations after anesthesia recovery in the POST group. Thus, the analgesic effect of the treatment in the postoperative period may be more pronounced in the POST group (reducing the difference between outcomes of the PRE and POST groups). Only one study specifically addressed this problem in the assessment of preemptive effect. Norman et al. (18) administered systemic ketorolac immediately after tourniquet inflation above the area of ankle surgery in the POST group (and before tourniquet inflation in the PRE group) so that the PRE and POST groups had similar systemic drug concentrations postoperatively. The authors demonstrated a significant preemptive effect.

8. Outcome Measures

Pain intensity is the most important outcome measure. Patient-rated pain scales (e.g., visual analog scale, numeric rating scale) are most commonly used for the measurement of spontaneous and movement-induced pain (standardized movement like sitting up from lying position). Measures of primary and secondary mechanical hyperalgesia (pressure algometry on or near the wound dressing, von Frey filaments at a distance from the wound) are also used. However, preemptive effect regarding mechanical hyperalgesia does not necessarily reflect preemptive effect regarding spontaneous pain. For example, Tverskoy et al. (19) demonstrated that fentanyl and ketamine preemptively decreased postoperative wound hyperalgesia, but not spontaneous pain.

The other outcome measure is analgesic (opioid) consumption. However, analgesic consumption is a less reliable index than pain intensity for assessing preemptive analgesia. There is no convincing evidence for proportionality between postoperative pain intensity and opioid requirements. Opioid plasma concentration-analgesic response curves are surprisingly steep (20). As a result, the within-patient difference between opioid concentration that is still ineffective and the concentration that provides complete analgesia may be too small to detect correct fractions of the response. In other words, it is impossible to distinguish between the doses of an opioid providing 50% and 100% pain relief in an individual patient.

Currently, patient-controlled analgesia (PCA) is commonly used in studies on preemptive analgesia. However, the use of PCA for algesimetry has several problems that undermine its usefulness. In addition to the problem of the quantal nature of analgesic response to opioids discussed above, the PCA method has another potential deficiency. Analgesic usage is significantly influenced by such factors as mood, anxiety, expectations of recovery, and perception of support (21). As a result, analgesic consumption reflects not only pain intensity but also other postoperative distress factors. If the administration of opioids is kept at the same level in all study groups, preemptive analgesia expresses itself only by a change in pain intensity. With the use of PCA, a change in opioid consumption is the main index of preemptive analgesia, but changes in pain intensity may also be in play. The balance of simultaneous changes in pain intensity and in analgesic consumption represents a difficulty for providing statistically significant results. In most studies, changes in one outcome measure counterbalance changes in another. As a result, changes of both measures often fail to reach a statistically significant level.

The main question of preemptive analgesia is how to demonstrate its *maximal* clinical benefits. It is clear that this cannot be done simply by comparing preincisional versus postincisional treatment groups. A number of requirements for adequacy of preemptive analgesia assessment should be observed to avoid potential study problems. The most important of them is providing effective suppression of the afferent input with sufficient duration of such treatment (that covers the initial postoperative period).

References

1. Crile GW (1913) The kinetic theory of shock and its prevention through anoci-association. Lancet 185:7–16
2. Woolf CJ (1983) Evidence for a central component of postinjury pain hypersensitivity. Nature 308:686–688

3. Wall PD (1988) The prevention of postoperative pain. Pain 33:289–290
4. Kissin I (2000) Preemptive analgesia. Anesthesiology 93:1138–1143
5. Kissin I (1994) Preemptive analgesia: terminology and clinical relevance. Anesth Analg 79:809–810
6. Katz J (2003) Timing of treatment and preemptive analgesia. In: Rowbotham DJ, Macintyre PE (eds) Acute pain. Arnold, London, pp 113–162
7. Moiniche S, Kehlet H, Dahl JB (2002) A qualitative and quantitative systematic review of preemptive analgesia for postoperative pain relief. Anesthesiology 96:725–741
8. Tverskoy M, Cozacov C, Ayache M, Bradley EL, Kissin I (1990) Postoperative pain after inguinal herniorrhaphy with different types of anesthesia. Anesth Analg 70:29–35
9. McQuay HJ (1992) Pre-emptive analgesia. Br J Anaesth 69:1–3
10. Ong KS, Lirk P, Seymour RA (2005) The efficacy of preemptive analgesia for acute postoperative pain management: a meta-analysis. Anesth Analg 100:757–773
11. Shir Y, Raja SN, Frank SM (1994) The effect of epidural versus general anesthesia on postoperative pain and analgesia requirements in patients undergoing radical prostatectomy. Anesthesiology 80:49–56
12. Gottschalk A, Smith DS, Jobes DR, Kennedy SK, Lally SE, Noble VE, Grugan KF, Seifert HA, Cheung A (1998) Preemptive epidural analgesia and recovery from radical prostatectomy: a randomized controlled trial. JAMA 279:1076–1082
13. Moller IW, Hjortso E, Kratz T, Wandall E, Kehlet H (1984) The modifying effect of spinal anesthesia in intra- and postoperative adrenocortical and hyperglycemic response to surgery. Acta Anaesthesiol Scan 28:266–269
14. Moller IW, Rem J, Brandt MR, Kehlet H (1982) Effect of posttraumatic epidural analgesia on the cortisol and hyperglycemic response to surgery. Acta Anaesthesiol Scand 26:56–58
15. Goto T, Marota JJA, Crosby G (1994) Nitrous oxide induces preemptive analgesia in the rat that is antagoinized by halothane. Anesthesiology 80:409–416
16. O'Connor TC, Abram SE (1995) Inhibitin of nociception-induced spinal sensitization by anesthetic agents. Anesthesiology 82:259–266
17. Jebeles JA, Reilly JS, Gutierrez JF, Bradley EL, Kissin I (1991) The effect of pre-incisional infiltration of tonsils with bupivacaine on the pain following tonsillectomy under general anesthesia. Pain 47:305–308
18. Norman PH, Daley MD, Lindsey RW (2001) Preemptive analgesic effects of ketorolac in ankle fracture surgery. Anesthesiology 94: 599–603
19. Tverskoy M, Oz Y, Isakson A, Finger J, Bradley EL, Kissin I (1994) Preemptive effect of fentanyl and ketamine on postoperative pain and wound hyperalgeisa. Anesth Analg 78:205–210
20. Austin KL, Stapleton JV, Mather LE (1980) Relationship between blood meperidine concentrations and analgesic response: A preliminary report. Anesthesiology 53:460–466
21. Jamison RN, Taft K, O'Hara JP, Ferrante FM (1993) Psychosocial and pharmacologic predictors of satisfaction with intravenous patient-controlled analgesia. Anesth Analg 77:121–125

Chapter 35

Standardization of Pain Measurements in Clinical Trials

William K. Sietsema

Abstract

Standardization of the measurement of pain in clinical trials will reduce variability, thus improving the quality of the data and reducing the number of patients needed to conduct pain trials. Standardization applies to the physical and psychosocial environment surrounding the patient, and there are many elements within this environment that can be effectively controlled. For example, the appearance of the examination room can be selected for neutrality and influences from visitors and staff can be minimized. Training is an important aspect of the standardization process and should be provided to all study staff. Staff training should first provide orientation on the protocol objectives and procedures and then a thorough discussion of the pain measures being used and how assessments will be conducted. Furthermore, as the patient is ultimately responsible for assessing his or her level of pain, it is important to train the patient to make reliable and accurate assessments of pain.

Key words: Analgesia, Pain, Measurement, Assessment, Clinical trial, Standardization, Variability, Environmental factors, Training, Pain relief, Visual analog scale, Dual stopwatch

1. Introduction

Despite intensive research into pain therapies over the last decade, there continue to be significant unmet patient needs (1–5). Thus, it is important that research into mechanisms as well as treatment of pain continue. Pain can be difficult to measure, and where there is a high degree of variability in the measurement of pain, the number of patients needed to evaluate a new treatment may be unreasonably large. Accordingly, consistent and accurate measurement of pain is critical to an efficient evaluation of new treatments (6). Standardization of the methods used and the environment in which pain is measured will help improve the quality of the data and reduce the number of patients needed to evaluate a new therapy. Due to elements of variability in pain

Arpad Szallasi (ed.), *Analgesia: Methods and Protocols*, Methods in Molecular Biology, vol. 617,
DOI 10.1007/978-1-60327-323-7_35, © Springer Science+Business Media, LLC 2010

measurements discussed below, clinical trials of new therapies for the treatment of pain will benefit from standardization and calibration of pain measurements (7).

2. Elements of Variability in Pain Assessments

One of the reasons why pain is difficult to measure is because it is not something the clinician can directly observe (8). The sensation of pain is internal to the patient, and something which only the patient can feel (9). The clinician, as an observer, is limited to interpreting outward signs, which may indicate pain that the patient feels.

The pain felt by a patient may vary, depending on factors of the patient's psychological makeup such as mood, attitude, and stoicism. For example, patients in a good mood (perhaps family has just been to visit) are likely to feel less pain than patients who are unhappy (perhaps it is a rainy day). Patients with a generally positive attitude may feel less pain than patients who feel hopeless or depressed (10). And stoic patients may feel less pain (or report less pain) than patients with less stoicism. There may also be cultural or social expectations related to the sensation or reporting of pain (11, 12). Perhaps the best example of this is gender difference, where, for example, in some cultures or societies, men are expected to be more tolerant to pain, thus leading to underreporting of pain (13).

Furthermore, the pain felt by patients may vary by other factors. The surrounding atmosphere will impact how pain is felt and reported (14). For example, if the examination room has graphic posters of medical procedures or abstract art, these may make the patient feel anxious and this can be manifested by an increase in pain felt or reported (15). On the contrary, peaceful pictures may reduce the sensation of discomfort and lessen the use of pain medication (15–17). Temperature, lighting (18), and color can have an impact on the reporting of pain, as can the presence of music (19). The behaviors and status of office personnel can also have a profound impact on how a patient feels and reports pain (20, 21). For example, if the study nurse is in a bad mood, this will most likely cause the patient to report greater levels of pain. Even tone of voice from the study nurse may have a significant affect on how the patient reports pain (22).

There are additional factors that may impact how a patient feels or reports pain. Patients have varying thresholds for pain, so those with a low threshold will report more pain while those with a high threshold will report less pain. In models of postsurgical pain, there may be differences among patients in the performance of the surgery (23). For example, in the dental pain model (Chapter 15), there can be differences in the amount of impaction of teeth or differences in the number of teeth that are impacted (24). Recent activity by the patient or movement may also impact the patient's pain. For example, if the nursing staff have just changed the bedding or have cleaned the surgical wound, the patient may report greater levels of pain. There may also be differences in a patient's biological response to a therapy, and these differences can have a neurologic basis or a metabolic basis.

3. Reasons for Standardizing Assessments

From the earlier discussion, it should be apparent that there are many factors, which may impact the way a patient feels or reports pain. One of the main reasons to standardize and calibrate pain assessment is to reduce the inherent variability in the measures. Standardization can reduce *intra*-observer variability. In most cases, this means reducing the variability with which the patient rates his or her level of pain and is accomplished by training the patient. The same training can reduce *inter*-observer variability if applied consistently to all the patients in the trial.

Standardization of the conditions can also reduce variability by reducing any positive or negative influence of the surrounding environment, as well as by reducing the influence caused by the study nurse and other site personnel.

The outcome of standardization of the measures and the environment will be reduced variability and increased statistical power to demonstrate a difference between treatment groups. Thus, standardization may allow a trial to be conducted with fewer patients. Standardization can also improve the reproducibility of the results, perhaps alleviating the need to conduct an extra clinical trial, which often occurs because one of the pivotal trials has failed due to inconsistency of the methods.

4. Standardizing Pain Measurements

Standardizing the measurement of pain focuses primarily on training clinical investigators and other site personnel on how to standardize the environment and how to train the patients to consistently and accurately assess their pain. There is no measurement device that the observer can directly apply in order to measure the patient's pain, so the best we can do is provide an appropriate measurement device for the patient to use, and train them in its optimal use. Accordingly, our role is to standardize the environment as much as possible and to train the patient to use the measurement device and then monitor how well he or she performs in his or her use of the measurement device.

4.1. Standardizing the Room

Whenever possible, it is desirable to have a patient assess his or her pain in a similar environment each time pain is assessed. Using the same room for each pain assessment would be ideal. In most clinical trial settings, the room being used would be an examination room or a hospital room. Ideally, the room should have neutral color paint, perhaps a soft pastel. Avoid paint schemes and décor that make the room look either commercial in nature or too home-like. The room should be in good repair and free of damage to walls. The floor should be hospital clean. Pictures on the wall are fine, but it would be best to avoid graphic medical posters or pictures that may evoke an emotional response. For example, paintings by Picasso would be ill-advised. The temperature of the room should be comfortable and stable. There should not be needles in sight, nor should there be any medical equipment that may be associated with a painful procedure. The level of lighting should be consistent, and because bright lights may reduce pain (17), lighting during a pain study should be moderate to dim so as to enhance the dynamic range of the measurement of pain.

4.2. Standardizing Study Personnel

Frequently, an observer, such as a study nurse, will be present while the patient is assessing his or her pain. This observer should be dressed in a neutral fashion, with loose-fitting clothes. A white lab coat is ideal so as to provide a clinical appearance. A clip board may improve the standardization of a clinical appearance. The observer should not wear revealing clothing. The observer should also avoid wearing any cologne or perfume, as many patients may be influenced by the odor, either because it is bothersome to the patient (25) or because it may create an attractive force between the patient and the observer.

The study nurse should also be standardized with respect to the way he or she approaches the patient and interacts with the patient (this is discussed further below).

4.3. Standardizing Other Environmental Factors

The surrounding environment can have a profound effect on the perception of pain (26). There are many environmental factors which may influence how a patient feels or reports pain. For example, guests can have a major influence on the patient's assessment of pain, either because the patient feels a need to meet their expectations or because of cultural pressures (27). Therefore, guests should be asked to leave the room prior to asking the patient to assess his or her pain. If it is possible for the patient to be alone for 5–10 min prior to pain assessment, this would be ideal.

Because recent painful procedures can have an impact on assessment of pain, it is important that pain assessments not be conducted shortly after an unpleasant procedure, such as drawing blood or cleaning a wound, or forced movement of the patient. Accordingly, the timing of pain assessments should be coordinated with other activities, especially in a hospital setting, so as to avoid such influences. In most cases, hospital personnel are quite happy to coordinate activities with the study nurse so as to optimize the quality of the clinical research.

If assessments are done in a hospital room with the patient in bed, the position of the bed should be for normal comfort, and the patient should not assess pain shortly after changing the bed position or shortly after performance of some painful procedure or forced movement.

5. Training

The objective of training is to reduce, as much as possible, any variability associated with measurement of pain. Training begins with education of the study personnel and should include training that will be given to the patient in order to standardize the way he or she measures his or her pain. Training of study personnel can be accomplished at an investigator meeting or during study initiation visits or both. Ideally, the study monitors should be able to provide such training so that they can recognize improper practice and provide additional training as needed to existing personnel or to new personnel who join the study team after formal training has been provided.

5.1. Training Site Personnel

Site personnel should first be well-trained on the protocol, including objectives of the research, study design, patient eligibility requirements, and nature and timing of pain assessments. Once study personnel have been trained on the basics of the protocol, it is advisable to have more focused and in-depth training in pain assessment for those study personnel (and their potential back-ups) who will serve as observers during the trial. This more in-depth training should begin with some of the basics of pain measurement but should also include a detailed discussion of each pain assessment instrument that will be used in the trial, especially with regard to elements of variability and how they can be reduced.

It may be argued that some study personnel are sufficiently experienced, so it is un-necessary to cover the basics of pain measurement. However, the high turnover of study personnel and the propensity for many sites to inject newly hired personnel directly into the clinical trial process suggests that this basic training should be provided, even if there is a risk of annoying a few of the more experienced study personnel. Highly experienced study personnel may even harbor mistaken concepts and basic training may be a useful way to refresh their understanding.

Some useful concepts to include in basic training include:

- *The difference between pain intensity and pain relief, and the scales used to measure each*

Pain intensity is how much pain a patient feels and can be the current level of pain or collected as pain felt over some recall period, such as a day, a week or even a month. In some variations of pain intensity, a patient is queried about the maximum pain, or the average pain, or even the minimum pain felt during the recall period. In contrast, pain relief is always measured in relation to a baseline level of pain and is an assessment of how much the pain has improved since the baseline reference.

- *Guidelines for differentiating between mild, moderate, and severe pain*

Study personnel and patients often benefit from some approximate definitions related to severity of pain. For example, these definitions have proven useful in clinical research settings:

> *Mild*: you cannot ignore the pain but it is not so bad that you would feel you need to treat it
>
> *Moderate*: the pain interferes with your concentration and you might have to stop and take some medication or treat it in some way
>
> *Severe*: not only does the pain interfere with your concentration, but you have to change your behavior to cope with it; you would definitely feel the need to treat the pain.

It may additionally be useful to translate these definitions into a guide on how they relate to choices on a visual analog scale. An example of this is shown in Fig. 1, which can be provided to the patient in order to improve the consistency of assessments made with a visual analog scale versus those made with a Likert scale. (A Likert scale provides text-based options for the subject to choose from, typically five items with two positive, two negative, and

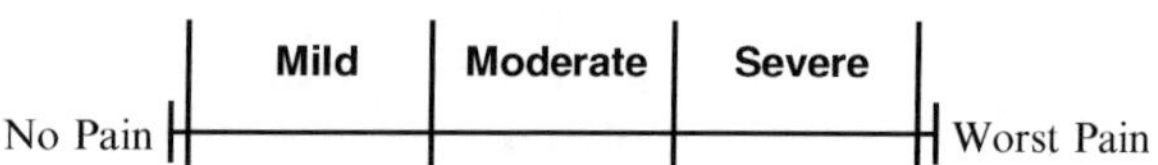

Fig. 1. Typical 100 mm Visual Analog Scale with guidance for definitions of mild, moderate, and severe pain

one neutral, for example, "strongly agree," "agree," "neither agree nor disagree," "disagree," and "strongly disagree.")

- *Use of the stopwatch technique for measuring time to onset of pain relief*

  The dual stopwatch technique can be used to assess the time to onset of pain relief. For this technique, the patient is given two stopwatches, which are both started at the time a treatment for pain is administered. The patient is asked to stop the first stopwatch when he or she feels any perceptible pain relief and to press the second stopwatch when the pain relief becomes meaningful.

- *Definitions of meaningful pain relief versus perceptible pain relief.*

  In order to standardize the way a patient uses the dual stopwatch, the following statements can be used:

  > "I would like you to stop the first stopwatch when you first feel any pain-relieving effect whatsoever from the drug. This does not necessarily mean that you feel completely better, although you might, but when you first feel any differences in the pain you have had."
  >
  > "I would like you to stop the second stopwatch when you have meaningful pain relief. That is, when the relief from the pain is meaningful to you."

- *Use of visual analog scales*

  It is surprising how frequently errors are made in the use of visual analog scales. Perhaps, the most frequent error is an incorrect length. VAS scales are generally designed to be 100 mm in length and the measurement is made in mm from the left anchor. Thus, if the scale is longer or shorter than 100 mm, the measurement will not accurately reflect the magnitude of the patient's pain. Length errors can occur when a form is printed, or if a form is copied. For this reason, any new supply of printed forms should be checked to ensure the length is correct. Copying of VAS scales is discouraged, but if necessary, the length should be checked since most copy machines do not reproduce the true length of the scale.

  Errors may also be made in the use of a VAS scale. Patients should be instructed to make a single vertical line on the scale to indicate their pain intensity. Circles, checks, and X-marks should not be used on a VAS as these would create uncertainty as to where the measure should be made.

  An additional common error is related to the placement of the scale descriptors. These should always be placed to the left or right of the scale anchors, never under the scale itself, as the presence of the descriptors under portions of the scale may inhibit full use of the scale by the patient.

5.2. Training Patients

Patients are generally quite capable of learning how to standardize their assessment of pain and are eager to be involved. Patients who lack interest in the quality of their pain assessment data may not be good candidates for a clinical trial so it may be worth excluding such patients.

Much of the same training that is used for study personnel can also be used for training patients. For example, patients need to know the difference between pain intensity and pain relief and the scales being used to measure each of these in the trial (28).

6. Addressing Patients and Working with Patients

There is much that can be done to standardize the way one addresses patients and works with them in the clinical setting:

1. Make sure outside influences, as discussed earlier in this chapter, are not affecting the patient.
2. Ask questions the same way to the patients each time you prompt them to conduct a pain assessment.
3. If there are apparent discrepancies in a patient's answers, for example, if the patient scores his or her pain intensity as severe in a Likert scale but as mild on the visual analog scale, repeat the definitions and ask the patient to clarify the responses.
4. Do not respond to patient's responses in a positive or negative way; patients often seek approval in the response that has been given, but any action construed as approval could influence the patient's subsequent responses.
5. Avoid socializing with patient; this can be difficult to avoid because it is human nature to converse with one another. It is important that the observer not be thought of as an acquaintance or "friend" of the patient as this can influence the responses that are given. If study personnel become too familiar with a patient, it might be worth considering whether to have a different observer work with the patient, though this in itself will create some variability in the data.
6. Do not be either cheerful or depressed; imagine the impact of being cheerful about a sunny day outside versus depressed about the constant rain – your attitude will influence the patient's response.
7. Avoid guiding or leading the patient; for example, do not ask the patient how much better he or she is feeling because the patient may feel that you are expecting him or her to feel better.
8. Do not discuss patient's condition, as this may create expectations that the pain will get worse or better.

9. Do come across as "neutral" and don't try to be encouraging or discouraging.
10. If a painful or uncomfortable activity is required, such as drawing blood, or cleaning a wound, schedule it shortly *after* a pain assessment.
11. Restrict ambulation during 15 min preceding pain assessment, especially if ambulation is likely to increase the intensity of pain.
12. Have the patient make assessments in his or her mind and share them with the observer before marking the worksheets. This will help solidify the assessments in the patient's mind and will avoid the need to make corrections to the worksheets.
13. For serial pain measurements, the observer should tell the patient when he or she will return for the next assessment and how to reach him or her in the meantime, if needed.

7. Summary

The best quality data will be obtained when the environment for assessment of pain has been standardized. This standardization can be achieved with careful attention to the room and surrounding environment in which assessments are made and with careful training of study personnel and patients so that pain measurements are made as consistently and as accurately as possible. Standardization of pain measures within a clinical trial will substantially reduce variability, thus improving the quality of data and increasing the chances of demonstrating statistically significant differences between treatment groups.

References

1. Holt DV, Viscusi ER, Wordell CJ (2007) Extended-duration agents for perioperative pain management. Curr Pain Headache Rep 11(1):33–37
2. O'Bryant SE, Marcus DA, Rains JC, Penzien DB (2005) Neuropsychology of migraine: present status and future directions. Expert Rev Neurother 5(3):363–370
3. Laufer S (2004) Osteoarthritis therapy–are there still unmet needs? Rheumatology (Oxford) 43(Suppl 1):i9–i15
4. Harden N, Cohen M (2003) Unmet needs in the management of neuropathic pain. J Pain Symptom Manage 25(5 Suppl):S12–S17
5. Dionne RA, Witter J (2003) NIH-FDA analgesic drug development workshop: translating scientific advances into improved pain relief. Clin J Pain 19(3):139–147
6. Caraceni A, Brunelli C, Martini C, Zecca E, De Conno F (2005) Cancer pain assessment in clinical trials. A review of the literature (1999–2002). J Pain Symptom Manage 29(5):507–519
7. Chapman CR (2005) Pain perception and assessment. Minerva Anestesiol 71(7–8):413–417
8. Sokka T (2005) Assessment of pain in rheumatic diseases. Clin Exp Rheumatol 23(5 Suppl 39):S77–S84

9. Collett B, O'Mahoney S, Schofield P, Closs SJ, Potter J, Guideline Development Group (2007) The assessment of pain in older people. Clin Med 7(5):496–500
10. Katona C, Peveler R, Dowrick C, Wessely S, Feinmann C, Gask L, Lloyd H, Williams AC, Wager E (2005) Pain symptoms in depression: definition and clinical significance. Clin Med 5(4):390–395
11. Fillingim RB, Edwards RR, Powell T (2000) Sex-dependent effects of reported familial pain history on recent pain complaints and experimental pain responses. Pain 86(1–2): 87–94
12. Arber A (2006) Forum for applied education and training: rethinking pain assessment. Eur J Cancer Care (Engl) 15(2):200–207
13. Miller C, Newton SE (2006) Pain perception and expression: the influence of gender, personal self-efficacy, and lifespan socialization. Pain Manag Nurs 7(4):148–152
14. Malenbaum S, Keefe FJ, Williams A, Ulrich R, Somers TJ (2008) Pain in its environmental context: implications for designing environments to enhance pain control. Pain 134:241–244
15. Ulrich R (1984) View through a window may influence recovery from surgery. Science 224:420–421
16. Tse MMY, Ng JKF, Chung JWY, Wong TKS (2002) The effect of visual stimuli on pain threshold and tolerance. J Clin Nurs 11:264–269
17. Ulrich RS, Lunden O, Etinge JL (1993) Effects of exposure to nature and abstract pictures on patient recovery from heart surgery. Psychophysiology. 30:S7
18. Walch JM, Rabin BS, Day R, Williams JN, Choi K, Kang JD (2005) The effect of sunlight on postoperative analgesic medication use: a prospective study of patients undergoing spinal surgery. Psychosom Med 67:156–153
19. Richards T, Johnson J, Sparks A, Emerson H (2007) The effect of music therapy on patients' perception and manifestation of pain, anxiety, and patient satisfaction. Medsurg Nurs 16(1):7–15
20. Williams DA, Park KM, Ambrose KR, Clauw DJ (2007) Assessor status influences pain recall. J Pain 8(4):343–348
21. Spiers J (2006) Expressing and responding to pain and stoicism in home-care nurse-patient interactions. Scand J Caring Sci 20(3):293–301
22. Griffith CH III, Wilson JF, Langer S, Haist SA (2003) House staff nonverbal communication skills and standardized patient satisfaction. Gen Intern Med 18(3):170–174
23. Olmedo-Gaya MV, Vallecillo-Capilla M, Galvez-Mateos R (2002) Relation of patient and surgical variables to postoperative pain and inflammation in the extraction of third molars. Med Oral 7(5):360–369
24. Levine JD, Gordon NC, Smith R, Fields HL (1982) Post-operative pain: effect of extent of injury and attention. Brain Res 234(2):500–504
25. Villemure C, Bushnell MC (2007) The effects of the steroid androstadienone and pleasant odorants on the mood and pain perception of men and women. Eur J Pain 11(2):181–191
26. Sharar SR, Carrougher GJ, Nakamura D, Hoffman HG, Blough DK, Patterson DR (2007) Factors influencing the efficacy of virtual reality distraction analgesia during post-burn physical therapy: preliminary results from 3 ongoing studies. Arch Phys Med Rehabil 88(12 Suppl 2):S43–S49
27. McCracken LM (2005) Social context and acceptance of chronic pain: the role of solicitous and punishing responses. Pain 113(1–2):155–159
28. Angst MS, Brose WG, Dyck JB (1999) The relationship between the visual analog pain intensity and pain relief scale changes during analgesic drug studies in chronic pain patients. Anesthesiology 91(1):34–41

Chapter 36

Procedural Sedation and Analgesia Research

James R. Miner

Abstract

The study of procedural sedation and analgesia has experienced significant development recently. As specific procedural sedation and analgesia agents have been developed and introduced into clinical practice, safety and efficacy studies have been conducted. The principle difficulty in conducting these studies has been the relatively low frequency of traditional outcome measures. As procedural sedation and analgesia research has expanded, measurement techniques have been refined to allow for precise comparisons between smaller groups of subjects to improve the capacity to compare these procedures. We have used capnography, bispectral EEG analysis, and subject perceptions of pain and recall as surrogate predictors of adverse events in order to compare agents and procedural techniques in procedural sedation and analgesia.

Key words: Procedural sedation and analgesia, Research methodology, Capnography, Level of consciousness, Oxygen saturation, Monitoring

1. Introduction

Although there have been a large number of procedural sedation and analgesia (PSA) studies, many questions remain about the optimal approach to research. Most of the procedural sedation and analgesia outcome factors relate to complications of the procedure. These include unplanned endotracheal intubation, bag mask ventilation, hypoxia, hypotension, or emesis. The rate of airway complications has been described at 1.4% for ketamine (1) and 5.0 to 9.4% for propofol (2–5), and the rate of serious complications (aspiration, anoxia with neurological impairment, death) is extremely rare. These low rates translate into outcome measures that need to be studied in very large trials, limiting the flexibility of research in this area. This can be compensated for by using more frequently occurring surrogate markers for complications. Surrogate markers such as the respiratory depression criteria we have used (3–6) or the adverse respiratory events criteria

Arpad Szallasi (ed.), *Analgesia: Methods and Protocols*, Methods in Molecular Biology, vol. 617,
DOI 10.1007/978-1-60327-323-7_36, © Springer Science+Business Media, LLC 2010

used by Burton (7) allow trends in respiratory depression to be compared using a relatively small number of patients. However, they have the disadvantage of having unclear clinical significance, limiting the external validity of the findings.

A similar approach can be extended to measures of the target depth of sedation. Commonly accepted measures of the depth of sedation, such as the Ramsey Sedation Scale (RSS) or the Observer's Assessment of Alertness Scale (OAAS) (8) are imprecise and subjective, and do not yield data that can be accurately compared. Objective measures such as the Bispectral Index (BIS) can yield more precise data that improves the comparison of achieved depths of sedation, allowing for the improved study of sedative dosing strategies and the sedation endpoints. Since the depth of sedation is likely to vary the chance of an adverse event, its precise determination has implications for the evaluation of the safety of various agents at given levels of sedation or in their likelihood to induce a given level of sedation.

Other outcome factors can be measured and compared, including medications used, procedure time, recovery time, subject pain, subject procedural recall, and procedural success. These outcomes can be difficult to relate to one another. Most procedural sedation and analgesia research has focused on the sedative, not the procedure for which the patient is being sedated, and studies have included a wide variety of procedures. If pain, recall, or procedure/sedation time is an outcome parameter, the complexity of the procedure for which the subject is being sedated will impact the measured parameter, resulting in a confounder that is difficult to quantify. Attempts to measure the complexity of the procedure (9) have been largely unsuccessful.

2. Materials

There are two types of monitoring used for PSA research: interactive monitoring by personnel and mechanical monitoring via specialized equipment.

2.1. Interactive Monitoring

Interactive monitoring is defined as the continuous observation of the subject by an individual capable of determining the subject's level of awareness and recognizing adverse events, including respiratory depression, apnea, upper airway obstruction, laryngospasm, and vomiting. This person must be able to continuously observe the patient's face, mouth, and chest wall motion in order to accomplish this.

Interactive monitor is also used to assess clinical signs of respiratory depression (CRD). CRD are defined as the addition of supplemental oxygen, an increase in supplemental oxygen, the

Score	Responsiveness
–4	Does not respond to mild prodding or shaking
–3	Responds only after mild prodding
–2	Responds only if name is called loudly
–1	Lethargic response to name
0	Responds readily to name spoken in normal tone
1	Anxious, restless
2	Anxious, Agitated
3	Very anxious, agitated
4	Combative, violent, or out of control

Fig. 1. Altered mental status scale

use of bag-valve-mask assisted ventilation, repositioning of the subject to improve ventilation, the use of a physical or verbal stimulus to induce breathing, the use of a reversal agent, the use of an oral airway, or intubation of the subject by the PSA operator. These criteria have been used in previous research to detect RD during PSA (7).

Interactive monitoring is also used to assess a subject's level of awareness using sedation scales. We have used the Altered Mental Status scale for this (Fig. 1), a subjective scale that we developed based on a combination of previously used scales accounting for agitation and sedation (10). In order to determine a subject's level of awareness, the observer must be able to interact with the subject to determine the response to verbal stimulation and mild prodding, which is defined as a glabellar tap (mid-forehead) with two fingers.

2.2. Mechanical Monitoring

2.2.1. Oxygenation

Pulse oximetry measures the percent of hemoglobin that is bound to oxygen via absorbance spectrometry of red and infrared light and is accurate to approximately 75% hemoglobin saturation. Pulse oximetry may be affected by numerous extrinsic factors, but a decrease from baseline is predictive of a decrease in subject oxygenation. Pulse oximetry has been found to be insensitive to changes in the respiratory status of subjects who receive supplemental oxygen (6, 11), and therefore we combine it with other measures of respiratory status.

2.2.2. Ventilation

Capnography is the measurement of the partial pressure of carbon dioxide (CO_2) in exhaled breath expressed over time. The relationship of CO_2 partial pressure to time is represented graphically by the CO_2 waveform or capnogram. Changes in the capnogram shape indicated changes in ventilatory status, while changes in end-tidal CO_2 ($EtCO_2$), the maximum CO_2 concentration at the end of each tidal breath, can be used to detect changes in the adequacy of ventilation. The capnogram sample is obtained using a nasal cannula positioned beneath the subject's nose.

The capnogram consists of four phases (Fig. 2) (12). Phase 1 (dead space ventilation, A–B) represents early exhalation when the dead space is cleared from the upper airway. Phase 2 (ascending phase, B–C) represents the increase in CO_2 concentration as air from the alveoli reaches the upper airway. Phase 3 (alveolar plateau, C–D) represents the CO_2 concentration reaching a stable value as alveolar air is expired. Point D, occurring at the end of the alveolar plateau, represents the maximum CO_2 concentration at the end of the breath ($EtCO_2$) and represents the number that appears on the monitor display of the capnograph. Phase 4 (D–E) represents inspiration.

The capnography waveform detects adverse respiratory events associated with PSA, including apnea, upper airway obstruction, laryngospasm, bronchospasm, and respiratory failure (4–7).

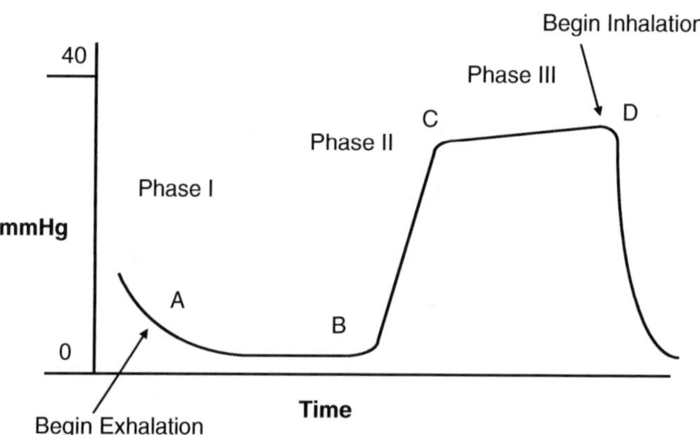

Fig. 2. Capnogram of Normal Ventilation. Phase I (points A–B) represents dead space ventilation. Phase II (points B–C) represents the ascending phase. Phase III (points C–D) represents the alveolar plateau. Point D represents the end-tidal CO_2. Phase IV (points D–E) represents inspiration

Normal physiologic variability results in changes in the amplitude of the waveform with no change in the respiratory rate or the $ETCO_2$ value. During hyperventilation, there is a decrease in the waveform amplitude, increase in respiratory rate, and a decrease in the $ETCO_2$ value. During hyponeic hypoventilation, there is a decrease in the waveform amplitude, a decrease in respiratory rate, and a decrease in the $ETCO_2$ value. During bradypneic hypoventilation, there is an increase in the amplitude of the waveform, a decrease in respiratory rate, and an increase in the $ETCO_2$ value. Bronchospasm results in a curved shape to phase II of the waveform, variable changes in respiratory rate, and an increase in the $ETCO_2$ value. Partial airway obstruction results in a normal waveform, a normal respiratory rate, and a decrease in $ETCO_2$ value due to increase in airway turbulence causing dilution of the expiratory sample with room air. Apnea and complete airway obstruction are represented by an absent waveform and an $ETCO_2$ value of 0. They are differentiated by the presence or absence of chest wall motion.

The unifying parameter associated with respiratory depression in these waveform descriptions is the change in $ETCO_2$ value from baseline. We have used a cutoff of 10 mmHg from baseline as a definition of respiratory depression using capnography for the purposes of comparison of all types of respiratory depression (2–6, 13, 14). This value was chosen in a post hoc analysis of PSA subjects, and likely will be refined as the use of capnography is better defined and further studied.

2.2.3. Hemodynamics

The three hemodynamic parameters of interest to PSA research include heart rate, blood pressure, and the electrocardiogram (ECG). Pulse oximetry and ECG both provide a continuous measure of heart rate. If pulse oximetry provides an adequate waveform, the heart rate will be accurate. A three lead ECG is used in order to detect dysrhythmias in addition to the heart rate.

Blood pressure may be measured by several methods. Manual auscultation using Korotkoff sounds is the most widely available method of measuring blood pressure, although automated noninvasive blood pressure (NIBP) machines can also be used. Manual auscultation is useful in situations where the automated monitors do not function well, such as when the subject is shivering, moving, or has an irregular heartbeat.

Automated NIBP monitors measure blood pressure based on oscillometry. The cuff pressure is raised above the systolic blood pressure, and then cuff pressure is gradually decreased while oscillations in cuff pressure due to arterial pulsations are sensed. The pressure at which the peak amplitude of oscillation occurs is the mean blood pressure; the systolic and diastolic pressures are then calculated internally.

2.2.4. Depth of Sedation/ Level of Consciousness Monitoring

Bispectral Index (BIS) monitoring is a continuous analog score (1–100) representing processed electroencephalogram (EEG) signals to measure a subject's level of awareness. It provides an objective measure of depth of sedation during PSA that varies with subjective sedation scales, the incidence of respiratory depression (4, 5) and a subject's ability to recall events during PSA (13). This monitor is very sensitive to subject motion and reports widely variable values (4, 15, 16). Motion artifact causes the monitor to give artificially high values. We therefore use the lowest score displayed over the monitor over each minute to represent a subject's level of sedation. It does not provide a measure of the dissociative sedation of ketamine, and cannot be used to study that drug.

3. Methods

3.1. Pre-procedure

1. Subject history obtained, including medical history, medication allergies, the nature of the procedure for which they are going to undergo PSA, and the time and nature of their last oral intake.
2. Subjects are placed on monitors: pulse oximetry, capnograph, BIS monitor, ECG monitor, and blood pressure monitor.
3. Interactive monitor begins to observe subject.
4. Baseline monitor measurements are obtained and repeated every one minute for the remainder of the procedure.
5. Pain is assessed using a 100 mm visual analog scale (VAS) with the indicators "no pain" on one side and "most pain possible" on the other.
6. Pre-procedure pain medication is given as needed for pain (morphine sulphate 0.1 mg/kg followed by 0.05 mg/kg every five minutes or fentanyl citrate 1.5 μg/kg followed by 0.75 μg/kg every 5 min until pain is relieved) (see Note 1).
7. Pain VAS is repeated after pain treatment is complete.
8. The patient is assigned to a study arm (see Note 2).

3.2. Procedure

1. Measurements are recorded every one minute during the procedure. The lowest BIS score over the previous minute is recorded. The $ETCO_2$ value with the largest absolute change from baseline is recorded each minute. Any absence of the capnograph waveform is noted.
2. The subject's AMS score is assessed by the interactive monitor every minute (see Note 3).

3. Adverse events and clinical signs of respiratory depression and the time at which they occur are noted by the interactive monitor (see Note 4).
4. The time of the start of the procedure is noted as the time the first dose of anesthetic is given.
5. All medication doses and their times are recorded (see Note 5).
6. The time of the start of the procedure for which the subject is receiving PSA is recorded.
7. The time of the completion of the procedure for which the subject was sedated is recorded. The success of the procedure is noted (see Note 6).
8. The time from the completion of the procedure for which the subject was sedated and from the start of the PSA procedure to the time the subject returns to the baseline AMS score is recorded.

3.3. Post-Procedure

1. Monitor measurements continue until 10 min after the subject has regained baseline mental status by the AMS scale.
2. The subject is asked to note whether or not they can recall any portion of the procedure for which they were sedated.
3. The subject is asked to recall whether or not they perceived any pain during the procedure (see Note 7).
4. A post procedure pain VAS is administered after a baseline AMS score has been achieved and before further pain medications are given.

4. Notes

1. The optimal method to treat pre-procedural pain has not been determined. There is evidence to support both weight-based protocols (3, 17, 18) and non-standardized dosing based on the patients level of complaint (19). These methods are described in the literature, and it is likely they result in different degrees of pre-procedural pain relief influencing the level of sedation needed and the amount of sedative used in the subsequent procedure. It is also likely that patients who receive more pre-procedural analgesia are more prone to respiratory depression during the sedation, confounding comparison between studies if different pain treatment end points are used.
2. Blinding has been a challenge in comparative trials and introduces potential bias. Given the dosing and titration

differences between medications (e.g., etomidate vs. propofol) and visible differences between medications (e.g., the physical appearance of propofol, the clinical appearance of dissociative sedation from ketamine), true blinding of agents and doses remains a challenge. Furthermore, given the importance of provider skill to sedative dosing, it is difficult to ethically blind the operator performing the sedation to the agent they are using. It is likely that physicians involved with a sedation study will have an opinion of which agent or protocol they prefer, or at least which they are more familiar with. This can affect how they dose the medication, the sedation depth they chose, and the point at which they chose to intervene for a possible adverse event. As a result, comparisons of sedation depth, interventions (e.g., bag mask ventilations or airway repositioning, or the physician's assessment of the patient) are difficult to interpret in these types of studies.

3. The principle limitation of sedation scales in PSA research is that they are subjective. Given the difficulty of blinding and the close association between the depth of sedation and respiratory depression (4), this limitation can have a great deal of influence on studies. There are several of these scales such as the observers assessment of alertness scale (OAAS), the Ramsey sedation scale (RSS), and the AMS scale (8, 10) that are based principally on whether or not the patient's eyes are closed and his/her response to stimuli. Essentially, these scales describe how asleep or awake a subject appears to be to the operator. The relationship of eye closing and the patient's response to stimuli to outcomes, such as success of the procedure, patient's recall of the procedure, and the incidence of adverse events during the procedure, is unclear (13).
4. Many of the obvious outcome criteria for respiratory depression, such as the use of a bag mask apparatus or the addition of supplemental oxygen, are dependent on the operator's style rather than an objective measure. There is no standard or uniform threshold for intervention, and intervention techniques for respiratory depression are numerous and can be variably applied. A subject exhibiting sonorous respirations after receiving a sedative bolus may respond to simple airway reposition, an oral airway, stimulation, bag mask ventilation, or may have spontaneous resolution of this abnormality with no intervention. Similarly, a subject with oxygen desaturation may receive supplemental oxygen, airway repositioning, or have spontaneous resolution with no intervention. All of these are appropriate interventions based on the judgment of the individual operator. However, if these interventions represent separate outcome points, then the operator's judgment

becomes the determining factor between detected differences rather than the agent or protocol that is being studied. We have used objective signs of unclear clinical significance, pulse oximetry and capnography, in place of the common indicators discussed above. Undefined aspects of these measurements make assessment of the data difficult. In the case of pulse oximetry, the degree to which transient hypoxia is harmful is unknown, though likely related to the degree of hypoxia and its duration. It is also not clear how to measure the degree of harm caused by hypoxia or what risk level is associated with harm. Capnography is more robust than oximetry as changes cannot be reversed or masked with the use of supplemental oxygen. It is not clear, however, what the inherent risks of increases or decreases in end-tidal CO_2 are, and what their clinical significance is. Furthermore, we do not know what the risk of transient apnea, as detected by the loss of the CO_2 waveform, is or how to best define it. The relative importance of these signs to significant complications and to each other is also not entirely clear. While they clearly demonstrate negative changes in a subject's ventilatory status and allow for the comparison of ventilatory effects between agents and protocols, the magnitude of the effect is difficult to extrapolate to actual clinical complication rates.

5. The dosing and timing of sedatives is difficult to study due to multiple confounding variables most notably the operators' relative tolerance of over-sedation and under-sedation. As studies typically include multiple operators, it is possible that one may stop giving medications to a subject who is still in visible discomfort but has begun to display respiratory depression (or another adverse event), while another clinician will give more medications and support the subject's ventilation. The varying responses to adverse events/complications make it difficult to describe, and limit the utility of descriptions of sedative doses during the procedure. Various adjuvant medications have also been used in PSA studies. Supplemental opioids are often given before, after, or with propofol, and midazolam is often given before, after, or with ketamine. Fentanyl and midazolam are strong respiratory depressants so their effects on measured outcome parameters, which usually include respiratory depression, are well described. In the case of fentanyl and propofol, the relative half lives of the two drugs differ by an order of magnitude. Therefore, the effects on outcomes such as time of sedation, as well as the effect on the outcome of the sedation relative to the timing of the opioid dose, are difficult to characterize and compare between studies due to their variable application and unclear potentiating effect to the agent being studied.

6. The success of sedation can be defined as a lack of recall, lack of response to pain, lack of an adverse event, lack of interference from the patient with the procedure, or successful completion of the procedure. However, the focus of the study and the specific outcome measures can influence the results. If the primary outcome measure is the adverse event rate and the principle concern of the procedure is to avoid respiratory depression, then patients may be sedated less deeply and there will be a lower rate of respiratory depression and a higher rate of recall or patient response to the procedure. Alternatively, if either the rate of recall or the success of the procedure is the primary measured outcome, the patient may be sedated more deeply with a higher rate of respiratory depression. Therefore, the success rate of the procedures will be difficult to compare since it will vary with the difficulty of the procedure and the depth of sedation.
7. Post procedure VAS scales to describe pain during the procedure have largely failed. Patients who do not recall the procedure do not report pain that occurred during the procedure since they cannot recall it. Since procedures for which patients are sedated are generally very painful, patients either report recall of the procedure and pain, or no recall of the procedure and no pain, making the two measures redundant. The question remains whether a lack of recall is sufficient to determine adequate sedation, or if unperceived pain needs to be evaluated and treated. Given the current understanding of pain, this could only be done outside the patient's realm of recall by asking the operator if the patient appeared as if he/she was in pain. This exposes studies of this type to problems of blinding, and does not address the question of the clinical importance of that finding. Defining the optimal level of sedation for a given procedure is difficult in the absence of further information on the relationship of pain and recall to outcome. Assuming that a lack of recall is a sufficient measure of procedural recall and pain, sedation levels (minimal, moderate, deep) can be compared relative to the success of the procedure and the rate of adverse events. The difficulty with this type of study will be the variable dosing requirements between patients of the varied sedative medications, causing these studies to rely on the operator to achieve the level of sedation under scrutiny if it is assigned in a random fashion. A nonrandomized comparison is unlikely to provide useful results, since the level may be chosen based on the patient's needs and apparent risk of having an adverse event. In the absence of accepted markers of stress or pain from brief painful encounters, it remains difficult to assess the optimal level of awareness other than with the patient's report of recall.

References

1. Green SM, Krauss B (2004) Clinical practice guideline for emergency department ketamine dissociative sedation in children. Ann Emerg Med 44:460–71
2. Miner JR et al (2007) The effect of the assignment of a pre-sedation target level on procedural sedation using propofol. J Emerg Med 32(3):249–55
3. Miner JR, Biros M, Krieg S, Johnson C, Heegaard W, Plummer D (2003) Randomized clinical trial of propofol versus methohexital for procedural sedation during fracture and dislocation reduction in the emergency department. Acad Emerg Med 10:931–7
4. Miner JR, Biros MH, Heegaard W, Plummer D (2003) Bispectral electroencephalographic analysis of patients undergoing procedural sedation in the emergency department. Acad Emerg Med 10:638–43
5. Miner JR, Biros MH, Seigel T, Ross K (2005) The utility of the bispectral index in procedural sedation with propofol in the emergency department. Acad Emerg Med 12:190–6
6. Miner JR, Heegaard W, Plummer D (2002) End-tidal carbon dioxide monitoring during procedural sedation. Acad Emerg Med 9:275–80
7. Burton JH, Harrah JD, Germann CA, Dillon DC (2006) Does end-tidal carbon dioxide monitoring detect respiratory events prior to current sedation monitoring practices? Acad Emerg Med 13:500–4
8. Avramov MN, White PF (1995) Methods for monitoring the level of sedation. Crit Care Clin 11:803–26
9. Miner JR, Danahy M, Moch A, Biros M (2007) Randomized clinical trial of etomidate versus propofol for procedural sedation in the emergency department. Ann Emerg Med 49(1):15–22
10. Miner JR, Gaetz A, Biros MH (2007) The association of a decreased level of awareness and blood alcohol concentration with both agitation and sedation in intoxicated patients in the ED. Am J Emerg Med 25:743–8
11. Deitch K, Chudnofsky CR, Dominici P (2007) The utility of supplemental oxygen during emergency department procedural sedation and analgesia with midazolam and fentanyl: a randomized controlled trial. Ann Emerg Med 49:1–8
12. Krauss B, Hess DR (2007) Capnography for procedural sedation and analgesia in the emergency department. Ann Emerg Med 50:172–81
13. Miner JR, Bachman A, Kosman L, Teng B, Heegaard W, Biros MH (2005) Assessment of the onset and persistence of amnesia during procedural sedation with propofol. Acad Emerg Med 12:491–6
14. Miner JR, Martel ML, Meyer M, Reardon R, Biros MH (2005) Procedural sedation of critically ill patients in the emergency department. Acad Emerg Med 12:124–8
15. Gill M, Green SM, Krauss B (2003) A study of the Bispectral Index Monitor during procedural sedation and analgesia in the emergency department. Ann Emerg Med 41:234–41
16. Agrawal D, Feldman HA, Krauss B, Waltzman ML (2004) Bispectral index monitoring quantifies depth of sedation during emergency department procedural sedation and analgesia in children. Ann Emerg Med 43:247–55
17. Bassett KE, Anderson JL, Pribble CG, Guenther E (2003) Propofol for procedural sedation in children in the emergency department. Ann Emerg Med 42:773–82
18. Guenther E, Pribble CG, Junkins EP Jr, Kadish HA, Bassett KE, Nelson DS (2003) Propofol sedation by emergency physicians for elective pediatric outpatient procedures. Ann Emerg Med 42:783–91
19. Vinson DR, Bradbury DR (2002) Etomidate for procedural sedation in emergency medicine. Ann Emerg Med 39:592–8

Chapter 37

Non-invasive Transcranial Direct Current Stimulation for the Study and Treatment of Neuropathic Pain

Helena Knotkova and Ricardo A. Cruciani

Abstract

In the last decade, radiological neuroimaging techniques have enhanced the study of mechanisms involved in the development and maintenance of neuropathic pain. Recent findings suggest that neuropathic pain in certain pain syndromes (e.g., complex regional pain syndrome/reflex sympathic dystrophy, phantom-limb pain) is associated with a functional reorganization and hyperexitability of the somatosensory and motor cortex. Studies showing that the reversal of cortical reorganization in patients with spontaneous or provoked pain is accompanied by pain relief stimulated the search for novel alternatives how to modulate the cortical excitability as a strategy to relieve pain. Recently, non-invasive brain stimulation techniques such as transcranial magnetic stimulation (TMS) and transcranial direct current stimulation (tDCS) were proposed as suitable methods for modulation of cortical excitability. Both techniques (TMS and tDCS) have been clinically investigated in healthy volunteers as well as in patients with various clinical pathologies and variety of pain syndromes. Although there is less evidence on tDCS as compared with TMS, the findings on tDCS in patients with pain are promising, showing an analgesic effect of tDCS, and observations up to date justify the use of tDCS for the treatment of pain in selected patient populations. tDCS has been shown to be very safe if utilized within the current protocols. In addition, tDCS has been proven to be easy to apply, portable and not expensive, which further enhances great clinical potential of this technique.

Key words: Transcranial direct current stimulation (tDCS), Neuropathic pain, Pain management

1. Introduction

In the last decade, radiological neuroimaging techniques have enhanced the study of mechanisms involved in the development and maintenance of neuropathic pain. Recent findings suggest that pain in certain neuropatic pain syndromes (e.g., complex regional pain syndrome/reflex sympathic dystrophy [CRPS/RSD], fibromyalgia, phantom-limb pain) is assoliated with functional reorganization of the somatosensory and motor cortices (1–9).

Arpad Szallasi (ed.), *Analgesia: Methods and Protocols*, Methods in Molecular Biology, vol. 617, DOI 10.1007/978-1-60327-323-7_37, © Springer Science+Business Media, LLC 2010

Cortical reorganization involves two main phenomena: (1) changes in somatotopic organization and (2) changes in excitability of the somatosensory and motor cortices. The observation that the reversal of cortical reorganization in patients with spontaneous or provoked pain is accompanied by pain relief (1–3) further stimulated the search for novel alternatives to modulate the cortical excitability as a strategy to relieve pain. In early studies, pain relief was achieved using invasive electrical stimulation with electrodes implanted over the motor cortex (10–12). Although promising results were reported with this approach, due to the invasive nature of this procedure, a clinical use of this technique as well as research studies remained to very specific patiem-populations limited. Recently, non-invasive brain stimulation techniques such as transcranial magnetic stimulation (TMS) and transcranial direct current stimulation (tDCS) were proposed as suitable methods for modulation of cortical excitability in patients with certain types of pain. Both TMS and tDCS have been studied in healthy volunteers (13–17), patients with various disorders (18–26), and in various pain syndromes (27–35). Although there is less evidence on the use of tDCS, as compared to TMS, the findings are very promising, and the observations up to date justify the use of tDCS for the treatment of pain in selected patient populations (27, 30, 34–39). The findings on tDCS safety suggest that the application of tDCS to motor and non-motor cortical areas is associated with relatively minor side effects if the safety recommendations are followed (40–53). In addition, tDCS has been proven to be easy to apply, portable, and not expensive, which further enhances great clinical potential of this technique.

This protocol and procedure describe the use of tDCS for the study and alleviation of spontaneous chronic pain and does not apply to experimentally induced or spontaneous acute pain.

2. Materials

1. tDCS device Phoresor® II Auto, Model No. PM850 or PM950 (IOMED, Salt Lake City, UT), consisting of the main battery-operated unit and a twin wire to connect the unit with electrodes (Fig. 1).
2. Two large saline-soaked sponge-electrodes (contact area 25 or 36 cm^2) and two cables, both with the ends "crocodile to banana".
3. An equipment for determining the proper position of the electrodes. Either an automated visual navigation system can be used, or the position can be determined manually using the 10–20 International system of the electroencephalographic electrode placement.

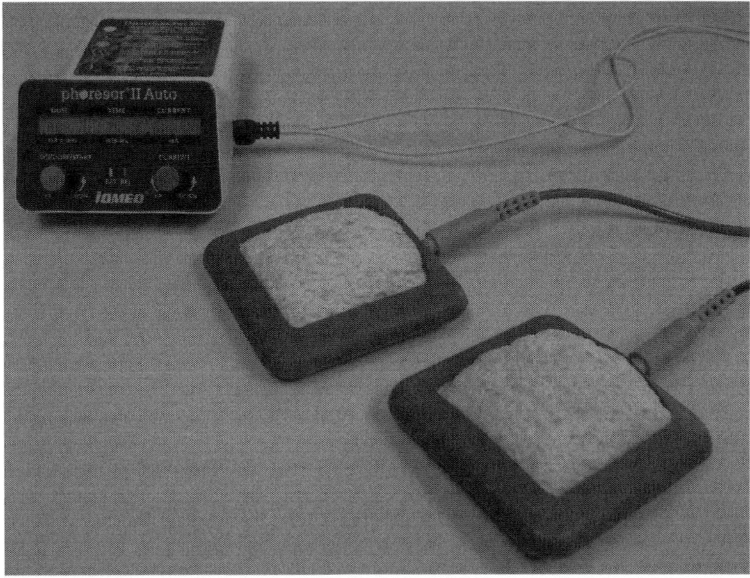

Fig. 1. The tDCS device. The tDCS device consists of the main battery-operated unit and two larger saline-soaked electrodes

4. Normal saline (9 g/liter).
5. Two elastic bands, medical tape, flexible plastic meter.

3. Methods

tDCS is based on influencing neuronal excitability and modulating the firing rates of individual neurons by a low amplitude direct current which is delivered non-invasively through the scalp to the selected brain structures (54, 55). The nature of tDCS-induced modulation of cortical excitability depends on polarity of the current. Animal studies suggest that cathodal stimulation decreases the resting membrane potential and therefore hyperpolarizes neurons, whereas anodal stimulation causes depolarization by increasing resting membrane potentials and spontaneous neuronal discharge rates (56–58). Generally, anodal tDCS increases cortical excitability, while cathodal tDCS decreases it (59, 60).

Anodal tDCS increases cortical excitability by reducing intracortical inhibition and enhancing intracortical facilitation. Cathodal tDCS diminishes excitability by reducing intracortical facilitation during stimulation and additionally by increasing intracortical inhibition after stimulation (54, 55, 60). Some of tDCS-induced changes occurs immediately during the stimulation (so called intra-tDCS changes), while others occur later as short-lasting and long-lasting after-effects.

The intra-tDCS effects which elicit no after-effects can be induced by a short (seconds) single application of tDCS. As suggested by recent pharmacological studies, intra-effects depend on the activity of sodium and calcium channels but not on efficacy changes of NMDA and GABA receptors, and thus are probably generated solely by polarity specific shifts of resting membrane potential (61–64). The intra-tDCS effect of cathodal tDCS is reduction of intracortical facilitation, while anodal tDCS has no intra-effect on intracortical facilitation or inhibition; all effects of anodal stimulation occur later as after-effects.

The short-lasting effects lasts 5–10 min after the end of stimulation and can be induced by application of 7 min of 1 mA tDCS, while to obtain long-lasting effects (about 1 h) at least 13 min of 1 mA tDCS is needed. As shown by Nitsche and colleagues (63), the after-effects critically depend on membrane potential changes, but have been demonstrated to involve also modulations of NMDA receptors efficacy (61). After-effects of anodal tDCS involve reduction of intracortical inhibition and enhancement of intracortical facilitation, while cathodal tDCS after-effect represent enhancement of intracortical inhibition (54, 55, 60).

Although data on the use of tDCS to alleviate pain are limited and large controlled studies need to be conducted, the findings (27, 30, 34–38) show that the anodal tDCS delivered over the motor cortex in patients with chronic pain can induce significant pain relief, as compared with baseline prior the tDCS and/or with a "placebo" sham tDCS.

Analgesic effects induced by tDCS outlast the period of stimulation and are cumulative, transient and site-specific.

Although the exact mechanisms responsible for underlying pain relief induced by the motor cortex stimulation have not yet been fully elucidated, some results suggests that the decrease in pain sensations that follows the motor cortex stimulation might be at least in part linked to changes in the thalamic activity (65, 66). PET scans performed in patients with neuropathic pain after motor cortex stimulation showed significant increase in cerebral blood flow in the ventral-lateral thalamus, medial thalamus, anterior cingulate/orbitofrontal cortex, anterior insula and upper brainstem (65). All of these areas are known to be involved in various mechanisms of transmission of pain. It is reasonable to speculate that the activation of the motor cortex in the hemisphere contralateral to the painful limb may trigger thalamic activity directly via cortico-thalamic projections, and this in turn might modulate the ascending nociceptive pathways, such as spinothalamic tract, which is considered to be the predominant pain-signaling pathway.

Further, there is an increasing evidence suggesting that changes in cortical excitability induced by motor cortex stimulation may be partially linked to the activity of dopaminergic neurons (67, 68). Recent insights have demonstrated a central role for dopaminergic neurotransmission in modulating pain perception and natural analgesia within supraspinal regions, including the basal ganglia, insula, anterior cingulate cortex, thalamus and periaqueductal gray, as well as in descending pathways (69). Decreased level of dopamine likely contributes to the painful symptoms that frequently occur in Parkinson's disease, and abnormalities in dopaminergic transmission have been objectively demonstrated in painful clinical conditions such as fibromyalgia (70).

Safety of tDCS has been evaluated in animal studies (41–44), as well as human studies (45–53, 71) involving healthy volunteers, and patients with various disorders. A recent study (71) looked at the prevalence of side-effects in a cohort of 102 subjects with a total of 567 tDCS sessions in which electrical current of 1 mA was applied over the primary motor cortex as well as other cortical areas (somatosensory, visual, dorsolateral prefrontal, parietal, and auditory cortex) (71). The pool of participants consisted of healthy subjects (75.5%), migraine patients (8.8%), post-stroke patients (5.9%), and tinnitus patients (9.8%). Results showed that during tDCS the most common reported side effect was a mild tingling sensation directly under the electrode (70.6%), a light itching sensation under the electrode (30.4%), and moderate fatigue (35.3%). In addition, headache (11.8%), nausea (2.9%), and insomnia (0.98%) were also reported. The overall findings on tDCS safety suggest that the application of tDCS to various cortical areas *is not* associated with occurrence of any serious side-effects.

The description of the procedure as appears below, relates to the use of anodal tDCS for alleviation of spontaneous chronic pain, and does not apply to experimentally induced- or spontaneous acute pain, or to the tDCS treatment of any other medical condition.

1. Using an elastic band, two saline-soaked sponge-electrodes are placed on the subject's head as follows: the anode over the motor cortex (see Note 1) of the hemisphere contralateral to the affected part of the body; the cathode over the supraorbital region of the ipsilateral hemisphere.
2. The area of the motor cortex can be determined either using the automated navigational system, or manually as the position of C4 (on the right hemisphere) or C3 (on the left hemisphere) (Fig. 2). C3/C4 respectively are located 7 cm from Cz point.
3. The main tDCS unit gets connected with electrodes.

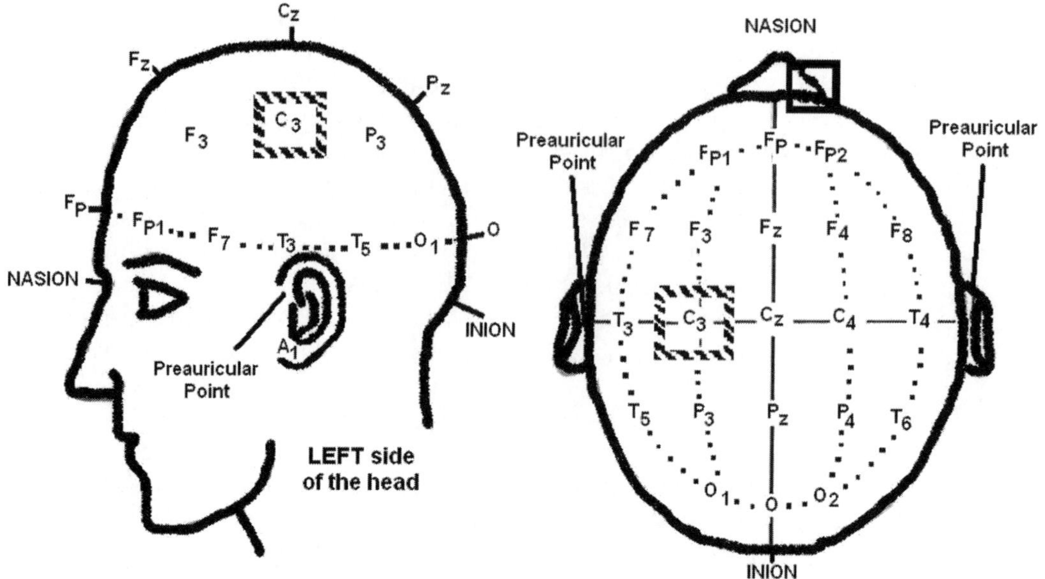

Fig. 2. The 10-20 EEG International System used for a manual positioning of the tDCS electrodes. To alleviate chronic spontaneous pain, the anode is placed at the position of C3 or C4 which lies in the area of the motor cortex on the left and right hemisphere respectively. In general, the anode has to be placed on the hemisphere contralateral to the affected part of the body, while the cathode is placed over the supraorbital region ipsilateral to the affected side

4. Desired intensity of the stimulation and time (see Note 2) is manually pre-set on the display. After the safety check (the right position of the electrodes, cable-connections, parameters on the display), the main unit is switched on.
5. The intensity of current increases automatically in the ramp manner over several seconds until reaching desired intensity.
6. At the end of stimulation, the intensity of the current gradually decreases to zero and the unit visually and acoustically signals the end of stimulation.
7. The tDCS procedure is usually delivered as a block of treatment, i.e., repeated on several consecutive days (see Note 3).
8. For long-term pain control, the block of tDCS treatment can be repeated (see Note 4).

4. Notes

1. Analgesic effects are site-specific. In a study by Roizenblatt and colleagues (30), thirty-two fibromyalgia patients were randomized into three arms to receive either sham or anodal tDCS (at the intensity of 2 mA for 20 min) delivered either over the primary motor cortex, or the dorsolateral prefrontal

cortex (DLPFC), on five consecutive days. The results indicated that neither sham nor real tDCS anodal stimulation over DLPFC produced significant pain relief. The stimulation over the primary motor cortex was the only parameter associated with a significant reduction of pain, with 59% pain relief after the last session. Up to date, published sham-controlled studies in population with chronic pain utilized the anodal tDCS delivered over the motor cortex. However, there is some preliminary evidence (39, 72) that analgesic effect can also be induced by targeting the somatosensory cortex provided that the *cathodal* stimulation is used.

2. The parameters utilized in clinical and research trials with tDCS in healthy volunteers and patients with various diagnoses vary highly and include differences in the position of the electrodes, polarity of the current (anodal or cathodal), intensity, and duration of the stimulation. In the studies using tDCS in patients with spontaneous chronic pain (27, 30, 34–38), anodal tDCS up to the intensity of 2 mA for up to 20 min over the motor cortex on up to five consecutive days has been safely applied, without eliciting any serious adverse effects.
3. The analgesic effects of tDCS are cumulative. Several independent observations indicated that repeated tDCS sessions on several (five) consecutive days can yield significantly better pain relief than a single application (27, 30, 35, 36). The findings showed that pain intensity after tDCS on Day-5 was substantially lower than pain intensity after Day-1 as compared to Baseline, and significant difference was also observed between pain intensity on Day-1 and Day-2 as compared with Baseline. For example, in the study in patients with central pain due to spinal cord injury (27), the results showed non-significant pain relief after Day-1, while after Day-2 the decrease in pain ratings reached significance $p<0.05$, and and after day 5 $p<0.001$, (27).
4. Analgesic effects of tDCS outlast the tDCS session but diminish with time. Evidence up to date in concordance indicate that although the pain relieving effect of tDCS outlasts the period of stimulation, the effect is not permanent (27, 30, 35–38). For example, in the study of patients with central pain due to spinal cord injury, the mean pain intensity after the active tDCS decreased from 6.2 at the baseline to 2.6 at the end of the fifth tDCS session, and the magnitude of this effect diminished somewhat at the follow up 16 days later (mean VAS pain intensity 3.9), but was still significant when compared with baseline (27). Similarly, in patients with fibromyalgia pain relief lasts beyond the fifth session, and although the effect diminished with time, three weeks after the last session, the pain relief was still highly significant when compared to baseline values (30, 36).

In a case obervation (45) of a patient with CRPS/RSD who received tDCS repeatedly in five blocks (each block consisting of five consecutive days) in "as needed" regimen, the duration of pain relief ranged between 3 and 11 weeks (35). No analgesic tolerance (a phenomenon often observed during opioid treatments, when the analgesic response to a specific dose declines with repeated use of the drug) was observed in the patient.

Acknowledgment

The authors thank Drs. Daniel Feldman and Veronika Stock for technical support during preparation of the manuscript.

References

1. Pleger B, Tegenthoff M, Ragert P, Forster AF, Dinse HR, Schwenkreis P, Nicolas V, Maier C (2005) Sensorimotor returning in complex regional pain syndrome parallels pain reduction. Ann Neurol 57(3):425–9
2. Maihöfner C, Handwerker HO, Neundorfer B, Birklen F (2003) Patterns of cortical reorganization in complex regional pain syndrome. Neurology 61(12):1707–15
3. Birbaumer N, Lutzenberger W, Montoya P, Larbig W, Unertl K, Topfner S, Grodd W, Taub E, Flor H (1997) Effects of regional anesthesia on phantom limb pain are mirrored in changes in cortical reorganization. J Neurosci 17(14):5503–5508
4. Flor H, Elbert T, Knecht S, Wienbruch C, Pantev C, Birbaumer N, Larbig W, Taub E (1995) Phantom limb pain as a perceptual correlate of cortical reorganization. Nature 357:482–4
5. Flor H (2003) Cortical reorganization and chronic pain: implications for rehabilitation. J Rehabil Med 41:66–72
6. Maihöfner C, Handwerker HO, Neundorfer B, Birklen F (2003) Patterns of cortical reorganization in complex regional pain syndrome. Neurology 61(12):1707–15
7. Schwenkreis P, Janssen F, Rommel O, Pleger B, Volker B, Hosbach I, Dertwinkel R, Maier C, Tegenthoff M (2003) Bilateral motor cortex disinhibition in complex regional pain syndrome(CRPS)type I of the hand. Neurology 61(4):515–9
8. Eisendberg E, Chystiakov AV, Yudashkin M, Kaplan B, Hafner H, Frensod M (2005) Evidence for cortical hyperexcitability of the affected limb representation area in CRPS: a psychophysical and transcranial magnetic stimulation study. Pain 113:99–105
9. Pleger B, Ragert P, Schwenkreis P, Forster AF, Wilimzig C, Dinse H, Nicoloas V, Maier C, Tegenthoff M (2006) Patterns of cortical reorganization parallel impaired tactile discrimination and pain intensity in complex regional pain syndrome. Neuroimage 32(2):503–10
10. Nguyen JP, Lefaucher JP, Le Guerinel C, Eizenbaum JF, Nakano N, Carpentier A, Brugieres P, Pollin B, Rostaining S, Keravel Y (2000) Motor cortex stimulation in the treatment of central and neuropatic pain. Arch Med Res 31(3):263–265
11. Brown J, Pilitsis J (2005) Motor cortex stimulation for central and neuropatic facial pain: a prospective study of 10 patients and observations of enhanced sensory and motor function during stimulation. Neurosurgery 56(2):290–297
12. Brown JA, Barbaro NM (2003) Motor cortex stimulation for central and neuropathic pain: Motor cortex stimulation for central and neuropathic pain: current status. Pain 104(3):431–5
13. Weiler F, Brandão P, de Barros-Filho J, Uribe CE, Pessoa VF, Brasil-Neto JP (2008) Low frequency (0.5 Hz) rTMS over the right (non-dominant) motor cortex does not affect ipsilateral hand performance in healthy humans. Arq Neuropsiquiatr S 66(3B): 636–640
14. Lang N, Siebner HR, Chadaide Z, Boros K, Nitshe MA, Rothwell JC, Paulus W, Antal A (2007) Bidirectional modulation of primary visual cortex excitability: a combined tDCS and rTMS study. Invest Ophthalmol Vis Sci 48(12):5782–7

15. Fecteau S, Knoch D, Fregni F, Sultani N, Boggio P, Pascual-Leone A (2007) Diminishing risk-taking behavior by modulating activity in the prefrontal cortex: a direct current stimulation study. J Neurosci 27(46):12500–5
16. Sparing R, Dafotakis M, Meister IG, Thirugnanasambandam N, Fink GR (2008) Enhancing language performance with non-invasive brain stimulation-A transcranial direct current stimulation study in healthy humans. Neuropsychologia 46(1):261–8
17. Yoo WK, You SH, Ko MH, Tae Kim S, Park CH, Park JW, Hoon Ohn S, Hallett M, Kim YH (2008) High frequency rTMS modulation of the sensorimotor networks: Behavioral changes and fMRI correlates. Neuroimage 39(4):1886–95
18. Celnik P, Hummel F, Harris-Love M, Wolk R, Cohen LG (2007) Somatosensory stimulation enhances the effects of training functional hand tasks in patients with chronic stroke. Arch Phys Med Rehabil 88(11):1369–76
19. Boggio PS, Ferrucci R, Rigonatti SP, Covre P, Nitsche M, Pascual-Leone A, Fregni F (2006) Effects of transcranial direct current stimulation on working memory in patients with Parkinson's disease. J Neurol Sci 249(1): 31–8
20. Boggio PS, Nunes A, Rigonatti SP, Nitsche MA, Pasual-Leone A, Fregni F (2007) Repeated sessions of noninvasive brain DC stimulation is associated with motor function improvement in stroke patients. Restor Neurol Neurosci 25(2):123–9
21. Chadaide Z, Arlt A, Nitsche MA, Lang N, Paulus W (2007) Transcranial direct current stimulation reveals inhibitory deficiency in migraine. Cephalalgia 27(7):833–9
22. Fregni F, Boggio PS, Nitsche MA, Marcolin MA, Rigonatti SP, Pascual-Leone A (2006) Treatment of major depression with transcranial direct current stimulation. Bipolar Disord 8:203–4
23. Fregni F, Boggio PS, Nitsche MA, Rigonatti SP, Pascual-Leone A (2006) Cognitive effects of repeated sessions of transcranial direct current stimulation in patients with depression. Depress Anxiety 23(8):482–4
24. Fregni F, Boggio PS, Santos MS, Lima M, Vieira AL, Rigonatti SP, Silva MT, Barbosa ER, Nitsche MA, Pascual-Leone A (2006) Noninvaisive cortical stimulation with transcranial direct current stimulation in Parkinson's disease. Mov Disord 21(10):1693–702
25. Fregni F, Marcondes R, Boggio PS, Marcolin MA, Rigonatti SP, Sanchez TG, Nitsche MA, Pascual-Leone A (2006) Transcranial tinnitus suppression induced by repetitive transcranial magnetic stimulation and transcranial direct current stimulation. Eur J Neurol 13(9):996–1001
26. Stanford AD, Sharif Z, Corcoran C, Urban N, Malaspina D, Lisanby SH (2008) rTMS strategies for the study and treatment of schizophrenia: a review. Int J Neuropsychopharmacol 1:1–14
27. Fregni F, Boggio PS, Lima MC, Ferreira MJ, Wagner T, Rigonatti SP, Castro AW, Souza DR, Riberto M, Freedman SD, Nitsche MA, Pascual-Leone A (2006) A sham-controlled, phase II trial of transcranial direct current stimulation for the treatment of central pain in traumatic spinal cord injury. Pain 122(1–2):197–209
28. André-Obadia N, Mertens P, Gueguen A, Peyron R, Garcia-Larrea L (2008) Pain relief by rTMS: differential effect of current flow but no specific action on pain subtypes. Neurology 71(11):833–40
29. Pleger B, Janssen F, Schwenkreis P, Volker B, Maier C, Tegenthoff M (2004) Repetitive transcranial magnetic stimulation of the motor cortex attenuates pain perception in complex regional pain syndrome type I. Neurosci Lett 356:87–90
30. Roizenblatt S, Fregni F, Gimenez R, Werzel T, Rigonatti SP, Tufik S, Boggio PS, Valle AC (2007) Site-specific effects of transcranial direct current stimulation on sleep and pain in fibromyalgia: a randomized, sham-controlled study. Pain Pract 7(4):297–306
31. Andre-Obadia N, Peyron R, Mertens P, Mauguiere F, Laurent B, Garcia-Larea L (2006) Transcranial magnetic stimulation for pain control. Double-blind study of different frequencies against placebo, and correlation with motor cortex stimulation efficacy. Clin Neurophysiol 117:1536–44
32. Khedr EM, Kotb H, Kamel NF, Ahmed MA, Sadek R, Rothwell JC (2005) Longlasting antalgic effects of daily sessions of repetitive transcranial magnetic stimulation in central and peripheral neuropathic pain. J Neurol Neurosurg Psychiatry 76:833–838
33. Rollnik JD, Wustefeld S, Dauper M, Karst M, Fink M, Kossev A, Dengler R (2002) Repetitive transcranial magnetic stimulation for the treatment of chronic pain- a pilot study. Eur Neurol 48:6–10
34. Fenton B, Fanning J, Boggio P, Fregni F (2008) A pilot efficacy trial of tDCS for the treatment of refractory chronic pelvic pain. Brain Stimulat 1(3):260
35. Knotkova H, Sibirceva U, Factor A, Feldman D, Ragert P, Flor H, Cohen H, Cruciani R (2008) Repetitive transcranial direct current stimulation(tDCS) for the treatment of

neuropathic pain due to complex regional pain syndrome(CRPS). Submitted for a poster presentation at the 12th World Congress on Pain, Glasgow, Scotland/U.K.

36. Fregni F, Gimenes R, Valle AS, Ferreira MJ, Rocha RR, Natalle L, Bravo R, Rigonatti SP, Freedman SD, Nitsche MA, Pascual-Leone A, Boggio PS (2006) A randomized, sham-controlled, proof of principle study of transcranial direct current stimulation for the treatment of pain in fibromyalgia. Arthritis Rheum 54(12):3988–98
37. Kuhnl S, Terney D, Paulus W, Antal A (2008) The effect of daily sessions of anodal tDCS on chronic pain. Brain Stimulat 1(3):281
38. Knotkova H, Feldman D, Factor A, Sibirceva U, Dvorkin E, Cohen L, Ragert P, Cruciani RA (2008) Repeated transcranial direct current stimulation improves hyperalgesia and allodynia in a CRPS patient. Brain Stimulat 1(3):254
39. Antal A, Brepohl N, Poreisz C, Boros K, Csifcsak G, Paulus W (2008) Transcranial direct current stimulation over somatosensory cortex decreases experimentally induced acute pain perception. Clin J Pain 24(1):56–63
40. Agnew WE, McGreery DB (1987) Considerations for safety in the use of extracranial stimulation for motor evoked potentials. Neurosurgery 20:143–147
41. Islam N (1994) Appearance of dark neurons following anodal polarization in the rat brain. Acta Med Okayama 48(3):123–130
42. Islam N (1995) Increase in the calcium level following anodal polarization in the rat brain. Brain Res 684(2):206–208
43. Moriwaki A (1991) Polarizing currents increase noradrenaline-elicited accumulation of cyclic AMP in rat cerebral cortex. Brain Res 544(2):248–252
44. Liebetanz D, Klinker F, Hering D, Koch R, Nitsche MA, Potschka H, Loscher W, Paulus W, Tergau F (2006) Anticonvulsant effects of transcranial direct-current stimulation (tDCS) in the rat cortical ramp model of focal epilepsy. Epilepsia 47(7):1216–1226
45. Nitsche MA, Paulus W (2000) Excitability changes induced in the human motor cortex by weak transcranial direct current stimulation. J Physiol 527:633–639
46. Nitsche MA, Paulus W (2001) Sustained excitability elevations induced by transcranial DC motor cortex stimulation in humans. Neurology 57:1899–1901
47. Nitsche MA, Fricke K, Henschke U, Schlitterlau A, Liebetanz D, Lang N, Henning S, Tergau F, Paulus W (2003) Pharmacological modulation of cortical excitability shifts induced by transcranial direct current stimulation in humans. J Physiol 553:293–301
48. Nitsche MA (2002) Transcranial direct current stimulation: a new treatment for depression. Bipolar Disord 4(Suppl 1):98–9
49. Nitsche MA, Liebetanz D, Lang N, Antal A, Tergau F, Paulus W (2003) Safety criteria for transcranial direct current stimulation (tDCS) in humans. Clin Neurophysiol 114(11):2220–2 author reply 2222–3
50. Priori A (2003) Brain polarization in humans: a reappraisal of an old tool for prolonged non-invasive modulation of brain excitability. Clin Neurophysiol 114(4):589–595
51. Antal A, Nitsche MA, paulus W (2001) External modulation of visual perception in humans. Neuroreport 12:3553–3555
52. Antal A, Kincses TZ, Nitsche MA, Paulus W (2003) Manipulation of phosphene thresholds by transcranial direct current stimulation in man. Exp Brain Res 150:375–378
53. Baudewig J, Siebner HR, Bestmann S, Tergau F, Tings T, Paulus W, Frahm J (2001) Functional MRI of cortical activations induced by transcranial magnetic stimulation (TMS). Neuroreport 12(16):3543–8
54. Nitsche MA, Paulus W (2000) Excitability changes induced in the human motor cortex by weak transcranial direct current stimulation. J Physiol 527(3):633–639
55. Nitsche MA, Paulus W (2001) Sustained excitability elevations induced by transcranial DC motor cortex stimulation in humans. Neurology 57(10):1899–1901
56. Bindman LJ, Lippold OC, Redfearn JW (1964) The action of brief polarizing currents on the cerebral cortex of the rat (1) during current flow and (2) in the production of long-lasting after-effects. J Physiol 172: 369–382
57. Creutzfeldt OD, From GH, Knapp H (1962) Influence of transcortical DC currents on cortical neuronal activity. Exp Neurol 5:436–452
58. Purpura DP, McMurry JG (1965) Intracellular activities and evoked potential changes during polarization of motor cortex. J Neurophysiol 28:166–185
59. Nitsche MA, Nitsche MS, Klein CC, Tergau F, Rothwell JC, Paulus W (2003) Level of action of cathodal DC polarization induced inhibition of the human motor cortex. Clin Neurophysiol 114(4):600–604
60. Paulus W (2004) Outlasting excitability shifts induced by direct current stimulation of the human brain. Suppl Clin Neurophysiol 57:708–714

61. Liebetanz D, Nitsche M, Tergau F, Paulus W (2002) Pharmacological approach to the mechanisms of transcranial DC-stimulation-induced after-effects of human motor cortex excitability. Brain 125:2238–2247

62. Nitsche MA, Jaussi W, Liebetanz D, Lang N, Tergau F, Paulus W (2004) Consolidation of human motor neuroplasticity by D-cycloserine. Neuropsychopharmacology 29:1573–1578

63. Nitsche MA, Seeber A, Frommann K, Klein CC, Rochford C, Nitsche MS, Fricke K, Liebetanz D, Lang N, Antal A, Paulus W, Tergau F (2005) Modulating parameters of excitability during and after transcranial direct current stimulation of the human motor cortex. J Physiol 568:291–303

64. Nitsche MA, Liebetanz D, Schlitterlau A, Henschke U, Fricke K, Frommann K, Lang N, Henning S, Paulus W, Tergau F (2004) GABAergic modulation of DC stimulation-induced motor cortex excitability shifts in humans. Eur J Neurosci 19:2720–2726

65. García-Larrea L, Peyron R, Mertens P, Gregoire MC, Lavenne F, Le Bars D, Convers P, Mauguière F, Sindou M, Laurent B (1999) Electrical stimulation of motor cortex for pain control: a combined PET-scan and electrophysiological study. Pain 83(2): 259–273

66. Wu CT, Fan YM, Sun CM, Borel CO, Yeh CC, Yang CP, Wong CS (2006) Correlation between changes in regional cerebral blood flow and pain relief in complex regional pain syndrome type 1. Clin Nucl Med 31(6): 317–320

67. Strafella AP, Paus T, Fraraccio M, Dagher A (2003) Striatal dopamine release induced by repetitive transcranial magnetic stimulation of the human motor cortex. Brain 126: 2609–2615

68. Lang N, Speck S, Harms J, Rothkegel H, Paulus W, Sommer M (2008) Dopaminergic potentiation of rTMS-induced motor cortex inhibition. Biol Psychiatry 63:231–233

69. Coffeen U, Lopez-Avilla A, Ortega-Legaspi JM, Del Angel R, Lopez-Munoz FJ (2008) Pellicer F. Eur J Pain 12(5):535–543

70. Wood PB (2008) Role of central dopamine in pain and analgesia. Expert Rev Neurother 8(5):781–797

71. Poreisz C, Boros K, Antal A, Paulus W (2007) Safety aspects of transcranial direct current stimulation concerning healthy subjects and patients. Brain Res Bull 72(4–6):208–14

72. Lnotkova H, Homel P, Crucian RA (2009) Cathodal TDCS over the somatosensory cortex relived chronic neuropathic pain in a patient with complex regional pain syndrome (CRPS/RSD). J pain manage 2(3) spec. Issue: 365–367

Chapter 38

Pain Imaging in the Emerging Era of Molecular Medicine

Christian S. Stohler and Jon-Kar Zubieta

Abstract

With the dawn of the twenty-first Century, imaging has assumed a new role in disease-oriented science. Regarding pain, the emphasis clearly turned from structural to functional imaging with functional molecular imaging assuming the leading edge. This trend parallels the efforts of biologists working to understand the molecular messages of cell and cell systems relevant to human disease processes. While originally imaging has been a stand-alone, documentary tool, today's metabolic and molecular imaging technologies provide quantitative insight into inter and intraindividual athogenetic processes relevant to human disease, complementing and expanding upon bench-type research. Imaging has become an indispensable tool in pain research.

Key words: Functional imaging, Metabolic imaging, Molecular imaging, fMRI, PET, SPECT, Complex disease

1. Introduction

This chapter focuses on the contemporary opportunities and emerging frontiers enabled by modern imaging technologies regarding the study of pain. Specifically, it is intended to provide a contemporary view of the role of current and future imaging opportunities with respect to advancing the research agenda in the field of pain. The goal is to link disease-oriented imaging science, with emphasis on pain, to the efforts of molecular biologists working to understand, by using experimental models, the behavior of cell and cell systems of relevance to human disease processes.

Contemporary imaging offers valuable understanding of complex human disease, providing much needed crosstalk between clinical phenomena and bench science where intra and intercellular systems are isolated, identified, and manipulated. While once purely documentary, a research field in isolation,

Arpad Szallasi (ed.), *Analgesia: Methods and Protocols*, Methods in Molecular Biology, vol. 617,
DOI 10.1007/978-1-60327-323-7_38, © Springer Science+Business Media, LLC 2010

today's imaging methodologies provide quantitative insight into complex disease phenomena that assist in assessing the relevance and utility of fundamental model systems used in bench research with respect to their validity for clinical pain phenomena encountered in humans.

2. Advancing Understanding Through Imaging

When it comes to the study of pain by means of imaging, the diversity of the pain phenotype needs to be recognized. Pain is experienced in the context of injury or disease. Its onset can be sudden or gradual and its presentation can be fleeting, continual, or recurrent and persistent. Although knowledge of the exact mechanistic underpinning is lacking, classifiers such as "persistent" or "chronic" are reserved for those nonterminal pain conditions that impose recurrent or persistent activity limitations upon the patient for prolonged times, typically months to years (1). Besides temporal descriptors, pain conditions also range in severity and the extent of bodily involvement with the most devastating forms of suffering often demonstrating little explanatory, notably structural findings. When it comes to the most distressing presentations, lack of knowledge of the pathogenesis and the absence of validated biomarkers mean that the pain condition is in effect syndromic in nature with the diagnostic assignment relying on a combination of clinically observable features, often limited to a particular anatomical domain. Given the phenomenological diversity of human pains, it is important to recognize that not all pains will show the same brain activation pattern (2).

Epidemiological data of most pain conditions further suggest that women are more susceptible to experience pain at greater frequency and severity than men, particularly beginning with and during the reproductive ages (3, 4). With respect to scientific opportunities, animal models of pain often exhibit limitations when it comes to modeling the complex processes unique to human function, particularly those in effect in pain conditions for which therapeutic options fall short. Given this background, strong interests exist in elucidating the complex regulation and individual vulnerabilities underlying the human experience of pain and for which imaging studies hold great promise in advancing the critical knowledge.

Beginning with the late 1990s, notably following the milestone paper published by the Bushnell group in Science in 1997 (5), imaging studies have greatly expanded the understanding of human brain function during pain. Recent imaging studies extended upon the earlier work and established the intriguing, functional neural underpinnings of pain, pleasure, and reward (6).

These manuscripts and related work point to a complex representation of the pain experience in the human brain. They highlight the concept that pain is not a simple sensory phenomenon but a complex experience, a stressor that threatens the homeostasis of the organism. As such, it has additional cognitive, emotional, and motivational components. Functional neuroimaging work has perhaps most clearly brought this concept forward, as various modalities of pain, whether experimental or clinical, are studied and their telencephalic correlates become clarified.

In contrast to animal experimentation, the psychophysical correlates provided by human subjects offer an unrivaled level of sensitivity and specificity in the assessment of pleasure, reward, and pain. As a result, new knowledge of higher order brain processing of humans has widened the range of research questions pursued in bench-type research, particularly applicable to the study of pain.

In the first decade of the twenty-first Century, in-vivo functional imaging in humans has reached a level of sophistication that complements and expands upon the bench research in cell systems, brain-slices, and animal models. In fact, today's ability to image, with metabolic or molecular measures the state of mind of the living human in response to a defined stimulus, even tackling mind–body interactions, opens the door to understanding complexly regulated disease phenomena at the level of systems' biology that are unparalleled by the opportunities offered by animal models. Imaging the awake, behaving human, experiencing complex behavioral states, such as pain, capturing feelings with validated psychophysical tools has become an indispensable research endeavor for advancing critically needed understanding at the system's level. This is exemplified by a series of recent imaging studies that elucidate the role of belief, anticipation, expectation, empathy, social loss, and distraction with respect to pain (7–12).

In this respect, imaging techniques and methodologies in living humans are expected to drive in a meaningful way further advances in the understanding of the complex and higher order regulation in effect in human pain conditions, which are believed to result from the combined action of many genes, risk-conferring behaviors and environmental factors and with expectations and beliefs greatly impacting on the individual experience of pain (13). Many brain areas are activated in pain (14). As far as the human brain in pain is concerned, evidence from imaging studies points to the involvement of the prefrontal cortex, insula, orbito-frontal cortex, anterior cingulate, dorsal striatum , nucleus accumbens and ventral striatum, ventral pallidum, thalamus, hypothalamus, midbrain, amygdala, hippocampus, cerebellum and brainstem (5, 12, 15–23). As noted above, this body of work points to the complex representation and integration of pain information in the human brain. As a result, intra-individual variations in the pain experience are likely to arise at multiple levels, from initial perception to integrative and complex behavioral levels.

In sum, enticed by technical advances and stimulated by the first demonstration in living humans of pain affect being encoded in the anterior cingulated but not somatosensory cortex (5), imaging tools became increasingly employed by clinician-scientists (24–26). With the turn of the century, not only have imaging technologies become less expensive, the number of institutions that have implemented respective services and the number of investigators taking advantage of the increased availability of such facilities has steadily increased over the past decade. As a consequence, publications utilizing imaging tools have sharply increased in numbers. The use of imaging in research also shifted from the purely descriptive documentation of event-related changes to adopting a more mechanistic, hypothesis-driven framework that has shaped much of the discovery process in the sciences at-large in past decades (27).

3. Each Tool Has Its Place

To gain insight into the unresolved questions linked to human pain conditions, and with pain being both a sensory and significant emotional experience, it is not surprising that the main focus has been on visualizing the brain – first its structure and more recently its function – much more than on depicting peripheral phenomena observable in the region reported in pain. Images of brain structures based on magnetic resonance imaging (MRI) and brain function, visualized by means functional magnetic resonance imaging (fMRI), positron emission tomography (PET) and single-photon emission computed tomography (SPECT) have emerged as the most notable imaging applications for gaining insight into the central neurobiology, the latter two applications being analogous to in vitro autoradiography and radioimmunoassays used in bench research. Today's in-vivo imaging techniques have matured to the point that enables the valid and reliable measurement of neuronal activity, neurochemistry and pharmacology in the living human brain, complementing and validating results obtained in bench-type research.

According to MEDLINE, taking into account the literature up to the third week of November, 2008, the number of hits involving *"pain"* and *"imaging"* reached 267 for years 1950–1980, 507 for years 1981–1990, 3,575 for years 1991–2000, and 7,001 for the remaining years of 2001–2008. Much of the growth is attributable to the expansive use of structural imaging modalities, notably computer-aided tomography (CT) and MRI that increasingly became available in the past three decades of the last

Century. While the trend looks great at first sight, a closer look identifies that the field of pain is not a leader when it comes to frontiers in imaging in the molecular age. The field of cancer with a literature body of about three times that of pain shows 1,295 publication that fit the descriptors of *"molecular imaging"* between 2001 and 2008; the field of pain only has 37 in the corresponding time window of which three overlap with cancer, although the number of publications fitting the generic terms "molecular" and "pain" has risen from 24 for years 1950–1980 to 60 for years 1981–1990, 560 for years 1991–2000, and 1,180 for the remaining period.

Overall, the overwhelming majority of the work is employing structural imaging methodologies. These have provided particular insight as to the changes in brain structure that take place in the context of chronic disease (28, 29). Newer technologies like functional imaging and even molecular functional imaging, the tools needed to complement laboratory research, make up the smallest portion of all imaging studies combined. It is increasingly understood that progress focusing on radiographically detectable change, captured by structural imaging modalities, represents the often late consequence of molecular processes, which, in turn, should be viewed as the clinically and therapeutically meaningful phenomenon to be captured (Fig. 1).

By no means should the various imaging tools, for both structural and functional imaging classes, be understood as interchangeable, particularly when it comes to their utility in the assessment of pain-related brain function. Differences exist in terms of the degree of the mechanistic specificity of the acquired data based upon the choice of the biological probes used for signal generation, and aspects of the inherent spatial and temporal limitations of the various imaging applications. Indication for one

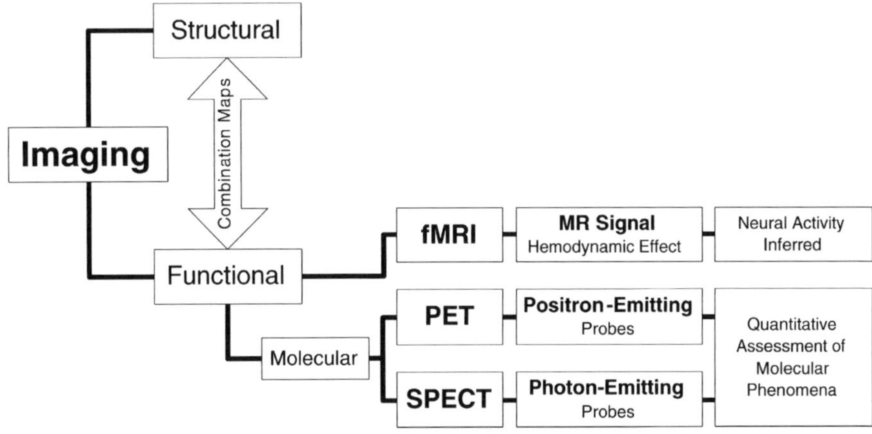

Fig. 1. Imaging literature classified by the nature of the imaged signal and explanatory yield

or the other imaging tool is determined by the scientific question under investigation and should not be made on the basis of the convenient availability of a particular imaging modality. For example, some pain effects are phasic in nature while others exert a tonic regulatory influence, e.g., long-lasting effects on neurotransmitter release, signal transduction and/or neurotransmitter interactions, necessitating imaging technologies with appropriately matched temporal resolution to answer the question posed.

In the case of lower spatial resolution, structural and functional imaging modalities are often combined by means of image co-registration techniques and processed using instrumentation-specific mathematical models to enhance the validity of assigning changes in biological brain function of lower spatial resolution to identifiable anatomical brain structures obtained using high-resolution MRI or CAT imaging. In fact, the newer classes of high-end imaging platforms incorporate multimodality imaging, e.g. PET-MRI or PET-CAT, permitting the convenient acquisition and fusion of multimodality images in the same recording session and without having to change the subject's head support with respect to the image focus.

Without any question, the evolutionary trend in medical imaging involves the migration from capturing structure to the visualization of specific molecular functions that are superimposed on detailed anatomical maps. Targeting and mapping the role of specific genes and their expressed and functional proteins in living humans, known or presumed to be of relevance to human disease, including the pain conditions, replacing nonspecific information with functional maps relevant to the mechanistic laboratory knowledge base constitutes the future of biomedical imaging (30). To compute inter-individual average response maps from individual data sets, validated spatial image normalization into internationally accepted standard stereotactic space using parametric mapping techniques (e.g., SPM, FSL) is required for which (linear and nonlinear) transformation algorithms are applied to match each individual image to a standard template (www.fil.ion.ucl.ac.uk/spm).

3.1. Functional Magnetic Resonance Imaging (fMRI)

Because of its noninvasiveness and widespread availability, fMRI constitutes the most used functional imaging modality to produce maps of human brain function. Its principle is founded on the hemodynamic response, the regional increase in blood flow that parallels neural activity, occurring with a delay of about 1–5 s after the onset of such activity. Regional changes in blood volume, blood flow, and the relative concentration of oxygenated (diamagnetic) and deoxygenated (paramagnetic) hemoglobin are the consequences.

Due to the increase in blood flow and volume without a corresponding increase in oxygen extraction from blood, deoxyhemoglobin concentration is lowered. The hemodynamic response is relatively short-lived, peaking after about 4 s before returning back to baseline again. Being an indirect measure of neuronal activity, other factors – regional or otherwise – have a bearing on the MR signal. With the MR signal being a measure of the hemodynamic response, it needs to be understood that activation involving excitatory or inhibitory neuronal networks is indistinguishable.

It is important to understand that the magnetic resonance (MR) signal captures the combined effect of arteries, veins, arterioles, venules, and capillaries with scanners producing magnetic fields of lesser strength being more influenced by events occurring in larger vessels. On the other hands, scanners with greater field strength (>4 tesla) emphasize the signal derived from smaller vessels and consequently capture information more closely to the source of neuronal activity. Blood oxygen-level-dependent (BOLD) fMRI, the most widely used assessment technique in research is based upon measurable differences of the magnetic resonance signal dependent upon the level of oxygenation and due to differences in the magnetic properties of oxyhemoglobin and deoxyhemoglobin. T1-weighted pulse sequences are better suited to detect changes in blood flow while T2-weighted images are more suited to detect changes in the local concentration of paramagnetic deoxyhemoglobin (Fig. 2).

3.2. Functional Molecular Imaging Using PET/SPECT

The rapid progress and new understanding gained by bench research using molecular probes, including the need to rapidly transfer findings into humans, calls for comparable tools to be

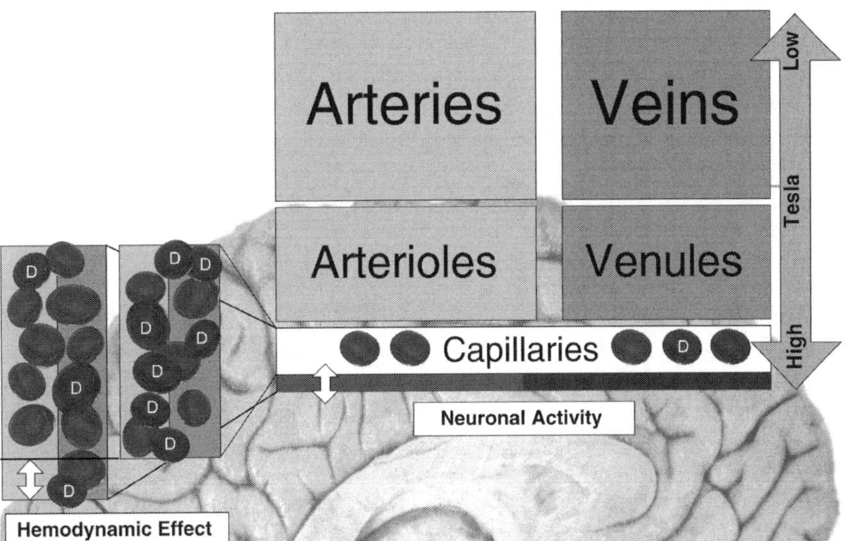

Fig. 2. Schematic illustration of the *bold* effect used for MR image generation based on the change in the ratio of oxyhemoglobin to deoxyhemoglobin (D). MR signals generated by scanners with high tesla value (>4 tesla) represent higher information content from relevant smaller vessels that are in the vicinity of active neurons

applied in the intact human, allowing in-vivo localization and quantification of specific molecules and their function in the human brain or other body regions of interest. Probes capable of monitoring the biological activity of enzymes, transporters, receptors, and other relevant target proteins will increasingly shape the future of medicine. Such methodologies require – optical imaging techniques excluded – attaching radioactive atoms to relevant molecules and observing the emitted radioactivity by a network of spatially arranged sensors around the subject, often referred to as "gamma camera". This sensor array defines the limitations of PET/SPECT in terms of spatial and temporal resolutions by its geometrical layout and sensor properties.

Suitable radioactive atoms for PET – positron emitters – include ^{15}oxygen, ^{11}carbon, or ^{18}fluorine, having a half-life of 2 min, 20 min, or 120 min, respectively. Radiotracers that are labeled with these atoms employed decay by positron emission. For SPECT, γ-ray emitters, such as ^{99}technetium, ^{123}iodine, and ^{133}xenon with a half-life of 6 h, 13 h, and 5 d, respectively, are used. Unlike radioligands suitable for PET, these compounds emit single or multiple uncorrelated γ-rays. Appropriate radioligands must show high selectivity for their target combined with low nonspecific binding to brain tissue devoid of the target. They must also exhibit rapid permeation of the compound through the blood–brain barrier and be metabolized in a way that does not interfere with the ongoing measurement process.

Compounds suitable for PET emit a positron that when colliding with an electron in its close vicinity results in the annihilation of the two particles and the generation of two photons, traveling in opposing directions, each with an energy of 511 keV. The phenomenon of two annihilation photons simultaneously traveling in opposing directions, hitting opposite γ-sensors within a very short time window (typically 5–7 ns) is taken advantage of to eliminate false-positive sensor hits and thereby improving the signal-to-noise ratio in PET data acquisitions. The acquisition of coincidence events over time forms the basis for the sinograms that, in turn, are used for PET 3-D image reconstruction.

After decay, isotopes used for SPECT imaging produce a single γ-ray (in case of some compounds, multiple, unrelated γ-rays) of varying, however lower energy than PET compounds, depending upon the type of radionuclide used. Although SPECT radionuclides are more readily available due their longer half-lives, radiopharmaceuticals with single emitting radionuclides are more difficult to prepare, limiting the current use of SPECT. On the other hand, the potential to radioactively label, biologically meaningful compounds with ^{11}carbon and ^{18}fluorine is substantial (Fig. 3).

When employing radiotracers, compounds that lend themselves to be radiolabeled and used in tracer amounts at occupancy

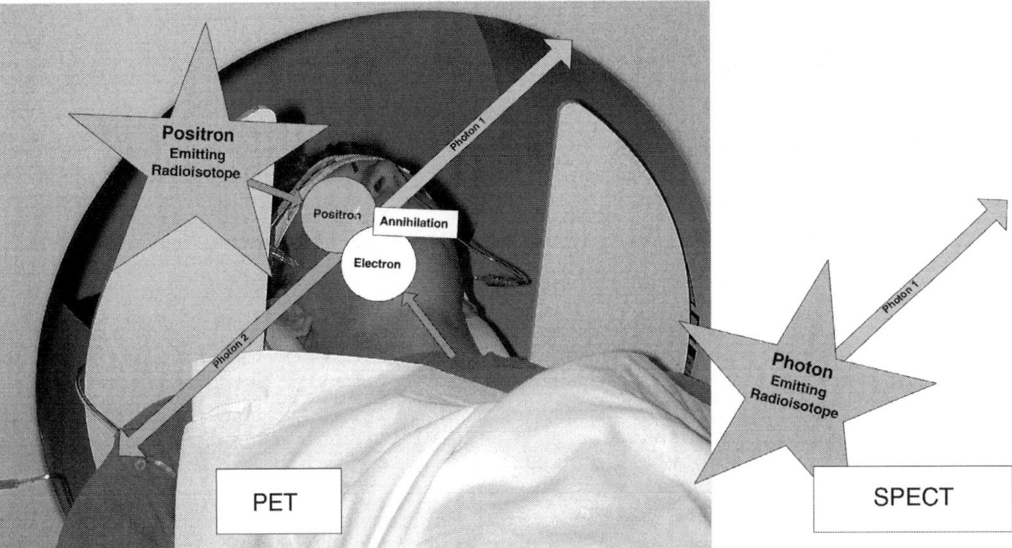

Fig. 3. Differences between PET and SPECT imaging (see text)

levels typically below 1% of the respective receptor sites, factors specific to the radioactive compound used for image generation, such as its metabolism and protein–binding properties require corrective adjustments for accurate assessment of the process of interest. The total radioactivity in a region of interest represents the sum of the radioactivity of the specifically bound compound and the presence of (1) nonspecifically bound and (2) any free compound in the region of interest. The latter two fractions are inferred from the radioactivity observed in a brain region known to be devoid of specific binding sites, or calculated using tracer kinetic analyses and the decay and metabolite corrected radiotracer concentrations in plasma. Reference region quantification models, as opposed to plasma input kinetic analyses, are currently favored if properly validated. Reasons for that include experimental and analytical convenience (without need for challenging arterial lines, and the collection and analysis of blood "on the fly" for the quantification of the parent compound and its radiolabeled metabolites in plasma), as well as the lesser statistical uncertainty in the quantification of the molecular process of interest (e.g., receptor binding sites, enzymatic activity).

PET or SPECT image data typically consist of time activity curves from which images are generated for a defined period of time following the administration of the radiotracer. As an example, Fig. 4 schematically illustrates the PET time activity curve using the radiotracer [^{11}C]carfentanil that binds to μ-opioid receptor for conditions of pain and the expectation of pain without actual pain to illustrate the methodological capability for functional assessments of the μ-opioid system at baseline and

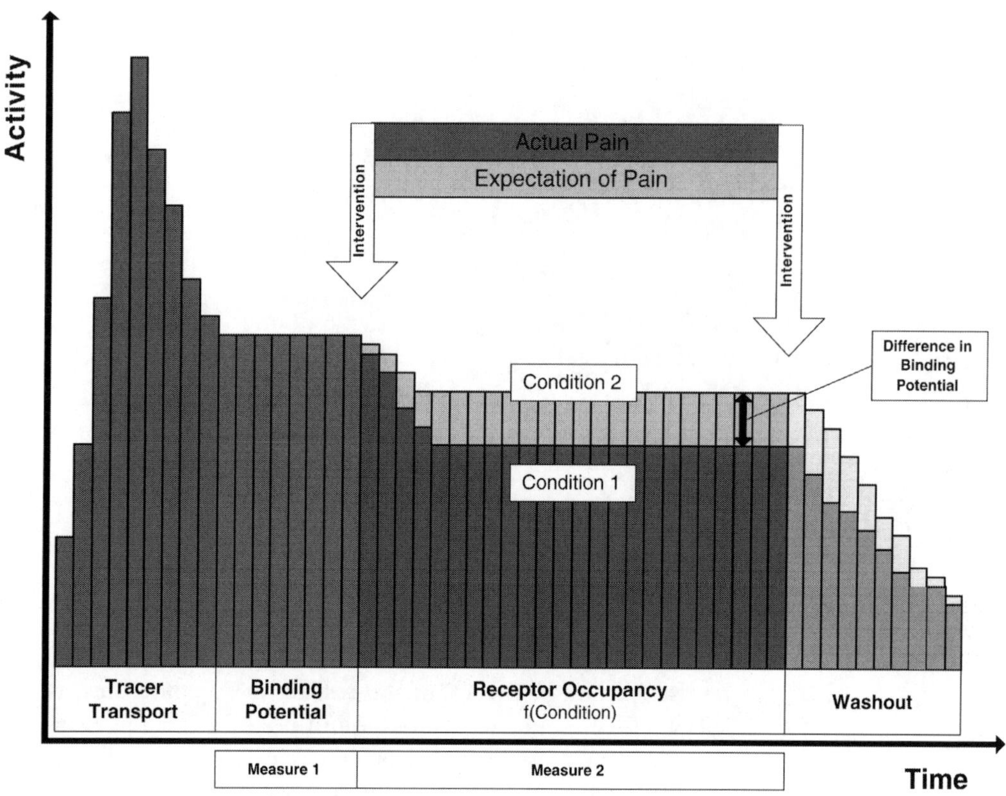

Fig. 4. Schematic time activity curve reflecting changes in regional radioactivity emitted from [^{11}C]carfentanil bound to the μ-opioid receptor when corrected for radioactivity due to unspecifically bound and free compound. Due to the greater availability of endogenous opioids in pain than in the saline control condition with the subject expecting pain but no pain is felt, less radioligand binding occurs because of the increased competition for available binding sites. Sequences are counterbalanced to control for order effects

when activated in pain and the expectation of pain (23). Carfentanil, a potent μ-opioid agonist, is preferred over ^{11}C-labeled morphine, heroin, or codeine because of metabolic complexities and high levels of unspecific binding encountered with these other compounds.

Suitable radioligands in combination with tracer kinetic models, representing the time-dependent local activity of the radiotracer in compartments, such as blood and brain tissue – free, unspecifically bound, and specifically bound – modeling equilibrium during timed data acquisition (e.g., using traditional compartment analyses or reference regions, such as in the Logan plots) turn a time sequence of PET images into a quantitative biological assay (31–34). Functional molecular imaging has matured to the point to permit unprecedented insight into the regulatory effect of systems visualized by highly selective molecular probes.

4. Cracking Complex Systems' Biology

With the turn of the Century, patient-oriented research has become more exciting than ever and imaging data, obtained by metabolic and molecular imaging studies started to play a major role in advancing the understanding of pain. Emerging biotechnologies, including the access, affordability, and experimental yield of various functional imaging modalities, offer unprecedented insight into the regulation of human disease and the mechanistic action of therapeutic interventions. Novel molecular methodologies support the discovery of explanations why certain treatments do not work and/or particular devices cause complications in individual patients. The specificity by which suitable biological probes, labeled with radioactive transmitters, are capable to dissect molecular processes in the intact human will increasingly influence laboratory investigations (35). For example, existing positron probes offer insight into the glucose metabolism by 2-[^{18}F]fluoro-2-deoxy-D-glucose (FDG), oxygen utilization by $^{15}O_2$, the function of neurotransmitter systems, such as the μ-opiate system by [^{11}C]carfentanil, the dopamine D2/D3 system by [^{11}C]raclopride and [^{18}F]fallypride, the serotonin transporter with [^{11}C]DASB, the serotonin receptor 5-HT_{1A} by [^{11}C]WAY-100635, benzodiazepine receptors by [^{11}C]flumazenil, or even enzyme functions, such as the monoamine oxidase (MAO) by [^{11}C]deprenyl, just to mention a few. However, development in this area has progressed slowly. Establishing accurate pharmacokinetics of the labeled molecule is not always simple, making only a few of the potentially suitable agents actually useful for molecular quantification in humans. In addition, the lack of access to existing molecular libraries (largely present in the drug industry) that includes ligands not necessarily destined to become therapeutic targets, limits the total number of compounds that could become available for molecular imaging.

Structural and functional imaging in humans, paired with psychophysics, brain biometry, bioinformatics and clinical, environmental and putative risk data enable clinician-scientists to pursue hypotheses for which animal model systems exhibit limitations in characterizing the psychophysical phenotype. With the dawn of the genomic age, molecular tools became available that combined with state-of-the-art imaging studies permit the modeling of complexly regulated processes in living humans down to the level of molecular function. Driven by the idea to link variations in brain biometry and function to behavioral differences of humans, this type of research is believed to generate knowledge of vulnerabilities to illnesses, including insight into the mechanisms by which genetic liability is conferred (Fig. 5). Traditional, single-laboratory-based

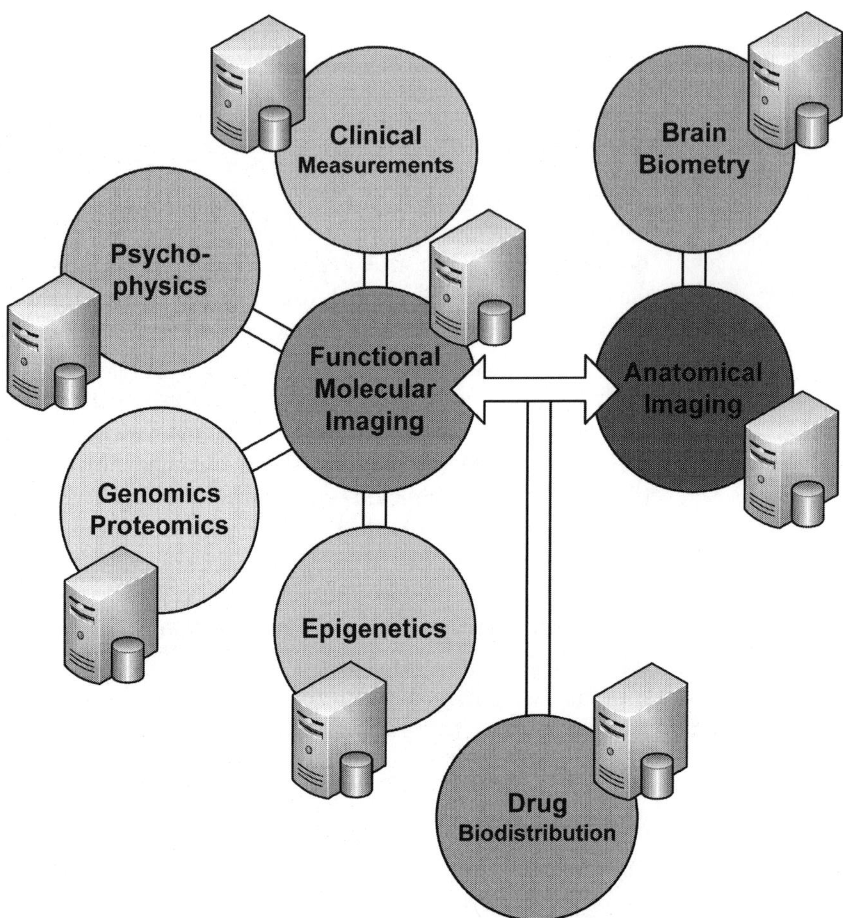

Fig. 5. Tackling biological complexity, linking phenotype to genotype using functional (molecular) brain imaging to explain complexly regulated phenomena, such as pain in humans

science is increasingly complemented by team science that addresses the organized problem complexities of interdisciplinary and multidisciplinary nature with imaging data playing a major role in modeling complexity. This is particularly true for those complex systems in which mind–body interactions influence outcomes.

The prevailing thinking states that clinical pain conditions are believed to develop from the combined action of many genes, risk-conferring behaviors and environmental factors, not understood from the function of each of these factors alone (36). Because traits, such as the sensitivity to a particular type of pain as well as the suppression of pain, are subject to considerable variation from subject to subject, the overall system response results from the interaction of a multitude of factors impacting upon the signal strength in pro- and anti-nociceptive signaling systems. Influences on these complexly regulated pro- and anti-nociceptive processes are difficult to resolve due to a multitude of inputs, which include endocrine signaling, genetic factors, neuroplastic changes linked to the persistence of pain, and even the lasting effects of prior treatments.

Besides untangling the regulatory complexity and difficulties that arise from defining the clinical phenotype, distinguishing between pro- and anti-nociceptive processes constitutes a challenge for conventional, nonmolecular imaging insofar that any regional activation could be due to either pro- or anti-nociceptive signaling. Given the need to further distinguish between excitatory and inhibitory neuronal activity in both pro- and anti-nociceptive systems, signal specificity greater than what is obtained from image generation based upon changes in hemodynamics is needed to resolve scientific questions with certainty, calling for highly selective radioligands. For this purpose, specific biological probes, capable of isolating receptor systems of interest, are required to unequivocally link changes in brain activity to one or the other process.

It should be understood that any kind of imaging study cannot occur in isolation. While on one hand, animal models and cell systems establish the scientific framework for hypothesis testing, results of imaging studies may call for novel lines of bench research. In particular, radioligands with high target specificity allow imaging of neurobiological and/or neuro-pharmacological processes in the functioning human brain, providing an exciting opportunity for the cross-validation of basic and clinical research findings.

4.1. Brain Receptor Imaging

Knowledge of the function of the human brain is fundamental to understanding the response to all types of injury and disease, not just neuropsychiatric conditions. Due to the pivotal role of receptors in neurotransmission and neuromodulation, in-vivo studies of receptor systems are gaining appeal (37). Using highly selective radioligands, the regional distribution, density, and activity of labeled receptor systems can be visualized (a) at rest and (b) in an experimental state that presumably involves the activation or deactivation of neurotransmission in the system under study. As stated by the law of mass action, free ligand binds to its receptor dependent on the concentration and affinity of both the ligand and the receptor. As noted above, receptor binding is quantified using suitable tracer kinetic models; receptor tracers for PET/SPECT imaging have been developed for dopamine, serotonin, cholinergic, γ-aminobutyric acid (GABA), adenosine, and the opioid systems. There is also growing understanding of the selective affinity of various ligands to receptor subtypes, including possible regional differences that may exist in terms of receptor affinity.

Regarding pain, quantifying neurotransmission at the neuroreceptor site using functional molecular assays permits the dissection of neural activity by assigning it to either a pro-nociceptive or anti-nociceptive regulatory phenomenon as the regional activation of a specific neurotransmission system can be correlated with psychophysical and/or clinical variables. As receptor-specific data of the neurotransmitter system under study are entered into statistical analyses (ANOVAs, correlations) – data unconfounded by unspecific activity in adjacent neural networks – such functional molecular imaging assays are expected to surge in popularity in neurobiological and neuro-pharmacological applications, notably by moving such imaging approaches into the early phases of drug development. This opens the door for drug activity – in a very early stage of testing – to be assessed down the level of receptor function in a dynamic assay in the phylogentically most relevant model system, the human, considering the powerful effects of emotions on the modulation of pain, or the modulation of emotions by neuro-pharmacological drugs on the experience of pain that remain a challenge to be untangled in animal models.

Competitive ligand–receptor assays are employed to visualize the degree to which radioligands are displaced by exogenously administered and endogenous ligands. The latter case, and in the instance of displaceable radiotracers, enables the study of the effect of physical or pharmacological challenges on neurotransmitter release in a particular neuroreceptor system and in turn, to modulate or to relate any changes to the clinical endophenotype. Such assays permit the study of the modulatory effect of a particular genetic makeup on neurotransmission (e.g., anti-nociceptive processes, presumably influencing a subject's ability (a) to suppress signaling in pro-nociceptive channels, or (b) to activate to a greater degree than average those circuits that influence pain suppression) (Fig. 6).

Rarely is reference given to the experimental complexity involved in imaging work, in particular the molecular imaging techniques. A host of problems, linked to equipment, instrumentation, research personnel, and subject selection can easily affect the successful completion of a functional imaging study. Patient movement is a common difficulty in fMRI studies that is difficult to correct for. In addition, molecular imaging adds elements related to cyclotron operation, such as the acquisition of enough "radiolabel" and factors related to the synthesis of the radiotracer, e.g., failure to synthesize the compound of sufficient purity, to achieve radiolabeling with low quantity of "cold" (unlabeled) compound, and to avoid physiological effects. Unlike fMRI studies, PET studies often require the acquisition of blood samples, particularly if traditional kinetic analyses using plasma radiotracer concentrations are contemplated. Needless to say, these types of imaging studies depend on a committed team where each member understands his/her role and everyone recognizes that their contribution counts.

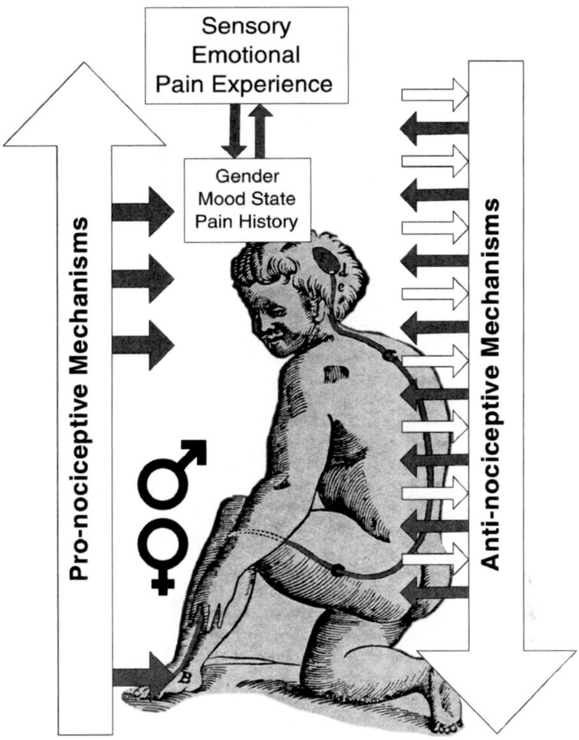

Fig. 6. The complex pain experience is shaped by pro-nociceptive and anti-nociceptive processes, which are influenced by a host of factors, including gender, present state of mood and pain history. To resolve questions whether neural activity is attributed to pro-nociceptive or anti-nociceptive signaling, specific molecular probes are required for image generation as unspecific neural activity, inferred by the hemodynamic effect for example, is not able to make the distinction with any degree of certainty

4.2. Imaging μ-Opioidergic Neurotransmission

The study of the opioidergic neurotransmission represents a good example to illustrate the scientific yield of target-specific neuroreceptor imaging for the study of the complex modulation of tissue-damaging signals at various levels of the pain system (38). Regarding opioidergic neurotransmission, four opioid receptor classes, OP_1 (δ_{1-2}), OP_2 (κ_{1-3}), OP_3, also referred to as μ-opioid receptors (μ_1, μ_2, and μ_3), and OP_4, known as the nociceptin receptor, represent potentially insightful radioligand binding sites for functional molecular studies of opioidergic neurotransmission. All opioid receptors consist of a seven transmembrane domain with a highly conserved amino acid sequence and belong to the family of G-protein-coupled receptors (39).

Of particular significance to pain regulation, μ-opioid receptors are widely distributed throughout the central and peripheral nervous system (40–43); μ-opioid receptors happen to be the binding site of endogenous opioid peptides, including endorphin, dynorphin, enkephalin, and, at normal therapeutic dosages, the principal receptor involved in morphine and in general, any exogenously administered opiate-induced analgesia (43). At higher dosages, and in the case of morphine and some of its derivatives, however, receptor selectivity is lost and opioid receptors other than the μ-opioid receptor are activated as well (44).

To assess the anti-nociceptive effects mediated by the μ-opioid system, we currently use [^{11}C]carfentanil in our laboratory for PET imaging. Regarding the selectivity of exogenous μ-opioid receptor agonists, fentanyl, followed by morphine and meperidine exhibit the highest receptor affinity (45–47). Carfentanil, a fentanyl derivative, is a potently selective μ-opioid receptors agonist, which when radiolabeled with [^{11}C] meets the requirements to act as a suitable radiotracer for the study of central μ-opioid receptor binding (48–51). Low occupancy of the receptors by the radioligand – typically only about 1% of receptors are labeled – is required to neglect, on a theoretical basis, any significant system's effect due to the presence of the radiotracer. Figure 7 illustrates the [^{11}C]carfentanil binding in humans at baseline, in the absence of any challenges, with binding regions and densities matching locations identified in postmortem studies (52, 53). Other commonly used compounds, such as [^{11}C]dyprenorphine and [^{11}C] cyclofoxy, display nonselective receptor pharmacology.

[^{11}C]carfentanil is also a compound that has demonstrated its capacity to be displaceable during endogenous opioid release in response to sustained or repetitive pain (23, 54). The reduction in the measured receptor signal during a noxious challenge is

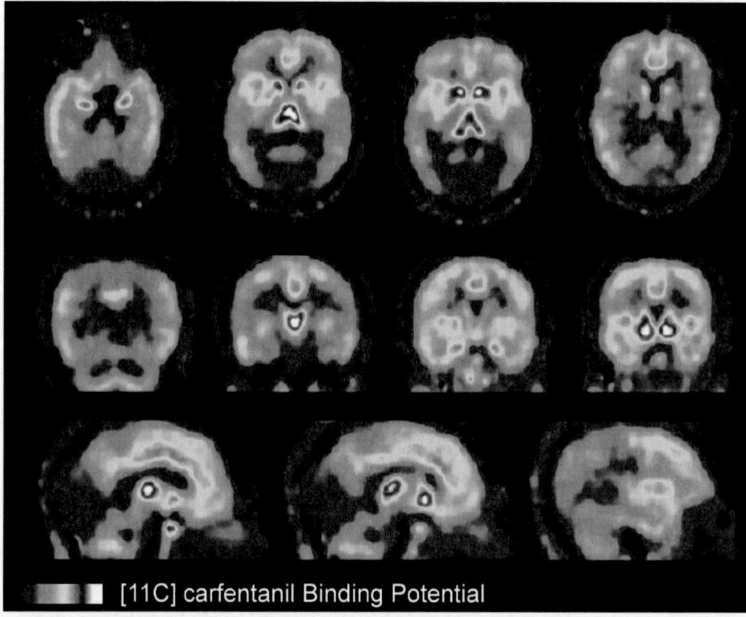

Fig. 7. In-vivo [^{11}C]carfentanil baseline binding in the human brain. Top, middle, and lower rows correspond to horizontal, frontal, and sagittal brain cuts. Binding values are represented by the pseudocolor scale in the lower part of the figure

interpreted as reflecting processes associated with the release of the endogenous neurotransmitter. These may include (a) competition between the endogenous neurotransmitter and the radiolabeled tracer; (b) changes in the conformational state of the receptors in the context of high concentrations of endogenous ligand in the synaptic cleft (a change from high to low affinity states, the latter being less capable of binding the agonist radioligand); and (c) receptor internalization and recycling (55). Activation of the endogenous neurotransmitter system results in the reduction of the externally acquired binding measure, often termed binding potential (Fig. 8).

Neuro-imaging studies in the human have shown the activation of μ-opioid neurotransmission during sustained pain in brain regions, most notably the insular cortex, both anterior and posterior, the anterior cingulate and prefrontal cortex, as well as the ventral basal ganglia (23, 56). These are regions respectively implicated in the representation of interoceptive states, emotional and cognitive integration, as well as motivation and reward processing. From the perspective of the regulation of the pain experience, present data point to a distributed network of regions regulated by the μ-opioid neurotransmitter system, with important implications for the understanding of the complexity of the pain experience and its relief. For example, it has been shown that during the administration of a placebo, expectancies of pain relief can activate endogenous opioid neurotransmission in a number

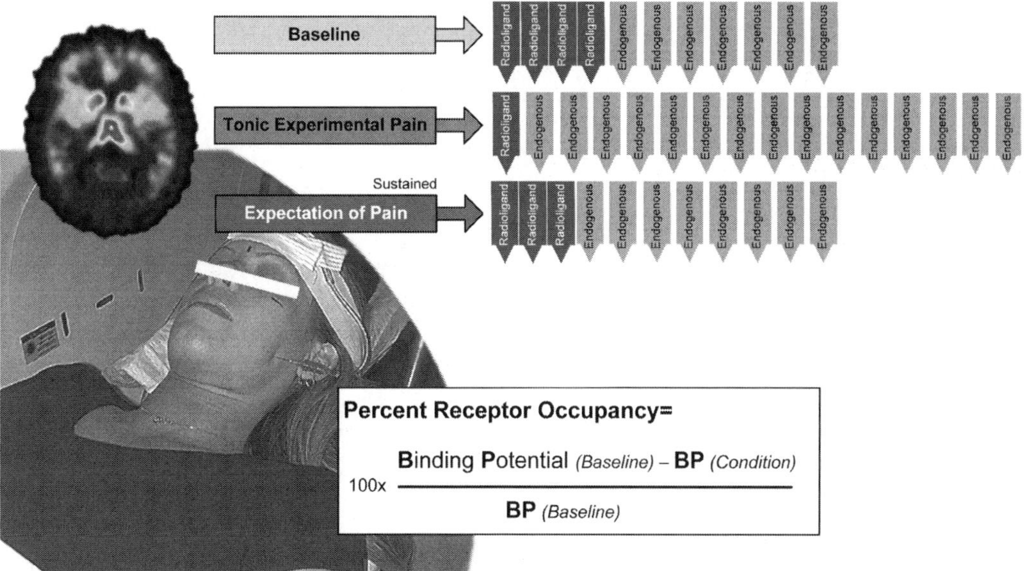

Fig. 8. Percent receptor occupancy (B_{max}/K_d) is used for the quantification of scans. It reflects the ratio of receptor concentration to its affinity for the radiotracer. Note the schematically captured different states of activation of the endogenous system as a function of the experimental condition, changing the availability of receptor sites for the competitive radioligand according to the law of mass action

of these regions (i.e., anterior cingulate, prefrontal cortex, insula, thalamus, ventral basal ganglia, amygdala, periaqueductal gray), with the magnitude of activation relating to the subjectively reported level of pain relief (12, 57).

Given the complex regulatory impact of the μ-opioid receptor system, it should be understood that (1) the number of available receptor sites, (2) the strength, and (3) the rate by which a subject activates his/her endogenous opioid system will have a bearing on the individual response to a pain-stressor. These parameters are quantified by recording the intra-individual binding potential (BP), the proportional receptor occupancy (a) before the initiation of the pain-stressor, and (b) during pain-stress.

Using this type of functional neuroreceptor imaging, the effect size of the changes in the in vivo μ-opioid receptor availability from the condition of (a) nonpainful control to (b) sustained pain of moderate intensity amounts to a reduction in the binding measure of as much as 20%, varying from subject to subject and with brain region (typically ranging from 8 to 20% for regions within which significant changes occur). Both sensory and affective components are modulated with the individual pain report being negatively correlated with the degree to which the μ-opioid system is activated on an individual basis (23). In this respect, genomic individuality – based upon the genetic variations that distinguish one person from another – is being explored to understand the individual response behavior to pain. The large effect size also makes the exploration of complex genetic effects (e.g., gene–gene interactions) feasible without extremely large sample sizes (19, 20).

5. Understanding Me

It is increasingly recognized that not all individuals are equally susceptible to encounter severe or lasting pain. In fact, individuality among humans (or animals) can no longer be dismissed as it appears to explain much of the variance in the response to an insult, disease, or any type of stressor in general. Just focusing on gender, women in their reproductive years represent the majority of those seeking care for a host of clinical pain conditions. Women also report greater pain severity on average (3).

In addition, molecular individuality appears to drive the subject-specific sensory, motor, affective and autonomic complaints, including those linked to stress-related illness and/or pain (23). Besides gender and age, different genotypes are increasingly studied with respect to their contribution in (a) the amplification of symptoms, (b) the susceptibility to a particular clinical course of the disease, and (c) the observation of a unique treatment response. The estimated >five million single nucleotide polymorphisms (SNPs) of the six billion bits of the human genetic code that exhibit a minor allele frequency of >10%, have become the target of investigation for select gene products that confer risk. The majority of SNPs, about fifteen million show minor allele frequencies of less than 10% of humans (http://www.hapmap.org).

To unravel the effect of common SNPs and their expressed and functional gene products, imaging, notably functional molecular imaging, will play a major role in examining differences in brain function as a consequence of SNP variants that either predispose to or protect from disease. As an example, in a PET radioligand study, a common functional polymorphism, homozygotes for the met^{158}met allele of the catechol-O-methyltransferase (COMT), shows significantly lower μ-opioid regional system activation in sustained pain-stress of 10 min and more when compared to subjects characterized as met^{158}val heterozygotes and val^{158}val homozygotes (19).

The fact that gender, age, and the genetic/molecular individuality influence the behavioral pain phenotype also impacts upon the design of imaging studies in terms of the assembly of matched control groups, particularly when study samples are small and differences in ancestry between experimental groups could confound results. Because molecular imaging studies are extremely resource-intensive and therefore study samples tend to be small, controlling for ancestry (more than just ethnicity) between contrasts, such as low and high responders, becomes necessary (18).

Acknowledgments

This work was supported by NIH RO1 DE15396 (CSS), NIH RO1 AT001415 (JKZ) and NIH RO1 DA016423 (JKZ)

References

1. Von Korff M, Dworkin SF, Le Resche L (1990) Graded chronic pain status: an epidemiologic evaluation. Pain 40:279–291
2. Lorenz J, Casey KL (2005) Imaging of acute versus pathological pain in humans. [Review] [15 refs]. Eur J Pain 9(2):163–165
3. Unruh AM (1996) Gender variations in clinical pain experience. [Review] [235 refs]. Pain 65(23):123–167
4. Von Korff M, Le Resche L, Dworkin SF (1993) First onset of common pain symptoms: a prospective study of depression as a risk factor. Pain 55:251–258
5. Rainville P, Duncan GH, Price DD, Carrier B, Bushnell MC (1997) Pain affect encoded in human anterior cingulate but not somatosensory cortex. Science 277(5328):968–971
6. Leknes S, Tracey I (2008) A common neurobiology for pain and pleasure. [Review] [124 refs]. Nat Rev Neurosci 9(4):314–320
7. Singer T, Seymour B, O'Doherty J, Kaube H, Dolan RJ, Frith CD (2004) Empathy for pain

involves the affective but not sensory components of pain. [see comment]. Science 303(5661):1157–1162
8. Panksepp J (2003) Neuroscience. Feeling the pain of social loss. [comment]. Science 302(5643):237–239
9. Petrovic P, Petersson KM, Ghatan PH, Stone-Elander S, Ingvar M (2000) Pain-related cerebral activation is altered by a distracting cognitive task. Pain 85(1–2):19–30
10. Petrovic P, Kalso E, Petersson KM, Ingvar M (2002) Placebo and opioid analgesia– imaging a shared neuronal network. Science 295(5560): 1737–1740
11. Ploghaus A, Tracey I, Gati JS, Clare S, Menon RS, Matthews PM et al (1999) Dissociating pain from its anticipation in the human brain. Science 284(5422):1979–1981
12. Scott DJ, Stohler CS, Egnatuk CM, Wang H, Koeppe RA, Zubieta JK (2008) Placebo and nocebo effects are defined by opposite opioid and dopaminergic responses. [see comment]. Arch Gen Psych 65(2):220–231
13. Ribeiro SC, Kennedy SE, Smith YR, Stohler CS, Zubieta JK, Ribeiro SC et al (2005) Interface of physical and emotional stress regulation through the endogenous opioid system and mu-opioid receptors. [Review] [250 refs]. Prog Neuropsychopharmacol Biol Psychiatry 29(8):1264–1280
14. Price DD (2002) Central neural mechanisms that interrelate sensory and affective dimensions of pain. [Review] [59 refs]. Mol Interv 2(6):392–403
15. Lorenz J, Minoshima S, Casey KL (2003) Keeping pain out of mind: the role of the dorsolateral prefrontal cortex in pain modulation. Brain 126(Pt:5):5–91
16. Wager TD, Rilling JK, Smith EE, Sokolik A, Casey KL, Davidson RJ et al (2004) Placebo-induced changes in FMRI in the anticipation and experience of pain. [see comment]. Science 303(5661):1162–1167
17. Rolls ET, O'Doherty J, Kringelbach ML, Francis S, Bowtell R, McGlone F (2003) Representations of pleasant and painful touch in the human orbitofrontal and cingulate cortices. Cereb Cortex 13(3):308–317
18. Zhou Z, Zhu G, Hariri AR, Enoch MA, Scott D, Sinha R et al (2008) Genetic variation in human NPY expression affects stress response and emotion. Nature 452(7190):997–1001
19. Zubieta JK, Heitzeg MM, Smith YR, Bueller JA, Xu K, Xu Y et al (2003) COMT val158met genotype affects mu-opioid neurotransmitter responses to a pain stressor. Science 299(5610):1240–1243
20. Zubieta JK, Smith YR, Bueller JA, Xu Y, Kilbourn MR, Jewett DM et al (2002) mu-opioid receptor-mediated antinociceptive responses differ in men and women. J Neurosci 22(12):5100–5107
21. Coghill RC, Talbot JD, Evans AC, Meyer E, Gjedde A, Bushnell MC et al (1994) Distributed processing of pain and vibration by the human brain. J Neurosci 14(7):4095–4108
22. Apkarian AV, Bushnell MC, Treede RD, Zubieta JK (2005) Human brain mechanisms of pain perception and regulation in health and disease. [Review] [241 refs]. Eur J Pain 9(4):463–484
23. Zubieta JK, Smith YR, Bueller JA, Xu Y, Kilbourn MR, Jewett DM et al (2001) Regional mu opioid receptor regulation of sensory and affective dimensions of pain. Science 293(5528):311–315
24. Casey KL (1999) Forebrain mechanisms of nociception and pain: analysis through imaging. [Review] [88 refs]. Proc Natl Acad Sci U S A 96(14):7668–7674
25. Casey KL (2000) Concepts of pain mechanisms: the contribution of functional imaging of the human brain [Review] [65 refs]. Prog Brain Res 129:277–287
26. Svensson P, Minoshima S, Beydoun A, Morrow TJ, Casey KL (1997) Cerebral processing of acute skin and muscle pain in humans. J Neurophysiol 78(1):450–460
27. Frost JJ (2008) Molecular imaging to biomarker development in neuroscience. Ann N Y Acad Sci 1144:251–255
28. Apkarian AV. Cortical pathophysiology of chronic pain. Novartis Foundation Symposium 245;261:239–45.
29. Apkarian AV, Sosa Y, Sonty S, Levy RM, Harden RN, Parrish TB et al (2004) Chronic back pain is associated with decreased prefrontal and thalamic gray matter density. J Neurosci 24(46):10410–10415
30. Cherry SR (2004) In vivo molecular and genomic imaging: new challenges for imaging physics. [Review] [145 refs]. Phys Med Biol 49(3):R13–R48
31. Joshi A, Fessler JA, Koeppe RA (2008) Improving PET receptor binding estimates from Logan plots using principal component analysis. J Cereb Blood Flow Metab 28(4):852–865
32. Naganawa M, Kimura Y, Yano J, Mishina M, Yanagisawa M, Ishii K et al (2008) Robust estimation of the arterial input function for Logan plots using an intersectional searching algorithm and clustering in positron emission tomography for neuroreceptor imaging. Neuroimage 40(1):26–34

33. Naganawa M, Kimura Y, Nariai T, Ishii K, Oda K, Manabe Y et al (2005) Omission of serial arterial blood sampling in neuroreceptor imaging with independent component analysis. Neuroimage 26(3):885–890
34. Kimura Y, Naganawa M, Shidahara M, Ikoma Y, Watabe H (2007) PET kinetic analysis – pitfalls and a solution for the Logan plot. [Review] [20 refs]. Ann Nucl Med 21(1):1–8
35. Jones T (1999) Present and future capabilities of molecular imaging techniques to understand brain function. [Review] [18 refs]. J Psychopharmacol 13(4):324–329
36. Cookson W, Liang L, Abecasis G, Moffatt M, Lathrop M (2009) Mapping complex disease traits with global gene expression. [Review] [109 refs]. Nat Rev Genet 10(3):184–194
37. Heiss WD, Herholz K (2006) Brain receptor imaging. [Review] [113 refs]. J Nucl Med 47(2):302–312
38. Henriksen G, Willoch F (2008) Imaging of opioid receptors in the central nervous system. [Review] [152 refs]. Brain 131(Pt:5):5–96
39. Probst WC, Snyder LA, Schuster DI, Brosius J, Sealfon SC (1992) Sequence alignment of the G-protein coupled receptor superfamily. [Review] [167 refs]. DNA Cell Biol 11(1):1–20
40. Voorn P, Brady LS, Berendse HW, Richfield EK (1996) Densitometrical analysis of opioid receptor ligand binding in the human striatum–I. Distribution of mu opioid receptor defines shell and core of the ventral striatum. Neuroscience 75(3):777–792
41. Nozaki-Taguchi N, Yaksh TL (2002) Spinal and peripheral mu opioids and the development of secondary tactile allodynia after thermal injury. Anesth Analg 94(4):968–974
42. Yaksh TL (1997) Pharmacology and mechanisms of opioid analgesic activity. [Review] [183 refs]. Acta Anaesthesiol Scand 41(1:Pt 2):111
43. Mansour A, Khachaturian H, Lewis ME, Akil H, Watson SJ (1988) Anatomy of CNS opioid receptors. [Review] [54 refs]. Trends Neurosci 11(7):308–314
44. Dykstra LA, Preston KL, Bigelow GE (1997) Discriminative stimulus and subjective effects of opioids with mu and kappa activity: data from laboratory animals and human subjects. [Review] [94 refs]. Psychopharmacology 130(1):14–27
45. Portoghese PS, el KR, Law PY, Loh HH, Le BB (2001) Affinity labels as tools for the identification of opioid receptor recognition sites. [Review] [18 refs]. Farmaco 56(3):191–196
46. Jacobs AM, Youngblood F (1992) Opioid receptor affinity for agonist-antagonist analgesics. [Review] [40 refs]. J Am Podiatr Med Assoc 82(10):520–524
47. Simonds WF (1988) The molecular basis of opioid receptor function. [Review] [164 refs]. Endocrine Rev 9(2):200–212
48. Sadzot B, Frost JJ (1990) Pain and opiate receptors: considerations for the design of positron emission tomography studies. Anesth Prog 37(2–3):113–120
49. Frost JJ, Mayberg HS, Sadzot B, Dannals RF, Lever JR, Ravert HT et al (1990) Comparison of [11C]diprenorphine and [11C]carfentanil binding to opiate receptors in humans by positron emission tomography. J Cereb Blood Flow Metab 10(4):484–492
50. Frost JJ, Douglass KH, Mayberg HS, Dannals RF, Links JM, Wilson AA et al (1989) Multicompartmental analysis of [11C]-carfentanil binding to opiate receptors in humans measured by positron emission tomography. J Cereb Blood Flow Metabolism 9(3):398–409
51. Frost JJ (1986) Measurement of neurotransmitter receptors by positron emission tomography: focus on the opiate receptor. NIDA Res Monogr 74:15–24
52. Gross-Isseroff R, Dillon KA, Israeli M, Biegon A (1990) Regionally selective increases in mu opioid receptor density in the brains of suicide victims. Brain Res 530(2):312–316
53. Gorelick DA, Kim YK, Bencherif B, Boyd SJ, Nelson R, Copersino ML et al (2008) Brain mu-opioid receptor binding: relationship to relapse to cocaine use after monitored abstinence. Psychopharmacology 200(4):475–486
54. Wager TD, Scott DJ, Zubieta JK (2007) Placebo effects on human mu-opioid activity during pain.[see comment]. Proc Natl Acad Sci U S A 104(26):11056–11061
55. Narendran R, Hwang DR, Slifstein M, Talbot PS, Erritzoe D, Huang Y et al (2004) In vivo vulnerability to competition by endogenous dopamine: comparison of the D2 receptor agonist radiotracer (-)-N-[11C]propyl-norapomorphine ([11C]NPA) with the D2 receptor antagonist radiotracer [11C]-raclopride. Synapse 52(3):188–208
56. Smith YR, Stohler CS, Nichols TE, Bueller JA, Koeppe RA, Zubieta JK et al (2006) Pronociceptive and antinociceptive effects of estradiol through endogenous opioid neurotransmission in women. J Neurosci 26(21):5777–5785
57. Zubieta JK, Bueller JA, Jackson LR, Scott DJ, Xu Y, Koeppe RA et al (2005) Placebo effects mediated by endogenous opioid activity on mu-opioid receptors. J Neurosci 25(34):7754–7762

Chapter 39

Current and Emerging Pharmacologic Therapies for Pain and Challenges Which Still Lay Ahead

Christopher Noto and Marco Pappagallo

Abstract

This chapter seeks to provide a concise overview of the pharmacologic armamentarium available to treat pain. Drugs will be discussed in terms of their indications, mechanisms of action, and major side effects. For the purposes of this chapter, analgesics will be divided into two groups: current and emerging; current analgesics will be further subdivided into older analgesics and newer analgesics. Older analgesics will refer to drugs that have had FDA approval or were used off label for pain before 1990. Newer analgesics will refer to drugs developed or approved for treating pain since 1990. Finally, emerging analgesics will refer to drugs that have pre-clinical data or phase I/II data to suggest efficacy in treating pain but have not been validated by larger Phase III clinical trials. The chapter concludes with a chart that seeks to highlight current problems involved in pain pharmacotherapy.

Key words: Current analgesics, Emerging analgesics, Opioids, Phase III clinical trials

1. Current Analgesics

1.1. Older Analgesics

1.1.1. Opioids

Opioids have been used to treat pain for centuries. While the term "opioid" has had different meanings over time, it now refers to agonists and antagonists that interact with one or more of the three opioid receptors: mu, kappa, and delta. The prototypical opioid is morphine; other opioids used to treat pain include hydrocodone, oxycodone, oxymorphone, hydromorphone, codeine, meperidine, tramadol, buprenorphine, methadone, fentanyl, propoxyphene, levorphanol, and buprenorphine. These drugs have differing affinities for one or multiple opioid receptors. Opioid receptors are rhodopsin-type G-protein-coupled receptors, which exist in the central and peripheral nervous system and in peripheral tissues. Binding of an opioid to its receptor results in the inhibition of adenylate cyclase which in turn causes

Arpad Szallasi (ed.), *Analgesia: Methods and Protocols*, Methods in Molecular Biology, vol. 617, DOI 10.1007/978-1-60327-323-7_39, © Springer Science+Business Media, LLC 2010

a decrease in the second messenger cyclic AMP (cAMP) (1, 2). In the central nervous system, mu opioid receptors are located in the brainstem and medial thalamus and serve to mediate supraspinal analgesia (3). Of note, the mu opioid receptor gene has been found to display genetic polymorphism (4). This may account for differences in patient response and development of tolerance to opioid therapy. Kappa receptors are found in the limbic system, brainstem, and spinal cord, and mediate spinal analgesia. Delta receptors are located mostly in the brain and their effects are less well known. Endogenous peptides to these receptors include endorphins, enkephalins, and dynorphins (3). In terms of sites of action, opioids act at peripheral, spinal, and supraspinal levels. In the dorsal horn, opioids inhibit release of substance P, calcitonin gene-related peptide, and glutamate from the presynaptic terminals of primary afferent nociceptive C-fibers and A-delta fibers. Activation of opioid receptors at these presynaptic sites results in decreased calcium influx through voltage dependent calcium channels and consequently, decreased neurotransmitter release. Postsynaptically, opioids hyperpolarize second-order dorsal horn spinal neurons by increasing membrane potassium conductance. The combination of effects at pre and postsynaptic levels results in a decrease in nociceptive transmission (2, 3). Also at the midbrain level, opioids activate a descending inhibitory control pathway on spinal neurons (5). Opioids have indications for acute pain, chronic pain, cancer pain, and neuropathic pain. In some settings such as neuropathic or chronic pain conditions, opioids are generally used when other pharmacologic interventions have proved unsuccessful or as adjunctive therapy. In the setting of acute pain or cancer pain, opioids are used to a greater extent as first-line agents. Side effects of opioid therapy include opioid bowel dysfunction (OBD), nausea, vomiting, dizziness, drowsiness, delirium, hypogonadism, and respiratory depression (2). OBD is a term which encompasses a variety of adverse gastrointestinal (GI) events including constipation, abdominal cramping, bloating, gastroesophageal reflux, and gastroparesis; these effects are mediated by binding of opioids to receptors located in the GI tract. Delirium frequently affects elderly patients, especially the cognitively impaired. Hypogonadism (low serum testosterone levels) may be seen in male patients. Respiratory depression is the most feared adverse event yet is uncommon if the opioid is titrated to accepted dosing guidelines. Other factors associated with opioid use are tolerance, dependence, addiction, and opioid-induced hyperalgesia. The mechanisms, prevention, and treatment of these phenomena are the subject of much of the ongoing research in opioid therapy (2).

1.1.2. NSAIDS

NSAIDS or nonsteroidal anti-inflammatory drugs are a class of drugs, which inhibit the synthesis of prostaglandins (e.g., PGE_2).

NSAIDs inhibit the enzyme cyclooxygenase (COX) of which there are two isoforms (COX-1 and COX-2) (6). As an aside, recent research has indicated the presence of a splice variant of COX-1 known as COX-3/COX-1b, which has been shown to be inhibited by NSAIDS such as aspirin, diclofenac, ibuprofen, and indomethacin (7). Inhibition of these enzymes decreases prostaglandin synthesis, which results in central and peripheral anti-inflammatory and analgesic effects (8). The class includes aspirin, ibuprofen, indomethacin, ketoprofen, naproxen, piroxicam, diclofenac, sulindac, and tolmetin, and ketorolac which are nonselective and inhibit both isoforms. Because of their anti-inflammatory effects, NSAIDS are useful in treating conditions such as osteoarthritis, rheumatoid arthritis, and skeletal muscle pain. They are also useful in acute pain settings as well as in cancer pain. Major side effects include gastrointestinal (GI) and renal complications. GI complications include ulcer formation, bleeding, perforation, and development of strictures. Chronic use of NSAIDS use may result in renal insufficiency (2). Celecoxib is a specific COX-2 inhibitor. COX-2 inhibitors were originally developed because they possess the anti-inflammatory effects of nonselective NSAIDS but have significantly reduced GI side effects. However, due to risk of serious cardiovascular events and concern over increased risk of severe skin reactions, all COX-2 inhibitors were removed from the market except celecoxib (2). There are also indications now that the nonselective NSAIDS can lead to increased risk of vascular events such as thrombosis. Interestingly, this effect appears to be drug-specific with studies showing that high-dose ibuprofen is associated with a moderate increase in atherothrombosis, while no such association is observed with high-dose naproxen. Reasons for this disparity are not yet fully understood (9).

1.1.3. Acetaminophen

Acetaminophen is widely used for the treatment of pain and to reduce fever. Studies indicate that acetaminophen exerts its analgesic effects via multiple mechanisms, which include inhibiting generation of prostaglandins, indirectly activating CB-1 (cannabinoid-1) receptors and activating CNS serotoninergic pathways (10–12). Because acetaminophen is generally well tolerated, it is often the first choice for treatment of mild acute or chronic pain and it can be used in combination with other classes of analgesics. The major adverse effect of acetaminophen is liver toxicity which can occur when daily dosing reaches 4 g/day (13).

1.1.4. Carbamazepine

Carbamazepine is an anti-epileptic drug, which decreases conductance through voltage-gated sodium channels and inhibits ectopic and repetitive action potentials (14). Its major use in neuropathic pain is for trigeminal neuralgia, for which it is FDA approved. However, side effects such as dizziness, ataxia, nausea, vomiting, somnolence, and in rare cases aplastic anemia have been major drawbacks to use of the drug (15). As a result, some physicians are now prescribing oxcarbazepine, a keto-analog of carbamazepine, which has fewer side effects. Studies indicate that oxcarbazepine blocks voltage-gated sodium channels (16). Oxcarbazepine has also been shown to modulate voltage-gated calcium channels and possibly enhance potassium conductance, which would further enhance its ability to stabilize neuronal membranes (17).

1.1.5. Tricyclic Antidepressants (TCAs)

Tricyclic antidepressents include amitriptyline, nortriptyline, desipramine, doxepin, and imipramine. Historically, TCAs have been used off label as the drugs of choice to treat neuropathic pain and studies support their efficacy in treating postherpetic neuralgia and diabetic neuropathy. These drugs inhibit serotonin and norepinephrine reuptake to differing degrees, but their exact analgesic mechanism is not fully understood. Some TCAs (amitrityline, doxepin, and imipramine) also have been shown to have local anesthetic properties. The major drawback to TCA use is the side effect profile, which includes dry mouth, urinary retention, constipation, sedation, and sexual dysfunction; the most serious side effects are those that affect the cardiovascular system such as arrhythmias, postural hypotension, and heart block (18, 19).

1.2. Newer Analgesics

1.2.1. Gabapentinoids (Gabapentin, Pregabalin)

Gabapentinoids are antiepilepsy drugs (AEDS) that have been shown in clinical trials to be effective agents in management of neuropathic pain (20). These drugs were designed to mimic the neurotransmitter GABA. However, studies have indicated that gabapentin and pregabalin do not interact with either the GABA-A or GABA-B receptors, are not metabolized to GABA, and do not block GABA reuptake or degradation. Current evidence indicates that gabapentin and pregabalin exert their antinociceptive effect by binding to the $\alpha 2\delta$ subunit of voltage-gated calcium channels in N-type spinal neurons (21, 22). These drugs are referred to as calcium channel "modulators" because binding decreases the amount of time the channel remains in an open state. Thus, they act by suppressing ectopic discharges in nociceptive dorsal root ganglia and dorsal horn neurons (23). In addition, they have relatively benign toxicity profiles without major drug interactions. As a result, gabapentinoids should be regarded as first-line treatment for neuropathic pain conditions rather than adjuvants (24).

Gabapentin has been shown to be effective for postherpetic neuralgia (for which it has FDA approval), painful diabetic neuropathy, and painful cancer neuropathies. Some studies suggest it is also effective for postamputation phantom limb pain, and for pain secondary to Guillain–Barré syndrome and spinal cord injury. Gabapentin is also useful as an adjuvant in acute pain conditions such as the postoperative setting where it has been shown to reduce opioid requirements. The most common side effects of gabapentin are dizziness, somnolence, and peripheral edema (25–31).

Pregabalin was given FDA approval for neuropathic pain associated with diabetic neuropathy and postherpetic neuralgia in December 2004. In June 2007, it was given FDA approval for the treatment of fibromyalgia. Pharmacology and side effect profile are similar to gabapentin; weight gain may also be seen with pregabalin (32–34).

1.2.2. Nongabapentinoid AEDS

Valproic acid received final FDA approval for migraine prophylaxis in 2008; it is also FDA approved for treating seizure disorders and bipolar disorder. There is consensus that valproic acid increases concentrations of the inhibitory neurotransmitter γ-aminobutyric acid (GABA) in various brain regions. Shortly after administration of valproic acid, significant increases in nerve terminal GABA concentrations can be observed in the midbrain. Cerebrospinal fluid concentration of GABA is also increased with administration of valproic acid (35). Common side effects of valproic acid include weight gain, hair loss, and dyspepsia. Valproic acid is contraindicated during pregnancy because it is a teratogen that can cause neural tube defects. A need to monitor serum drug levels is another downside of its use (36).

Topiramate is an anti-epileptic drug that has several proposed mechanisms of action: (1) modulation of voltage-gated sodium channels, (2) enhancing GABA-ergic inhibition, (3) blocking excitatory glutamate activity via AMPA and kainate receptors, and (4) blocking voltage-gated calcium channels (37). Topiramate was thought to be effective for painful diabetic neuropathy; however, subsequent studies failed to show a benefit. Topiramate has shown efficacy for migraine prophylaxis in some studies. Side effects of topiramate include psychomotor slowing, dizziness, confusion, memory impairment, somnolence, and fatigue. Kidney stones were also found at a rate of 1.5% in clinical trials. These adverse effects limit compliance with topiramate (37, 38).

Zonisamide is another AED that has been shown to be beneficial in migraine prophylaxis. Its mechanism of action is unknown but may be due to T-type calcium channel blockade, sodium channel blockade, free radical scavenging, and inhibition of nitric oxide formation. Side effect profile is similar to topiramate (38, 39).

Lamotrigine likely acts by stabilizing a slow inactivated conformation of voltage-gated sodium channels and inhibiting glutamate release from presynaptic neurons (37). Lamotrigine has shown some efficacy in treating trigeminal neuralgia that is resistant to carbamazepine treatment. Additionally, some studies suggest that it may be useful in migraine, HIV neuropathy, and poststroke pain. However, recent studies have called into question its effectiveness for painful diabetic neuropathy. Dermatologic side effects may be seen with lamotrigine; in rare cases, Stevens–Johnson Syndrome and Toxic Epidermal Necrolysis have been observed (37, 38, 40, 41).

1.2.3. Newer Antidepressants

Duloxetine, milnacipram, and venlafaxine act as both serotonin and norepinephrine reuptake inhibitors. They also weakly inhibit the reuptake of dopamine. Unlike TCAs, they show low affinity for histamine and cholinergic muscarinic receptors (42). Duloxetine received FDA approval for painful diabetic neuropathy in 2004. Milnacipram was recently approved for fibromyalgia. Venlafaxine has also been shown to be effective for painful diabetic neuropathy and studies support efficacy for other forms of neuropathic pain. Common side effects of duloxetine, milnacipram, and venlafaxine include nausea, dizziness, and restlessness. Bupropion is a dopamine reuptake inhibitor, which has weak norepinephrine and serotonin reuptake inhibition properties. Some studies indicate potential efficacy of bupropion for neuropathic pain. Bupropion is not associated with sexual dysfunction as are other antidepressants (43).

1.2.4. Transdermal Lidocaine and Other Local Anesthetics

Local anesthetics bind to sodium channels in neuronal membranes of primary sensory fibers and block propagation of action potentials to second-order neurons. In neuropathic pain, they exert their effects by inhibiting ectopic and paroxysmal discharges. Lidocaine is a local anesthetic and antiarrythmic that is commonly used as a topical agent. Transdermal lidocaine received FDA approval for the treatment of postherpetic neuralgia in 1999 and has been shown to alleviate pain in postherpetic neuralgia without serious adverse effects (43, 44).

Of note, mexiletine is a local anesthetic and antiarrythmic, available in an oral form and administered systemically. It has shown efficacy in neuropathic pain and central pain states. However, it is contraindicated in patients with second- or third-degree atrioventricular blocks and has a high incidence of GI side effects (2).

1.2.5. Triptans

Triptans are a class of drugs, which are used as an abortive treatment for migraine and cluster headaches. Triptans are agonists for $5HT_{1B}$, $5HT_{1D}$, and $5HT_{1F}$ serotonin receptor subtypes. The mechanism of action is thought to be inhibition of the activation of trigeminal sensory neurons and a reduction in the release of "pain" neurotransmitters centrally. Drugs in this class include sumatriptan, rizatriptan, almotriptan, zolmitriptan, naratriptan, eletriptan, and frovatriptan. Sumatriptan was the first triptan developed and received FDA approval in 1992; it is also the only triptan available in an injectable form. Tritpans usually have few side effects. However, there is a risk of life-threatening serotonin syndrome in patients who are concurrently taking selective serotonin uptake inhibitors or selective serotonin/norepinephrine reuptake inhibitors (45, 46).

1.2.6. Ziconotide

Ziconotide is a synthetic peptide that blocks N-type calcium channels located on primary afferent nociceptive neurons in the superficial layers of the dorsal horn. Animal studies suggest that ziconotide works by blocking calcium influx into the presynaptic nerve terminal, thus decreasing the release of excitatory neurotransmitters in the synapse. Ziconotide is an intrathecal therapy, which received FDA approval in December 2004. It is indicated for the management of severe chronic pain in patients for whom intrathecal therapy is warranted, and who are intolerant of or refractory to other treatments, such as systemic analgesics, adjunctive therapies, or intrathecal morphine. Thus, ziconotide is to be used only after less invasive or more conservative treatment regimens have failed to adequately reduce pain levels or have caused intolerable side effects for patients (47). Common side effects of ziconotide include dizziness, nausea, headache, and confusion. Psychiatric consultation before use of ziconotide is prudent as the drug may cause hallucinations and its use is contraindicated in patients with a history of psychosis. No withdrawal or other side effects are seen after ziconotide is discontinued. The results of clinical trials with ziconotide have spawned interest in the development of other selective N-type calcium channel blockers, particularly those that can be administered orally (48).

1.2.7. α_2-Adrenergic Agonists

α_2-adrenergic receptor agonists have effects in the peripheral nervous system, spinal cord, and brain. Clonidine is the most commonly used α_2 agonist for the treatment of pain. In the periphery, clonidine binds to α_2 autoreceptors of sympathetic endings resulting in a decrease in release of further norepinephrine. Studies have shown topical clonidine to be effective in treating hyperalgesia in patients with sympathetically maintained pain (49). α_2-adrenergic receptor agonists also have a spinal antinociceptive effect through action of α_2 receptors in the dorsal horn of the spinal cord (50). Clonidine has been shown to potentiate the effect of opioids when given intrathecally. Intrathecal clonidine may cause hypotension, dizziness, and somnolence. Tizanidine is a short acting oral α_2-agonist, which has a lower hypotensive effect than clonidine and has shown effectiveness for a variety of pain states (49).

2. Emerging Analgesics

2.1. Bone Metabolism Modulators

Bisphosphonates are synthetic analogs of pyrophosphate, which bind with high affinity to bone hydroxyapatite crystals and inhibit bone resorption by osteoclasts. Bisphosphonates can be divided into two classes: nitrogenous bisphosphonates and nitrogen-deficient bisphosphonates. Nitrogenous bisphosphonates (e.g., pamidronate, ibandronate, zoledronate) bind and block the enzyme farnesyl pyrophosphate synthase in the mevalonate pathway. This enzyme is necessary for synthesis of isoprenoid compounds, which are responsible for posttranslational modification of GTPases such as Rho, Rab, and Rac. Inhibition of these enzymes is likely responsible for disruption of osteoclast activity and apoptosis. Nitrogen-deficient bisphosphonates (etidronate) are older, first-generation bisphosphonates, which are incorporated into nonhydrolyzable analogs of ATP that inhibit ATP-dependent intracellular events (51). However, in clinical use, these drugs have largely been replaced by nitrogenous bisphosphonates. Bisphosphonates are valuable for treating disorders associated with bone pain such as metastatic disease, hypercalcemia, osteoporosis, Paget's disease, and multiple myeloma (2). Although use of bisphosphonates for these conditions is certainly not new, there is emerging evidence that bisphosphonates may be useful in treating complex regional pain syndrome (CRPS). While the mechanism of analgesia in this disease is not understood, it may be due to inhibition of osteoclasts and other activated cells involved in inflammation and immune responses such as macrophages. Inhibition of these cells would result in a decrease in the release of proinflammatory cytokines in the area of inflammation in CRPS (52–54). Interestingly, in an animal model of neuropathic pain from nerve injury due to sciatic nerve ligature, bisphosphonates decreased the number of activated macrophages infiltrating the ligated nerve, reduced Wallerian nerve fiber degeneration, and decreased experimental hyperalgesia (55). The bioavailability of bisphosphonates when used orally is poor. Therefore, when used for bone pain, research and clinical use has often focused on intravenous therapy. Osteonecrosis of the jaw has been seen in a small number of oncologic patients who received intravenous, high-dose bisphosphonates on a monthly basis usually for more than 1 year. These patients also had a history of poor dental hygiene, or a recent history of dental extraction or dental implants (24).

Calcitonin is a polypeptide hormone synthesized by the parafollicular cells of the thyroid gland. The receptor for calcitonin is a member of the class B family of G-protein-coupled receptors (56). Binding of calcitonin to its receptor inhibits osteoclastic bone resorption making calcitonin a useful adjuvant for treating bone pain in conditions such as metastatic bone disease (2). Although its analgesic mechanism is not fully understood, calcitonin has been shown to inhibit prostaglandin E2 synthesis and elevate endogenous β-endorphin levels. Phase II trials of oral salmon calcitonin have shown significant benefit in relieving osteoarthritic pain. Currently, a Phase III trial is underway for oral salmon calcitonin and pain associated with osteoarthritis (57).

2.2. TRPV1 Agonists

Capsaicin is the natural molecule, which gives chili peppers their pungent taste. TRPV1 is a neuronal membrane protein found on a subset of nociceptive primary sensory afferents which is activated by heat, low pH, endogenous ligands, and capsaicin (58). Topical application of capsaicin to the skin initially causes an excitation of primary sensory afferents, which express TRPV1. This is followed by a state of nociceptor function deactivation, called desensitization. In this state, the neuron enters a refractory phase and is unresponsive to further stimulation. Capsaicin-induced fiber desensitization is dose-dependent. Studies of topical capsaicin have shown mild benefit for patients with neuropathic pain. However, noncompliance likely limits effectiveness of capsaicin as the drug causes a burning sensation when it is applied to the skin. Preliminary observations have indicated that high-dose topical capsaicin, (doses of 5–10% preparation) when used as a one-time treatment under regional anesthesia provided some degree of relief in patients with neuropathic pain; the benefit lasted as long as 18 weeks in some patients (59). Another study demonstrated efficacy for high-dose capsaicin in patients with HIV neuropathy. Currently, there is a transdermal patch Qutenza™ containing high-concentration capsaicin (8% w/w) for treatment of postherpetic neuralgia (60). An injectable TRPV1 agonist preparation based on capsaicin known as ADLEA™ is undergoing trials for pain after knee replacement surgery and bunionectomy (61).

2.3. Cannabinoids

Cannabinoid receptors are G-protein-coupled receptors, which are coupled negatively to adenylate cyclase and positively to mitogen-activated protein kinase (MAP). Two cannabinoid receptors have been identified, CB_1 and CB_2. CB_1 is mostly found in brain tissue, but is also present in the dorsal horn of the spinal cord. CB_2 is located mostly on immune cells and on microglia in the brain. There is some evidence that a third cannabinoid receptor may exist, which has yet to be cloned (43, 62). Both animal and clinical studies suggest that cannabinoids have analgesic properties through effects on the peripheral and central nervous systems as well as peripheral anti-inflammatory effects. However, strong clinical evidence of the efficacy of cannabinoids to treat pain is not available. Synthetic Δ[9]-trans-tetrahydrocannabinol also known as dronabinol is used to increase appetite in patients with cancer, AIDS, and wasting syndromes (24). In chronic neuropathic pain, a compound known as CT-3, a THC-11-oic analog has been shown to be more effective than placebo (63). Cannabinoids also have been shown to have an anti-allyodynic/antihyperalgesic effect (64). These observations have led to interest in development of other drugs, which will bind to cannabinoid receptors.

2.4. NMDA Antagonists

N-methyl-D-aspartate (NMDA) receptors are ionotropic receptors for glutamate located in the central and peripheral nervous system (43). Studies have indicated that after tissue or nerve injury, NMDA receptors in the spinal cord may mediate central sensitization and play an important role in the development of hyperalgesia, allodynia, and chronic pain (65, 66). NMDA antagonists include dextromethorphan, D-methadone, memantine, amantadine, and ketamine. Ketamine can be used as an adjuvant to opioid therapy, allowing 20–30% greater pain relief and opioid dose reduction of 25–50%. However, ketamine has a narrow therapeutic window and its use can cause hallucinations and memory impairment in patients. Despite potential adverse effects and failure of randomized clinical trials of dextromethorphan, there is a renewed interest in the development of NMDA receptor antagonists/modulators for the treatment of neuropathic pain states. Currently, several clinical trials in various phases are underway. There is also interest in the possibility that NMDA antagonists could be used to counteract or prevent opioid analgesic tolerance when used in combination with opioids (2, 67, 68).

2.5. Neuroimmunomodulatory Agents and Microglial Inhibitors

Studies show that proinflammatory cytokines, such as TNF-α (tumor necrosis factor), have a significant role in generating and maintaining neuropathic pain in inflammatory diseases such as autoimmune conditions. Nerve growth factor (NGF), IL-1β, IL-6, and leukemia inhibitory factor are such molecules upregulated in inflammatory states (69). Anti-NGF therapy has been demonstrated to be effective in reducing bone cancer pain (70). Studies in rats indicate that thalidomide, an inhibitor of TNF-α, may prevent hyperalgesia in nerve constriction injury (71). Development of thalidomide analogs may be another approach to controlling hyperalgesia in neuropathic pain. A recent area of research involves inhibiting microglial activation. Studies have shown that microglial activation in the medullary dorsal horn can contribute to the development of tactile hypersensitivity in a model of trigeminal nerve injury. Minocycline, an inhibitor of microglial activation, was shown to decrease pain hypersensitivity in this model (72). A recent study involving a phosphodiesterase inhibitor, which also suppresses glial-cell activation, demonstrated effectiveness in rat models of neuropathic pain (73).

2.6. Botulinum Toxin

Botulinum Toxin type A (BoNT-A) is a neurotoxin protein produced by the bacterium *Clostridium botulinum*. BoNT-A exerts its effect by preventing exocytotic release of acetylcholine into the neuromuscular junction. The protein has a heavy chain region and a light chain region. The heavy chain region targets the toxin to specific motor neuron axon terminals. The light chain possesses metalloproteinase activity through a zinc endopeptidase located in the middle of the chain. Once inside the terminal, the light chain cleaves a type of SNARE protein known as SNAP-25 (synaptosomal-associated protein 25). SNAP-25 is a membrane-bound protein anchored to the cytosolic side of the neuronal plasma membrane that is involved in docking neurotransmitter containing synaptic vesicles at nerve terminals. Cleavage of SNAP 25 prevents neurosecretory vesicles of acetylcholine from docking and fusing with the plasma membrane of the axon terminal, thus preventing release of acetylcholine and inhibiting muscle contraction (74). BoNT-A has therefore been used to treat disorders involving increased muscle tone, such as dystonia, which also have pain as an associated symptom. However when used in these disorders, analgesic effects were noted to exceed improvements in muscle contraction, suggesting that BoNT-A might have pain relieving effects independent of its effects on muscle tone. Further studies showed that BoNT-A decreased release of neurotransmitters such as substance P, calcitonin gene-related peptide, and glutamate, which have roles in nociceptor sensitization and the development of neuropathic pain (75). As a result, there is now interest in using BoNT-A in the management of neuropathic pain. Recently, a randomized, double-blind, placebo-controlled study of BoNT-A demonstrated long-lasting analgesic effect when injected in 29 patients who had focal chronic neuropathic pain. In particular, a reduction in intensity of mechanical allodynia and a decrease in cold pain thresholds were observed (76). Larger studies will need to be performed to confirm these findings and investigate whether BoNT-A may be useful in a variety of neuropathic pain conditions.

2.7. Potassium Channel Openers

One of the most novel areas of development in the area of pain pharmacotherapeutics is development of neuronal potassium channel activators (77). Retigabine's mechanism of action involves opening of neuronal $K_v7.2$-7.5 voltage activated K^+ channels. These channels are responsible for generation of the M-current. The M-current is a subthreshold, noninactivating potassium current found in many neuronal cell types. It is dominant in controlling membrane excitability because it is the only sustained current in the range of action potential initiation. M-current modulation has profound effects on neuronal excitability, which underlies the potential for potassium channel openers to be effective in neuropathic pain. Retigabine has also been shown to increase synthesis of GABA in rat hippocampal neurons and to allosterically potentiate GABA-induced chloride currents in cultured rat cortical neurons. Behavioral studies have shown retigabine can reduce pain behaviors involving animal models of neuropathic pain (78–81). Potassium channel openers may soon become another class of ion channel regulators in the pharmacologic armamentarium for pain control.

2.8. Free Radical Scavengers

Studies have indicated that the presence of reactive oxygen species contribute to the development of neuropathic pain and that antioxidant therapy may be effective in preventing or treating neuropathic pain (82). Vitamin C (ascorbic acid) has been reported to decrease the incidence of complex regional pain syndrome following wrist fractures (83). There is also evidence that alpha lipoic acid is effective in the management of painful diabetic neuropathy (84). Further studies are needed to clarify the role of antioxidants to treat chronic pain.

2.9. Current and Future Challenges

See Table 39.1 for further information.

Table 1
Current and future challenges in pain pharmacotherapy

Challenge	Background
Chronic pain is a complex phenomenon, which continues to remain undertreated in the majority of affected patients.	Pain medicine is a new field; research efforts focused on the understanding of pain mechanisms and adequate treatments are also new, but fast growing; the psychosocial aspects affecting the patient with chronic pain add to the intricacy of pharmacotherapy outcomes. Of note, treatment outcome is based on functional and pain improvement.
Multiple mechanisms account for chronic pain.	No specific drug may appropriately target every mechanism involved. Combination of treatments or "broad-spectrum" drugs are likely necessary in patients with refractory pain to a single-drug approach. Despite the variety of classes of pain drugs, only 40–60% of patients with neuropathic pain obtain partial relief of their pain (85).
Disease modifying drugs as therapeutic analgesics	Increased knowledge of specific diseases that cause pain and their mechanisms may lead to breakthrough discoveries for treatments that will have the potential not only for reversing the course of the disease but also for pain control. These drugs would not necessarily inhibit nociception, but rather decrease factors involved in inflammation and tissue damage which in turn lead to sensitization and activation of nociceptors.
Variability in drug-related side effects; variability in the analgesic effects of drugs	Drugs may reach their maximal efficacy yet still not adequately relieve pain. Some drugs may also need to be discontinued due to intolerable or unmanageable side effects. Pharmacogenomic studies of pain and headache are necessary.

(continued)

Table 1 (continued)

Challenge	Background
Noncompliance	Noncompliance is a major barrier to effective pain management. Pain medicine requires a comprehensive, longitudinal assessment of the patient with chronic pain. This starts with patient education on treatments and discussion of treatment expectations; the whole process adds to the complexity of treating chronic pain.
Analgesic tolerance (e.g., opioid tolerance) and opioid induced hyperalgesia	Tolerance and opioid-induced hyperalgesia may hamper successful treatment of pain. More research on the mechanisms of these entities is needed. There is also interesting research being done on agents (such as NMDA antagonists) that may prevent or counteract opioid analgesic tolerance.
Individual vulnerability to drug addiction	This is a complex task for the physician who needs to screen and treat a patient affected by chronic pain as well as psychiatric co-morbidities, abnormal behaviors, and addiction. Addiction is a primary, chronic, neurobiological disease with genetic, psychosocial, and environmental factors influencing its development. Research into addiction is both clinically and socially relevant. When drugs with addiction potential are used, risk management expertise and expensive structured programs will be needed.

References

1. Davis M (2005) Opioid Therapy. In: Pappagallo M (ed) The neurological basis of pain. McGraw-Hill, New York, pp 559–580
2. Pappagallo M, Werner M (2008) Chronic pain a primer for physicians. Remedica, Chicago, pp 154–98
3. Trescot AM, Sukdeb D, Lee M, Hans H (2008) Opioid pharmacology. Pain Physician 11(2 suppl):S133–153
4. Bond C, LaForge KS, Tian M et al (1998) Single-nucleotide polymorphism in the human mu opioid receptor gene alters beta-endorphin binding and activity: possible implications for opiate addiction. Proc Natl Acad Sci U S A 95:9608–13
5. Dickenson AH, Kieffer B (2006) Opiates: basic mechanism. In: McMahon SB, Koltzenburg M (eds) Wall and Melzack's textbook of pain. Churchill Livingstone, London, pp 427–442
6. Golden BD, Abramson SB (2005) Nonsteroidal anti-inflammatory medications and acetaminophen. In: Pappagallo M (ed) The neurological basis of pain. McGraw-Hill, New York, pp 545–558
7. Chandrasekharan NV, Dai H, Roos KL et al (2002) COX-3, a cyclooxygenase-1 variant inhibited by acetaminophen and other analgesic/antipyretic drugs: cloning, structure, and expression. Proc Natl Acad Sci U S A 99: 13926–31
8. Cashman JN (1996) The mechanisms of action of NSAIDS in analgesia. Drugs 52: 13–23
9. Kearney PM, Baigent C, Godwin J et al (2006) Do selective cyclo-oxygenase-2 inhibitors and traditional non-steroidal anti-inflammatory drugs increase the risk of atherothrombosis? Meta-analysis of randomised trials. BMJ 332:1302–08

10. Graham GG, Scott KF (2005) Mechanism of action of paracetamol. AM J Ther 12:46–55
11. Bertolini A, Ferrari A, Ottani A et al (2006) Paracetamol: new vistas of an old drug. CNS Drug Rev 12:250–75
12. Bonnefont J, Daulhac L, Etienne M et al (2007) Acetaminophen recruits spinal p42/p44 MAPKs and GH/IGF-1 receptors to produce analgesia via the serotonergic system. Mol Pharmacol 71:407–15
13. Watkins PB, Kaplowitz N, Slattery JT et al (2006) Aminotransferase elevations in healthy adults receiving 4 grams of acetaminophen daily: a randomized controlled trial. JAMA 296:87–93
14. Tremont-Lukats IW, Megeff C, Backonja MM (2000) Anticonvulsants for neuropathic pain syndromes: mechanisms of action and place in therapy. Drugs 60:1029–52
15. Tegretol (Carbamazepine): Prescribing information. Novartis, Inc.
16. Schmutz McLean MJ, Wamil AW et al (1994) Oxcarbazepine: mechanisms of action. Epilepsia 35:S5–9
17. Schmidt D, Elger C (2004) What is the evidence that oxcarbazepine and carbamazepine are distinctly different antiepileptic drugs? Epilepsy & Behav 5:627–35
18. Saarto T, Wiffen PJ (2007) Antidepressants for neuropathic pain. *Cochrane Database Syst Rev* 4: CD005454.
19. Gerner P, Haderer AE, Mujtaba M et al (2003) Assessment of differential blockade by amtriptyline and its N-methyl derivative in different species by different routes. Anesthesiology 98:1484–90
20. Backonja M, Glanzman RL (2003) Gabapentin dosing for neuropathic pain: evidence from randomized placebo-controlled clinical trials. Clin Ther 25:81–104
21. Sills GJ (2006) The mechanisms of action of gabapentin and pregabalin. Curr Opin Pharmacol 6:108–13
22. Maneuf YP, Luo ZD, Lee K (2006) $\alpha 2\delta$ and the mechanism of action of gabapentin in the treatment of pain. Semin Cell Dev Biol 17:565–70
23. Wallace MS (2006) Ziconotide: a new nonopioid intrathecal analgesic for the treatment of chronic pain. Expert Rev Neurother 6:1423–28
24. Knotkova H, Pappagallo M (2007) Adjuvant analgesics. Med Clin N Am 91:113–124
25. Turan A, Karamanlioglu B, Memis D et al (2004) Analgesic effects of gabapentin after spinal surgery. Anesthesiology 100:935–38
26. Eckhardt K, Ammon S, Hofmann U et al (2000) Gabapentin enhances the analgesic effect of morphine in healthy volunteers. Anesth Analg 91:185–89
27. Rowbotham M, Harden N, Stacey B et al (1998) Gabapentin for the treatment of postherpetic neuralgia: a randomized control trial. JAMA 280:1837–42
28. Rice AS, Maton S (2001) Gabapentin in postherpetic neuralgia: a randomized, double blind, placebo controlled study. Pain 94:215–24
29. Bone M, Critchley P, Buggy DJ (2002) Gabapentin in postamputation phantom limb pain: a randomized, double blind, placebo-controlled, cross over study. Reg Anesth Pain Med 27:481–86
30. Pandey CK, Bose N, Garg G et al (2002) Gabapentin for the treatment of pain in Guillain-Barré syndrome: a double blinded, placebo-controlled, crossover study. Anesth Analg 95:1719–23
31. Tai Q, Kirshblum S, Chen B et al (2002) Gabapentin in the treatment of neuropathic pain after spinal cord injury: a prospective, randomized, double blind, crossover trial. J Spinal Cord Med 2005:100–5
32. Lesser H, Sharma U, Lamoreaux L et al (2004) Pregabalin relieves symptoms of painful diabetic neuropathy: a randomized controlled trial. Neurology 63:2104–10
33. Crofford LJ, Rowbotham MC, Mease PJ et al (2005) Pregabalin for the treatment of fibromyalgia syndrome: results of a randomized, double blind, placebo-controlled trial. Arthritis Rheum 52:1264–73
34. Dworkin RH, Corbin AE, Young JP Jr et al (2003) Pregabalin for the treatment of postherpetic neuralgia: a randomized, placebo-controlled trial. Neurology 60:1274–83
35. Owens MJ, Nemeroff CB (2003) Pharmacology of valproate. Psychopharmacol Bull 37(Suppl 2):17–24
36. Depakote ER (Divalproex Sodium): Prescribing Information. Abbott Laboratories. Physician Desk Reference® PDR Network publisher, Mondale NJ, 2009
37. Jensen TS (2002) Anticovulsants in neuropathic pain: rationale and clinical evidence. Eur J Pain 6(Suppl A):61–8
38. Pappagallo M (2003) Newer antiepileptic drugs: possible uses in the treatment of neuropathic pain and migraine. Clin Ther 25:2506–38
39. Leppik IE (2004) Zonisamide: chemistry, mechanism of action, and pharmacokinetics. Seizure 13(Suppl 1):S5–9

40. Zakrzewska JM, Chaudry Z, Nurmikko TJ et al (1997) Lamotrigine (Lamictal) in refractory trigeminal neuralgia: results from a double-blind placebo controlled crossover trial. Pain 73:223–30
41. Vinik AI, Tuchman M, Sairstein B et al (2007) Lamotrigine for treatment of pain associated with diabetic neuropathy: results of two randomized, double blind, placebo-controlled studies. Pain 128:169–179
42. Mattia C, Coluzzi F (2003) Antidepressants in chronic neuropathic pain. Mini Rev Med Chem 3:773–784
43. Coluzzi F, Mattia C (2005) Antidepressant, anticonvulsants, and miscellaneous agents. In: Pappagallo M (ed) The neurological basis of pain. McGraw-Hill, New York, pp 581–598
44. Rowbotham MC, Davies PS, Verkempinck C et al (1999) Topical lidocaine patch relieves postherpetic neuralgia more effectively than a vehicle topical patch: results of an enriched enrollment study. Pain 80:533–38
45. Mauskop A (2005) Migraine and cluster headaches. In: Pappagallo M (ed) The neurological basis of pain. McGraw-Hill, New York, pp 391–399
46. Nikai T, Basbaum AI, Ahn A (2008) Profound reduction of somatic and visceral pain in mice by intrathecal administration of the anti-migraine drug, sumatriptan. Pain 139:533–540
47. Wallace S (2006) Ziconotide: a new nonopioid intrathecal analgesic for the treatment of chronic pain. Expert Rev Neurothe 6:1423–28
48. Prialt (Ziconotide) Prescribing Information. Elan Pharmaceuticals, Inc. Physician Desk Reference® PDR Network publisher, Mondale NJ, 2009
49. Pappagallo M (2005) Peripheral neuropathic pain. In: Pappagallo M (ed) The Neurological basis of pain. McGraw-Hill, New York, pp 321–337
50. Fukuda T, Furukawa H, Setsuji H, Hidenori T (2006) Systemic clonidine activates neurons of the dorsal horn, but not the locus ceruleus (A6) or the A7 area, after a formalin test: the importance of the dorsal horn in the antinociceptive effects of clonidine. J Anesth 20:279–283
51. Russell RG (2007) Bisphosphonates: mode of action and pharmacology. Pediatrics 119(Suppl 2):S150–62
52. Breuer B, Pappagallo M, Ongseng F (2008) An open-label pilot trial of ibandronate for complex regional pain syndrome. Clin J Pain 24:685–9
53. Varenna M, Zucchi F, Ghiringhelli D et al (2000) Intravenous clodronate in the treatment of reflex sympathetic dystrophy syndrome: a randomized, double blind, placebo-controlled study. J Rheumatol 27: 1477–1483
54. Cortet B, Flipo RM, Coquerelle P et al (1997) Treatment of severe, recalcitrant reflex sympathetic dystrophy: assessment of efficacy and safety of the second generation bisphosphonate pamidronate. Clin Rheumatol 16:51–56
55. Liu T, van Rooijen N, Tracey DJ (2000) Depletion of macrophages reduces axonal degeneration and hyperalgesia following nerve injury. Pain 86:25–32
56. Dong M, Pinon DI, Cox RF et al (2004) Importance of the amino terminus in secretin family G protein-coupled receptors. Intrinsic photoaffinity labeling establishes initial docking constraints for the calcitonin receptor. J Biol Chem 279:2894–903
57. Read SJ, Dray A (2008) Osteoarthritic pain: a review of current, theoretical and emerging therapeutics. Expert Opin Investig Drugs 17(5):619–640
58. Caterina MJ, Schumacher MA, Tominaga M et al (1997) The capsaicin receptor: a heat-activated ion channel in the pain pathway. Nature 389:816–24
59. Robbins WR, Staats PS, Levine J et al (1998) Treatment of intractable pain with topical large-dose capsaicin: preliminary report. Anesth Analg 86:579–83
60. Simpson DM, Brown S, Tobias J (2008) NGX-4010C107 Study Group. Controlled trial of high-concentration capsaicin patch for treatment of painful HIV neuropathy. Neurology 70:2305–13
61. "Adlea™". Anesiva. http://www.anesiva.com/wt/page/adlea. Accessed Oct 2008.
62. Cabral GA, Marciano-Cabral F (2005) Cannabinoid receptors in microglia of the central nervous system: immune functional relevance. J Leukoc Biol 78:1192–97
63. Karst M, Salim K, Burstein S et al (2003) Analgesic effect of synthetic cannabinoid CT-3 on chronic neuropathic pain: a randomized controlled trial. JAMA 290:1757–62
64. Richardson JD, Aaononsen L, Hargreaves KM (1998) Antihyperalgesic effects of spinal cannabinoids. Eur J Pharmacol 345: 145–53
65. Bennett AD, Everhart AW, Hulsebosch CE (2000) Intrathecal administration of an NMDA or a non NMDA receptor antagonist reduces mechanical but not thermal allodynia in a rodent model of chronic central pain after spinal cord injury. Brain Res 859:72–82
66. Dickenson AH, Chapman V, Green GM (1997) The pharmacology of excitatory and

inhibitory amino acid-mediated events in the transmission and modulation of pain in the spinal cord. Gen Pharmacol 28:633–8

67. Fitzgibbon EJ, Viola R (2005) Parenteral ketamine as an analgesic adjuvant for severe pain: development and retrospective audit of a protocol for a palliative care unit. J Palliat Med 8:49–57
68. Price DD, Mayer DJ, Mao J et al (2000) NMDA-receptor antagonists and opioid receptor interactions as related to analgesia and tolerance. J Pain Symptom Manage 19(Suppl 1):S7–S11
69. Marchand F, Perretti M, McMahon SB (2005) Role of the immune system in chronic pain. Nat Rev Neurosci 6:521–32
70. Sevcik MA, Ghilardi JR, Peter CM et al (2005) Anti-NGF therapy profoundly reduces bone cancer pain and the accompanying increase in markers of peripheral and central sensitization. Pain 115:128–41
71. Sommer C, Marziniak M, Myers RR (1998) The effect of thalidomide treatment on vascular pathology and hyperalgesia caused by constriction injury of rat nerve. Pain 74:83–91
72. Piao ZG, Cho IH, Park CK et al (2006) Activation of glia and microglial p38 MAPK in medullary dorsal horn contributes to tactile hypersensitivity following trigeminal sensory nerve injury. Pain 121:219–31
73. Ledeboer A, Liu T, Schumilla JA et al (2006) The glial modulatory drug AV411 attenuates mechanical allodynia in rat models of neuropathic pain. Neuron Glia Biol 2:279–91
74. Schiavo G, Matteoli M, Montecucco C (2000) Neurotoxins affecting neuroexocytosis. Physiol Rev 80:717–766
75. Aoki KR (2005) Review of a proposed mechanism for the antinociceptive action of botulinum toxin type A. Neurotoxicology 26:785–93
76. Ranoux D, Attal N, Marain F (2008) Botulinum toxin type a induces direct analgesic effects in chronic neuropathic pain. Ann Neurol 64:274–83
77. Valeant Pharmaceuticals Starts Phase 2 Retigabine Study For Treatment Of Postherpetic Neuralgia. Medical News Today. 30 Nov. 2007. http://www.medicalnewstoday.com/articles/90315.php. Accessed 25 Oct 2008
78. Wickenden A, Weifeng Y, Zou, A (2000) Retigabine, a novel anti-covulsant, enhances activation of KCNQ2/Q3 potassium channels. *Mol Pharmacol* 58:591–600.
79. Wuttke T, Seebohm G, Bail S (2005) The new anticonvulsant Retigabine favors voltage-dependent opening of Kv7.2(KCNQ2) channel by binding to its activation gate. Mol Pharmacol 67:1009–17
80. Marrion NV (1997) Control of M-current. Annu Rev Physiol 59:483–504
81. Blackburn-Munro G, Jensen BS (2003) The anticonvulsant retigabine attenuates nociceptive behaviours in rat models of persistent and neuropathic pain. Eur J Pharmacol 460:109–16
82. Gao X, Kim HK, Chung JM et al (2007) Reactive oxygen species (ROS) are involved in enhancement of NMDA-receptor phosphorylation in animal models of pain. Pain 131:262–71
83. Zollinger PE, Tuinebreijer WE, Breederveld RS et al (2007) Can vitamin C prevent complex regional pain syndrome in patients with wrist fractures? J Bone Joint Surg Am 89:1424–31
84. Ziegler D (2008) Treatment of diabetic neuropathy and neuropathic pain: how far have we come? Diabetes Care 31(Suppl 2):S255–61
85. Dworkin RH, O'Connor AB, Backonja M et al (2007) Pharmacologic management of neuropathic pain: evidence-based recommendations. Pain 132:237–51

Concluding Remarks

It is a great pleasure for me to write the concluding remarks for the book *Analgesia*, Methods in Molecular Biology Series, edited by Arpad Szallasi.

Arpad Szallasi is very well known in the pain research field, especially with his description of the vaniloid receptor VR1 or now better known as TRPV1 receptor, which may be a major novel target for analgesic drugs.

Clinicians are not very familiar with (or interested in) basic research in pain medicine. However, the infrastructure of basic knowledge in pain medicine begins with research and fundementals of biology. The problem for clinicians also may arise from how basic knowledge and research of pain medicine is presented to the readers.

I am very happy to see in this book that all topics have been presented and they have a systematic approach for the readers. The book opens with experimental pain models (Chapters 1–10) which is also very important to conduct studies even for clinical purpose. This section gives detailed information about animal models for acute, chronic, inflammatory, neuropathic, orofacial pain, and migraine.

The second step (Chapters 11–15) deals with human pain models. The chapters (Chapters 17–30) on genetic determinants of pain sensitivity and gene expression changes during pain, which is a new and interesting area in pain medicine, may be very influential in the near future. These chapters also give insights into drug discovery and development. Methods for the study of mechanism of action of anesthetic (Chapters 1 and 31) and analgesic drugs (Chapters 16–19) are also presented. The chapter (Chapter 33) on "Proteomics and metabolomics and their application to analgesia research" is new to us. Future therapies are described including gene-based approaches (Chapter 22) and stem cell therapy (Chapter 25) which may be speculative for today but has a future. Last, methods are described for clinical studies in pain management (Chapters 35–38) which also have important input for clinicans.

This book is a comprehensive coverage of research methods in analgesia from target discovery through target validation and drug development to preclinical trials, and from in silico methods and cell lines through drosophilia and mice to patients.

I congragulate Arpad Szallasi and all contributing authors for their great efforts for this book. I do believe it is a great contribution to pain medicine.

Serdar Erdine, MD, FIPP
President
World Institute of Pain

Index

M

N

O

P

R

S

T

U

V

W

Z